SOUTH COLLEGE
709 Mall Blvd.
Savannah, GA 31406

DO NOT REMOVE FROM LIBRARY

REFERENCE

PREGNANCY and BIRTH SOURCEBOOK

Health Reference Series

Volume Thirty-one

PREGNANCY and BIRTH SOURCEBOOK

∎

Basic Information about Planning for Pregnancy, Maternal Health, Fetal Growth and Development, Labor and Delivery, Postpartum and Perinatal Care, Pregnancy in Mothers with Special Concerns, and Disorders of Pregnancy, Including Genetic Counseling, Nutrition and Exercise, Obstetrical Tests, Pregnancy Discomfort, Multiple Births, Cesarean Sections, Medical Testing of Newborns, Breastfeeding, Gestational Diabetes, and Ectopic Pregnancy.

Edited by
Heather E. Aldred

Omnigraphics, Inc.

Penobscot Building / Detroit, MI 48226

BIBLIOGRAPHIC NOTE

This volume contains individual publications and excerpts from documents produced by the National Institutes of Health (NIH), its sister agencies and subagencies. Numbered publications are: 97-4189, HRSA-M-DSEA-96-5, 96-0007, HRSA-MCH-95-1, 95-3929, 94-8087, 93-1998, 93-2788, 93-2011, 93-0564, 93-3464, 93-3279, 92-2256S, HRSA-MCCHB-92-4-A, 92-0064, 91-3029, 90-3182, 90-3174, and 88-1587. Unnumbered publications included: "Every Child Deserves a Healthy Start," "Before You Get Pregnant: Planning is the Key," and "Facts about Cesarean Childbirth." Numbered publications from the Centers for Disease Control and Prevention are: 244002, 245002, 246003, 242002, and 248002. Selected articles from *FDA Consumer, Morbidity and Mortality Weekly,* and *Research Resources Reporter* are also included. Other documents include copyrighted articles from Group Health Cooperative, Information Network Inc., and the Mayo Foundation for Medical Education and Research. These are used by permission. Full citation information is located on the first page of each article.

Edited by Heather E. Aldred
Karen Bellenir, Series Editor, *Health Reference Series*
Peter D. Dresser, *Managing Editor, Health Reference Series*

Omnigraphics, Inc.

Matthew P. Barbour, *Production Manager*
Laurie Lanzen Harris, *Vice President, Editorial*
Peter E. Ruffner, *Vice President, Administration*
James A. Sellgren, *Vice President, Operations and Finance*
Jane J. Steele, *Marketing Consultant*

Frederick G. Ruffner, Jr., Publisher

Copyright ©1997, Omnigraphics, Inc.

Library of Congress Cataloging-in-Publication Data

Library of Congress Cataloging-in-Publication Data
Pregnancy and birth sourcebook ; basic about planning for
 pregnancy, maternal health, fetal growth and development . . . /
 edited by Heather E. Aldred.
  p. cm. -- (Health reference series ; v. 31)
 Includes bibliographical references and index.
 ISBN (invalid) 0078080082 (lib. bdg. ; alk. paper)
  1. Pregnancy. 2. Childbirth. 3. Pregnancy--Complications.
 I. Aldred, Heather E. II. Series
 RG525.P676   1997   97-36154
 618.2--dc21   CIP

∞

This book is printed on acid-free paper meeting the ANSI z39.48 Standard. The infinity symbol that appears above indicates that the paper in this book meets that standard.

Printed in the United States

Contents

Preface xi

Part I: Planning for Pregnancy

Chapter 1—Before You Get Pregnant 3

Chapter 2—Information about Immunizations 7
      Section 2.1—Chickenpox 8
      Section 2.2—Rubella 10
      Section 2.3—Mumps 12
      Section 2.4—Hepatitis B 13
      Section 2.5—Pertussis 15
      Section 2.6—Tetanus 16
      Section 2.7—Diphtheria 16

Chapter 3—Genetic Counseling for Couples with Concerns 17
      Section 3.1—Understanding DNA Testing 18
      Section 3.2—Genetic Screening 26

Chapter 4—Home Pregnancy Tests 37

Part II: Maternal Care During Pregnancy

Chapter 5—Taking Care of Yourself During Pregnancy 41
      Section 5.1—Your Health During Pregnancy 42
      Section 5.2—X-Rays, Pregnancy, and You 46

Chapter 6—Nutrition 49
    Section 6.1—All about Eating for Two 50
    Section 6.2—Recommendations for Weight
                     Gain During Pregnancy 56
    Section 6.3—Prenatal Vitamin
                     Recommendations 59
    Section 6.4—How Folate Can Help
                     Prevent Birth Defects 60
    Section 6.5—Knowledge and Use of Folate
                     in the United States 68

Chapter 7—Prenatal Exercise Plans 73

Chapter 8—Prenatal Care: What to Expect at Obstetrical
               Visits 79

Chapter 9—Medical Tests Sometimes Used During
               Pregnancy 93
    Section 9.1—Maternal Urinalysis and
                     Blood Sampling 94
    Section 9.2—Diagnostic Ultrasound
                     Imaging in Pregnancy 95
    Section 9.3—Amniocentesis and Chorionic
                     Villus Sampling (CVS) 104
    Section 9.4—Alpha-Fetoprotein and Triple
                     AFP Screening 116
    Section 9.5—Fetal Monitoring: Stress and
                     Non-Stress Tests 117

Chapter 10—Coping with Common Discomforts of
                Pregnancy 119

Part III: Fetal Development During Gestation

Chapter 11—Fetal Growth and Development 129

Chapter 12—Cautions about Drugs and Their Impact on
                the Developing Fetus 135
    Section 12.1—Drugs and Pregnancy: Often the
                      Two Don't Mix 136
    Section 12.2—Prescription and Over-the-
                      Counter Medications 141
    Section 12.3—Tobacco and Pregnancy 148

Section 12.4—Caffeine and Pregnancy 149
Section 12.5—Alcohol and Pregnancy 151
Section 12.6—Illegal Drugs and Pregnancy .. 157

Chapter 13—Infectious Organisms and Fetal Development .. 205
Section 13.1—Sexually Transmitted Diseases
and Your Baby 206
Section 13.2—Toxoplasmosis 212
Section 13.3—Group B Streptococcal
Infections 221
Section 13.4—Listeriosis During Pregnancy . 225

Part IV: Labor and Delivery

Chapter 14—Stages of Labor and Delivery 231

Chapter 15—Pre-Term Labor 239
Section 15.1—Management of Pre-Term
Labor 240
Section 15.2—Cervix Length: A Predictor
of Pre-Term Labor 245
Section 15.3—Common Vaginal Condition
Increases Risk of Pre-Term
Delivery and Low Birth
Weight 247
Section 15.4—Treatment of Pre-Term
Labor with Corticosteroids 250
Section 15.5—Pre-Term Babies 262

Chapter 16—Medical Care During Labor and Delivery 269
Section 16.1—Pain Relief Options 270
Section 16.2—Epidural 272
Section 16.3—Use of Forceps 273
Section 16.4—Episiotomy 275
Section 16.5—Electronic Fetal Monitoring
During Labor 277

Chapter 17—Cesarean Childbirth 291

Part V: Postpartum and Perinatal Care

Chapter 18—Postpartum Concerns 305
Section 18.1—Taking Care of Yourself
after the Baby Is Born 306

Section 18.2—Childbirth and Bladder
        Control 313
Section 18.3—Postpartum Depression 317
Section 18.4—Planning Your Family 320

Chapter 19—Breastfeeding.. 331
Section 19.1—Breastfeeding Statistics 332
Section 19.2—Feeding Baby: Nature and
        Nurture 334
Section 19.3—Lactation Suppression:
        Safer without Drugs................. 341
Section 19.4—Breastfeeding and the
        Working Mother 346
Section 19.5—Potential Health Care Cost
        of Not Breastfeeding 352
Section 19.6—Recent Advances in Maternal
        and Infant Nutrition 355

Chapter 20—Routine Medical Testing of Newborns 361

Part VI: Pregnancy in Mothers with Special Concerns

Chapter 21—Information for Rh-Negative Women 377

Chapter 22—Pregnancy in Women with Asthma 389

Chapter 23—Pre-Gestational Diabetes................................. 435

Chapter 24—Pre-Gestational Hypertension 451

Chapter 25—Multiple Pregnancy 465
Section 25.1—Twins or More 466
Section 25.2—Rates of Twin Birth 481

Chapter 26—Pregnancy in Women with Sickle Cell Anemia . 485

Chapter 27—Pregnancy in Women with Lupus 497

Chapter 28—Breast Cancer and Pregnancy 505

Chapter 29—Pregnancy in Women with Hodgkin's Disease .. 511

Chapter 30—AIDS and Pregnancy 515
Section 30.1—HIV Testing and Counseling
        for Pregnant Women 516

Section 30.2—Pregnancy and HIV: Is AZT the Right Choice for You and Your Baby? 530

Part VII: Disorders of Pregnancy

Chapter 31—Ectopic Pregnancy 537
    Section 31.1—Ectopic Pregnancy Explained .. 538
    Section 31.2—Ectopic Pregnancy in the United States, 1990-1992 542

Chapter 32—Molar Pregnancy 547

Chapter 33—Understanding Gestational Diabetes 553

Chapter 34—Gestational Hypertension and Preeclampsia-Eclampsia 593

Chapter 35—Disorders of the Placenta 621

Chapter 36—Intrauterine Growth Retardation 627

Chapter 37—Post-Term Birth 631

Chapter 38—Maternal Death 635

Chapter 39—Pregnancy Loss 643
    Section 39.1—Infant Mortality 644
    Section 39.2—Miscarriage (Spontaneous Abortion) 651
    Section 39.3—Early Pregnancy Loss 656
    Section 39.4—Grieving a Loss 660

Part VIII: Glossary

Chapter 40—Glossary of Medical Terms 679

Index **695**

Preface

About This Book

Pregnancy is a time of major physiological and emotional change. Some of the discomforts women endure are normal. For example, an estimated 50 to 90 percent of all pregnant women experience morning sickness during the first trimester. Although doctors do not know what causes morning sickness, researchers have noted that women who suffer from the condition are 30 percent less likely to miscarry or deliver prematurely than women who do not.

Other problems that may develop during pregnancy can be serious—even life threatening. These include gestational diabetes, hypertension, preeclampsia, and disorders of the placenta. Some women with pre-existing conditions, such as asthma, sickle cell anemia, lupus, breast cancer, Hodgkin's Disease, and AIDS, require special care to decrease the risk of childbirth and to improve infant health.

This book was designed to help women as they plan for pregnancy, implement a program of prenatal care, and prepare for childbirth. It offers suggestions to help mothers make informed decisions about lifestyle questions and to distinguish between the normal discomforts of pregnancy and the symptoms that may signal more serious problems.

Pregnancy and Birth Sourcebook contains numerous publications produced by a wide variety of government and private agencies including the National Institutes of Health (NIH), the Department of Health and Human Services (DHSS), the Food and Drug Administration, Centers for Disease Control and Prevention, Group Health Care

Cooperative, the Mayo Foundation for Medical Education and Research, and Information Network, Inc. The documents chosen present basic medical information for the layperson regarding the health of the mother and her unborn child.

How to Use This Book

This book is divided into parts, chapters, and sections. Parts focus on broad areas of interest, and individual chapters present topics within those areas. To help the reader locate specific information, some chapters are further subdivided into sections.

Part I: *Planning for Pregnancy* provides information about factors to be considered prior to conception. Recommended immunizations are identified, genetic counseling is explained, and lifestyle decisions that may impact health are presented. Part I concludes with a chapter about home pregnancy tests.

Part II: *Maternal Care During Pregnancy* focuses on care during pregnancy. Subjects include nutritional guidelines for pregnant women, coping with the discomforts of pregnancy, and prenatal exercise. The content of prenatal care, including information about tests such as amniocentesis and ultrasound, is also presented.

Part III: *Fetal Development During Gestation* describes the growth of the fetus throughout the gestational period and identifies factors that may influence development. Potential problems related to specific over-the-counter and prescription drugs are discussed along with the effect of substance abuse on fetal outcome. The impact of infectious organisms including toxoplasmosis, streptococcal B, and a variety of sexually transmitted diseases, is also explained.

Part IV: *Labor and Delivery* describes what to expect during the different stages of childbirth. It includes information regarding medical care and intervention. The risks, management, and fetal outcome of pre-term labor are also examined.

Part V: *Postpartum and Perinatal Care* considers areas of concern after the baby is born. These include the routine medical testing of newborns, breastfeeding, postpartum depression, and future family planning decisions.

Part VI: *Pregnancy in Mothers with Special Concerns* provides information regarding pregnancy and birth specific to particular maternal situations. Women with pre-existing conditions such as asthma, AIDS, breast cancer, lupus, and sickle cell anemia will find individual chapters focused on their unique needs.

Part VII: *Disorders of Pregnancy* focuses on specific medical conditions that may arise during pregnancy. The chapters in this section provide a description of each condition, their diagnoses, treatment, and expected maternal and fetal outcome.

Part VIII: *Glossary of Medical Terms* provides a listing and short explanation of some common medical terms used throughout this volume.

Acknowledgements

The editor wishes to thank Group Health Care Cooperative, Information Network Inc., the Mayo Foundation for Medical Education and Research, and Matria Healthcare Inc. for granting permission to reprint their useful and important articles; researcher Mary Margaret Missar for locating the documents included in this volume; and Karen Bellenir and Peter Dresser for their technical assistance and advice.

Note from the Editor

This book is part of Omnigraphics' Health Reference Series. The series provides basic information about a broad range of medical concerns. It is not intended to serve as a tool for diagnosing illness, in prescribing treatments, or as a substitute for the physician/patient relationship. All persons concerned about medical symptoms or the possibility of disease are encouraged to seek professional care from an appropriate health care provider.

Part One

Planning for Pregnancy

Part One

Planning for Pregnancy

Chapter 1

Before You Get Pregnant

Planning is the Key

The best start for your future baby begins right now, before you are pregnant. There are many things you and your partner can do to give your baby the best possible start. Did you know that all of your baby's important organs form very early. Birth defects may happen before a woman has missed a period and knows she is pregnant.

You can lower the risk of birth defects and pregnancy problems by making good health choices before and during your pregnancy.

Time

Choosing **when** you get pregnant is important.

- **Family Planning.** Planning your future is important. Family Planning lets you decide if you want a child, when that will happen, and helps you have a healthy baby. If you are having sex, it's important to use a method of birth control until you are ready to have a baby.

- **Age.** Women under 18 and over 34 who have babies are more likely to have problems with pregnancy or have small babies.

- **Before You Stop Your Birth Control.** Go to a clinic or health care provider for a physical exam and counseling. Go in for this

---

State Family Planning Administrators, July 1994

visit at least three months before you want to become pregnant. Ask your clinic or doctor about taking vitamins like folic acid.

Habits

Habits before you get pregnant may be good or bad.

- **Eating.** Eat healthy food and regular meals. It's important for you and your baby. Dieting may be harmful. Use less caffeine.

- **Exercise.** Regular exercise will help you feel better and get your body ready for pregnancy.

- **Smoking.** Smoking or being around others' smoke can cause your baby to be born too small or too soon to be healthy. Smoking marijuana can cause these problems too.

- **Drugs and Medicines.** Using illegal drugs or even some medicines (prescribed or bought over-the-counter) can cause miscarriage, brain damage, addiction, and/or death to your baby.

- **Alcohol.** Drinking alcohol (beer, wine, wine coolers, hard liquor and even cough and cold medicines) can cause birth defects, mental retardation and even death to your baby.

Smoking, drugs, medicines and alcohol...all of these can be harmful depending how much and how often you use them.

- **Other Hazards.** Working with certain metals and chemicals such as lead, paint, oven cleaners, bug killers, gasoline and car exhaust can cause pregnancy problems. They also could harm your baby. Other hazards include eating raw meats, handling used cat litter or being around animals or people with certain diseases.

Health

Before you get pregnant, talk to your nurse, doctor or clinic about:

- **Medical Conditions.** Medical problems (such as diabetes, epilepsy, high blood pressure, heart or kidney disease, infections, hepatitis or anemia) need to be treated before pregnancy.

- **Immunizations.** Make sure your immunizations are up to date. They can prevent some diseases like German Measles (rubella) which can cause serious birth defects.

Before You Get Pregnant

- **Family Health.** Does anyone in your family have a birth defect, inherited disease, or mental retardation? Some diseases and birth problems can run in families.

- **STD.** You or your partner may have a sexually transmitted disease (STD) that you don't know about. All STDs (such as chlamydia, syphilis, and HIV/AIDS) can cause serious problems.

- **Emotional Health.** Get help if you have violence or abuse in your life, high levels of stress, or not enough personal support. Pregnancy can cause money problems or interfere with school or work.

Now That You Have Planned

Getting Pregnant. An average woman can become pregnant for a short period of time about 2 weeks before her next period. However, some women can get pregnant at very different times in their menstrual cycles. Talk to your health care provider or clinic about when you are most likely to get pregnant. Get a pregnancy test if you think you are pregnant or if you miss your period. Usual signs of pregnancy include sore or enlarged breasts, urinating more often, nausea and tiredness. It's important to get care as early as possible when you are pregnant.

Plan Ahead

There are many things you need to think about before you get pregnant. What will you need to know, and do, to plan for your pregnancy and parenthood?

You may find it useful to get more information from:

- Family planning services.
- Pre-pregnancy books at your local library, bookstore or clinic.
- Exercise classes.
- Stop smoking programs.
- Food programs.
- Counseling and mental health centers.
- Religious leaders.
- School counselors and nurses.
- Alcohol/drug treatment programs.
- Medical insurance plans.
- Social services.
- Health department.
- Health care providers: doctors, nurses, clinics and hospitals.

Chapter 2

Information about Immunizations

Chapter Contents

Section 2.1—Chickenpox 8
Section 2.2—Rubella 10
Section 2.3—Mumps 12
Section 2.4—Hepatitis B 13
Section 2.5—Pertussis 15
Section 2.6—Tetanus 16
Section 2.7—Diphtheria 16

Section 2.1

Chickenpox

CDC Doc. No. 248002, July 1995

More than 90% of the adult U.S. population is immune to chickenpox because of an infection during childhood. Therefore, for the vast majority of pregnant women, being exposed to chickenpox should pose little concern to either the pregnant woman or the unborn child

Pregnant women who are not immune to chickenpox, and who have been significantly exposed may be at increased risk. Both the pregnant woman and the unborn child have risks including:

1. A pregnant woman has an increased risk of complications associated with a chickenpox illness. However, remember that while chickenpox is usually a mild infection with few complications for normal children, for normal adults the infection can be more severe, and complications are a little more frequent. Therefore, normal adults, including pregnant women, may have an infection with symptoms somewhat more severe than children, and these adults are also at increased risk of complications.

    Pregnant women who are not immune to chickenpox and who have significant exposure to a person with chickenpox can be evaluated by their doctor for possible treatment with Varicella-Zoster Immune Globulin, also known as VZIG. Treatment with VZIG, if given within 96 hours of exposure, can prevent or moderate a chickenpox infection in the pregnant women. There is, however, no evidence that VZIG can prevent or moderate a chickenpox infection in the unborn child. A treatment dose of VZIG costs between $400 and $500 and physicians can obtain VZIG from The American Red Cross.

2. The unborn child is at a low risk of birth defects if the pregnant woman is infected with chickenpox during the first 16 weeks of pregnancy. Infants whose mother was infected with chickenpox during the first 16 weeks of pregnancy rarely develop congenital varicella syndrome, which can include eye, skin, or limb defects in the child. The risk of having congenital varicella is low (around 2 to 3 percent), and is similar to the

Information about Immunizations

risk of developing birth defects in general. Unborn children whose mother is infected with chickenpox after the first 16 weeks do not appear to develop congenital varicella syndrome.

3. The newborn child is at increased risk of serious infection if the pregnant woman is infected with chickenpox close to the time of delivery. If the mother develops chickenpox between 5 days before delivery and 48 hours after delivery, the newborn infant may develop serious infection. Infants whose mothers develop chickenpox outside the "5 days before to 48 hours after delivery" window do not appear to be at increased risk of serious illness.

4. Premature infants who have significant exposure after birth may be at increased risk for serious illness, especially those infants born before 28 weeks of gestation, or whose mothers are not immune to chickenpox.

If there is concern that a pregnant woman has been exposed to chickenpox, there are 3 ways to figure out if she is already immune to chickenpox.

1. By asking her parents or relatives if they remember whether she had chickenpox.
2. Check the medical records of her family or pediatric physician.
3. Have a laboratory test performed that would indicate whether she was already infected and thus is immune.

If the pregnant woman is not known to be immune to chickenpox, it is important to figure out whether she was significantly exposed to a person with chickenpox. Significant exposure means being in the presence or having prolonged contact with someone who is developing or currently has a chickenpox infection. For example, significant exposure to chickenpox can include:

- continuous household contact,
- playmate contact of greater than one hour,
- hospital contact involving the same bedroom, or adjacent beds in a large ward, or
- prolonged face-to-face contact.

If a woman is pregnant <u>and</u> had a significant exposure to chickenpox, she should consult with her physician about the risk to herself and her unborn child.

Section 2.2

Rubella

CDC Document Numbers 243005 and 243002.

For the developing unborn baby, rubella can be a devastating illness with consequences that last a lifetime. Infants born to mothers who become ill with rubella during pregnancy have an increased risk of birth defects that include hearing loss, loss of sight, heart defects, mental retardation, and even death. By receiving the rubella vaccine, a woman can protect her unborn child from rubella. Therefore, all women of childbearing age should be immunized against rubella. Because it is not recommended that rubella vaccine be given during pregnancy, vaccination should occur at least three months before conception.

Pregnancy and the Rubella Vaccine

While it is not recommended that pregnant women receive the rubella vaccine, some women have been inadvertently vaccinated while pregnant. When rubella vaccine was licensed, this situation was of concern. Therefore, from 1971-1989, the Centers for Disease Control maintained a list of reported women vaccinated during pregnancy to determine the vaccination effects, if any, on the infants of such mothers. This list of women was called the Vaccine in Pregnancy Registry. Because enough reports had been received and analyzed, CDC discontinued the VIP registry on April 30, 1989.

Based on data in the Vaccine in Pregnancy Registry (VIP), there is no evidence that defects consistent with congenital rubella syndrome have occurred in offspring of women vaccinated during or close to the time of pregnancy. Therefore, the observed risk of birth defects for vaccination in pregnancy is zero. However, since the vaccine consists of a weakened live virus, it is theoretically possible that the vaccine could rarely damage the unborn child, although such an effect has never been observed. It is believed that if vaccination occurs within 3 months before or after conception, there is a theoretical risk of CRS, but it is so small as to be negligible. Inadvertent vaccination of a pregnant woman should not be a reason in itself to consider interruption of pregnancy. However, the patient and her physician should make the final decision about continuing the pregnancy.

Information about Immunizations

In summary, rubella vaccine is not known to cause special problems for pregnant women and their unborn babies. However, doctors usually avoid giving any drugs or vaccines to pregnant women unless there is a specific need. Therefore to be safe, pregnant women should not be vaccinated with rubella vaccine.

Congenital Rubella Syndrome (CRS)

Rubella can be a disastrous disease early in pregnancy, leading to miscarriages, stillbirths, or birth defects. The severity and risk of the effects of rubella virus on the unborn baby depend on the time during pregnancy when the rubella infection occurs. Up to 85% of infants infected in the first three months of pregnancy (first trimester) will be found to be affected after birth. Even an inapparent rubella infection in the mother can result in birth defects. While infection in the unborn child may occur throughout pregnancy, defects are rare when infection occurs after the 20th week of pregnancy. The overall risk of defects during the third trimester is probably no greater than that associated with normal pregnancies.

Common manifestations of congenital rubella include deafness, which is the most common of the defects, eye problems including cataracts, and glaucoma; congenital heart disease; mental retardation; and many other defects. Some manifestations of CRS may not be apparent for up to 2-4 years after birth.

Infants infected with rubella before birth often shed the virus for as long as 12 months after birth, or, rarely, longer. Infants with congenital rubella syndrome, who were infected with rubella before birth, may be able to infect others for usually about a year and can therefore transmit rubella to those susceptible persons caring for them.

After an attack of rubella or vaccination against rubella most mothers are protected against the disease for their whole life. However, reinfection with rubella virus can occur. The overwhelming majority of these reinfections occur without symptoms, but occasionally a rash or joint pain have been observed. Rubella reinfection during pregnancy rarely results in transmission of the virus to the unborn child. Rare cases <u>have</u> been reported in which infants with congenital rubella syndrome were born to mothers who were reinfected during pregnancy.

Section 2.3

Mumps

CDC Doc. No. 242002, July, 1995

Natural mumps infection during pregnancy has not been associated with an increased risk of premature delivery or birth defects. However, mumps infections during the first trimester may increase the rate of miscarriages. Birth defects have rarely been reported among children of women who had mumps while they were pregnant, but mumps has not been proven to be the cause of the defects. This is in contrast to rubella (sometimes called German Measles) which does cause birth defects particularly if rubella is contracted during the first three months of pregnancy.

Despite the fact that neither natural mumps nor mumps vaccine are known to cause birth defects, mumps-containing vaccine should not be given to a woman known to be pregnant or who is considering becoming pregnant within three months.

A pregnant woman who inadvertently receives a dose of mumps vaccine, should consult with a doctor. The precaution against vaccinating a pregnant women is based on the theoretical risk of infection in the unborn child, however, there is no actual evidence that mumps or mumps vaccine can harm the developing unborn child. Mumps vaccination during pregnancy is not a reason in itself to consider interruption of the pregnancy, however, the decision to continue a pregnancy is always a personal and medical decision which can only be made by the pregnant woman and her physician.

Children of a pregnant women can receive the vaccine. This will pose no risk to the pregnant mother.

Information about Immunizations

Section 2.4

Hepatitis B

CDC Division of Viral and Rickettsial Diseases, July 1994.

What Is Hepatitis B?

Hepatitis B is a serious disease of the liver caused by hepatitis B virus, or HBV. All people—no matter how old they are or where they live may be at risk for hepatitis B.

HBV attacks and destroys the liver, which is such an important organ that you cannot live without it.

Hepatitis B may cause:

- scarring (cirrhosis) of the liver
- liver cancer
- lifelong (chronic) HBV infection
- liver failure
- death

Why Is Hepatitis B a Problem for Pregnant Women and Their Babies?

Pregnant women may have HBV in their blood without knowing it and can pass it on to their babies at birth. Many of these babies develop lifelong HBV infections and can pass the virus on to others through out their lives. At first, babies may not look or feel sick, but as they grow up, they may have liver damage. About 25% of babies who develop lifelong HBV infections die of liver disease or liver cancer.

How Can You Get Hepatitis B?

HBV is spread from person to person by direct contact with infected blood or body fluids. Even small amounts of infected blood can cause infection.

HBV infection can be spread by:

- an infected mother to her baby during birth
- sharing needles for injecting drugs
- having sex with an infected person

You are at increased risk for hepatitis B if:

- you live in the same household with someone who has lifelong HBV infection
- you have a job that exposes you to human blood.

If You Feel Healthy, Can You Still Have Hepatitis B?

Some people who have hepatitis B have no symptoms and may not know they are infected. Others who are infected with HBV never fully recover and carry the virus in their blood for the rest of their lives. These people are known as carriers, and they can infect other household and sexual contacts throughout their lives.

How Do You Find Out If You Have Hepatitis B?

Get a blood test at your clinic or doctor's office.

All pregnant women should get a blood test for hepatitis B early in their pregnancy.

If the test is positive, the doctor or nurse will tell you how to take care of yourself and how to prevent infecting your baby and others.

How Do You Protect Your Baby If Your Hepatitis B Blood Test Is Positive?

A safe vaccine has been used since 1982 to prevent hepatitis B. The vaccine is given in a series of three shots. If you have HBV infection, your baby will get the first shot within 12 hours of birth, along with another shot, hepatitis B immune globulin. The next two shots of hepatitis B vaccine will be given along with other baby shots. All other members of your household should get a blood test for hepatitis B. If the blood test is negative, hepatitis B vaccine should be given to the other household members.

Do You Need to Protect Your Baby If the Hepatitis B Blood Test Is Negative?

Hepatitis B vaccination is recommended for all infants to protect them from becoming infected with HBV. If your blood test for hepatitis B is negative, your baby will still receive the hepatitis B vaccine series with other baby shots, but will not need a shot of hepatitis B immune globulin. The baby may get the first shot either

Information about Immunizations

before leaving the hospital or with the first baby shots at the doctor's office or clinic. Ask your doctor or nurse when the next shots need to be given.

Protect Your Baby Against Hepatitis B

- Get a blood test
- Vaccinate your baby

For more information on hepatitis B and pregnancy, contact your local health department or call the **CDC Hepatitis Hotline (404) 332-4555**.

Section 2.5

Pertussis

CDC Document No. 246003, June 1995

Pertussis vaccine is usually given in combination with diphtheria and tetanus toxoids as DTP vaccine. This DTP vaccine contains inactivated bacteria and toxoids which can not be transmitted from the person receiving vaccine to another person. Therefore, it is safe to vaccinate children of pregnant women with DTP vaccine.

There is no convincing evidence of risk to the fetus from vaccinating a pregnant women with inactivated bacteria or toxoic vaccines. However, pertussis vaccine should not be given to anyone older than 7 years because the person over 7 years receiving vaccine may have more side effects than someone less than 7 years old. Tetanus and Diphtheria toxoids, combined as Td, should be given every 10 years to adolescents and adults. A pregnant women who has not received Td vaccine within the last 10 years should receive a dose of Td, preferably past the first trimester.

Section 2.6

Tetanus

CDC Document No. 245002, March 1993

A pregnant women should not be concerned if she inadvertently received a dose of tetanus toxoid. In fact a previously unimmunized pregnant women who may deliver her child under unhygienic circumstances should receive two doses of the adult formulated tetanus and diphtheria vaccination. The doses should be spaced as usual, 4 to 8 weeks apart, during the last two trimesters. Incompletely immunized pregnant women should complete the 3 dose series. Those immunized more than 10 years previously should have a booster dose.

The children of pregnant women can receive tetanus toxoid. This will pose no risk to the pregnant women.

Section 2.7

Diphtheria

CDC Document No. 244002, June 1995

A pregnant women should not be concerned if she inadvertently received a dose of diphtheria toxoid. Diphtheria toxoid is usually available only in combination with tetanus toxoid in a vaccine called Td, spelled with a capital T and small d. If possible, waiting until the second trimester of pregnancy to administer Td is a reasonable precaution for minimizing any theoretical possibility of any reactions.

Children living in the same household as a pregnant women can receive diphtheria toxoid, and this will pose no risk to the pregnant women.

Diphtheria illness during pregnancy may be associated with an increased risk of miscarriages, premature delivery, or harmful effects to the unborn child.

Chapter 3

Genetic Counseling for Couples with Concerns

Chapter Contents

Section 3.1—Understanding DNA Testing.................................. 18
Section 3.2—Genetic Screening... 26

Section 3.1

Understanding DNA Testing

Southeastern Regional Genetics Group, January 1991

This text will explain how DNA analysis can be performed for families. It is meant to help you explain to other family members why certain testing is done and why we may need blood from many members of the family, as well as discussing some of the procedures used in testing. This text is designed to supplement counseling that you receive from your doctor or genetic specialist. If you have or any family member has questions or concerns, contact your physician or genetic center.

In the past, physicians have diagnosed diseases by studying changes in the body, especially body fluids such as blood and urine. We know that some of these changes can result from abnormal genes. In recent years, new ways to test for certain inherited traits have been developed which use a person's DNA.

What is an inherited trait?

An inherited trait is any feature such as blue eyes, dark hair or a disease which can be passed from parent to child. For any feature or disease to be passed to the next generation, the code for that trait must be in the DNA. Since we receive half of the total amount of DNA from each of our parents, we share ethnic and family characteristics, while retaining our own unique combination of features. Because we share DNA in common with other relatives, certain inherited diseases can be traced through families.

What is DNA?

DNA (deoxyribonucleic acid) is a compound found at the center (nucleus) of almost every cell. It carries the code for nearly all inherited traits. We receive DNA from each parent in packages called **chromosomes.**

Normally, each person should have 23 pairs of chromosomes and a pair of genes for every feature or trait. The father gives one set of 23 chromosomes with its DNA in his sperm. The mother gives another set of 23 chromosomes with its DNA in her egg. The egg and sperm combine at fertilization. Thus we get one or more genes from **each parent** for every inherited trait, feature, or characteristic.

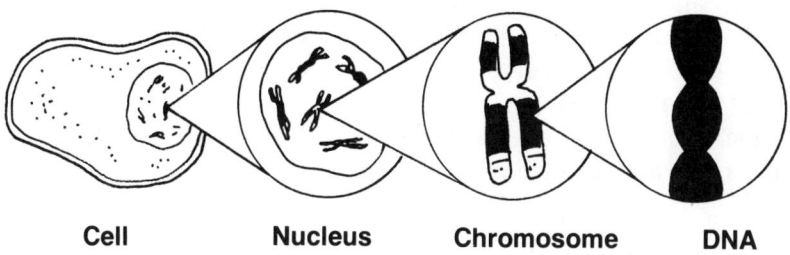

Cell   Nucleus   Chromosome   DNA

Figure 3.1. Inside the cell. The nucleus of each human cell contains a complete genetic blueprint for that person. The information is housed on 46 chromosomes, made mostly of long chains of DNA. DNA is the master chemical that controls the development and functioning of all living things. A segment of the DNA chain which codes for inherited traits is called a GENE.

What is a gene?

A gene is a tiny portion of DNA that has the code for an inherited trait. Remember, each chromosome has thousands of genes, hooked together something like beads on a string. Each gene is identified by its unique sequence of DNA.

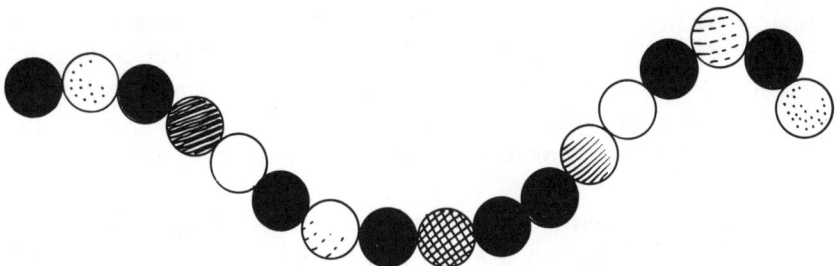

Figure 3.2. Each chromosome has thousands of genes, hooked together something like beads on a string.

Who might want DNA testing?

When a specific inherited disease occurs within a particular family, family members often want to know if they might develop the same disease or if they might be carriers and pass on that inherited trait to their children. DNA technology provides new tests for some of these inherited traits. In certain situations DNA can be analyzed and the results can be used to determine who has a risk for developing a particular inherited problem or for passing it on to their children. Each test looks for a specific genetic change. **There is no test which can determine all genetic risks in a family.**

What kinds of DNA studies are available?

There are two main types of DNA studies. They are direct and indirect detection methods.

What is direct detection?

Direct detection is the best type of DNA study, but it is only useful for a few diseases. To use this type of study we must know what kind of change has occurred in the structure of the DNA and exactly where this change is located. We can then study a particular section of DNA and determine whether a change is present. The change is distinct and will identify a precise genetic condition.

For example, pretend you are in a strange city and are looking for a particular house. You have a map, a description of the house and the complete address, including street number and zip code. You can drive directly to that house without other landmarks.

In the same way, when the location of the change in the DNA is known, methods can be employed which allow us to identify the problem gene without other DNA landmarks. There are several methods for direct detection. In every case, however, when direct detection is possible, DNA testing can be done using blood or tissue samples from a single individual. Direct detection does not require blood samples from affected relatives or any previous family history of the disease.

A Direct Detection Example. One of the earliest and best examples of direct detection is sickle cell anemia. In sickle cell anemia we know where the exact defect is located. A special enzyme (called a restriction endonuclease) will recognize the normal gene and will cut DNA at a particular site, producing a shorter fragment (piece of DNA).

Genetic Counseling for Couples with Concerns

In sickle cell anemia the DNA is altered and the enzyme will no longer be able to cut at this site.

The various size fragments can be measured in the laboratory. If there are shorter fragments, the hemoglobin is encoded as normal and the patient is not a "carrier." If there is one longer piece, the patient has sickle cell anemia. If there are all three sizes of DNA fragments, the patient is a carrier, i.e., has one normal gene and one abnormal gene for hemoglobin.

What is indirect detection or linkage analysis?

For most diseases we do not know the exact location of the gene or the precise change that has occurred to the DNA. When this is the case we must use a test that requires family studies. This is called indirect or linkage analysis.

How is indirect detection used?

Remember that genes are small pieces of information that are hooked together in a long chain of DNA on the chromosome. Genes or DNA regions which are close together are usually inherited together—they are "linked." To use linkage analysis we need families that have normal variations in their DNA makeup. These differences are called polymorphisms. Another term that is often used is "marker." Markers are normal variations of DNA regions that are close enough to the problem gene to be inherited as a group. We can use the markers as landmarks.

For example, suppose that we are looking for a particular house. We know the general neighborhood but do not have a street address. We do know that a red brick house and a house with blue shutters are nearby. If we can find those landmarks we will know we are on the right street. In the same manner the markers help us locate the area close to the problem gene.

What is a Polymorphic Site?

A polymorphic site is a recognizable variation along the string of DNA. These variations or differences occur many times within the DNA and the patterns are "family specific." It is estimated that about 1% of all genes are polymorphic. This means that for any person the markers on one chromosome may be different enough from the markers on the other chromosome for us to recognize this difference. By looking at the DNA from parents and other relatives, we can usually tell which side of the family passed on a certain polymorphism.

Why is this important?

Polymorphic sites are important if they are close to the disease-related gene. If the disease-related gene is linked to a known polymorphism, the inheritance of this polymorphism can be used to track the transmission of a disease gene within a family. The certainty of this prediction, or "probability," depends on how closely the disease gene is linked to the polymorphism.

Remember the example of genes arranged like beads on a string.

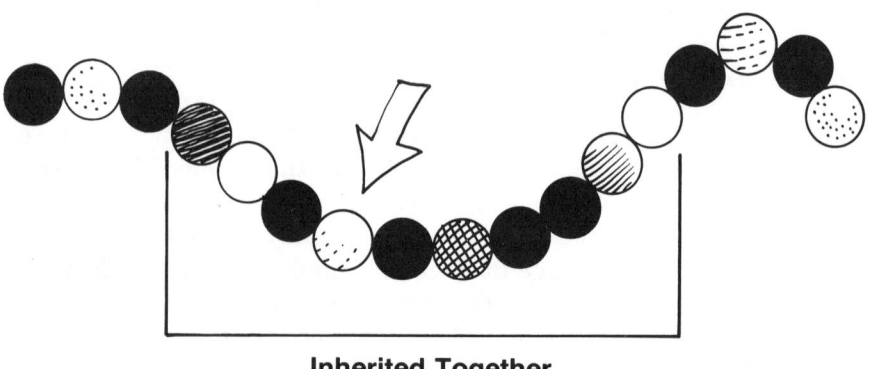

Inherited Together

Figure 3.3

Genes which are close together are more likely to be inherited together. Let's use the house example again. If you were looking for a particular white frame house, it would be easier if the landmarks were right next door. If the landmarks were three blocks away, they might help you find houses, but not your particular white frame house. However, if a blue shuttered house and a red brick house were on either side of the white frame house, it would be easy to find the house you were seeking.

In the same way, polymorphisms on either side of the problem gene are most useful.

Genetic Counseling for Couples with Concerns

Why are extended family studies important?

Useful polymorphisms are those markers from the mother's family which are different from the markers found in the father's family. Linkage analysis requires samples from several close relatives and at least one affected family member to try to locate some of the important marker regions. If family members have differences in their DNA that allow us to associate a few polymorphisms and the problem gene, the family is informative. If no polymorphism is identified and the gene cannot be traced through a family, the test will be non-informative. For those families, continued research and identification of new polymorphisms may be helpful in DNA diagnosis at a later time.

How is DNA testing done?

1. Your physician or counselor will ask questions about your family. This is usually done by taking a careful family history and drawing a family tree, called a pedigree. A pedigree helps us identify people in the family who may have the disease or be carriers of the disease. Other close relatives also need to be studied to learn if the particular part of the DNA is informative.

2. The laboratory will obtain a sample of blood or other tissue and remove the DNA from the cells. Blood will be collected from an affected child, as well as from brothers or sisters, the mother, the father, and perhaps other close relatives. Sometimes a DNA sample may be obtained from an unborn baby by using special prenatal tests.

3. The laboratory will purify the DNA. This step separates the DNA from other parts of the blood or tissue sample which are not needed for this test.

4. The laboratory will process the DNA. This involves the use of special proteins called restriction enzymes to precisely cut the DNA into small pieces, creating specific fragments. Restriction enzymes recognize the DNA polymorphism—those differences discussed earlier in this text.

5. Technicians will "label and study" the DNA. Special materials are used to "label" markers or gene regions so the DNA fragment of importance can be recognized. This is done with the aid of X-ray film and produces a picture of the DNA fragments being studied.

6. The laboratory director will interpret the results and genetic counseling will be provided. The laboratory director, together with the genetic specialist, will evaluate the possible pattern of inheritance and decide which chromosome might carry the gene with the particular problem. The results will be discussed with you so that you can understand what the results mean for you and your family. This usually requires an appointment with a genetic specialist.

What are the advantages of DNA studies

- Testing is accurate and specific.

- People in the family who are at risk for the disease can sometimes be identified before symptoms occur.

- Carriers of a problem gene can be identified and given appropriate genetic counseling. Non-carriers can also be identified and reassured.

- If no DNA tests are currently available for the particular disease, family members who are potentially at risk can still have their DNA saved for the future. This is called "DNA banking."

- Any tissue (blood, skin, etc.) that has DNA can be used.

- Carrier testing can be performed at any time.

What are the disadvantages of DNA studies?

- **Family Participation:** DNA studies need family cooperation since most tests require samples from several people in one family, including affected family members.

- **Time for Study:** DNA studies are complicated and will require time and care by specialized laboratories. Some results may be available in a few days, but, more often, it will take several weeks. Therefore, it is very important to try to arrange testing prior to pregnancy! If you are not pregnant now, but are considering prenatal tests in the future, complete the DNA studies now and call your genetic specialist as soon as you learn you are pregnant. If you are pregnant now, tell your genetic specialist immediately!

- **Non-informative Family Studies:** You may not receive an answer because the polymorphisms in your family do not permit

Genetic Counseling for Couples with Concerns

distinction of individual chromosomes carrying the disease gene. These are special problems that are not related to laboratory competence. Your genetic specialist will discuss some of these with you.

- **Inadequate Family History:** Sometimes no answer is possible because of an inadequate or incorrect family history. Problems such as adoption, the death of important affected family members, or lack of contact with certain branches of the family may all contribute to inadequate history.

- **Nonpaternity:** The test might show that the father in the household is not the "biological" (natural) father of the person who needs DNA testing. To complete the test, we must have DNA samples from both natural parents. If nonpaternity is a possibility in your family, it is important to tell your genetic specialist prior to DNA testing.

- **Recombination:** Markers are used to predict the inheritance of a disease gene because regions close to each other are inherited together. There is a very small possibility that the genes we want to study will become switched from one chromosome pair to another. When this type of scrambling occurs, we call it recombination. Recombination is a normal genetic process that occurs during the formation of an egg or sperm cell. However, this "switching" may destroy the ability to track the inheritance of a particular gene.

What diseases can be diagnosed through DNA studies?

Some of the more common disease for which DNA tests are available include:

- Cystic Fibrosis
- Duchenne Muscular Dystrophy
- Fragile X Syndrome
- Hemophilia
- Myotonic Muscular Dystrophy
- Adult Polycystic Kidney Disease
- Sickle Cell Anemia
- Thalassemia

New developments occur every day. It is important to check with your genetic specialist for an updated list of available tests.

Section 3.2

Genetic Screening

FDA Consumer, December 1990

A worldwide effort to understand all our genes is well under way. Along this journey of discovery, tests are being developed to identify both healthy people who can pass a genetic disorder to a child (carriers) as well as those, including fetuses, who will actually develop symptoms.

In the past few years, scientists have identified the genes responsible for several major disorders, including cystic fibrosis, Duchenne's muscular dystrophy, and a few inherited cancers. Applying this new and complex information to the practice of medicine will require education of health professionals, patients, and their families.

How will physicians, medical consumers, and, ultimately, the Food and Drug Administration deal with this coming avalanche of information? Fortunately, experts can turn to past experience with genetic screens to guide then, in planning the programs of the future.

Urine: Clues to PKU

The age of genetic screening dawned in 1934, when a mother of two retarded children in Oslo, Norway, commented to a relative who was a chemist that her children's diapers had an odd smell. The curious chemist analyzed the urine and found too much of one biochemical yet none of another, an enzyme (a protein that speeds a biochemical reaction).

The children had an "inborn error of metabolism" called phenylketonuria (PKU), each inheriting a defective gene from each carrier parent. The combined deficit blocked production of the enzyme (phenylalanine hydroxylase) that normally breaks down phenylalanine, a protein building block. This genetic roadblock caused the mental retardation.

Knowing precisely what a faulty gene does (or doesn't do) is half the battle in conquering an inherited disease. The story of PKU indeed has a very happy ending. In 1963, a test was approved to detect the enzyme deficiency at birth, making it possible to prevent retardation if the child follows a very low phenylalanine diet for the first 8 years. Thanks to the observant mother, today every newborn in the

Genetic Counseling for Couples with Concerns

United States is tested for PKU, and often other inborn errors, such as sickle cell disease, hypothyroidism, galactosemia, biotinidase deficiency, and homocystinuria.

Even though PKU is rare (affecting 1 in 14,000 whites and 1 in 300,000 blacks), genetic screening makes economic sense—it costs $3.3 million a year to screen newborns, but $189 million to care for the PKU patients who would be retarded if not for the screen.

PKU screening got off to a rocky start In the early 1960s, a few children who had transiently high levels of phenylalanine, but not PKU, were inappropriately placed on the diet. Some of them died. But PKU testing and treatment have since been perfected.

Sickle Cell Confusion

Another genetic screening program was initially disastrous. In the early 1970s, mass screening of blacks to identify carriers of sickle cell disease, a painful inherited anemia, began in earnest. (Although sickle cell disease affects other populations, notably Arabs, in the United States, it is overwhelmingly predominant among blacks.)

Semantics led to mass misunderstanding. Sickle cell disease carriers are referred to as having "sickle cell trait," although these people in fact have no symptoms. Quite understandably, people told they had sickle cell trait feared they would develop symptoms—and also often did not understand the genetic odds their children would face. If two carriers have a child, the child has a 1 in 4 chance of having full-blown sickle cell disease, a 1 in 2 chance of being a carrier like each parent, and a 1 in 4 chance of being completely free of the sickle cell gene.

Discrimination against carriers was widespread. In Massachusetts, black children had to be screened for sickle cell trait before they would be admitted to public school. In New York, the test was mandated when applying for a marriage license. Carriers were denied health and life insurance and entrance to the U.S. Air Force Academy. As geneticists began to recognize in the late 1970s that being a sickle cell disease carrier does not adversely affect health, these restrictions were lifted.

Newborn screening is useful when early diagnosis is coupled with treatment. Screening newborns for sickle cell disease is now mandatory, because it is known that daily penicillin can ward off life-threatening infections.

Marilyn Gaston, M.D., deputy chief of the sickle cell disease branch of the National Heart, Lung, and Blood Institute, explains, "Infection is what kills kids with sickle cell disease. A fever can progress to death in under nine hours, and we can't treat an infection that moves that fast. But we can diagnose the disease at birth, and then give oral penicillin daily. The test is easy, it's quick, it works, and it's cheap." Blood taken for the PKU test is used.

Adds Kenneth Pass, Ph.D., and director of the newborn screening program in New York, "With early diagnosis and prophylactic penicillin, mortality can be reduced to zero."

Tay Sachs Success

Ironically, at the same time that the sickle cell carrier screening program was causing unwarranted panic, another screen for a genetic disease—Tay Sachs—was quite successful.

In a child with Tay Sachs disease, a missing enzyme (hexosaminidase) leads to buildup of fat on nerve cells, destroying the nervous system. The child begins to lose developmental skills from about the age of 6 months, and by 2 years of age can no longer see or hear. Death comes by age 4. Like PKU and sickle cell disease, a Tay Sachs child usually comes as a surprise to two healthy parents who each carry the gene.

Tay Sachs disease is 100 times more prevalent among Jewish people of eastern European descent than in other populations. In this ethnic group, 1 in 3,000 newborns has the disease, and 1 person in 27 is a carrier. A pilot screening program in the early 1970s searched for carriers among the Jewish community in the Washington, D.C., area, and other programs followed. Because most couples found to be at risk of having a Tay Sachs child (that is, both parents were carriers) chose not to have children, the number of children born with Tay Sachs disease has since dropped by 90 percent.

The secret to the success of Tay Sachs screening, experts agree, was education. Community and religious leaders were first informed by the physicians in charge, and they informed the public. Testing was widely available on college campuses and in synagogues, community centers, and shops, and offered at times convenient for young people.

Clues in DNA

The sequence of a gene's building blocks (called bases) instructs the cell to string together amino acids to build a particular protein. Screens for PKU, sickle cell disease, and Tay Sachs disease were possible because the abnormal proteins causing the symptoms were known.

Genetic Counseling for Couples with Concerns

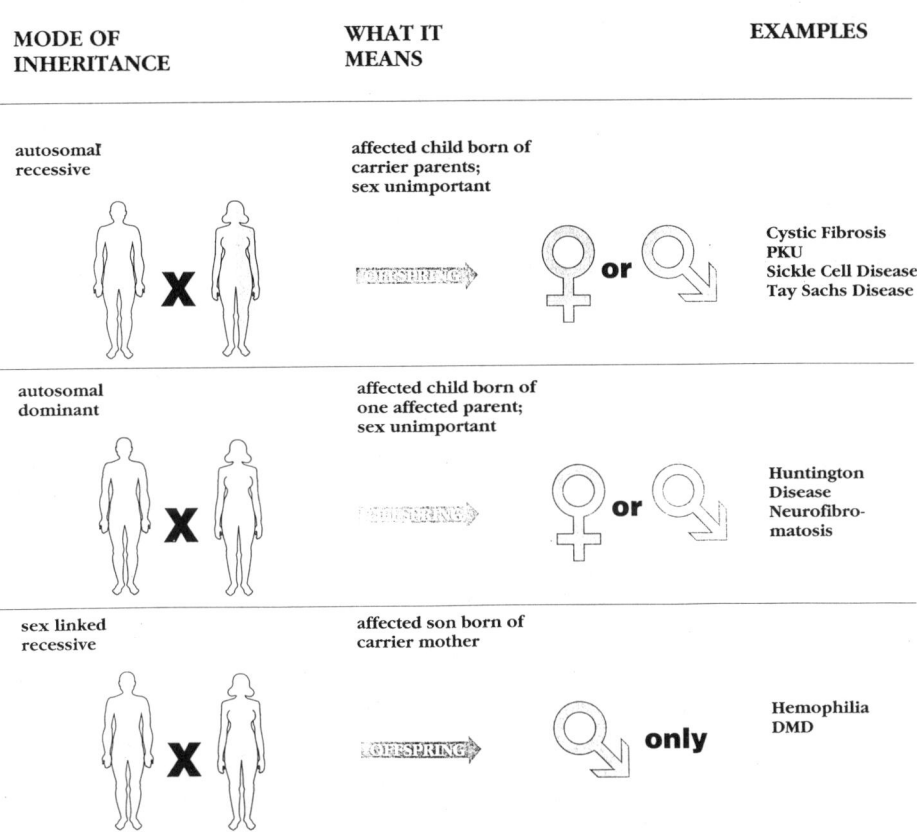

Figure 3.4. *How Diseases are Inherited*

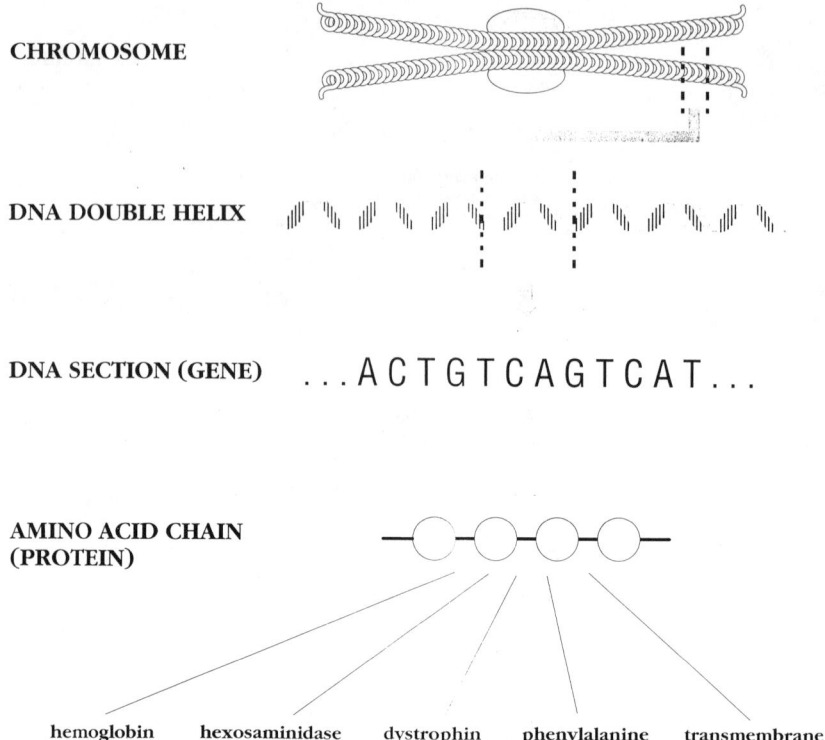

Figure 3.5. From Gene to Protein

Genetic Counseling for Couples with Concerns

But knowing which protein lurks behind a genetic disease is rare. Still, with much work and luck, researchers can pinpoint the stretch of DNA that causes a disease, even if its corresponding protein is not known. Zeroing in on the few thousand DNA bases whose activity causes a disease, among the 3 billion bases wound into every human cell, is a needle-in-a-haystack quest of daunting proportions. Even narrowing the gene search down to a specific chromosome is a tall order. (Chromosomes are rod-shaped bodies that carry the genes.) Often, this search can be expedited by very special patients.

In the 1970s, for example, a few young people with Duchenne's muscular dystrophy (DMD) and similarly broken X chromosomes (the X chromosome and Y chromosome determine sex; females are XX, and males are XY) led researchers to the precise location of the DMD gene—the site of the chromosome break. Then, in 1985, a boy was found who not only had DMD, but two other diseases linked to his X chromosome. In addition, his X chromosome had a tiny gap in it. The gap corresponded to the region of the break in the already-known unusual chromosomes.

It wasn't long before Louis Kunkel, Ph.D., at Harvard Medical School used a technique called "chromosome walking" to find that these patients' X chromosomes were missing a huge gene. That gene normally encodes a protein called dystrophin, which is present, sparingly, just beneath the surfaces of muscle cells and is essential for their activity. Because boys inheriting DMD from carrier mothers lack dystrophin, they become wheelchair bound by puberty, and die by their 20s. Thanks to the discovery of dystrophin's role, cell transplants are now being tested to treat DMD.

Patients with unusual chromosomes have also helped to unravel the genes behind Wilms' tumor (a childhood kidney cancer) and neurofibromatosis (also known, erroneously, as Elephant Man disease), which causes benign tumors to grow beneath the skin.

Genetic Markers

Even without unusual chromosomes as clues, some genes can be tracked by studying the DNA neighboring them—a little like judging a party by surveying the guests, even if the host is not in sight. The neighboring DNA is called a genetic marker, and it provides an indirect glimpse of a gene.

A genetic marker is an unusual sequence of DNA located near an unknown disease-causing gene. In certain families, a marker is found in every person who has the disease, but not in healthy relatives. Finding a marker is a laborious process, involving cutting DNA from many family members and meticulously searching for a piece of an unusual size found only among the ill.

A genetic marker allows detection of a disease-causing gene before symptoms arise. It can be tracked in a person of any age, as well as a fetus, because all genes are present from conception. For "marked" genes whose associated diseases are currently untreatable, such as those that cause the uncontrollable movements and personality changes of Huntington disease and the mental deterioration of inherited Alzheimer's disease, the value of predicting future ills may be questionable. Some healthy individuals, told they have such genetic diseases in their futures, may become suicidal. Others, however, may want to know the prognosis so they can plan their lives.

The promise of a genetic marker, though, is that it tells investigators where to hunt for the disease-causing gene. Once that is known, the gene's protein can be deduced from the gene's sequence and the biochemical basis of the symptoms revealed. Treatment may follow.

For example, in 1988 a marker for neurofibromatosis was found, and the gene was identified in July 1990. In August 1990, a University of Utah team led by Ray White, Ph.D., deciphered the gene's product. It is a protein that normally suppresses certain cancer-causing genes (oncogenes). White says that "future experiments ... may suggest new means of therapy. It may become possible, for example, to develop a blocking agent to halt the stimulation of cell growth in a developing neurofibroma [tumor]. Or, it might also be possible to deliver the gene product locally, likewise inhibiting development of neurofibromas".

Cystic Fibrosis and Beyond

Soon, mass population screening may begin for cystic fibrosis, the most common inherited disease of whites. In cystic fibrosis, glands in the lungs and pancreas secrete abnormally thick mucus that obstructs these structures. Also, sweat is very salty. The protein behind cystic fibrosis normally forms a channel in certain cells that controls passage of salts.

A marker for cystic fibrosis was found in 1985, but, like all marker tests, it requires that several family members participate so that the unusual sequence of DNA that travels with the disease-causing gene in that family can be traced. A marker test cannot be used on people who have no relatives with the disorder. For a population-based test (one on people who do not have cystic fibrosis in the family), the gene

Genetic Counseling for Couples with Concerns

itself must be in hand. This was indeed accomplished in 1989 by Francis Collins, Ph.D., M.D., at the University of Michigan at Ann Arbor and Lap-Chee Tsui, Ph.D., M.D., at the Hospital for Sick Children in Toronto.

But carrier screening for cystic fibrosis is complicated, because the specific alteration, or mutation, in the gene that led to its identification causes the disorder in only 75 percent of whites of AngloSaxon origin—and in less than 40 percent of Jews, blacks, Asians, Italians, and other population groups. This means that a carrier test based only on this one mutation will give many false negatives—people who have a genetic glitch slightly different from the first, who will erroneously be told that they are not carriers.

Scientists are finding dozens of other mutations that cause cystic fibrosis, and additional screening tests for carriers are being developed. With these tests, more carriers can be identified. "Testing for [the four most common mutations] will still detect only 80 to 85 percent of carriers in the United States. It is not yet time for population screening, but it is the time for pilot projects," says Collins.

For now, carrier testing is recommended only for people with cystic fibrosis in the family, says Tom Tsakeris, director of FDA's division of clinical laboratory devices. In these cases, markers can be used along with identifying the mutation, increasing accuracy to close to 100 percent. Demand for population-based carrier testing is likely to be great, because 1 in 25 of all whites—8 million to 12 million people—carries the gene.

While cystic fibrosis carrier tests are being refined, Robert Williamson, M.D., of St. Mary's Hospital in London is already combining technologies to diagnose the disease in a fetus in a single day. The diagnostic duo includes chorionic villus sampling of cells surrounding an 8-week fetus and the polymerase chain reaction, a new method to rapidly copy genes. PCR is applied to a body fluid sample, and the component of interest (such as a gene or marker) is amplified to a level at which it can be detected for a diagnosis.

Says P. Michael Conneally, Ph.D., medical geneticist at the Indiana University School of Medicine and co-discoverer of the marker for Huntington disease: "A pregnant woman comes into St. Mary's Hospital early in the morning. They do a chorionic villus sampling right away, and send the material to Dr. Williamson to do the PCR. They know the results by early afternoon, and the couple is counseled right away."

Like the tests themselves, FDA's role in regulating genetic tests is constantly evolving. For now, tests to detect recently revealed genes or markers are offered by reference laboratories, which are not regulated by FDA unless they market kits to physicians. Physicians send patient samples to these labs, which return the results along with interpretations. Tighter scrutiny of reference labs is beginning. "A new law, the Clinical Laboratory Improvement Act of 1988, will regulate reference labs, except tests for research purposes only. This act will have a tremendous impact on clinical laboratory testing and gene tests," says Tsakeris.

He predicts that screening the general population for cystic fibrosis will be trend-setting. "Cystic fibrosis presents the kind of situation that will emerge for other types of tests. There will be lots of conditions and caveats applied to the use of these tests. It will be a real challenge, and FDA will be caught in the middle. On the one hand, there is a strong push to get new cutting edge tests on the market. Yet, as we all know, as tests are used and experiences collected, tests often do not meet their initial promise. This is true for all clinical tests. For gene tests, the implications will be more profound," Tsakeris says.

Various organizations are rallying to ensure that the mistakes of the past are not repeated in future genetic screens. The National Institutes of Health has called for informed consent, confidentiality, equal access, education and counseling, quality control of reference labs, and voluntary testing as guidelines.

As genetic researchers work their way through human genetic material, their discoveries are expected to spawn many diagnostic tests and, ultimately, treatments. What scientists have learned from experience will enable them to make the best use of this new information. Genetic screening, then, promises to be very much a part of FDA's—and the consumer's—future.

Treating the Fetus and Child

Blake Schultz' life was saved seven weeks before he was born. Early in 1990, ultrasound revealed a hole in his diaphragm, the muscle sheet dividing the chest from the abdomen. His stomach, intestines and spleen protruded into his chest, squashing his lungs. He would probably have suffocated shortly after birth, were it not for experimental surgery performed by Michael Harrison, M.D., and colleagues at the University of California at San Francisco.

They exposed part of the fetus, opened his left side, gently tucked the organs back into place, and repaired the hole with a patch of Goretex, a synthetic material used in warm-up suits. Blake was the first human success, following six others who didn't make it.

Genetic Counseling for Couples with Concerns

Other fetal treatments are more routine. For hydrocephalus ("water on the brain"), a shunt can drain the fluid buildup into the digestive tract, where it exits harmlessly. For too little amniotic fluid caused by a blocked fetal bladder, a catheter can be inserted to drain off the accumulating urine.

"Left untreated, this causes a backup of urine into the fetal genitourinary system, which leads to fetal kidney damage, too little amniotic fluid, and destruction of the lungs—which kills the baby," says Frank Craparo, M.D., who performs such surgery at Pennsylvania Hospital in Philadelphia.

Craparo samples fetal blood to detect anemia and rapidly analyze chromosomes, and can also enter the blood vessels of the umbilical cord to deliver drugs directly to the fetus while bypassing the mother. Called PUBS (percutaneous umbilical blood sampling), the procedure can also be used to provide a lifesaving transfusion when blood between mother and child is incompatible.

"In these cases, the fetus becomes severely anemic, and may die in utero, or be born prematurely," Craparo says. He is working on expanding the capabilities of PUBS. "We will be able to study blood gases, and perhaps see how well oxygenated a fetus is in cases of growth retardation. There are a whole host of tests on the horizon. Anything we can do on adult blood, we may be able to do on a fetus' blood." Still experimental, PUBS carries a risk of 1 to 1.5 percent of harming the fetus.

Treating inherited illness after birth is an option following prenatal diagnosis or newborn screening. Like Blake Schultz, Sam Looper is a trailblazer. One spring morning in 1990, Sam wiggled the big toe of his left foot and, in so doing, made medical history. The 9-year-old suffers from Duchenne's muscular dystrophy, and because of a missing protein called dystrophin, his muscles have been slowly wasting away since toddlerhood.

When the gene behind DMD and its errant protein were discovered in 1986, Peter K. Law, M.D., professor of neurology at the University of Tennessee in Memphis, began reversing DMD-like symptoms in mice by injecting them with immature muscle cells (myoblasts) that produce dystrophin. By 1989, he felt ready to try the approach in humans. To do it as safely as possible, he injected Sam's left big toe with healthy, dystrophin-producing myoblasts from his father.

The boy's body accepted his father's cells, and two months after the transplant, he could wiggle the toe. Still, the approach needs a great deal of refinement to treat major muscles before it enters medical practice.

Sometimes, ideas for new treatments come from existing data. Steve Shak, a molecular biologist at Genentech Inc. in South San Francisco, was intrigued by papers from the 1950s describing a cow enzyme that could dissolve some of the sticky mucus that clogs the lungs of cystic fibrosis patients. But too many patients were allergic to the cow enzyme for it to be developed. Shak applied state-of-the-art genetic technology to locate the human version of the gene that specifies the human version of the enzyme. He hopes that it will clear lungs without triggering allergic reactions, and has applied to FDA to begin testing with patients.

—by Ricki Lewis

Chapter 4

Home Pregnancy Tests

Many women use home pregnancy tests if they suspect they're pregnant. Regulated by the Food and Drug Administration, pregnancy tests have come far since the early to mid-1900s when toads, rats and rabbits were used in testing. Now, over-the-counter home pregnancy kits provide privacy and fast results, and can detect pregnancy as early as six days after conception, or one day after a missed menstrual period. This gives an early advantage for vital prenatal care.

All pregnancy tests are based on the presence of a hormone, human chorionic gonadotropin (HCG), that the pregnant woman produces after conception. The first self tests of the 1970s used ring, or "tube agglutination," tests consisting of prepackaged red blood cells to detect HCG in urine. A ring at the bottom of the tube indicated a positive result. Sensitive to movement and human error, ring tests are now rarely used.

Today's brands, such as e.p.t. and First Response, contain monoclonal antibodies that detect minute traces of HCG. These antibodies are molecules coated with a substance that bonds to the pregnancy hormone, if it's present, to produce either a positive or negative result. (Each test manufacturer uses a different "trade secret" chemical formula for the bonding substance.) The user collects urine and combines it with the antibodies provided in the package. The test is timed, and a color change indicates the result.

Although most manufacturers claim 99 percent accuracy in laboratory tests, inaccurate results may be more frequent in actual use,

Excerpt from FDA Consumer, November 1990

Pregnancy and Birth Sourcebook

due to such factors as improper use of the test, using a product past its expiration date, exposure of the test to the sun, and cancers. The procedures outlined in the instructions must be followed exactly for results to be accurate.

Whitehall Laboratories markets the newest one-step brand, Clearblue Easy. It gives results in three minutes and informs the user when the test hasn't been done properly. This new testing method, called rapid assay delivery system, combines a biochemical process with monoclonal antibodies in one pen-like instrument.

Whatever the result or the brand used, most manufacturers recommend repeating the process a few days later to confirm the results. After conception, a woman produces a minimal amount of HCG. The strength of each test varies, and although a woman may be pregnant, the test may not pick up the amount of HCG hormone present the first time.

Part Two

Maternal Care During Pregnancy

Chapter 5

Taking Care of Yourself During Pregnancy

Chapter Contents

Section 5.1—Your Health During Pregnancy............................ 42
Section 5.2—X-Rays, Pregnancy and You 46

Pregnancy and Birth Sourcebook

Section 5.1

Your Health During Pregnancy

Excerpt from DHSS publication entitled "Every Child Deserves a Healthy Start", September 1992 and excerpts from DHSS Publication No. HRSA-MCHB-92-4-A, 1994

Doesn't the United States have the healthiest babies in the world?

No. Not by a long shot. About 36,500 infants die each year in the U.S. And there are 21 countries where babies have a better chance of living to celebrate their first birthday than babies born here.

Why are babies dying?

Most often, it is because they are born too soon and too small—less than 5 1/2 lbs. (called "low birthweight"). Each year about 284,000 underweight babies are born in the U.S.

How does this affect me?

It means that you or someone you know may give birth to a baby too small and too sick to make it through the first year of life. We all share in paying the high medical care costs—more than $2,000 each day—for these babies.

How can we help more babies get a healthy start?

The best way to make sure babies are healthier is for all pregnant women to get early and continual health care (called "prenatal care") and the necessities of life—nutritious food, adequate housing, and support from family and friends.

Also, it's especially important for a woman who is pregnant—or even planning to become pregnant—not to smoke, drink alcohol, or take drugs, and to talk to her health care provider about prescription drugs.

Taking Care of Yourself During Pregnancy

Is anything being done to help women have healthy babies?

Absolutely. In fact, there are many people who care, and many programs for women and babies that are working to make sure that all babies have a strong and healthy beginning.

Take Care of Yourself

Take care of yourself so that you feel good and your baby grows normally. Some things to do:

- eat a variety of healthful foods each day.
- eat 3 meals at regular times during the day.
- drink 6-8 glasses of water and other liquids each day.
- exercise regularly. Ask your health care giver about starting or continuing to exercise.
- wear your seat belt every time you ride in a car, van or truck.
- brush and floss your teeth at least once a day. Continue to see your dentist on a regular basis.
- tell all your health care givers that you are pregnant before getting any X-rays (see next section).
- read the label for directions and warnings before you use any paint, cleaner, bug spray, or other chemical.
- keep all of your health care appointments. If you miss an appointment, make another right away. Don't wait until the next month.
- ask your health care giver if you have questions about what you should be doing to have a healthy baby!

Some things you might do when you are pregnant can harm your baby. Some things not to do:

- Don't smoke. Tobacco of any kind will harm you and your baby. Smoking increases the chances that your baby may be born too soon and too small. Quitting at any time during your pregnancy helps. There are programs to help a pregnant woman stop smoking. Ask your health care giver about them. Quit as soon as you can.

- Don't drink alcohol (beer, wine, wine coolers, liquor). Drinking alcohol can cause birth defects. No one knows whether drinking even a little is safe. The best advice is don't drink when you are pregnant. Programs to help you stop drinking are available.

- Don't use any street drugs (such as crack, cocaine, marijuana, PCP). Street drugs can hurt you and your baby. Your baby can be born too small to live, or have severe mental or physical problems that can last for years. Tell your health care givers about any drugs you use so they can help you stop.

- Don't take any medicine—even an aspirin—anything prescribed before you were pregnant without first asking your health care providers if it is safe.

Pregnancy is a time of physical and emotional change. Having mixed feelings is normal. Doctors , nurses and other medical staff understand these mixed feelings. They can help you understand that these feelings are normal. They are always ready to listen to your questions and concerns.

Who can you contact?

American Academy of Pediatrics
P.O. Box 927
Elk Grove Village, IL 60009-0927
for additional information on access to health care.

The American College of Obstetricians and Gynecologists (ACOG)
Attention: Resource Center
409 12th Street SW
Washington, DC 20024
for single free copies of pamphlets on prenatal care.

Children's Defense Fund
25 E Street, NW,
Washington, DC 20001
for information on public policy affecting children's health.

Taking Care of Yourself During Pregnancy

Healthy Mothers, Healthy Babies Coalition
409 12th Street, SW,
Washington, DC 20024-2188
202-863-2458
to find out how to link up with local coalitions and mobilize your community to promote quality prenatal care.

March of Dimes Birth Defects Foundation
1275 Mamaroneck Avenue
White Plains, NY 10605
about volunteer activities and for referrals to prenatal care and community programs.

National Maternal and Child Health Clearinghouse
8201 Greensborough Drive, Suite 600
McLean, VA 22102
for a free single copy of Infant Care, a guide for new parents.

National Coalition of Hispanic Service Organizations (COSSMHO)
1501 16th Street, NW
Washington, DC 20036
for information on Hispanic maternal health and child health.

National Commission to Prevent Infant Mortality
Switzer Building, 330 C Street, SW, Room 2014
Washington, DC 20201
about the health and education policies and services every community should have for mothers and children.

Call your state health department (usually in the capital city) and ask for the office that handles maternal and child health issues. Every state has a toll free phone line for prenatal care referrals for low income women. Also check with your local health department to see if there are activities they know of in your area.

Call your local community hospital. They may have a range of programs and services for pregnant women and newborns. As part of its commitment to serve the community, a hospital has classes, materials, and other services often for free or for a small fee.

Section 5.2

X-Rays, Pregnancy and You

DHSS Publication No. (FDA) 94-8087, 1994

Pregnancy is a time to take good care of yourself and your unborn child. Many things are especially important during pregnancy, such as eating right, cutting out cigarettes and alcohol, and being careful about the prescription and over-the-counter drugs you take. Diagnostic x-rays and other medical radiation procedures of the abdominal area also deserve extra attention during pregnancy. This text is to help you understand the issues concerning x-ray exposure during pregnancy.

Diagnostic x-rays can give the doctor important and even life-saving information about a person's medical condition. But like many things, diagnostic x-rays have risks as well as benefits. They should be used only when they will give the doctor information needed to treat you.

You'll probably never need an abdominal x-ray during pregnancy. But sometimes, because of a particular medical condition, your physician may feel that a diagnostic x-ray of your abdomen or lower torso is needed. If this should happen don't be upset. The risk to you and your unborn child is very small, and the benefit of finding out about your medical condition is far greater. In fact, the risk of not having a needed x-ray could be much greater than the risk from the radiation. But even small risks should not be taken if they're unnecessary.

You can reduce those risks by telling your doctor if you are, or think you might be, pregnant whenever an abdominal x-ray is prescribed. If you are pregnant, the doctor may decide that it would be best to cancel the x-ray examination, to postpone it, or to modify it to reduce the amount of radiation. Or, depending on your medical needs, and realizing that the risk is very small, the doctor may feel that it is best to proceed with the x-ray as planned. In any case, you should feel free to discuss the decision with your doctor.

Taking Care of Yourself During Pregnancy

What kind of X-rays can affect the unborn child?

During most x-ray examinations—like those of the arms, legs, head, teeth, or chest—your reproductive organs are not exposed to the direct x-ray beam. So these kinds of procedures, when properly done, do not involve any risk to the unborn child. However, x-rays of the mother's lower torso abdomen, stomach, pelvis, lower back, or kidneys—may expose the unborn child to the direct x-ray beam. They are of more concern.

What Are the Possible Effects of X-Rays?

There is scientific disagreement about whether the small amounts of radiation used in diagnostic radiology can actually harm the unborn child, but it is known that the unborn child is very sensitive to the effects of things like radiation, certain drugs, excess alcohol, and infection. This is true, in part, because the cells are rapidly dividing and growing into specialized cells and tissues. If radiation or other agents were to cause changes in these cells, there could be a slightly increased chance of birth defects or certain illnesses, such as leukemia, later in life.

It should be pointed out, however, that the majority of birth defects and childhood diseases occur even if the mother is not exposed to any known harmful agent during pregnancy. Scientists believe that heredity and random errors in the developmental process are responsible for most of these problems.

What if I'm X-rayed before I know I'm pregnant?

Don't be alarmed. Remember that the possibility of any harm to you and your unborn child from an x-ray is very small. There are, however, rare situations in which a woman who is unaware of her pregnancy may receive a very large number of abdominal x-rays over a short period. Or she may receive radiation treatment of the lower torso. Under these circumstances, the woman should discuss the possible risks with her doctor.

How You Can Help Minimize the Risks

- Most important, tell your physician if you are pregnant or think you might be. This is important for many medical decisions, such as drug prescriptions and nuclear medicine procedures, as well as x-rays. And remember, this is true even in the very early weeks of pregnancy.

- Occasionally, a woman may mistake the symptoms of pregnancy for the symptoms of a disease. If you have any of the symptoms of pregnancy—nausea, vomiting, breast tenderness, fatigue—consider whether you might be pregnant and tell your doctor or x-ray technologist (the person doing the examination) before having an x-ray of the lower torso. A pregnancy test may be called for.

- If you are pregnant, or think you might be, do not hold a child who is being x-rayed. If you are not pregnant and you are asked to hold a child during an x-ray, be sure to ask for a lead apron to protect your reproductive organs. This is to prevent damage to your genes that could be passed on and cause harmful effects in your future descendants.

- Whenever an x-ray is requested, tell your doctor about any similar x-rays you have had recently. It may not be necessary to do another. It is a good idea to keep a record of the x-ray examinations you and your family have had taken so you can provide this kind of information accurately.

- Feel free to talk with your doctor about the need for an x-ray examination. You should understand the reason x-rays are requested in your particular case.

For further information, write to:

CDRH (HFZ-210)
Rockville, MD 20857

Chapter 6

Nutrition

Chapter Contents

Section 6.1—All About Eating for Two 50
Section 6.2—Recommendations for Weight Gain During
 Pregnancy 56
Section 6.3—Prenatal Vitamin Recommendations 59
Section 6.4—How Folate Can Help Prevent Birth Defects 60
Section 6.5—Knowledge and Use of Folate in the U.S.A. 68

Section 6.1

All About Eating for Two

Excerpts from DHSS Publication No. (FDA) 90-2183, 1990

"Pickles and ice cream" conjures up a picture of a woman whose pregnancy has caused her food preferences to become a bit off-beat.

Although the tastes of mothers-to-be usually run along far more normal lines, the "pickles and ice cream" image is accurate in portraying the food cravings—and aversions—that sometimes accompany pregnancy. These tastebud changes often reflect changes in nutritional needs.

Such changes are partly due to the nourishment demands of the fetus and partly to other physiological variations that affect absorption and metabolism of nutrients. These changes help insure normal development of the baby and fill the subsequent demands of lactation, or nursing.

Exactly how nutrients are exchanged between mother and fetus is not understood. In the past it was viewed as a host-parasite relationship, with the fetus in the role of the parasite, taking whatever nourishment it required from the host mother. But recent research has shown that the fetus is not a perfect parasite. The fetus is sometimes more affected than the mother by lack of nourishment, and there is a relationship between maternal weight gain and growth and development of the fetus.

Pedro Rosso, M.D., of Columbia University's Institute of Human Nutrition, wrote in *Nutritional Disorders of American Women* that "contrary to the idea of fetal parasitism, there seem to be feedback mechanisms operating in the mother that would reduce the maternal supply line to the fetus when nutrients are in short supply."

Writing in *Nutritional Impacts on Women,* two English researchers, Frank E. Hytten, M.D., and Angus Thomson, said that changes in nutritional needs in pregnancy appear to be related to the body's adaptation to pregnancy because the changes occur too early to be responding solely to fetal needs. Such changes include a reduction of

Nutrition

electrolytes, proteins, glucose, vitamin B12, folate, vitamin B6, and a rise in lipids, triglycerides, and cholesterol in blood.

The consequences of maternal malnourishment may include health problems for the mother and an infant of low birth weight who may have nutritional and other deficiencies.

Nutrients for the fetus come from the mother's diet, stored nutrients in the mother's bones and tissues, and synthesis of certain nutrients in the placenta. The placenta facilitates the transfer of nutrients, hormones, and other substances from mother to fetus.

According to a booklet by Roslyn B. Alfin-Slater, Ph.D., titled *Nutrition and Motherhood,* if the mother is poorly nourished, the placenta does not perform its functions as well.

The Food and Nutrition Board of the National Academy of Sciences specifies certain increases in the Recommended Daily Dietary Allowances (RDAs) for pregnant and lactating women.

Iron

More iron is needed not only because of fetal demands, but also because the mother's blood volume may be increased as much as 30 percent. Because the additional requirement for iron cannot be met by the usual American diet nor by existing stores in many women, iron supplements of 30 to 60 milligrams under supervision of a healthcare professional are recommended.

The main effect of inadequate iron during pregnancy is iron deficiency anemia, which makes the mother less able to fight off an infection and less able to tolerate hemorrhaging during childbirth. It has been suggested that pica, the craving for substances with little or no nutritional value, may be associated with iron deficiency. Although pica occurs during pregnancy in a number of ethnic groups and geographic areas, in this country it is most prevalent among southern blacks. The most common substances eaten are dirt, clay, starch, and ice. The National Research Council has noted that as many as 75 percent of the pregnant women attending southern health department clinics consumed starch and 50 percent ate clay. Concerns about the practice are several. First, eating these substances may take the place of eating nutritionally adequate food. Second, some pica substances, such as starch, are high in calories and may contribute to obesity. Third, some pica substances (such as charcoal, air fresheners, and mothballs) contain toxic substances. Fourth, the chemical makeup of some of these substances interferes with the absorption of minerals. Although it is not known

Table 6.1.

Recommended Daily Dietary Allowances for Women (Revised 1989)

From the Food and Nutrition Board of the National Academy of Sciences/National Research Council

Age	Weight	Height	Protein	Fat-Soluble Vitamins				Water-Soluble Vitamins							Minerals						
				Vit. A	Vit. D	Vit. E	Vit. K	Vit. C	Thia-mine	Ribo-flavin	Niacin	Vit. B_6	Folate	Vit. B_{12}	Cal-cium	Phos-phorus	Mag-nesium	Iron*	Zinc	Iodine	Selenium
(years)	(lbs)	(inches)	(g)	(mcg)	(mcg)	(mg)	(mcg)	(mg)	(mg)	(mg)	(mg)	(mg)	(mcg)	(mcg)	(mg)	(mg)	(mg)	(mg)	(mg)	(mcg)	(mcg)
11-14	101	62	46	800	10	8	45	50	1.1	1.3	15	1.4	150	2.0	1200	1200	280	15	12	150	45
15-18	120	64	44	800	10	8	55	60	1.1	1.3	15	1.5	180	2.0	1200	1200	300	15	12	150	50
19-24	120	65	44	800	10	8	60	60	1.1	1.3	15	1.6	180	2.0	1200	1200	280	15	12	150	55
25-50	120	64	44	800	5	8	65	60	1.1	1.3	15	1.6	180	2.0	800	800	280	15	12	150	55
Pregnant			60	1300	10	10	65	70	1.5	1.6	17	2.2	400	2.2	1200	1200	320	30	15	175	65
Lactating																					
1st 6 months			65	1300	10	12	65	95	1.6	1.8	20	2.1	280	2.6	1200	1200	355	15	19	200	75
2nd 6 months			62	1200	10	11	65	90	1.6	1.7	20	2.1	260	2.6	1200	1200	340	15	16	200	75

*The increased requirement during pregnancy cannot be met by the iron content of typical American diets nor by the existing iron stores of many women; therefore, the use of 30 to 60 mg of supplemental iron is recommended. Iron needs during lactation are not substantially different from those of non-pregnant women, but continued supplementation for mothers of two to three months after parturition is advisable to replenish stores depleted by pregnancy.

Key:
g = grams
mcg = micrograms
mg = milligrams

whether anemia is the cause of or the effect of pica, the craving abates when the anemia is corrected.

To a certain extent, Mother Nature lends a hand in pregnancy by improving iron absorption. A woman who is not pregnant absorbs about 10 percent of the iron present in food consumed. A pregnant woman, however, can absorb up to twice as much. In addition, the fetus stores iron during the last month or two of gestation. Some good sources of iron are meat (especially liver and other organs), egg yolks, and legumes.

Folate

Pregnancy doubles a woman's need for folate (folic acid or folacin). However, there is not universal agreement on the necessity of folate supplements for all pregnant women. Women can get additional folate by eating more green leafy vegetables, certain fruits, and liver and other organ meats. Severe folate deficiency can result in a condition called megaloblastic anemia, which occurs most often in the last trimester of pregnancy. In this condition the mother's heart, liver and spleen may become enlarged, and the life of the fetus may be threatened.

Because folic acid is crucial to cell multiplication, the fetus's needs are met before those of the mother. Therefore, the mother's health is more adversely affected at first. In contrast to the increased absorption of iron in pregnancy, folic acid absorption may be impaired by hormonal changes in pregnancy. For more information read further in this Chapter.

Calcium

Pregnant adult women need an extra 400 milligrams of calcium daily. That's about 50 percent more than recommended for women 25 and older. Nearly all of the extra calcium goes into the baby's bones. This need can usually be met by consuming more dairy products. If there is not enough calcium in the mother's diet, the fetus may draw calcium from the mother's bones. Calcium deficiency in pregnancy may result in osteopenia (decreased bone density) in the mother.

Nature also helps supply the extra calcium needed in pregnancy by improving calcium absorption. Less is lost in urine and feces, and passage of calcium through the placenta to the fetus is facilitated.

A pregnant woman needs three or more servings of milk or other dairy products a day to get 1,200 milligrams of calcium. For women who are lactose intolerant, there are a variety of low-lactose and reduced-lactose food products available. Sometimes calcium supplements are recommended by a woman's doctor. But pregnant women should not take calcium supplements such as bone meal and dolomite. FDA surveys have shown that some bone meal and dolomite products contain substantial amounts of lead. Lead can be harmful to both mother and fetus.

Other Nutritional Concerns

Pregnancy is a natural, healthy state, and most changes in pregnant women occur without harmful effects. But some physiological changes have been topics of particular medical concern. In past years, the tendency of pregnant women to retain water has led to restriction of sodium intake. When water retention was severe, diuretics were frequently prescribed to avoid toxemia. However, views on sodium restriction have changed. Today, there is considerable medical opinion that pregnancy is a "salt-wasting" condition—that is, one in which the body can use more salt than usual. Further, sodium deprivation may be harmful to the fetus. The sodium intake usually recommended in pregnancy is 2,000 to 8,000 milligrams a day, compared to the normally recommended 1,100 to 3,300 milligrams per day. However, pregnant women should be careful that their sodium intake does not greatly exceed this allowance.

Sugar is also an occasional concern in pregnancy. Virtually all women excrete more glucose (a form of sugar) in their urine when they are pregnant. This is one of the normal physiological adjustments to pregnancy and is not a cause for concern in the majority of women. It is significant only in the few women who have a tendency towards diabetes and who may thus become diabetic during pregnancy.

Diabetic women should be closely monitored to make sure their blood sugar values are at or near normal. If maternal blood sugar rises too high, the increased sugar crossing the placenta can result in a large, overdeveloped fetus and an infant with blood sugar level abnormalities. Diabetic women may also suffer from a greater loss of some nutrients.

Nausea in early pregnancy is another condition that often can be managed nutritionally. Dr. Alfin-Slater's booklet suggests the following:

- Keep meals small, and avoid long periods without food.
- Drink fluids between, but not with, meals.
- Avoid foods that are greasy, fried or highly spiced.

Nutrition

Current Research into Diet and Fetal Development

Improvements in the technological ability to diagnose birth defects early in pregnancy have focused attention on ways to correct certain fetal defects by manipulating the mother's diet. For example, researchers are investigating the use of vitamin-mineral supplements to prevent neural tube defects—that is, failure of the fetus's neural tube to close because of spinal cord abnormalities. Other investigators are researching ways maternal nutrition can help fetuses with inherited birth defects, usually inborn errors of metabolism, in which certain nutrients are not processed normally.

The effects of a woman's diet on her children start long before she becomes pregnant. Stores of fat, protein, and other nutrients built up over the years are called upon during pregnancy for fetal nourishment.

According to Roy M. Pitkin, M.D., of the University of Iowa College of Medicine, in *Nutritional Impacts on Women,* pre-pregnant weight and pregnancy weight exert independent and added influences on the infant's birth weight.

To what extent pregnancy affects a woman long after she has given birth is another subject under investigation. FDA's Jean Pennington, Ph.D., says it is known that a woman who has a large number of children may deplete calcium stores. Walter H. Glinsmann, M.D., chief of FDA's clinical nutrition branch, counsels that having babies should be considered a major life effort that begins long before conception.

"Getting pregnant is like running a race," Dr. Glinsmann says. "You have to get yourself in condition."

—by Judith Levine Willis

Section 6.2

Recommendations for Weight Gain During Pregnancy

Excerpts from DHSS Publication No. (FDA) 90-2183 (1990), DHSS Publication No. HRSA-MCHB-92-4-A (1994) and FDA Consumer, November 1990 by Lisa Iannucci

Attitudes have changed about weight gain in pregnancy. In the past, pregnant women were told to limit gain to about 15 pounds. Higher weight gain was thought to be related to a number of problems. The most worrisome of these problems was toxemia (also called Pregnancy Induced Hypertension—PIH), a condition of unknown origin occurring after the 20th week of pregnancy and involving high blood pressure and protein in the urine or water retention or both. Although sudden large weight gain, water retention, and blood pressure elevation continue to be recognized danger signs of toxemia, most physicians have come to agree that weight gain does not cause toxemia. The consequences of restricting weight gain, in fact, appear to be potentially more harmful, particularly to the fetus, than unrestricted weight gain, even in women who are overweight before becoming pregnant.

Studies have shown that underweight women, or those who gain fewer than 20 pounds during pregnancy, are at an increased risk of delivering low-birth-weight babies. If a woman's calorie intake is restricted in pregnancy, she may not get enough protein, vitamins and minerals to adequately nourish her unborn child. Low-calorie intake can result in a breakdown of stored fat in the mother, leading to the production of substances called ketones in her blood and urine. The production of ketones is a sign of starvation or a starvation-like state. Chronic production of ketones can result in a mentally retarded child.

For these reasons, the National Academy of Sciences recommends that pregnant women eat an average of 150 calories more per day in the first trimester and 350 calories more per day in the two subsequent trimesters than they did before becoming pregnant. A total

Nutrition

weight gain of about 25 to 30 pounds is usually recommended, with the actual pattern of gain considered more important than the number of pounds. Adolescents and black women, who often have smaller babies, are now strongly advised to gain greater amount. Weight gain should be at its lowest during the first trimester, and should steadily increase, with the mother-to-be gaining the most weight in her third trimester, when the fetus and placenta are growing the most.

The recommended increase in weight gain does not give a green light for mothers-to-be to overeat. Although the extra nutrients are required, an increase of only 300 calories per day is recommended. Weight gain during pregnancy should be gradual. The American College of Obstetricians and Gynecologists recommends 3 to 4 pounds in the first three months and 3 to 4 pounds per month during the rest of the pregnancy.

Your weight will be checked each time you go to your health provider. How much you gain is related to your weight before you became pregnant. Usually:

- If you were underweight, you should gain 28 to 40 pounds.
- If your weight was normal, you should gain 25 to 35 pounds.
- If you were very heavy, you should gain 15 to 25 pounds.

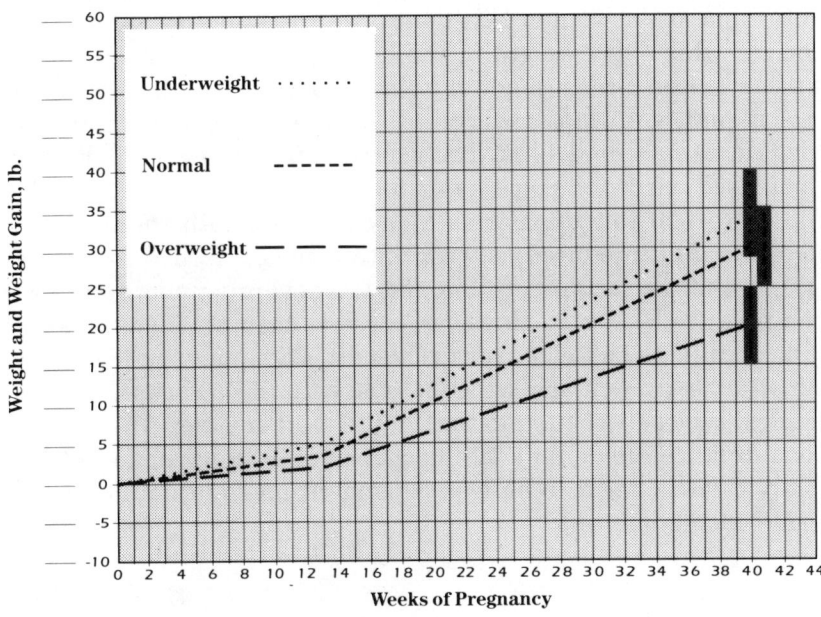

Figure 6.2. Prenatal Weight Gain Chart

Pregnancy and Birth Sourcebook

Your health care provider may advise you to gain more or less, depending on your size and weight before you became pregnant. This is not the time to lose weight, no matter how heavy you are. Your steady weight gain is a sign that your baby is growing. Gaining weight is what sometimes makes pregnant women most unhappy and uncomfortable. But if you remember how important it is to the health of your baby, it may be easier for you to handle. Besides most women lose all the extra weight they have gained by 2 or 3 months after their baby is born, and even sooner if they breastfeed.

The effects of undernutrition on infant size is greatest when nutritional deprivation occurs during the final three months. Weight gain in the second trimester is due mostly to increases in tissue, blood volume, and fat stores, and enlargement of the uterus (womb) and breasts.

Arthur Alfin-Slater estimates that a 25-pound weight gain breaks down as follows: baby, 8 pounds; placenta, 1 pound; amniotic fluid, 1.5 pounds; breasts, 3 pounds; uterus, 2.5 pounds; and stored fat and protein, water retention, and blood volume, 8 pounds.

Along with increased total calories, pregnant women need high-quality protein daily, the approximate amount contained in two large eggs and 2 ounces of cheese or a 4-ounce serving of meat.

During pregnancy, fat deposits may increase by more than a third the total amount a women had before she became pregnant. Most women lose this extra weight in the birth process or within several weeks thereafter. Breast-feeding helps to deplete the fat deposited during pregnancy. A woman who breast-feeds expends 600 to 800 more calories than one who doesn't. The woman who nurses her baby also has increased needs for specific nutrients.

The extra 600 to 800 calories a day includes both the nutritive value of the milk produced as well as the energy needed to synthesize the milk from lactose, protein and fat. Severely undernourished women produce less milk. However, obese women produce the same amount of milk as those of average weight. The amount of vitamins in human milk, particularly water-soluble vitamins such as C and the B complex, is closely related to that in the mother's diet. The concentrations of trace elements such as copper and fluoride, and of fat-soluble vitamins, seem to be less dependent on the fluctuations in maternal eating habits.

Nutrition

Section 6.3

Prenatal Vitamin Recommendations

Excerpt from DHSS Publication No. (FDA) 90-21833, 1990 and FDA Consumer, November 1990 by Lisa Iannucci

Pregnant women also have an increased need for vitamin B6 and B12. B6 requirements usually can be met by eating more whole grains, milk, egg yolks, and organ meats. Vitamin B12 is found in foods of animal origin, including eggs and milk products. Because B12 occurs only in such foods, vegetarians who eat no eggs or cheese (vegans) should ask their health-care professionals about the necessity of B12 supplements. Severe vitamin B12 deficiency in pregnancy is rare.

A word about using vitamin and mineral supplements in pregnancy: If taken, they should be at about RDA levels. Large doses of vitamins and minerals should be avoided. In animal studies, megadoses of vitamins A and D have resulted in fetal defects. The same is likely to be true in humans.

Research questions whether there may be some benefit from multivitamins in preventing neural tube defects. The U.S. Centers for Disease Control reported a study of women who took multivitamin pills three months before and three months after conception. Researchers found a slightly higher incidence of birth defects in babies of women who were not multivitamin users. However, it is unclear whether the increase in defects was due to a lack of vitamins or to other factors that were not measured.

Although some subsequent studies showed that taking a daily multivitamin helped decrease birth defects, other studies showed multivitamin intake had no relationship to the incidence of birth defects.

While research continues, the Institute of Medicine recommends supplements only for pregnant women who are smokers, drug users, alcohol drinkers, or strict vegetarians. Obstetricians will continue to make the decision to recommend supplements based on individual requirements and will not recommend megavitamins without a specific medical reason.

Section 6.4

How Folate Can Help Prevent Birth Defects

FDA Consumer, September 1996 by Paula Kurtzweil and excerpts from
FDA Consumer, May 1994 by Rebecca Williams

If you plan to have children some day, here's important information for the future mother-to-be: Think folate now.

Folate is a B vitamin found in a variety of foods and added to many vitamin and mineral supplements as folic acid, a synthetic form of folate. Folate is needed both before and in the first weeks of pregnancy and can help reduce the risk of certain serious and common birth defects called neural tube defects, which affect the brain and spinal cord.

The tricky part is that neural tube defects can occur in an embryo before a woman realizes she's pregnant. That's why it's important for all women of childbearing age (15 to 45) to include folate in their diets: If they get pregnant, it reduces the chance of the baby having a birth defect of the brain or spinal cord.

"Adequate folate should be eaten daily and throughout the childbearing years," said Elizabeth Yetley, Ph.D., a registered dietitian and director of FDA's Office of Special Nutritionals.

There are several ways to do this:

- Eat fruits, dark-green leafy vegetables, dried beans and peas, and other foods that are natural sources of folate.

- Eat folic acid-fortified breakfast cereals.

- Take a vitamin supplement containing folic acid.

Folate's potential to reduce the risk of neural tube defects is so important that the Food and Drug Administration is requiring that by 1998 food manufacturers fortify enriched grain products with folic acid. This will give women another way to get sufficient folate: by eating fortified breads and other grains.

Nutrition

Nutrition information on food and dietary supplement labels can help women determine whether they are getting enough folate which is 400 micrograms (0.4 milligrams) a day before pregnancy and 800 micrograms a day during pregnancy.

Neural Tube Birth Defects

Neural tube malformations are serious birth defects that cause disability or death. They are the most common disabling birth defects, affecting between one and two infants out of every 1,000 births in the United States.

There are two main kinds of neural tube defects: anencephaly and spina bifida. A baby with anencephaly does not develop a brain, and dies shortly after birth.

Spina bifida is a defect of the spinal column. If the vertebrae (bones of the spinal column) surrounding the spinal cord do not close properly during the first 28 days after fertilization, the cord or spinal fluid bulge through, usually in the lower back.

While once all these children died, with proper medical treatment, about 85 to 90 percent of them now live to adulthood, according to the Spina Bifida Association of America. Depending on the severity of the condition, they have varying degrees of paralysis and incontinence.

There are two major forms of the condition. The mild form, spina bifida occulta ("hidden") is only a small gap in the spine, with a dimple in the skin covering it. There are usually no symptoms. Some Americans have spina bifida occulta and don't even know they have it, according to the National Information Center for Children and Youth with Disabilities.

The more disabling form is spina bifida aperta, which produces a noticeable sac on the infant's back. A small sac, called a meningocele, produces little or no muscle paralysis or incontinence once it is repaired.

But in 90 percent of all spina bifida cases, a portion of the undeveloped spinal cord itself protrudes through the spine and forms a sac protruding on the baby's back. Any portion of the spinal cord outside the vertebrae is undeveloped or damaged, causing paralysis and incontinence. This is called a myelocele (or meningomyelocele), and it is what most people refer to as spina bifida.

The location of the sac determines how severely disabled the child will be. In general, the higher it is on the spinal column, the more paralysis there is.

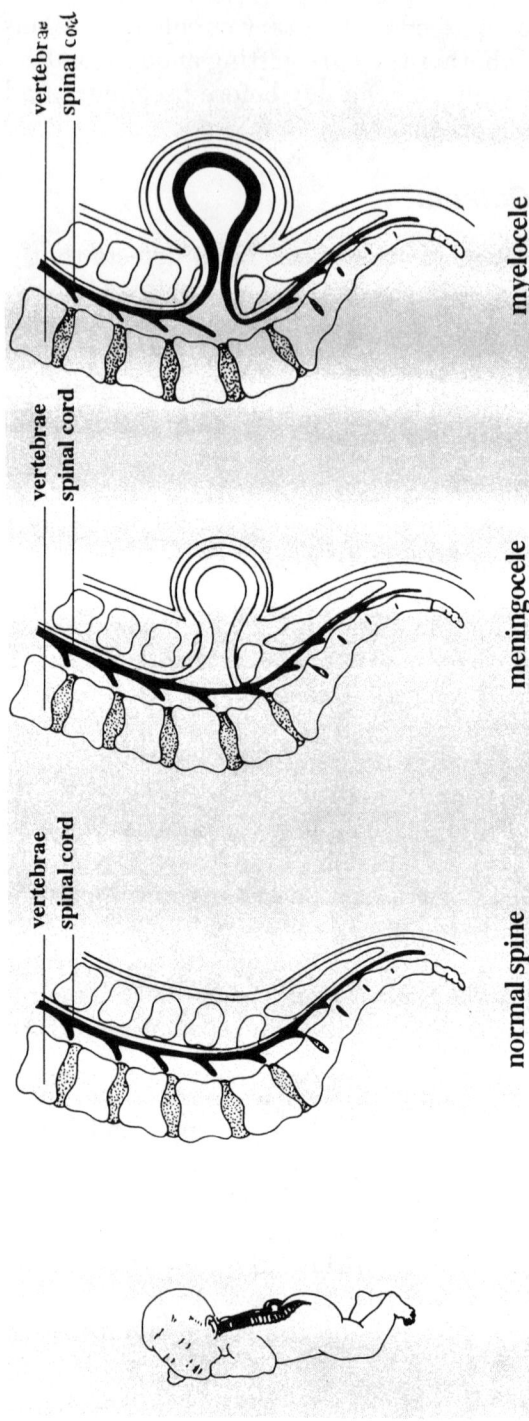

Figure 6.3. Spina Bifida Aperta. Compared to the normal spine (left), the spine of a baby with spina bifida aperta has a noticeable sac. When the sac is small (center), it can be repaired and there will be no muscle paralysis. But in 90 percent of cases, a portion of the undeveloped spinal cord protrudes through the spine and in to the sac (right), causing paralysis and incontinence.

Nutrition

Doctors must repair the opening of the spine shortly after birth or the child will die. Other major surgeries often follow in the child's first years. About 85 percent of children with spina bifida develop hydrocephalus, an accumulation of cerebrospinal fluid surrounding the brain. This fluid must be drained to the abdomen or bloodstream with a surgically implanted tube.

Some children with spina bifida develop foot and knee deformities caused by an interruption of spinal nerve circuits. Many patients require leg braces, crutches, and other devices to help them walk. They may have learning disabilities, and about 30 percent of children have slight to severe mental retardation, especially if they have chronic hydrocephalus. Chronic bladder infections and kidney problems require lifelong medical attention.

Despite their need for medical attention, children with spina bifida can learn to care for many of their own needs. They often learn to catheterize themselves, for instance, so they can attend regular schools. With proper medical care, a person with spina bifida can live a long and productive life. Maternal factors also may contribute to the development of neural tube defects. These include:

- family history of neural tube defects
- prior neural tube defect-affected pregnancy
- use of certain anti-seizure medications
- severe overweight
- hot tub use in early pregnancy
- diabetes.

Any woman concerned about these factors should consult her doctor.

Folate Link

Scientists first suggested a link between neural tube birth defects and diet in the 1950s. The incidence of these conditions has always been higher in low socioeconomic groups in which women may have poorer diets. Also babies conceived in the winter and early spring are more likely to be born with spina bifida, perhaps because the mother's diet lacks fresh fruits and vegetables—which are good sources of folate—during the early weeks of pregnancy.

In 1991 British researchers found that 72 percent of women who had one pregnancy with a neural tube birth defect had a lower risk of having another child with this birth defect when they took prescription doses of folic acid before and during early pregnancy.

Another study looked at folic acid intake in Hungarian women. The evidence indicated that mothers who had never given birth to babies with neural tube defects and who took a multivitamin and mineral supplement with folic acid had less risk in subsequent pregnancies for having babies with neural tube defects than women given a placebo.

These studies led the U.S. Public Health Service in September 1992 to recommend that all women of childbearing age capable of becoming pregnant consume 0.4 mg of folate daily to reduce their risk of having a pregnancy affected with spina bifida or other neural tube defects.

That corresponds to FDA's Daily Value for folic acid, which is 400 micrograms for nonpregnant women, as well as children 4 and older and adult men. For pregnant women, the Daily Value jumps to 800 micrograms. Daily Values are dietary reference numbers used on the Nutritional Facts panel on food labels to show the amounts of various nutrients in a serving of food.

Many women between 19 and 50 get only 200 micrograms of folate a day, according to the U.S. Department of Agriculture.

Folate Sources

Folate occurs naturally in a variety of foods, including liver; dark-green leafy vegetables such as collards, turnip greens, and Romaine lettuce; broccoli and asparagus; citrus fruits and juices; whole-grain products; wheat germ; and dried beans and peas, such as pinto, navy and lima beans, and chickpeas and black-eyed peas.

Under FDA's folic acid fortification program, the agency is requiring manufacturers to add from 0.43 mg to 1.4 mg of folic acid per pound of product to enriched flour, bread, rolls and buns, farina, corn grits, cornmeal, rice, and noodle products. A serving of each product will provide about 10 percent of the Daily Value for folic acid. Whole-grain products do not have to be enriched because they contain natural folate. Some of the natural folate in non-whole-grain products is lost in the process of refining whole grains.

The fortification regulations become effective Jan. 1, 1998, although manufacturers may begin folic acid fortification immediately, as long as they adhere to the regulations.

Folate also can be obtained from dietary supplements, such as folic acid tablets and multivitamins with folic acid and from fortified breakfast cereals.

A study reported in the March 9, 1996, issue of *The Lancet,* suggested that folic acid, the synthetic form of folate, may be better absorbed than folate found naturally in foods. Christine Lewis, Ph.D.,

Nutrition

a registered dietitian and special assistant in FDA's Office of Special Nutritionals, said, "This is a complex and poorly understood issue, and more data are needed."

Food	Serving Size	Amount (Micrograms)	% Daily Value*
Chicken liver	3.5 oz	770	193
Breakfast cereals	1/2 to 1 1/2 cup	100 to 400	25 to 100
Braised beef liver	3.5 oz	217	54
Lentils, cooked	1/2 cup	180	45
Chickpeas	1/2 cup	141	35
Asparagus	1/2 cup	132	33
Spinach, cooked	1/2 cup	131	33
Black beans	1/2 cup	128	32
Burrito with beans	2	118	30
Kidney beans	1/2 cup	115	29
Baked beans with pork	1 cup	92	23
Lima beans	1/2 cup	78	20
Tomato juice	1 cup	48	12
Brussels sprouts	1/2 cup	47	12
Orange	1 medium	47	12
Broccoli, cooked	1/2 cup	39	10
Fast-food French fries	large order	38	10
Wheat germ	2 tbsp	38	10
Fortified white bread	1 slice	38	10

* based on Daily Value for folate of 400 micrograms
(Source: *Food Values of Portions Commonly Used*, 16th edition)

Table 6.4. Some Good Sources of Folate

Finding Foods with Folate

Certain information on food and dietary supplement labels can help women spot foods containing substantial amounts of folate. Some labels may claim that the product is "high in folate or folic acid," which means a serving of the food provides 20 percent or more of the Daily Value for folic acid. Or the label may say the food is a "good source" of folate, which means a serving of the food provides 10 to 19 percent of the Daily Value for folic acid. The exact amount will be given in the label's Nutrition Facts panel.

Some food and dietary supplement labels may carry a longer claim that says adequate folate intake may reduce the risk of neural tube birth defects. Products carrying this claim must:

- provide 10 percent or more of the Daily Value for folic acid per serving

- not contain more than 100 percent of the Daily Value for Vitamins A and D per serving because high intakes of these vitamins are associated with other birth defects.

- carry a caution on the label about excess folic acid intake, if a serving of food provides 100 percent of the Daily Value for folic acid. FDA has set 1 mg (or 1,000 micrograms) of folate daily as the maximum safe level. There are limited data on the safety of consuming more than 1 mg daily, and there may be a risk for people with low amounts of vitamin B-12 in their bodies—for example, older people with malabsorption problems, and people on certain anticancer drugs or drugs for epilepsy whose effectiveness can diminish when taken with high intakes of folate.

- list on the label's Nutrition or Supplement Facts panel the amount by weight in micrograms and the %Daily Value of folate per serving of the product. This information, which appears toward the bottom of the panel, along with the listing of other vitamins and minerals, can be used to compare folate levels in various food supplements.

Optional information may appear with the health claim to let consumers know about other risks associated with neural tube birth defects, when to consult a doctor, other foods that are good sources of folate, and other important messages about neural tube defects.

Other Considerations

The claim about folate cannot imply that adequate folate intake alone will ensure a healthy baby, since so many factors can affect a pregnancy.

Women should bear this in mind when contemplating pregnancy, advises Jeanne Latham, a registered dietitian and consumer safety officer at FDA's Office of Special Nutrition. "Folate can make a significant contribution," she said, "but it's no guarantee of a healthy baby."

Genetics plays a role, as do other healthful prenatal practices, such as eating an all-around good diet. But unlike genetics, diet is a risk factor women can modify to their—and their baby's—advantage, said Jeanne Rader, Ph.D., director of the division of science and applied technology in FDA's Office of Food Labeling.

"Folic acid is one of many nutrients needed in a healthy diet for women of childbearing age," she said. "A well-balanced diet with a variety of foods can provide all those nutrients, including adequate amounts of folate."

Women have options for reaching the folate intake goal: They can get the necessary nutrients and calories both before and during pregnancy by eating a well balanced diet, keeping in mind folate-rich foods, nutritions experts say. Folic acid-fortified grain products, including breakfast cereals, will help too. Dietary supplements are another source of folate. Any one or a combination of these options for ensuring adequate folate can help assure women of childbearing age that, if they become pregnant, their babies will be off to a healthy start.

More Information

For more information on having a healthy baby contact:

Maternal and Child Health Clearinghouse
5600 Fishers Lane, Room 18A-55
Rockville, MD 20857
(703) 821-8955

March of Dimes Birth Defects Foundation
1275 Mamaroneck Ave.
White Plains, NY 10605
(914) 428-7100
Voice mail only: (914) 997-4750
World Wide Web:
http://server.triplesoft.com//marchofdimes/index.html

Section 6.5

Knowledge and Use of Folic Acid by Women of Childbearing Age—United States, 1995

Morbidity and Mortality Weekly, September 1995

Each year in the United States approximately 2500 infants are born with spina bifida and anencephaly, and an estimated 1500 fetuses affected by these birth defects are aborted. Recent studies indicate that the B vitamin folic acid can reduce the risk for spina bifida and anencephaly by at least 50% when consumed daily before conception and during early pregnancy. In September 1992, the Public Health Service (PHS) recommended that all women of childbearing age who are capable of becoming pregnant consume 0.4 mg of folic acid daily. Folic acid can be obtained from multivitamins or other supplements containing folic acid and some breakfast cereals. This report summarizes the results of a survey conducted during January-February 1995 regarding knowledge and practices of women of childbearing age in the United States about consumption of folic acid from supplements and breakfast cereals.

During January-February 1995, The Gallup Organization conducted for the March of Dimes Birth Defects Foundation a proportionate, stratified random-digit-dialed telephone survey of a national sample of 2010 women aged 18-45 years. The response rate was 50%. Respondents were asked, "Have you ever heard or read anything about folic acid?" Respondents also were asked, "From what you know, is there anything a woman can do to reduce her risk of having a baby with birth defects?" and "To the best of your knowledge, can consuming vitamins during pregnancy reduce the risk of birth defects?" For this analysis, estimates were statistically weighted to reflect the total population of women aged 18-45 years in the continental United States residing in households with telephones. The margin of error for estimates based on the total sample size within 95% confidence intervals is 2%.

Nutrition

Overall, 52% of women reported ever hearing of or reading about folic acid. Of these, 9% answered that folic acid helps to prevent birth defects and 6% that folic acid helps reduce the risk for spina bifida; 45% were unable to recall what they had heard or read. Fifteen percent of respondents reported having knowledge of the PHS recommendation regarding the use of folic acid; 4% reported that the recommendation was for prevention of birth defects and 1%, for prevention of spina bifida.

A total of 88% of respondents reported that a woman can help reduce the risk for having an infant with birth defects. The most common responses about how to reduce risk were avoiding alcohol and drugs (73%), and not smoking (63%); 1% reported that folic acid could reduce risk. Overall, 56% reported that consumption of vitamins during pregnancy can reduce the risk for having an infant with birth defects, and 78% reported that women should take multivitamins before pregnancy. The most frequently mentioned supplements respondents believed to be especially important to women of childbearing age and to pregnant women were iron (27%), calcium (26%), multivitamins (20%), vitamin C (14%), and folic acid (6%).

Overall, 25% of nonpregnant women of childbearing age reported taking a daily vitamin supplement containing folic acid. Of women who had been pregnant during the 2 years preceding the survey, 20% reported taking the vitamins before pregnancy. Among women who did not take vitamin or mineral supplements daily, the most frequently cited reasons for not taking them were "Don't feel I need them," (22%); "Forget to take them," (18%); and "Get balanced nutrition from foods," (12%).

Overall, 77% of women surveyed reported eating at least one serving of breakfast cereal each week; 14% reported eating at least seven servings per week. The average number of servings per week was three. Most cereals eaten contained 0.1 mg folic acid per serving, and few (6%) respondents who included cereals in their diets reported eating a cereal that contains 0.4 mg folic acid per serving.

A convenient method for a woman to achieve the PHS recommendation for the use of folic acid to reduce the risk for spina bifida and anencephaly is to take daily a vitamin supplement that contains 0.4 mg folic acid or eat a breakfast cereal containing 0.4 mg folic acid per serving. The findings in this report indicate that only 25% of nonpregnant women in the United States regularly consumed a vitamin supplement containing 0.4 mg folic acid, and only a small proportion ate a breakfast cereal containing 0.4 mg folic acid per serving. A previous report indicated that among women in South Carolina who had given birth during October 1992-September 1994, only 12% had used folic acid-containing vitamin supplements during the periconceptional period. In addition to consumption of folic acid-containing supplements or breakfast cereals, women can increase their consumption of folates by choosing foods consistent with the U.S. Dietary Guidelines for Americans and the U.S. dietary pyramid (e.g., orange juice and green leafy vegetables).

An important limitation of this telephone survey was the low response rate (50%). In particular, knowledge and behavior patterns of nonparticipants may have been different from those of participants. Because participating women were more highly educated than the total U.S. population, the prevalence of use of vitamin supplements may have been higher among these women than U.S. women in general because vitamin usage increases with education. Additional surveys of a more representative sample of women of childbearing age in the United States will be necessary to obtain more precise estimates of the use of vitamin supplements among such women. Nonetheless, the findings in this report and the South Carolina study suggest the need to increase knowledge of the importance of consuming folic acid among women of childbearing age and to heighten awareness among women about the potential benefits of taking folic acid on a daily basis.

Strategies for educating women about folic acid include reporting the issues in the news media, widely distributing informational materials (e.g., in physicians' offices, clinics, schools, and health clubs), and encouraging health-care providers to emphasize consistently the importance of daily consumption of folic acid when speaking to women of childbearing age. The most effective and efficient methods for increasing knowledge of the benefits of increased folic acid consumption and for changing behavior to increase use should be determined by additional research and demonstration projects. In addition, because folic acid consumption also could be increased by the addition of folic acid to staple foods, the Food and Drug Administration has proposed requiring the addition of folic acid to a variety of enriched cereal grain products.

References

CDC. Recommendations for the use of folic acid to reduce the number of cases of spina bifida and other neural tube defects. MMWR 1991;41(no. RR-14): 1-7.

Nutrition

CDC. Prevention program for reducing risk for neural tube defects—South Carolina, 1992-1994. MMWR 1995;44: 141-3, 149-50.

Block G, Cox C, Madans J, et al. Vitamin supplement use by demographic characteristics. Am J Epidemiol 1988;127: 297-309.

FDA. Proposed rule. Food standards: amendment of the standards of identity for enriched grain products to require addition of folic acid. Federal Register 1993;58: 53305-12.

Chapter 7

Prenatal Exercise Plans

Keeping fit and staying healthy are important during pregnancy. In general, it is safe to continue activities you like and participated in prior to pregnancy such as swimming, walking, or tennis. If you never exercised before, you may want to try walking. Walking is one of the easiest and healthiest forms of exercise for you and your baby. Always use common sense and stop before you get too tired. Unless your healthcare provider says otherwise, you may choose to join a prenatal exercise program.

If you have any medical problems (such as bleeding, spotting, low placenta, high blood pressure, or underlying medical problems), you may be advised not to exercise. Be sure to tell your healthcare provider what kind of exercise you are doing or want to start doing.

Precautions

- Always check with your healthcare provider before starting any exercise program.

- Do not start vigorous activities like skiing or horseback riding while you're pregnant.

Reprinted with permission from Group Health Cooperative of Puget Sound, copyright 1996. *Disclaimer of Warranties:* This publication was developed by Group Health for use in communicating with our enrollees. Group Health specifically disclaims any warranties, implied or expressed, including the warranty of merchantability and the warranty of fitness for a particular purpose. Information at the end of this chapter under the subtitle "Further Recommendations" is an excerpt from NIH Publication No. 93-2788, 1993

- Begin and end exercise with a warm up and cool down time.
- Do not get overheated.
- Drink water before, during, and after exercise. Do not get dehydrated.
- Stop if you feel dizzy or faint.
- Avoid deep bending motions and vigorous stretches.
- After the 4th month, do not exercise lying flat on your back.

Special Prenatal Exercises

The muscles in your lower abdomen, lower back, and around the vagina (the birth canal) come under great strain during pregnancy. Doing some simple exercises will help you strengthen the muscles that hold up your growing uterus and relax and stretch during delivery.

- Kegel squeeze
- Pelvic tilt
- Tailor stretch

Kegel Squeeze

The Kegel muscles are the ones you use to stop the flow of urine. This exercise is done by tightening, holding, and then relaxing these muscles.

An easy way to learn this exercise is to do it while you urinate. Squeeze the muscles to stop the flow of urine. Hold it tight for a short while, relax, and squeeze again. Once you feel how the Kegel squeeze feels, you can do it anywhere and no one will know.

Repeat this exercise 10 times a day. This is a good exercise for all women to do. It helps keep the vagina, bladder, and rectum in place as women get older.

Pelvic Tilt

This exercise relieves back pain as well as maintains and improves abdominal muscle tone. Many women find it helpful during labor, too.

- Get on your hands and knees on the floor with your back straight.

Prenatal Exercise Plans

- Breathe in and relax your back.
- Breathe out, tighten your stomach muscles and tuck in buttocks. (Think of a dog that's frightened and tucks its tail between its legs.) Your back will arch.
- Hold and count 1-2-3-4-5.
- Then breathe in again and relax.
- Repeat 8 to 10 times.

Pelvic Tilt Variation. You can also do a pelvic tilt against the wall. Stand with your back against a wall. Tighten your abdomen and tuck in your buttocks until your lower back is flat against the wall. Hold it while you count 1-2-3-4-5, then relax.

Tailor Stretch

This exercise stretches your inner thighs.

- Sit on the floor with the soles of your feet together.
- Gently let your knees open down toward the floor until you feel a mild stretch. Do not push down on your legs with your hands.
- Hold and slowly count to five, relax.
- Repeat five times twice a day.

Posture and Body Mechanics During Pregnancy

During the second trimester, you may find that you'll need to change how you get up, sit, and lie down. The following suggestions can help prevent strain and low back pain.

Sitting

- When sitting down, keep your back straight and use your leg muscles to lower yourself onto the seat.
- Slide back into the chair.
- Sit tall with your weight evenly distributed. Your back, buttocks, and shoulders should be supported by the back of the chair.

- Rest your feet flat on the floor or on a footstool right in front of the chair.

Getting Out of a Chair

- Press your upper back against the chair and slide your bottom forward (pulling on the arms of the chair).

- Turn sideways so you're sitting on the edge of the chair.

- Push on the arms of the chair and rise.

Lying Down

It's OK to lie on your back during the early part of your pregnancy, but you'll feel more comfortable lying on your side or in the "three-quarter position" during late pregnancy and labor.

Lying on your back:

- Use pillows to support your head and shoulders.

- Place an additional pillow or folded blanket under your thighs to help keep your knees bent for greater relaxation. (Do not place it under your knees where it may slow circulation.)

- Let your legs and feet roll outward. Roll one or both legs back and forth to relieve lower back pain.

- Bend your elbows slightly. Let your hands rest on your thighs or on the bed. If you feel dizzy, faint, or nauseated, turn onto your left side.

Lying on your side:

- Lie on your side with a pillow under your head.

- Place a pillow or blanket between your legs.

- Place another pillow or rolled up blanket behind your back for additional support.

Prenatal Exercise Plans

Three-quarter lying position:

This is an excellent position for sleeping, and as your pregnancy progresses you may find it the most comfortable.

- Lie on your left side with your left arm behind you and the bottom leg straight down. Bend your upper leg and rest it on a firm, fat pillow and bend your upper arm up. In this position you'll need only a flat pillow for your head.

Getting Up from a Lying Position

From the bed:

- Roll to one side and roll up your knees.
- Move your knees and feet to the edge of the bed.
- Push up to a sitting position with your arms and swing your legs over the side of your bed.
- Pause for a moment before standing.

From the floor:

- Bend knees up, feet on the floor.
- Roll onto your side.
- Roll over onto your hands and knees.
- Bring one knee forward and use it to push yourself up to a standing position.

Lifting

Don't lift very heavy objects.

- Stand facing the object you want to lift.
- Bend your knees and lower yourself slowly to a squatting position.
- Keep your back straight and your knees and feet well apart.
- If the object is heavy, bring it close to your body before lifting.
- Rise using your leg muscles to avoid back strain.

Further Recommendations

A daily exercise program is an important part of a healthy pregnancy. Daily exercise helps you feel better and reduces stress. In addition, being physically fit protects against back pain, and maintains muscle tone, strength, and endurance.

Talk with your doctor about what exercise program is right for you. Your doctor can advise you about limitations, warning signs, and any special considerations. Generally, you can continue any exercise program or sport you participated in prior to pregnancy. Use caution, however, and avoid sports or exercises where you might fall, or that involve jolting. Pre-pregnancy bicycling, jogging, and cross-country skiing are good exercises to continue during pregnancy. If you plan to start an exercise program during pregnancy, talk to your doctor before beginning and start slowly. Vigorous walking is good for women who need to start exercising and have not been active before pregnancy.

Don't omit a warm-up period of 5 to 10 minutes and a cool-down period of 5 to 10 minutes. Always stop exercising if you feel pain, dizziness, shortness of breath, faintness, palpitations, back or pelvic pain, or experience vaginal bleeding. Also, avoid vigorous exercise in hot, humid weather or if you have a fever. It is important to prevent dehydration during exercise, especially during pregnancy. The American College of Obstetricians and Gynecologists (ACOG) recommends drinking fluids prior to and after exercise, and if necessary, during the activity to prevent dehydration.

An ACOG report(*Home Exercise Program: Exercise During Pregnancy and the Postnatal Period.* American College of Obstetricians and Gynecologists May 1985, 6 pp.) issued in 1985, warned that target heart rates for pregnant and postpartum women should be set approximately 25 to 30 percent lower than rates for non-pregnant women. It may be that exercising too vigorously will direct blood flow away from the uterus and fetus. ACOG recommends that pregnant women measure their heart rate during activity and that maternal heart rate not exceed 140 beats per minute.

Chapter 8

Prenatal Care: What to Expect at Obstetrical Visits

In this century, the health care service most relied upon to assure positive pregnancy outcomes has been prenatal care (Thompson et al. 1990). In general, women who receive prenatal care during the first trimester have better pregnancy outcomes than women who have little or no prenatal care (National Center for Health Statistics 1988). Major improvements in the quality of life have resulted from the use of the present prenatal care system, and the birth of an infant is an important and happy event in most families. The Panel reaffirms that prenatal care provides a foundation for improving the health of the pregnant woman, infant, and family, and that the prenatal care system is a cornerstone of health care delivery in our society.

Objectives of Prenatal Care

In the past, prenatal care focused on the prevention of eclampsia and other maternal correlations of toxemia. In recent years, prenatal care has become more concerned with the identification and management of high-risk conditions for the fetus and newborn. A broader, contemporary view of prenatal care, however, sees pregnancy as an opportunity to promote the health and well-being of the family. In addition to assuring the health of the pregnant woman and the birth of a healthy infant, the objectives of prenatal care apply to the family during the pregnancy and the infant's first year of life.

Excerpts from NIH Publication No. 90-3182, and DHSS Publication Numbers HRSA-M-DSEA-96-5, September 1996, and HRSA-MCH-95-1, July 1995

Objectives of Prenatal Care for the Pregnant Woman

- to increase her well-being before, during, and after pregnancy and to improve her self-image and self-care;

- to reduce maternal mortality and morbidity, fetal loss, and unnecessary pregnancy interventions;

- to reduce the risks to her health prior to subsequent pregnancies and beyond childbearing years; and

- to promote the development of parenting skills.

Objectives of Prenatal Care for the Fetus and the Infant

- to increase well-being;

- to reduce preterm birth, intrauterine growth retardation, congenital anomalies, and failure to thrive;

- to promote healthy growth and development, immunization, and health supervision;

- to reduce neurologic, developmental, and other morbidities; and

- to reduce child abuse and neglect, injuries, preventable acute and chronic illness, and the need for extended hospitalization after birth.

Objectives of Prenatal Care for the Family

The objectives of prenatal care for the family during pregnancy and the first year of the infant's life are:

- to promote family development, and positive parent-infant interaction;

- to reduce unintended pregnancies; and

- to identify for treatment behavior disorders leading to child neglect and family violence.

Prenatal Care: What to Expect at Obstetrical Visits

Enriching Prenatal Care

The broad objectives of prenatal care are to promote the health and well-being of the pregnant woman, the fetus, the infant, and the family up to 1 year after the infant's birth. The prenatal period provides an opportunity to look beyond pregnancy and delivery to identify the resources essential for further healthy development of parents and infant. The objectives of prenatal care are concerned with more than the prevention of maternal and neonatal morbidity and mortality; these objectives include other aspects of the woman's health prior to, during, and after pregnancy and include the promotion of healthy child development, positive family relationships, and family planning.

For prenatal care to be effective, it must be available and it must be used. Every woman of reproductive age in the United States should participate in a basic program of prenatal health care and family planning-care that is augmented according to her needs and risk status. In planning, using, and evaluating prenatal care and services, the active participation of a woman and her support persons is essential; professionals can meet the prenatal care objectives only with their cooperation and partnership.

The three basic components of prenatal care are (1) early and continuing risk assessment, (2) health promotion, and (3) medical and psychosocial interventions and followup. Risk assessment includes a complete history, a physical examination, laboratory tests, and assessment of fetal growth and well-being. Health promotion consists of counseling to promote and support healthful behaviors, general knowledge of pregnancy and parenting, and information on proposed care. Interventions include treatment of existing illness, modifications of behavior, provision of social and financial resources, and referral to and consultation with other specialized providers.

To ensure the health of the woman and the developing fetus, preconception care should be an integral part of prenatal care. Many of the medical conditions, personal behaviors, and environmental hazards associated with the negative outcomes of pregnancy can be identified and should be modified or treated prior to conception. Care begun before pregnancy has great potential to assure health and ameliorate disease conditions for women. Such care would also avoid possible negative effects on the fetus of maternal treatment. The three components of prenatal care should begin prior to pregnancy in a preconception visit and should continue during prenatal visits, educational sessions, and other contacts with prenatal care providers. Pregnancy is often the impetus for a woman to seek health care following a period of either no care or episodic care. Every woman (and, when possible, her partner) contemplating pregnancy within 1 year should consult a prenatal care provider. Because many pregnancies are not planned, providers should include preconception counseling, when appropriate, in contacts with women and men of reproductive age.

Prenatal care should add to the traditional medical concerns a new emphasis on the psychosocial dimensions of that care, maintaining a balance among all factors. During the latter half of the 20th century, the approach to prenatal care has been a continuation of a medical model based primarily on the detection and treatment of preeclampsia and, more recently, the prevention of preterm birth. The content of prenatal care should include all necessary psychological, social, educational, and general medical assessments and interventions. Comprehensive prenatal care such as this has considerable potential for improving the health of the woman, infant, and family. Medical, psychological, and social risks often interact with each other and consequently require a multidisciplinary strategy for success.

Because significant change in risk status can arise at any time during pregnancy, continuing risk assessment throughout pregnancy is necessary for all women. Pregnancy is considered to be a healthy, normal state for most women, and a large number of women are healthy during pregnancy. Yet not all women remain so throughout pregnancy or begin pregnancy free of risk, because of preexisting medical, psychological, or social conditions. Those women who have increased risk of adverse pregnancy outcome can, to a considerable extent, be identified either before pregnancy begins or early in pregnancy, enabling treatment to be initiated early to minimize adverse outcome.

The specific content and timing of prenatal visits, contacts, and education should vary depending on the risk status of the pregnant woman and her fetus. For women considered to be healthy, visits with prenatal care providers should be scheduled for specific risk assessment or planned health promotion. The information obtained from

Prenatal Care: What to Expect at Obstetrical Visits

continuing risk assessment will determine the content and frequency of prenatal care. When possible, risk assessment and health promotion should be integrated into a single visit to minimize inconvenience for the pregnant woman for whom transportation or child care may be a problem. To minimize stress while adequately addressing women's pregnancy care needs, the timing of prenatal visits should be flexible and the information provided should be substantive. One prenatal care provider should be in charge of and coordinate the team providing each woman's prenatal care.

A comprehensive prenatal care record facilitates continuous documentation of all risk assessment, health promotion, and intervention activities, including those done preconceptionally, as well as facilitating information transfer for intrapartum care. As risk assessment changes the content of prenatal care in the attempt to reach prenatal care objectives, the prenatal record serves as a vehicle of communication among the health care team members and institutions as well as among the patient and her care providers. It functions as an instrument for evaluating and enhancing the quality of care. A universal prenatal care record will promote continuity of care and allow comparable analyses from diverse settings and populations.

The effectiveness of prenatal care will be improved by additional research on the specific content of prenatal care. As in other health care systems, many prenatal care practices have not been studied. Further, many practices that have been studied were not evaluated rigorously or with an adequate research design. Finally, new patient-care practices will need evaluation as clinicians, families, and health policy personnel seek to attain the broad objectives of prenatal care.

Prenatal Visits for Healthy Women

For many women, pregnancy is a planned event filled with joyous expectation. These women are generally in good health with no apparent medical or psychosocial risks. Ideally, these women are identified as free from risk at a preconception visit. Consequently, prenatal care for healthy pregnant women focuses on health promotion. Because risk may arise at any time during pregnancy, however, continuing assessment is essential. This text contains lists of the risk assessment and health promotion activities for each prenatal visit.

It must be emphasized that there should be a single prenatal care provider with primary and comprehensive responsibility. It is that provider who should be available to support the woman if unexpected pregnancy-related problems occur or are detected by risk assessment. Care may be delivered in an office, clinic, or through a home visit when necessary.

Recommended content and timing results in a core schedule of nine visits for the healthy nulliparous woman and seven for the healthy parous woman; one visit occurs prior to conception in each case.

First Pregnancy Visit for Healthy Women (6-8 Weeks Gestation)

Risk Assessment

- History of pregnancy to date; medical and psychosocial

- Physical examination for uterine size

- Laboratory tests:

  1. hematocrit or hemoglobin
  2. rubella titer (if no preconception visit)
  3. blood/Rh, Rh titer (if no preconception visit), antibody screen
  4. HIV offered
  5. gonorrhea culture
  6. pap smear (unless obtained during last year)
  7. urinalysis—protein, glucose, no microanalysis urine culture

- Dating pregnancy

Health Promotion

- Counseling to promote and support healthful behaviors: smoking cessation, alcohol avoidance, illicit drug and teratogen avoidance, nutrition, safer sex.

- General knowledge of pregnancy and parenting: physiologic and emotional changes in pregnancy, sexuality, self-help for discomforts, general health habits—hygiene, exercise and muscle toning, rest and sleep patterns, early pregnancy classes—encouragement of good nutrition, exercise, and fitness.

Prenatal Care: What to Expect at Obstetrical Visits

- Information on proposed care: need for early entry into prenatal care, preparation for screening and diagnostic tests, content and timing of prenatal visits, need to report danger signs.

Second Pregnancy Visit (Within Four Weeks of Previous Visit)

Risk Assessment

- Review of laboratory results

Health Promotion

- Counseling to promote and support healthful behaviors such as smoking cessation, alcohol avoidance, illicit drug and other teratogen avoidance, nutrition, maternal seatbelt use, and work patterns.
- General knowledge of pregnancy and parenting: physiologic and emotional changes in pregnancy, self-help for discomforts, general health habits—hygiene, exercise and muscle toning, rest and sleep patterns, early pregnancy classes—encouragement of good nutrition, exercise, and fitness.
- Information on proposed care: preparation for screening and diagnostic tests, content and timing of prenatal visits, need to report danger signs.

Third Pregnancy Visit Nulliparous Women; Second Pregnancy Visit Parous Women (14-16 Weeks)

Risk Assessment

- Partial history
- Vaginal bleeding
- Psychosocial factors
- Partial physical: auscultation, FHR (Doppler), fundal height, weight, Laboratory tests—MSAFP

Health Promotion

- Counseling to promote and support healthful behavior: smoking cessation, alcohol avoidance, illicit drug and other teratogen avoidance, nutrition.

- General knowledge of pregnancy and parenting: physiologic and emotional changes in pregnancy, sexuality, fetal growth and development, self-help for discomforts, general health habits—hygiene, exercise and muscle toning, rest and sleep patterns.

- Information on proposed care: preparation for screening and diagnostic tests, content and timing of prenatal visits, need to report danger signs, signs and symptoms of preterm labor.

Fourth Pregnancy Visit Nulliparous Women; Third Pregnancy Visit Parous Women (24-28 Weeks)

Risk Assessment

- Partial history—fetal movement, general health, nutrition, signs or symptoms of preterm labor, psychosocial factors.

- Partial physical exam—same as 14-16 weeks plus blood pressure.

- Laboratory tests: hematocrit or hemoglobin, glucose screen for diabetes, antibody screen for Rh women with negative titers.

Health Promotion

- Counseling to promote and support healthful behaviors: smoking cessation, alcohol avoidance, illicit drug and other teratogen avoidance, nutrition.

- General knowledge of pregnancy and parenting: physiologic and emotional changes in pregnancy, sexuality, fetal growth and development, self-help for discomforts, general health habits—hygiene, exercise and muscle toning, rest and sleep patterns), promotion of breastfeeding, need for prepared childbirth classes, perineal exercises.

- Information on proposed care, preparation for screening, and diagnostic tests, content and timing of prenatal visits, need to report danger signs, signs and symptoms of preterm labor.

Prenatal Care: What to Expect at Obstetrical Visits

Fifth Pregnancy Visit Nulliparous Women; Fourth Pregnancy Visit Parous Women (32 Weeks)

Risk Assessment

- Partial history—same as 24-28 weeks

- Partial physical exam—same as 24-28 weeks including blood pressure, abdominal exam.

Health Promotion

- Counseling to promote and support healthful behaviors: smoking cessation, alcohol avoidance, illicit drug and other teratogen avoidance, nutrition.

- General knowledge of pregnancy and parenting: physiologic and emotional changes in pregnancy, sexuality, fetal growth and development, self-help for discomforts, general health habits—hygiene, exercise and muscle toning, rest and sleep patterns, promotion of breastfeeding, childbirth education enrollment, infant car seat use, perineal exercises, family roles and adjustment.

- Information on proposed care: content and timing of prenatal visits, signs and symptoms of preterm labor.

Prepared Childbirth Classes

A formal series of prepared childbirth classes is recommended for all women. These are recommended at 32-38 weeks for first-time attenders and at 36-38 weeks if attended previously. For women who have never attended, the full series of sessions is recommended. For parous women who have attended during a previous pregnancy, a refresher series of one or two classes is recommended. These classes, at minimum, should educate women about the physiology of labor and birth, exercises and self-help techniques for labor, the role of support persons, family roles and adjustments, and preferences for care during labor and birth. The birth settings should be discussed and the woman's or couple's questions about the prenatal care provider and setting answered. This is a time when information relating to cesarean childbirth and vaginal birth after cesarean birth can be reviewed.

Timing

These classes are best placed during the third trimester of pregnancy, when interest in labor is evident and conditioned responses that are being learned will be used relatively soon. For classes to be completed before term labor (38 to 42 weeks), they should begin about 31 to 32 weeks so that they will be completed no later than 38 weeks. The refresher course is often only one or two classes and can be done at any time between 36 and 38 weeks.

Provider and Setting

The usual provider of prepared childbirth education is a childbirth educator with formal preparation in teaching such classes. Knowledge of the several kinds of childbirth education programs will help the prenatal provider assist the woman in choosing the series that best meets her needs. Choice of educator and setting will depend on what is available and accessible in the woman's community.

Sixth Pregnancy Visit Nulliparous Women; Fifth Pregnancy Visit Parous Women (36 Weeks)

Risk Assessment

- Partial history—same as 24-28 weeks

- Partial physical exam—same as 32 weeks

Health Promotion

- Counseling to promote and support healthful behaviors: smoking cessation, alcohol avoidance, illicit drug and other teratogen avoidance, nutrition, safer sex.

- General knowledge of pregnancy and parenting; physiologic and emotional changes in pregnancy, sexuality, fetal growth and development, self-help for discomforts, general health habits—hygiene, exercise and muscle toning, rest and sleep patterns, preparation for parenting classes, promotion of breastfeeding, signs and symptoms of labor, infant car seat use.

- Information on proposed care: content and timing of prenatal visits, need to report danger signs, signs and symptoms of preterm labor, preparation for labor and birth, birth planning when to call, where to go in labor.

Prenatal Care: What to Expect at Obstetrical Visits

Seventh Pregnancy Visit Nulliparous Women (38 Weeks); Sixth Pregnancy Visit Parous Women (39 Weeks)

Risk Assessment

- Partial history—same as 24-28 weeks.

- Partial physical—blood pressure, fetal lie, presentation, descent.

Health Promotion

- Counseling to promote and support healthful behaviors: smoking cessation, alcohol avoidance, illicit drug and other teratogen avoidance, nutrition.

- General knowledge of pregnancy and parenting: physiologic and emotional changes in pregnancy, sexuality, fetal growth and development, self-help for discomforts, general health habits—hygiene, exercise and muscle toning, rest and sleep patterns, promotion of breastfeeding, signs and symptoms of labor, infant car seat use, postpartum activity—including family planning, newborn care, family roles and adjustment.

- Information on proposed care: content and timing of prenatal visits, need to report danger signs, signs and symptoms of preterm labor, review of preparation for labor and birth, review of birth plan, when to call, where to go in labor.

Eighth Pregnancy Visit Nulliparous Women (40 Weeks)

Risk Assessment

- Partial history—fetal movement counts, signs and symptoms of labor.

- Partial physical—same as 38 weeks.

Health Promotion

- Counseling to promote and support healthful behaviors: smoking cessation, alcohol avoidance, illicit drug and other teratogen avoidance, nutrition.

- General knowledge of pregnancy and parenting: physiologic and emotional changes in pregnancy, sexuality, fetal growth and development, self-help for discomforts, general health habits—hygiene, exercise and muscle toning, rest and sleep patterns, promotion of breastfeeding, signs and symptoms of labor, infant car seat use, postpartum activity—including family planning, newborn care, family roles and adjustment.

- Information on proposed care: need to report danger signs, signs and symptoms of preterm labor, review of preparation for labor and birth, review of birth plan, preparation for postterm tests, when to call, where to go in labor.

The nulliparous woman is at increased risk for pregnancy induced hypertension and therefore needs to be followed more closely at the end of pregnancy. Weekly visits were not supported by the literature. Nonetheless, the Panel has concluded that weekly visits are appropriate.

Ninth Pregnancy Visit Nulliparous Women; Seventh Pregnancy Visit Parous Women (41 Weeks)

Risk Assessment

- Partial history

- Partial physical—same as 40 weeks

- Cervical check

Health Promotion

- Counseling to promote and support healthful behaviors: smoking cessation, alcohol avoidance, illicit drug and other teratogen avoidance, nutrition.

- General knowledge of pregnancy and parenting: physiologic and emotional changes in pregnancy, sexuality, fetal growth and development, self-help for discomforts, general health habits—hygiene, exercise and muscle toning, rest and sleep patterns, promotion of breastfeeding, signs and symptoms of labor, infant car seat use, postpartum activity—including family planning, newborn care and family roles and adjustment.

Prenatal Care: What to Expect at Obstetrical Visits

- Information on proposed care: content and timing of prenatal visits, need to report danger signs, signs and symptoms of preterm labor, review of preparation for labor and birth, review of birth plan, when to call, where to go in labor.

Indications for genetic counseling, chorionic villus sampling (CVS), amniocentesis, fetal testing, and postterm management fall outside the content and schedule of visits for healthy women. Once women carry their pregnancies beyond 41 weeks, more active intervention may be indicated.

Statistical Information

Early Prenatal Care

Overall, 78% of all mothers received prenatal care in the first trimester of pregnancy in 1992. In 1994 80% of all mothers received prenatal care in the first trimester of pregnancy.

There is substantial racial disparity in the timely receipt of prenatal care. In 1994, 83% of white mothers, as compared to 68% of black mothers, received early prenatal care.

Women younger than 20 years of age are less likely than older women to receive early prenatal care.

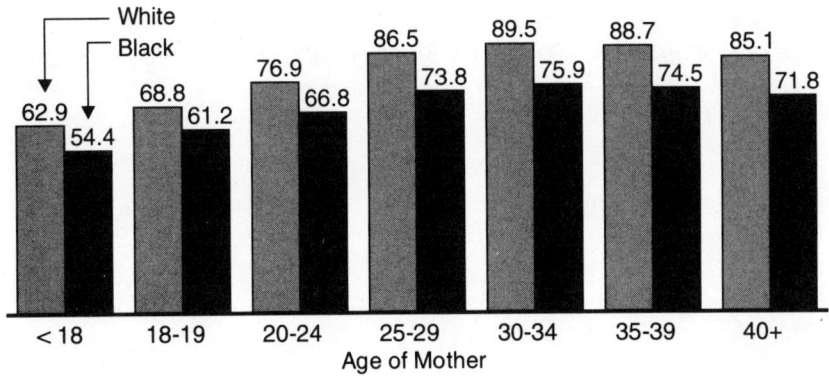

Figure 8.1. Percentage of Women with Early Prenatal Care, by Age and Race of Mother: 1994. Source (IV.8) National Center for Health Statistics.

No Prenatal Care

Every year from 1983 to 1991, 6% of infants were born to mothers who initiated care during the third trimester or received no prenatal care. In 1992, however, that figure dropped to 5% and was 4% in 1994.

Regardless of age, black women are less likely to receive prenatal care than are white women.

Risk factors for not receiving prenatal care include being less than 18 years of age, unmarried status, low educational attainment and being in a minority group.

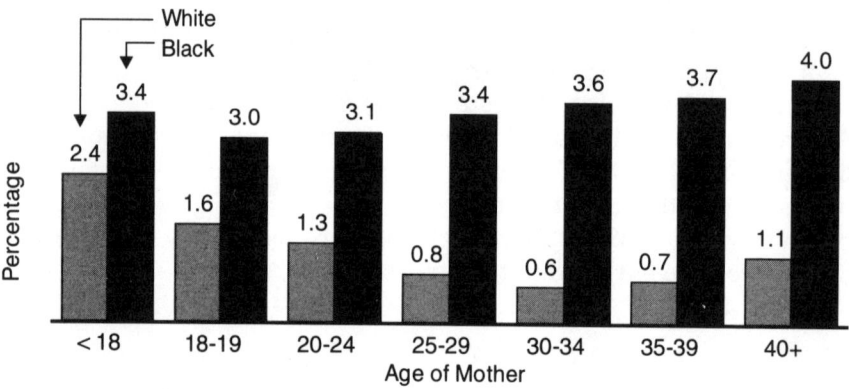

Figure 8.2. Percentage of Women with No Prenatal Care, by Age and Race of Mother: 1994. Source (IV.8): National Center for Health Statistics.

Chapter 9

Medical Tests Sometimes Used During Pregnancy

Chapter Contents

Section 9.1—Maternal Urinalysis and Blood Sampling 94
Section 9.2—Diagnostic Ultrasound Imaging in Pregnancy 95
Section 9.3—Amniocentesis and Chorionic Villus Sampling
    (CVS) 104
Section 9.4—Alpha-fetoprotein and Triple AFP Screening..... 116
Section 9.5—Fetal Monitoring: Stress and Non-Stress Tests . 117

Section 9.1

Maternal Urinalysis and Blood Sampling

From DHSS Publication No. HRSA-MCHB-92-4-A and
NIH Publication No. 90-3182

You will have your urine checked via dipstick at every prenatal visit for sugar and protein. These tests check for diabetes, infection, and problems related to your kidneys and blood pressure.

Blood tests are performed to see if you have certain conditions which might affect your pregnancy or your baby. Below is a list of the laboratory blood tests that are recommended as a part of all prenatal care (see Chapter 8).

- Hemoglobin or Hematocrit for testing anemia (low blood count)
- Rh factor
- Syphilis
- HIV
- Hepatitis B
- Check protection against rubella (German measles)

The following tests are recommended for some individuals:

- Toxoplasmosis
- CMV
- Herpes simplex
- Varicella
- Hemoglobinopathies
- Tay-Sachs
- Parental karotype
- Illicit drug screen

Medical Tests Sometimes Used During Pregnancy

Section 9.2

Diagnostic Ultrasound Imaging in Pregnancy

NIH Consensus Statement, Volume 5, Number 1, 1984
and excerpt from FDA Consumer, December 1990

Introduction

In an ultrasound exam, a device called a transducer passed over the abdomen or inserted into the vagina bounces sound waves off the fetus, much like sonar locating a submarine. A computer converts the sound waves into an image. Many studies show it is very safe to mother and fetus.

Ultrasound can establish the date of conception, the presence of twins, and monitor development. By 8 weeks, an image resembling a lima bean with a pulsating blip in the middle is an assurance that a "viable fetus"—with its blip of a heartbeat—is there.

By 15 weeks, a trained eye can discern major organs. While the parents happily count toes and fingers, a physician may measure the length of the leg bones or check facial features for signs of Down syndrome.

By 20 weeks, a penis—or lack of one—may be apparent. By 35 weeks, calcium deposits in the placenta, the organ linking mother to child, signal lung maturity. As the birth day nears, ultrasound reveals the fetal position.

Technological Developments

From crude initial studies in the 1950s, ultrasonography in pregnancy has become a highly developed technology capable of detecting many fetal structural and functional abnormalities. It has found application in detecting ectopic pregnancy and multiple pregnancy, assessing fetal life and function, diagnosing physical anomalies, and guiding physicians as they make efforts to treat the fetal patient. The advent of ultrasound has overcome many of the diagnostic limitations of X-ray and has virtually eliminated the need for fetal exposure to ionizing radiation.

With these advantages and marked improvements in the technology and equipment, the use of ultrasound in obstetric practice has grown rapidly. The procedure is available in nearly all hospitals, and many physicians have acquired equipment for use in their offices. Further, because of the absence of clinically perceived risk of ultrasound and its usefulness in assessing structural anomalies, multiple pregnancy, and fetal size and gestational age, many practitioners have begun to advocate its routine use as a screening device in all pregnancies.

Lack of risk has been assumed because no adverse effects have been demonstrated clearly in humans. However, other evidence dictates that a hypothetical risk must be presumed with ultrasound. Likewise, the efficacy of many uses of ultrasound in improving the management and outcome of pregnancy also has been assumed rather than demonstrated, especially its value as a routine screening procedure. The marked increase in the use of ultrasound, coupled with concerns regarding its safety and efficacy, prompted three NIH components—the National Institute of Child Health and Human Development (NICHD), the Office of Medical Applications of Research (OMAR), and the Division of Research Resources (DRR)—and the FDA National Center for Devices and Radiological Health to join in sponsoring a Consensus Development Conference to assess the use of diagnostic ultrasound imaging in pregnancy.

What types of ultrasound scanning are currently used in obstetric practice? How extensive is this use? What is known about the dose/exposure to the fetus and the mother from each type?

On the basis of the collective experience of members of the panel, the material presented, and the literature review that was conducted, we conclude that in obstetric practice in the United States, use of diagnostic ultrasound imaging has an expanding role, and its use is becoming widespread. Information on the extent of use of diagnostic ultrasound in pregnancy was available from single institutions and states, marketing studies, the office survey conducted by the American College of Obstetricians and Gynecologists, and the 1980 National Natality Survey. These data lead to estimates of the percentage of pregnant women exposed to at least one ultrasound examination ranging from a low of 15 percent to a high of 40 percent. There is reason to believe that all of these data sources seriously underestimate the true extent of exposure to ultrasound since they do not necessarily include exposure via Doppler devices, including those used to listen to fetal heart tones and in antepartum and intrapartum fetal heart rate monitoring.

Medical Tests Sometimes Used During Pregnancy

Exposure to imaging devices in the recent past has been to static scanners, real-time equipment of the linear array type, and mechanical sector scanners. The quantity used most often to report instrumentation output is intensity. Typical time average value ranges of intensity are 0.1-60 mW/cm2 (spatial average, temporal average intensity) and 1-200 mW/cm2 (spatial peak, temporal average intensity). The spatial peak, pulse average intensity typically ranges from 1-200 W/cm2 for such pulsed ultrasound equipment.

The time average intensities of the typical obstetrical Doppler devices used to listen to the fetal heart and for fetal heart rate monitoring in the antepartum and intrapartum period are within the same range as for pulsed equipment. These systems operate in the continuous wave mode, *viz*, 0.2-20 mW/cm2 (spatial average, temporal average intensity) and 0.6-80 mW/cm2 (spatial peak, temporal average intensity). As new technologies and applications evolve, for example, measurement of blood flow using pulsed Doppler, exposure levels may be substantially higher.

Manufacturers of ultrasound equipment introduced into U.S. commerce are required to report outputs to the FDA. We recommend that these quantities be measured and reported to the user in a form consistent with the requirements of the AIUM/NEMA Safety Standard for Diagnostic Ultrasound Equipment.

Dose is a quantitative measure of an agent that is given or imparted and combines quantities such as intensity and exposure time. No dose quantity has been identified for ultrasound. Variation in tissue properties between individuals as well as scanning conditions influence dose in an unpredictable way. For all practical purposes, fetal dose cannot be quantitated precisely. For this reason, there are no data on the dose to either the mother or the fetus in the clinical setting. Documentation of dwell time and type of machine and transducer used would begin to address this problem. It is recommended that at least this specific exposure information be recorded for each examination. Thus, it is important that each exposure to ultrasound by all Doppler and imaging devices be recorded.

For what purposes is ultrasound now used in pregnancy? For each use, what is the evidence that ultrasound improves patient management and/or outcome of pregnancy?

Ultrasound has been used in a wide variety of clinical situations to aid in managing pregnancy. For each of these applications, there is literature recording the clinical experience from various centers, with evidence of benefits ultrasound has had in each respective application, although these applications have not been subjected to the rigorous evaluation provided by a randomized, controlled clinical trial. The following should not be considered circumstances in which use of diagnostic ultrasound imaging is mandatory. Rather, where significant clinical questions exist, the resolution of which would alter the remainder of prenatal care, ultrasound can be of benefit for:

- *Estimation of gestational age for patients with uncertain clinical dates, or verification of dates for patients who are to undergo scheduled elective repeat cesarean delivery, indicated induction of labor, or other elective termination of pregnancy.* Ultrasonographic confirmation of dating permits proper timing of cesarean delivery or labor induction to avoid premature delivery.

- *Evaluation of fetal growth* (e.g., when the patient has an identified etiology for uteroplacental insufficiency, such as severe preeclampsia, chronic hypertension, chronic renal disease, severe diabetes mellitus, or for other medical complications of pregnancy where fetal malnutrition, i.e., IUGR or macrosomia, is suspected). Following fetal growth permits assessment of the impact of a complicating condition on the fetus and guides pregnancy management.

- *Vaginal bleeding of undetermined etiology in pregnancy. Ultrasound often allows determination of the source of bleeding* and status of the fetus.

- *Determination of fetal presentation* when the presenting part cannot be adequately determined in labor or the fetal presentation is variable in late pregnancy. Accurate knowledge of presentation guides management of delivery.

- *Suspected multiple gestation* based upon detection of more than one fetal heartbeat pattern, or fundal height larger than expected for dates, and/or prior use of fertility drugs. Pregnancy management may be altered in multiple gestation.

- *Adjunct to amniocentesis.* Ultrasound permits guidance of the needle to avoid the placenta and fetus, to increase the chance of obtaining amniotic fluid, and to decrease the chance of fetal loss.

Medical Tests Sometimes Used During Pregnancy

- *Significant uterine size/clinical dates discrepancy.* Ultrasound permits accurate dating and detection of such conditions as oligohydramnios and polyhydramnios, as well as multiple gestation, IUGR, and anomalies.

- *Pelvic mass detected clinically.* Ultrasound can detect the location and nature of the mass and aid in diagnosis.

- *Suspected hydatidiform mole* on the basis of clinical signs of hypertension, proteinuria, and/or the presence of ovarian cysts felt on pelvic examination or failure to detect fetal heart tones with a Doppler ultrasound device after 12 weeks. Ultrasound permits accurate diagnosis and differentiation of this neoplasm from fetal death.

- *Adjunct to cervical cerclage placement.* Ultrasound aids in timing and proper placement of the cerclage for patients with incompetent cervix.

- *Suspected ectopic pregnancy* or when pregnancy occurs after tuboplasty or prior ectopic gestation. Ultrasound is a valuable diagnostic aid for this complication.

- *Adjunct to special procedures,* such as fetoscopy, intrauterine transfusion, shunt placement, in vitro fertilization, embryo transfer, or chorionic villi sampling. Ultrasound aids instrument guidance that increases safety of these procedures.

- *Suspected fetal death.* Rapid diagnosis enhances optimal management.

- *Suspected uterine abnormality* (e.g., clinically significant leiomyomata, or congenital structural abnormalities, such as bicornuate uterus or uterus didelphys, etc.). Serial surveillance of fetal growth and state enhances fetal outcome.

- *Intrauterine contraceptive device localization.* Ultrasound guidance facilitates removal, reducing chances of IUD-related complications.

- *Ovarian follicle development surveillance.* This facilitates treatment of infertility.

- *Biophysical evaluation for fetal well-being* after 28 weeks of gestation. Assessment of amniotic fluid, fetal tone, body movements, breathing movements, and heart rate patterns assists in the management of high-risk pregnancies.

- *Observation of intrapartum events* (e.g., version/extraction of second twin, manual removal of placenta, etc.). These procedures may be done more safely with the visualization provided by ultrasound.

- *Suspected polyhydramnios or oligohydramnios.* Confirmation of the diagnosis is permitted, as well as identification of the cause of the condition in certain pregnancies.

- *Suspected abruptio placentae.* Confirmation of diagnosis and extent assists in clinical management.

- *Adjunct to external version from breech to vertex presentation.* The visualization provided by ultrasound facilitates performance of this procedure.

- *Estimation of fetal weight and/or presentation in premature rupture of membranes and/or premature labor.* Information provided by ultrasound guides management decisions on timing and method of delivery.

- *Abnormal serum alpha-fetoprotein value* for clinical gestational age when drawn. Ultrasound provides an accurate assessment of gestational age for the AFP comparison standard and indicates several conditions (e.g., twins, anencephaly) that may cause elevated AFP values.

- *Followup observation of identified fetal anomaly.* Ultrasound assessment of progression or lack of change assists in clinical decision making.

- *Followup evaluation of placenta* location for identified placenta previa.

- *History of previous congenital anomaly.* Detection of recurrence may be permitted, or psychologic benefit to patients may result from reassurance of no recurrence.

Medical Tests Sometimes Used During Pregnancy

- *Serial evaluation of fetal growth in multiple gestation.* Ultrasound permits recognition of discordant growth, guiding patient management and timing of delivery.

- *Evaluation of fetal condition in late registrants for prenatal care.* Accurate knowledge of gestational age assists in pregnancy management decisions for this group.

The information presented in the material reviewed by the panel, including the studies of Bennett, Eik-Nes, Bakketeig, Grennert, and others, allowed no consensus that routine ultrasound examinations for all pregnancies improved perinatal outcome or decreased morbidity or mortality. There was, however, evidence that there was a higher rate of detection of twins and congenital malformations, as well as more accurate dating of pregnancy, but without significant evidence of improved outcome. The evidence with respect to the number of antepartum days of hospitalization and induction rates was contradictory among trials. The data on perinatal outcome were inconclusive. The panel recognized the inadequacy of the clinical trials on which these conclusions are drawn. Furthermore, it is acutely aware of the difficulty associated with conducting ideally controlled clinical trials and the large numbers of patients that must be included to uncover differences between control and experimental groups, where a morbid event occurs infrequently and spontaneously in the control population.

The panel concludes that diagnostic ultrasound for pregnant women improves patient management and pregnancy outcome when there is an accepted medical indication. Randomized, controlled clinical trials would be the best way in the United States to determine the efficacy of routine screening of all pregnancies.

What are the theoretical risks of ultrasound to the fetus and the mother? What evidence exists from animal, tissue culture, and human studies on the actual extent of the risk?

The panel conducted an extensive review of the primary literature on this subject and of reports by the Bureau of Radiological Health (1976), Food and Drug Administration (1982), World Health Organization (1982), and the National Council on Radiation Protection and Measurements (1984).

A number of epidemiological studies tend to support the safety of diagnostic ultrasound exposure in humans. In particular, in the three randomized clinical trials in which half of the women were exposed routinely to ultrasound, there was no association of routine ultrasound exposure with birth weight. In the two studies that addressed the subject, no association of ultrasound exposure with hearing loss was observed. On the other hand, many of the studies reporting on the safety of diagnostic ultrasound in humans were considered inadequate to address many other important issues because of technical problems in conducting such research.

Some of the more than 35 published animal studies suggest that *in utero* ultrasound exposure can affect prenatal growth. When teratological effects have been found, energies capable of causing significant hyperthermia have usually existed.

A number of biological effects have been observed following ultrasound exposure in various experimental systems. These include reduction in immune response, change in sister chromatid exchange frequencies, cell death, change in cell membrane functions, degradation of macromolecules, free radical formation, and reduced cell reproductive potential. It should be noted that (a) some of the studies employed energy levels greater than would be expected to exist in clinical use; (b) in vitro exposure conditions to ultrasound used in many of the experiments are hard to place in perspective for risk assessment; (c) some of the observations, for example, sister chromatid exchange frequency changes and induction of chromosomal abnormalities, have not been reproducible, tending to refute the original findings. Nevertheless, some of the reported effects cannot be ignored or overlooked and deserve further study. The existence of these studies is one of the factors that contributed to our decision that routine ultrasound screening cannot be recommended at this time.

Based on the available evidence, what are the appropriate indications for, and the limitations on, use of ultrasound in obstetrics today?

From the body of information reviewed, taking into account the available bioeffects literature, data on clinical efficacy, and with concern for psychosocial, economic, and legal/ethical issues, it is the consensus of the panel that ultrasound examination in pregnancy should be performed for a specific medical indication. The data on clinical efficacy and safety do not allow a recommendation for routine screening at this time.

Ultrasound examinations performed solely to satisfy the family's desire to know the fetal sex, to view the fetus, or to obtain a picture

Medical Tests Sometimes Used During Pregnancy

of the fetus should be discouraged. In addition, visualization of the fetus solely for educational or commercial demonstrations without medical benefit to the patient should not be performed.

Prior to an ultrasound examination, patients should be informed of the clinical indication for ultrasound, specific benefit, potential risk, and alternatives, if any. In addition, the patient should be supplied with information about the exposure time and intensity, if requested. A written form may expedite this process in some cases. Patient access to educational materials regarding ultrasound is strongly encouraged. All settings in which these examinations are conducted should assure patients' dignity and privacy.

Given that the full potential of diagnostic ultrasound imaging is critically dependent on examiner training and experience, the panel recommends minimum training requirements and uniform credentialing for all physicians and sonographers performing ultrasound examinations. All health care providers who use this modality should demonstrate adequate knowledge of the basic physical principles of ultrasound, equipment, recordkeeping requirements, indications and safety.

What further studies are needed of efficacy and safety of use of ultrasound in pregnancy?

It is critical, in view of the existing data and the special considerations affecting fetal and embryonic development, to encourage and support a sustained research effort aimed specifically at test systems that can help provide a better data base for developing reasonable estimates of bioeffects and of risk. In particular, we recommend:

1. The study of fundamental mechanisms leading to bioeffects.
2. Laboratory experiments that focus especially on those cellular processes that are most likely to be affected during embryonic and fetal development.
3. Postnatal studies in animals after *in utero* exposure to ultrasound.
4. Exploration of interactions between administered ultrasound and such developmentally significant agents as drugs, nutrition, ionizing radiation, hyperthermia, and hypoxia.
5. Development of improved dosimetry.

A long-term followup of infants involved in a randomized clinical trial would help clarify questions about the effect of ultrasound on

Pregnancy and Birth Sourcebook

development in humans, and other epidemiologic studies using a wide variety of methods should be considered. Studies of the psychosocial, ethical, and legal aspects of ultrasound use are also needed.

Further non-experimental studies that seek to establish the clinical efficacy of ultrasound should address the question of its contribution to reducing morbidity and mortality. Randomized, controlled clinical trials of routine ultrasound screening in pregnancy should be conducted in the United States.

Section 9.3

Amniocentesis and Chorionic Villus Sampling (CVS)

Excerpts from FDA Consumer, December 1990 and Morbidity and Mortality Weekly Report, July 21, 1995

Chorionic villus sampling (CVS) and amniocentesis are prenatal diagnostic procedures used to detect certain fetal genetic abnormalities.

What is Amniocentesis?

Through amniocentesis, the amniotic fluid surrounding the fetus is sampled with a needle inserted into the woman's abdomen. This fluid contains cells that are shed primarily from the fetal skin, bladder, gastrointestinal tract, and amnion. Typically, amniocentesis is done at 15-18 weeks' gestation.

Fetal cells floating in the fluid are grown and examined for chromosomal abnormalities, such as the extra chromosome 21 that causes Down syndrome. Biochemicals in the fluid also provide diagnostic clues to several inborn errors of metabolism. Approved since 1967, amniocentesis is offered to women over 35, the age when the risk of the procedure causing a miscarriage is equal to the risk of the woman carrying a fetus with a detectable chromosomal problem (this risk

Medical Tests Sometimes Used During Pregnancy

increases with age). Women younger than 35 may have the procedure if a relative has a detectable abnormality. Amniocentesis can rule out many disorders, but it cannot guarantee a healthy baby.

The major drawback of amniocentesis at present is that it cannot safely be performed until the 16th week of pregnancy, and it takes 10 days or longer for fetal cells to be cultured and results to be known. However, several medical centers are experimenting with performing amniocentesis as early as 12 weeks.

Another advance is the use of automated, computerized chromosome sorters that are programmed to scan for abnormalities. This replaces technicians cutting up photographs of chromosomes and arranging them into a standard chart, then searching visually for aberrations—a time-consuming process.

Yet another new approach to viewing chromosomes is "in situ hybridization," a technique that uses DNA probes (bits of DNA tagged with a chemical) to locate and highlight specific chromosomes with no need to culture them first. This approach, still for research use only, can identify the extra chromosome of Down syndrome in hours.

What is Chorionic Villus Sampling (CVS)?

In CVS, a catheter inserted through the vagina samples chorionic villi, finger-like structures that form the placenta by 10 weeks of prenatal development. Because villi cells descend from the fertilized egg, their chromosomes match those of the fetus. Typically, CVS is done at 10-12 weeks' gestation.

The great advantage of CVS is that it can be performed as early as 8 weeks, and results are ready within days.

In the March 9, 1989, *New England Journal of Medicine,* George G. Rhoads, M.D., and co-workers at the National Institute of Child Health and Human Development reported on a seven-center study comparing CVS to amniocentesis. They conclude, "CVS is a safe and effective technique for the early prenatal diagnosis of cytogenetic abnormalities, but it probably entails a slightly higher risk of procedure failure and fetal loss than does amniocentesis." The risk of amniocentesis causing miscarriage is 0.5 percent; that of CVS is 1.3 percent. Miscarriages are more often associated when CVS is performed more than twice.

Both procedures increase the risk for miscarriage. In addition, concern has been increasing among health-care providers and public health officials about the potential occurrence of birth defects resulting from CVS.

Use of CVS and Amniocentesis

In the United States, the current standard of care in obstetrical practice is to offer either CVS or amniocentesis to women who will be older than 35 years of age when they give birth, because these women are at increased risk for giving birth to infants with Down syndrome and certain other types of aneuploidy. Karyotyping of cells obtained by either amniocentesis or CVS is the standard and definitive means of diagnosing aneuploidy in fetuses. The risk that a woman will give birth to an infant with Down syndrome increases with age. For example, for women 35 years of age, the risk is 1 per 385 births (0.3%), whereas for women 45 years of age, the risk is 1 per 30 births (3%). The background risk for major birth defects (with or without chromosomal abnormalities) for women of all ages is approximately 3%.

Before widespread use of amniocentesis, several controlled studies were conducted to evaluate the safety of the procedure. The major finding from these studies was that amniocentesis increases the rate for miscarriage (i.e., spontaneous abortions) by approximately 0.5%. Subsequent to these studies, amniocentesis became an accepted standard of care in the 1970s. In 1990, more than 200,000 amniocentesis procedures were performed in the United States.

In the 1960s and 1970s, exploratory studies were conducted revealing that the placenta (i.e., chorionic villi) could be biopsied through a catheter and that sufficient placental cells could be obtained to permit certain genetic analyses earlier in pregnancy than through amniocentesis. In the United States, this procedure was initially evaluated in a controlled trial designed to determine the miscarriage rate. The difference in fetal-loss rate was estimated to be 0.8% higher after CVS compared with amniocentesis, although this difference was not statistically significant. Because that study was designed to determine miscarriage rates, it had limited statistical power to detect small increases in risks for individual birth defects.

CVS had become widely used worldwide by the early 1980s. The World Health Organization (WHO) sponsors an international Registry of CVS procedures; data in the International Registry probably represent less than half of all procedures performed worldwide. More than 80,000 procedures were reported to the International Registry from 1983-1992; approximately 200,000 procedures were registered from 1983-1995. CVS is performed in hospitals, outpatient clinics, selected obstetricians' offices, and university settings; these facilities are often collectively referred to as prenatal diagnostic centers. Some investigators have reported that the availability of CVS increased the

Medical Tests Sometimes Used During Pregnancy

overall utilization of prenatal diagnostic procedures among women over 35 years of age, suggesting that access to first-trimester testing may make prenatal chromosome analysis appealing to a larger number of women. Another group of obstetricians did not see an increase in overall utilization when CVS was introduced. The increase in CVS procedures was offset by a decrease in amniocentesis, suggesting that the effect of CVS availability on the utilization of prenatal diagnostic testing depends on local factors. In the United States, an estimated 40% of pregnant women over 35 years of age underwent either amniocentesis or CVS in 1990.

Indications for Amniocentesis and CVS

Although maternal age-related risk for fetal aneuploidy is the usual indication for CVS or amniocentesis, prospective mothers or fathers of any age might desire fetal testing when they are at risk for passing on certain mendelian (single-gene) conditions. In a randomized trial conducted in the United States, 19% of women who underwent CVS were younger than 35 years of age. DNA-based diagnoses of mendelian conditions, such as cystic fibrosis, hemophilia, muscular dystrophy, and hemoglobinopathies, can be made by direct analysis of uncultured chorionic villus cells (a more efficient method than culturing amniocytes). However, amniocentesis is particularly useful to prospective parents who have a family history of neural tube defects, because alpha-fetoprotein (AFP) testing can be done on amniotic fluid but cannot be done on CVS specimens.

When testing for chromosomal abnormalities resulting from advanced maternal age, CVS may be more acceptable than amniocentesis to some women because of the psychological and medical advantages provided by CVS through earlier diagnosis of abnormalities. Fetal movement is usually felt and uterine growth is visible at 17-19 weeks' gestation, the time when abnormalities are detected by amniocentesis; thus, deciding what action to take if an abnormality is detected at this time may be more difficult psychologically. Using CVS to diagnose chromosomal abnormalities during the first trimester allows a prospective parent to make this decision earlier than with amniocentesis.

Maternal morbidity and mortality associated with induced abortion increase significantly with increasing gestational age; thus, the timing of diagnosis of chromosomal abnormalities is important. Results of studies of abortion complications conducted by CDC from 1970 through 1978 indicated that the risk for major abortion complications (e.g., prolonged fever, hemorrhage necessitating blood transfusion, and injury to pelvic organs) increases with advancing gestational age. For example, from 1971 through 1974, the major complication rate was 0.8% at 11-12 weeks' gestation, compared with 2.2% at 17-20 weeks' gestation. However, the risk for developing major complications from abortion at any gestational age decreased during the 1970s. More contemporary national morbidity data based on current abortion practices are not yet available. CDC surveillance data also indicate an increase in the risk for maternal death with increasing gestation. From 1972 through 1987, the risk for abortion-related death was 1.1 deaths per 100,000 abortions performed at 11-12 weeks' gestation compared with 6.9 deaths per 100,000 abortions for procedures performed at 16-20 weeks' gestation. The lower risk associated with first-trimester abortions may be an important factor for prospective parents who are deciding between CVS and amniocentesis.

Amniocentesis is usually performed at 15-18 weeks' gestation, but more amniocentesis procedures are now being performed at 11-14 weeks' gestation. "Early" amniocentesis (defined as earlier 15 weeks' gestation) remains investigational, because the safety of the procedure is currently being evaluated with controlled trials.

Miscarriage Risk

Risk estimates for miscarriage caused by either CVS or mid-trimester amniocentesis have been adjusted to account for spontaneous fetal losses that occur early in pregnancy and are not procedure-related. Although one randomized trial indicated that the amniocentesis-related miscarriage rate may be as high as 1%, counselors usually cite risks for miscarriage from other amniocentesis studies ranging from 0.25%-0.50% (1/400-1/200). Rates of miscarriage after CVS vary widely by the center at which CVS was performed. Adjusting for confounding factors such as gestational age, the CVS-related miscarriage rate is approximately 0.5%-1.0% (1/200-1/100).

Although uterine infection (i.e., chorioamnionitis) is one possible reason for miscarriage after either CVS or amniocentesis, infection has occurred rarely after either procedure. In one study, no episodes of septic shock were reported after 4,200 CVS procedures, although less severe infections may have been associated with 12 of the 89 observed fetal losses. Overall infection rates have been less than 0.1% after either CVS or amniocentesis.

Cytogenetically ambiguous results caused by factors such as maternal cell contamination or culture-related mosaicism are reported

Medical Tests Sometimes Used During Pregnancy

more often after CVS than after amniocentesis. In these instances, follow-up amniocentesis might be required to clarify results, increasing both the total cost of testing and the risk for miscarriage. However, ambiguous CVS results also may indicate a condition (e.g., confined placental mosaicism) that has been associated with adverse outcomes for the fetus. Thus, in these situations, CVS may be more informative than amniocentesis alone.

Limb Deficiencies Among Infants Whose Mothers Underwent CVS

Certain congenital defects of the extremities, known as limb deficiencies or limb reduction defects, have been reported among infants whose mothers underwent CVS. This section addresses:

1. the expected frequency and classification of these birth defects and
2. the physical features of reported infants in relation to the timing of associated CVS procedures, and
3. cohort and case-control studies that have been done to systematically examine whether CVS increases the risk for limb deficiencies.

Population-Based Rates and Classification of Limb Deficiencies

Population-based studies indicate that the risk for all limb deficiencies is from 5-6 per 10,000 live births. Limb deficiencies usually are classified into distinct anatomic and pathogenetic categories. The most common subtypes are transverse terminal defects, which involve absence of distal structures with intact proximal segments, with the axis of deficiency perpendicular to the extremity. Approximately 50% of all limb deficiencies are transverse, and 50% of those defects are digital, involving the absence of parts of one or more fingers or toes. Transverse deficiencies occur as either isolated defects or with other major defects. The rare combination of transverse limb deficiencies with either absence or hypoplasia of the tongue and lower jaw—usually referred to as oromandibular-limb hypogenesis or hypoglossia/hypodactyly—occurs at a rate of approximately 1 per 200,000 births. Although the cause of many isolated limb deficiencies and multiple anomalies that include transverse deficiencies is unknown, researchers have hypothesized that these deficiencies are caused by vascular disruption either during the formation of embryonic limbs or in already-formed fetal limbs.

Limb Deficiencies Reported in Infants Exposed to CVS

Reports of clusters of infants born with limb deficiencies after CVS were first published in 1991. Three studies illustrate the spectrum of CVS-associated defects. Data from these studies suggest that the severity of the outcome is associated with the specific time of CVS exposure. Exposure at >70 days' gestation has been associated with more limited defects, isolated to the distal extremities, whereas earlier exposures have been associated with more proximal limb deficiencies and orofacial defects. For example, in a study involving 14 infants exposed to CVS at 63-79 days' gestation and examined by a single pediatrician, 13 had isolated transverse digital deficiencies. In another study in Oxford of five infants exposed to CVS at 56-66 days' gestation, four had transverse deficiencies with oromandibular hypogenesis. In a review of published worldwide data, associated defects of the tongue or lower jaw were reported for 19 of 75 cases of CVS-associated limb deficiencies. Of those 19 infants with oromandibular-limb hypogenesis, 17 were exposed to CVS before 68 days' gestation. In this review, 74% of infants exposed to CVS at 270 days' gestation had digital deficiencies without proximal involvement.

Cohorts of CVS-Exposed Pregnancies

Cohort studies usually measure rates of a specified outcome in an exposed group compared with an unexposed group. Ideally, both groups should be selected randomly from the same study population. The three largest collaborative trials of CVS in Europe, Canada, and the United States were designed originally in this way; however, in these studies, the outcome of interest was fetal death. The report of the first U.S. collaborative trial included no mention of any structural defects; such outcomes were reported later.

After the initial case reports in 1991, neonatal outcomes from the collaborative trials were analyzed more intensively. However, rather than comparing rates for limb defects in the CVS-exposed cohorts with those of amniocentesis-exposed cohorts from the same study population, the rates in the CVS groups were compared with population-based rates. Consequently, these comparisons must be interpreted with caution because population-based rates are derived differently (i.e., usually from birth-defect registries). CVS-associated risk for limb

Medical Tests Sometimes Used During Pregnancy

deficiencies could be underestimated by these comparisons if followup of pregnancies in the exposed cohort is incomplete. Other epidemiologic issues must also be considered when interpreting comparisons of crude rates. Unless a formal meta-analysis is performed, these comparisons neither account for heterogeneity between studies nor assign individual "weights" to studies. Comparisons of crude rates also do not adjust for potential confounding variables, such as maternal age. Methods of anatomic subclassification also vary between registries and can differ from methods applied to CVS-exposed cohorts. In addition, comparing overall rates of limb deficiency in groups exposed to CVS with groups unexposed to CVS might overlook an association with a specific phenotype, such as transverse deficiency.

Published CVS cohort studies of greater than 1,000 CVS procedures include data from 65 CVS centers. (Table 9.1)

Location[†]	No. of Centers	CVS		Rate
		No. of Cases	No. of Procedures	
U.S. (NICHD[§]) (22,23)	10	7	9,588	7.3
U.S. (24)	9	3	4,105	7.3
Netherlands—Rotterdam (25)	1	3	3,973	7.6
Italy—Sardinia (26)	1	3	3,082	9.7
U.S.—Beverly Hills, CA (27)	1	1	3,016	3.3
Germany—Münster (28)	1	2	2,836	7.1
Italy (GIDEF[¶]) (29)	5	3	2,759	10.9
U.S.—Philadelphia, PA (30)	1	1	2,710	3.7
Denmark (31)	2	0	2,624	0.0
Australia—Victoria (32)	2	3	2,071	14.5
Europe (MRC[**]) (33)	31	2	1,609	12.4
U.S.—Evanston, IL (34)	1	1	1,048	9.5
Total	65	29	39,421	7.4

*Per 10,000 CVS procedures.
[†]Excluded were centers (i.e., collaborating hospitals or other health-care facilities) reporting either ≤1,000 procedures or incomplete information about birth-defect outcomes.
[§]National Institute of Child Health and Human Development (combined data from two trials [5,10]).
[¶]Gruppo Italiano Diagnosi Embrio-Fetali.
[**]Medical Research Council, United Kingdom.

Table 9.1. *Rates of transverse terminal limb-deficiencies at 65 centers CVS centers—selected geographical locations, 1984-1992.*

These rates include studies that describe affected limbs in sufficient detail to exclude non-transverse defects. Rates calculated for the smaller cohorts (i.e., centers performing less than 3,500 procedures) are less stable, but the overall rate of non-syndromic transverse limb deficiency from these centers was 7.4 per 10,000 procedures.

Case-Control Studies

Case-control approaches with a minimum of 100 case and 100 control patients have greater statistical power than cohort studies of 10,000 or fewer births to detect a fourfold increase in risk for transverse deficiencies (the degree of relative risk suggested by data from the 65 CVS centers). Investigators participating in multicenter birth-defect studies have used this case-control approach both to measure the strength of the association between CVS and limb deficiency and to determine if a dose-response (or gradient) effect of risk exists. The latter effect would be indicated by an increased relative risk for limb deficiency after earlier procedures, suggested in case reports of CVS-associated limb deficiencies by the high frequency of early exposures to CVS. Three case-control studies have used infants with limb deficiencies registered in surveillance systems and control infants with other birth defects to examine and compare exposure rates to CVS.

The U.S. Multistate Case-Control Study and the study of the Italian Multicentric Birth Defects Registry both indicated a significant association between CVS exposure and subtypes of transverse limb deficiencies. The EUROCAT study did not analyze risk for transverse limb deficiencies; the risk for all limb deficiencies (odds ratio [OR]=1.8, 95% confidence interval [CI]=0.7-5.0) was similar to that measured in the U.S. Multistate Case-Control Study for all limb deficiencies (OR=1.7, 95% CI=0.4-6.3). Analysis of subtypes in the U.S. study indicated a sixfold increase in risk for transverse digital deficiencies. In the U.S. study, no association between limb deficiencies and amniocentesis was observed.

Gestational Age at CVS

The lower risk observed in the United States may be related to the later mean gestational age of exposure. Increased risk was associated with decreased gestational age at the time of exposure. The risk for transverse deficiencies was greatest at less than 9 weeks' gestation. An analysis of cohort studies regarding the timing of CVS indicated a similar gradient with a relative risk for transverse deficiencies of 6.2 at less than 10 weeks' and 2.4 at later than 10 weeks' gestation. Because of reports of high rates of severe limb deficiencies after CVS at 6-7 weeks' gestation, a WHO-sponsored committee recommended that CVS be performed at 9-12 weeks after the last menstrual period.

Possible Mechanisms of CVS-Associated Limb Deficiencies

Several biological events have been proposed to explain the occurrence of limb deficiency after CVS, the variation in severity, and the risk associated with the timing of the procedure. These mechanisms, which include thromboembolization or fetal hypoperfusion through hypovolemia or vasoconstriction, are based on the assumption that the defects associated with CVS were caused by some form of vascular disruption. The limbs and mandible are susceptible to such disruption before 10 weeks' gestation; however, isolated transverse limb deficiencies related to fetal hypoperfusion have been reported at 11 weeks' gestation.

The rich vascular supply of chorionic villi can potentially be disrupted by instrumentation. Data from one study of embryoscopic procedures demonstrated fetal hemorrhagic lesions of the extremities following placental trauma, which produced subchorionic hematomas. Placental hemorrhage following CVS could lead to substantial fetal hypovolemia with subsequent hypoperfusion of the extremities. Because animal models show that limb deficiencies have been produced by either vasoconstrictive agents or occlusion of uterine vessels, some researchers have hypothesized that CVS-associated defects might be caused by uteroplacental insufficiency. Although the period of highest embryonic susceptibility appears to be when CVS is performed before 9 weeks' gestation (i.e., early CVS), these mechanisms also can disrupt limb structures at later gestational ages.

Absolute Risk for Limb Deficiency

Subtypes of limb deficiencies rarely occur in the population of infants not exposed to CVS. Thus, even a sixfold increase in risk for such types as digital defects (the finding of the U.S. Multistate Case-Control Study) is comparable to a small absolute risk (i.e., 3.46 cases per 10,000 CVS procedures [0.03%]). The upper 95% confidence limit for this absolute risk estimate is approximately 0.1%. A range of absolute risk from 1 per 3,000 to 1 per 1,000 CVS procedures (0.03%-0.10%) for all transverse deficiencies is consistent with the overall increase in risk reported by the

65 centers (Table 9.1). In cohort studies that reported the timing of the CVS, the absolute risk for transverse limb deficiencies was 0.20% at less than 9 weeks, 0.10% at 10 weeks, and 0.05% at later than 11 weeks (0.07% at more than 10 weeks of gestation).

The absolute risk for CVS-related birth defects is lower than the procedure-related risk for miscarriage that counselors usually quote to prospective parents (i.e., 0.5% to 1.0%) and also is lower than the risk for Down syndrome at age 35 (0.3%). Data from a decision analysis study supported the conclusion that, weighing a range of possible risks associated with prenatal testing, amniocentesis was preferred to CVS. This study was published in 1991 and did not consider risk for limb deficiency. Data indicate that publication of the initial case reports of limb deficiency decreased subsequent utilization of CVS. However, one study demonstrated that prospective parents who were provided with formal genetic counseling, including information about limb deficiencies and other risks and benefits, chose CVS at a rate similar to a group of prospective parents who were counseled before published reports of CVS-associated limb deficiencies.

Recommendations

An analysis of all aspects of CVS and amniocentesis indicates that the occasional occurrence of CVS-related limb defects is only one of several factors that must be considered in counseling prospective parents about prenatal testing. Factors that can influence prospective parents' choices about prenatal testing include their risk for transmitting genetic abnormalities to the fetus and their perception of potential complications and benefits of both CVS and amniocentesis. Prospective parents who are considering the use of either procedure should be provided with current data for informed decision making. Individualized counseling should address the following:

Indications for Procedures and Limitations of Prenatal Testing

- Counselors should discuss the prospective parents' degree of risk for transmitting genetic abnormalities based on factors such as maternal age, race, and family history.

- Prospective parents should be made aware of both the limitations and usefulness of either CVS or amniocentesis in detecting abnormalities.

Medical Tests Sometimes Used During Pregnancy

Potential Serious Complications from CVS and Amniocentesis

- Counselors should discuss the risk for miscarriage attributable to both procedures: the risk from amniocentesis at 15-18 weeks' gestation is approximately 0.25%-0.50% (1/400-1/200), and the miscarriage risk from CVS is approximately 0.5%-1.0% (1/200-1/100).

- Current data indicate that the overall risk for transverse limb deficiency from CVS is 0.03%-0.10% (1/3,000-1/1,000). Current data indicate no increase in risk for limb deficiency after amniocentesis at 15-18 weeks' gestation.

- The risk and severity of limb deficiency appear to be associated with the timing of CVS: the risk earlier than 10 weeks' gestation (0.20%) is higher than the risk from CVS done earlier than 10 weeks' gestation (0.07%). Most defects associated with CVS at <10 weeks' gestation have been limited to the digits.

Timing of Procedures

- The timing of obtaining results from either CVS or amniocentesis is relevant because of the increased risks for maternal morbidity and mortality associated with terminating pregnancy during the second trimester compared with the first trimester.

- Many amniocentesis procedures are now done at 11-14 weeks' gestation; however, further controlled studies are necessary to fully assess the safety of early amniocentesis.

Section 9.4

Alpha-fetoprotein and Triple AFP Screening

Excerpt from FDA Consumer, December 1990

In 1975, scientists found a link between high levels of alpha-fetoprotein (AFP) in pregnant women's blood and a type of fetal abnormality called a neural tube defect, which includes spina bifida (an open spine) and anencephaly (lack of higher brain structures). The open lesions of such defects allow AFP to leak faster than normal from the fetus' liver into the mother's bloodstream, causing the elevated levels.

In 1984, studies linked too little of the substance to Down syndrome. After this discovery, measuring AFP at 15 weeks for use as a prenatal warning greatly expanded. This helps in spotting Down syndrome in women under 35, who would usually not have amniocentesis. Abnormal AFP levels may also be associated with other birth defects and with late miscarriage, low birth weight, toxemia (very high blood pressure in a woman in the last trimester of pregnancy), premature delivery, and other birth defects.

How can one substance show so much? "We think the abnormal readings reflect something wrong with the placenta," says Washington Hill, M.D., director of maternal-fetal medicine at the Creighton University School of Medicine in Omaha.

AFP testing has a very high false-positive rate, because the level of AFP can be thrown off by such factors as a miscalculated due date, obesity, twins, or being black or diabetic. In 1987 accuracy was improved by considering levels of human chorionic gonadotropin, too, which is high in Down syndrome. The recent addition of a third measurement—unconjugated estriol—may make readings even more accurate.

By indicating a low risk, the use of this "triple test" could spare some women over 35 from amniocentesis recommended only because of their age. However, this is a screening test, not a diagnostic test, cautions George J. Knight, Ph.D., of the Foundation for Blood Research in Scarborough, Maine, where the test was developed. Women with abnormal results must undergo more definitive tests, such as ultrasound and amniocentesis, before the diagnosis is considered final.

Medical Tests Sometimes Used During Pregnancy

Section 9.5
Fetal Monitoring: Stress and Non-Stress Tests

Excerpt from NIH Publication No. 93-2788, 1993

Non-Stress Test

The "non-stress" test refers to the fact that no medication is given to the mother to cause movement of the fetus or contraction of the uterus. It is often used to confirm the well-being of the fetus based on the principle that a healthy fetus will demonstrate an acceleration in its heart rate following movement. Fetal activity may be spontaneous or induced by external manipulation such as rubbing the mother's abdomen or making a loud noise above the abdomen with a special device. When movement of the fetus is noted, a recording of the fetal heart rate is made. If the heart rate goes up, the test is normal. If the heart rate does not accelerate, the fetus may merely be "sleeping"; if, after stimulation, the fetus still does not react, it may be necessary to perform a "stress test" (oxytocin challenge test).

Stress Test (oxytocin challenge test)

Labor represents a stress to the fetus. Every time the uterus contracts, the fetus is momentarily deprived of its usual blood supply and oxygen. This is not a problem for most babies. However, some babies are not healthy enough to handle the stress and demonstrate an abnormal heart rate pattern. This test is often done if the non-stress test is abnormal. It involves giving the hormone oxytocin (secreted by every mother when normal labor begins) to the mother to stimulate uterine contractions. The contractions are a challenge to the baby, similar to the challenge of normal labor. If the baby's heart rate slows down rather than speeds up after a contraction, the baby may be in jeopardy. The stress test is considered more accurate than the non-stress test. Nevertheless, it is not 100 percent fool-proof and your obstetrician may want to repeat it on another occasion to ensure its accuracy. Most women describe this test as mildly uncomfortable but not painful.

Chapter 10

Coping with Common Discomforts of Pregnancy

Morning Sickness

The illness was described as early as 2000 B.C. It affects between 50 percent and 90 percent of all pregnant women. It is a major reason for visits to the obstetrician. Yet doctors don't know what causes it or how to cure it. And even in this day of high-tech medical care, treatment often must rely simply on saltine crackers and sips of hot tea.

Morning sickness—the bane of most pregnant women—is so common in the first trimester of pregnancy that it has been accepted as a given. Little research has been conducted; since 1950, according to one estimate, only about 30 articles have been published on nausea and vomiting during pregnancy.

"I suspect there's little motivation to research an illness from which women rarely die and which disappears in a few weeks of its own accord," says Dr. Mark A. Klebanoff, an obstetric epidemiologist with the National Institute of Child Health and Human Development.

Morning sickness usually begins about six weeks after the start of the last menstrual period, and then the nausea and vomiting disappear seemingly magically six to eight weeks later.

The cause of morning sickness still eludes doctors. Although various hormones have been implicated nothing has been proved. In some cases, blood levels of estrogen in pregnant women who had morning sickness were found to be higher than those of pregnant women who

---

FDA Consumer, November 1988 by Judy Folkenberg and excerpts from DHSS Publication No. HRSA-MCHB-92-4-A, 1994.

were not sick. But these differences have not been consistent. Also levels of human chorionic gonadotropin increase in the first trimester of pregnancy and then diminish about the 14th or 15th week of pregnancy—just about the time morning sickness diminishes in most women. But certain tumors also secrete this hormone, and people with these tumors do not have nausea.

Because doctors don't know what causes the illness, they can only try to ease the symptoms. So, even though morning sickness plagues most pregnant women, little can be done to hasten its demise. Time seems to be the only cure, and even in this age of sophisticated drugs and high-tech medicine, treatment consists of the simple, the tried, and the true. Most doctors and nurse-midwives admit that treating morning sickness is a trial-and-error process of figuring out what foods are least upsetting for the pregnant woman. Technology is no help at all.

"Most physicians recommend a bland diet, frequent small meals to keep the stomach filled but not overfilled, breakfasting in bed before arising, and drinking beverages between meals rather than with meals," says Dr. Phil Price, an obstetrician with the Food and Drug Administration.

Dry toast, crackers, tea, peppermint-flavored water, chicken noodle soup, rice, and pasta without spicy sauces seem to be the most easily tolerated foods for women who are sick, he says. Large meals, greasy foods, fried foods, and spicy foods such as peppers, chili and garlic on the other hand may worsen morning sickness. And Emetral, a nonprescription syrup similar to cola syrup, assuages nausea in some women.

"It's the only kind of nausea that gets better with food on the stomach, and I suspect this may be nature's way of getting the pregnant woman to eat," says Deborah Bopp, a certified nurse-midwife with the Group Health Association in Washington, D.C.

Treatment is mostly palliative—a variation on the theme of doing whatever gets you through the night. If food odors are bothersome, then open the windows or get someone else to do the cooking, says one obstetrician.

Only one drug has been specifically formulated for morning sickness—Bendectin. FDA approved the drug in 1956, and approximately 900,000 pregnant women—or 1 in 10—took the drug annually at the height of its use. But in 1983, Merrell Dow Pharmaceuticals, the drugs manufacturer, voluntarily took Bendectin off the market in this country because of a number of lawsuits against the company from women who claimed that the drug caused birth defects. The company's insurance premiums had soared so high because of the lawsuits that it was no longer profit able to sell the drug, according to the firm.

Coping with Common Discomforts of Pregnancy

Whether or not Bendectin caused birth defects was never resolved. (The drug remains on the market in Europe.) In 1980, an FDA panel reviewed the available data and found no association between the drug and birth defects. However, because it is nearly impossible to prove the absolute safety of any drug under every circumstance, the panel said there must remain a "residual uncertainty" about the drug's effects on the unborn child.

The removal of Bendectin meant there were no longer any drugs formulated specifically for the nausea of pregnancy. It's a void that has not been filled, nor is it likely that any new drugs will be forthcoming.

"No U.S. company wants to take the medical or legal risk that one of their drugs might harm a fetus, so there is little incentive to research and develop a morning sickness pill," says FDA's Price.

For a small minority of women, morning sickness becomes very serious. In most cases, this condition, known as hyperemesis gravidarum (or, simply, hyperemesis), requires hospitalization. Dehydration and weight loss are major worries, as are such possible complications as electrolyte imbalance, pulse irregularities, and kidney or liver damage.

During hospitalization a woman suffering from hyperemesis is kept from dehydrating with an intravenous (through the vein) solution of water, glucose and vitamins. Sometimes anti-nausea drugs such as promethazine hydrochloride, trimethobenzamide hydrochloride, or prochlorperazine are prescribed to stop the vomiting. (These drugs are usually administered later in the pregnancy so the fetus's neurological system is less likely to be harmed.) Some physicians have reported that acupuncture, behavioral therapy, and hypnosis relieve nausea and vomiting in some women.

The fetus can also be harmed by the mother's continuing nausea. When the body can't keep food in the stomach, it looks elsewhere for nourishment and starts breaking down or metabolizing carbohydrates, fats and proteins that have already been stored by the body. The breakdown products of fat are called "ketone bodies." Ketones can damage the neurological development of the fetus.

Although doctors don't know what causes hyperemesis gravidarum, it is thought that emotional factors, such as ambivalence about pregnancy, may play a role if vomiting persists into the second trimester.

There is a bright side to morning sickness. Women who suffer from this condition are less likely to miscarry or deliver prematurely. In a recent study of 9,098 pregnancies, researchers at the National Institute of Child Health and Human Development (NICHHD) and National Institute of Allergy and Infectious Diseases discovered that:

- Queasy women had a 17 percent lower chance of delivering prematurely (before 37 weeks), and

- Women who vomited during their first trimester had a 3.4 percent rate of miscarriages and stillbirths, compared with 5.3 percent for women with calmer stomachs.

"This means that women who vomit have a 30 percent lower chance of miscarriage or stillbirths than women who don't," says NICHHD's Mark Klebanoff, who led the study. Researchers aren't sure why vomiting has this positive effect but hypothesize that nauseated women have higher levels of pregnancy-related hormones—a sign that the pregnancy is progressing normally.

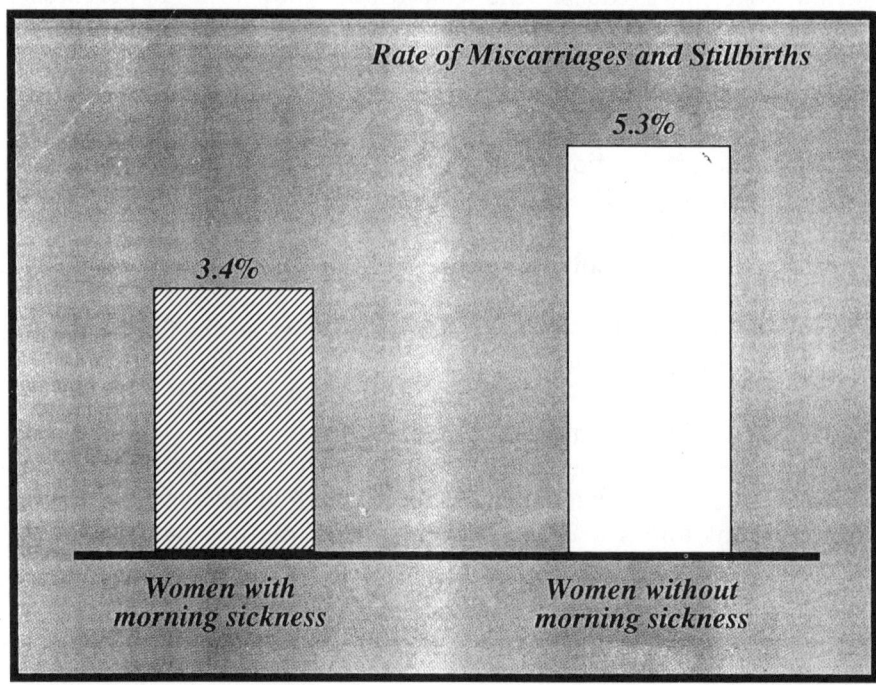

Figure 10.1. *A Bright Side to Morning Sickness.* Based on a study of 9,098 pregnancies, this chart shows that women who experience morning sickness during their first trimester had a 3.4 percent rate of miscarriages and stillbirths, compared with a 5.3 percent rate for women who did not experience morning sickness. Source: National Institute of Child Health and Human Development.

Coping with Common Discomforts of Pregnancy

So, while morning sickness may cause pregnant women much discomfort, it just might also bode well that a healthy baby waits to be born.

Exotic Remedies of the Past

For centuries, pregnant women with morning sickness cursed their lots while their doctors cursed their inability to come up with very effective treatments. Frustrated and puzzled by the seeming intractability of morning sickness during the first trimester, doctors nevertheless plunged ahead trying remedy after remedy.

Their inability to cure was matched by an endless imagination to try virtually everything under the sun. For instance, in the first century the Roman physician Soranus recommended that a pregnant woman with morning sickness punch a leather bag, and if the vomiting persisted he advised that her arms and legs be bound and immersed in hot water.

By the 19th century, the situation had not improved. Medical journals from the 1800s featured a ponderous exchange of letters as doctors traded advice on their methods of curing morning sickness. This was medicine by trial and error, and if one treatment didn't work, others were tried. In a case study reported in the 1878 British journal *Lancet,* one physician had tried over 20 remedies, including leeches and opium, to curb one woman's vomiting. But nothing worked, and the woman finally died.

Nineteenth century remedies seemed to fall into two categories: treating the cervix or giving oral medications. Various doctors applauded "Dr. Copeman's method"—the forced dilation of the cervix, which seemed to stop the vomiting in many women. Dilating the cervix also increased the woman's chance of miscarriage. Doctors also reported success with silver nitrate, carbolic acid, bromide of potash (all burning agents), cocaine, or opium applied to the cervix.

Some doctors also recommended that women consume whiskey, belladonna (a drying agent that reduces saliva), popcorn, swamp dogwood, wild yams, wine of ipecac, and morphine.

Perhaps the most novel method was reported in the *Journal of the Medical Society of North Carolina* in 1874. The woman's physician was stumped. His patient could not keep any food down during her pregnancy. She was reduced to a virtual skeleton with large painful bedsores and was on the brink of the grave.

"What was to be done?" asked her physician. "We had exhausted all the methods of nourishment known, except one, and that one inunction [anointing]. Having previously observed how very speedily mercurial ointment was absorbed by some patients, I proposed that we should anoint her three times a day with fresh lard, rubbing it on the inside of the thighs, the groins and under the arms. By thus applying about a half a pound of lard three times a day, rubbing it carefully and persistently, it left a soft, silky delightful state of the skin . . . although at first she thought it very foolish; with iced tea, and milk in it, given internally, we not only supported life for eight weeks, but it was evident after a while that the patient was gaining some flesh and strength."

The physician ends his report with good news: The woman recovered from morning sickness and rapidly gained back her strength.

Heartburn

Later in your pregnancy, you may feel some "heartburn", because as the baby grows bigger, there is more pressure on your stomach. There are several causes of heartburn including food choices, quantity of food eaten, and tight clothing.

Prevention.

- Avoid irritating your stomach: Eat less greasy, fried or highly seasoned foods. Figure out which give you heartburn and don't eat them.

- Avoid both coffee and cigarettes: They increase the acidity in your stomach and may irritate.

- Eat several small meals a day rather than 3 large ones.

- Drink plenty of liquids (six 8-ounce glasses daily).

- Wear clothing that is loose around your waist. Tight clothing will put pressure on your stomach.

- Do not lie down right after eating.

- Sleep or rest with your head slightly elevated.

Useful Remedies. When you have heartburn:

- Sip water, milk, carbonated water, or have a tablespoon of yogurt, heavy cream, or half-and-half.

Coping with Common Discomforts of Pregnancy

- Try the "flying" exercise. Sit cross-legged or tailor fashion, and quickly raise and lower your arms, bringing the backs of your hands together over your head. Repeat several times.

- Sit-up. Lying down can make your heartburn worse.

- Try taking a leisurely walk or sitting quietly and breathing deeply.

- Antacids [Tums (R), Maalox (R), Mylanta (R), Riopan (R), Gelusil (R)] may bring relief by reducing stomach acid. Ask your doctor/midwife or nurse for antacids which are low in salt. Use antacids only occasionally. they contain minerals which may be harmful in large amounts. Some heartburn medicines contain aspirin [Alka-Seltzer (R), Fizrin (R)] which should not be taken during pregnancy. Do not take heartburn medicines that contain large amounts of salt [such as baking soda, Soda Mint (R), Eno (R), Fizrin (R), Rolaids (R), Alka-Seltzer (R)].

Other Discomforts

Headaches

You have headaches because there is more blood in your body now that you are pregnant, or because you are tired, tense, hungry or thirsty. It may help to:

- Lie down and try to relax all the muscles in each part of your body.

- Eat more protein-rich foods.

- Try to rest and relax more.

- Stroke your forehead gently and put a cold cloth on it.

- Take a walk outside.

- Take Tylenol (**not** Aspirin) if you need to. Take two tablets (regular strength) every 6 hours, but no more than 3 times a day for 3 days. Tell your doctor.

Frequent Urination

Most women need to urinate more often when they are pregnant. The growing baby presses on your bladder making you need to urinate. It may help to:

- Urinate when you feel the need to. Holding it in can cause more problems.

- Drink less after dinner so that you won't have to urinate as often after you go to bed.

- Tell the doctor/midwife if you have any burning when you urinate. This can be a sign of infection.

Rest if you feel tired. It is normal to feel tired in the first months of pregnancy.

You may have develop darker areas on your face, stomach, or other places on your skin. These are normal. They will go away after your baby is born.

If you become constipated, drink more fruit juices and water and eat high fibre foods such as raw fruits and vegetables, whole grain breads and cereals.

As your baby gets big it may be harder for you to breathe. Slow down, stretch your arms over your head, breathe deeply.

Part Three

Fetal Development During Gestation

Chapter 11

Fetal Growth and Development

Your baby starts out a as a tiny fertilized egg in side your uterus. Each day your baby grows and changes. Your baby gets its food through a cord ("umbilical cord") which connects your baby to a special organ called the "placenta". The placenta is attached to the wall of your uterus. The food you eat goes from your body to your baby through the placenta and the cord.

It will take about 40 weeks before your baby is ready to be born.

First Three Months

The first three months is the time when all of your baby's big organs and limbs are formed, like the arms, legs, brain and heart. Your baby moves in the first three months, but it is so small that you don't feel it yet. You may be able to hear your baby's heart beat at the doctors office at the end of your third month.

Second Three Months

Now the organs are developing more. Fine hair covers your baby's body. Even nails are growing. You will probably begin to feel your baby move between the 4th and 5th month. Also, your baby begins to hear.

Excerpts from DHSS Publication No. HRSA-MCHB-92-4-A, 1994

Third Three Months

The baby gains most of its weight during the last three months. The skin is covered with a cream which protects it (vernix). You may see this when your baby is born. In the last few weeks, the baby is getting ready to live outside you.

Your Baby Month By Month

8 Weeks

Your baby is about 1 inch long and weight less than 1 ounce. All organs are developing. Your baby's tiny heart will beat by the 25th day.

12 Weeks

Your baby is now about 3 inches long and weighs about 1 ounce. Your baby is starting to open and close its mouth and move its tiny hands, legs, and head.

16 Weeks

Your baby weighs about 6 ounces, is 6-8 inches long, and the organs, such as, the heart and lungs, are formed. For the rest of your pregnancy your baby will be growing and gaining weight. You may look pregnant now. You will soon need maternity (or larger sized) clothes. You may want to wear lighter weight clothes. It is normal to be warmer and perspire more when you are pregnant.

20 Weeks

Your baby weighs about 1/2 to 1 pound, is 8-12 inches long, and is much more active now, moving from side to side or turning around.

24 Weeks

You are now carrying a fully formed, but tiny baby, with wrinkled skin, about 14 inches long, and 1-1 1/2 pounds. Your baby still needs to grow and fully develop vital organs such as the lungs and brain. Your baby will grow quickly during the rest of your pregnancy. Your baby's size will put pressure on your bladder. You may need to go to the bathroom more often.

Fetal Growth and Development

28 Weeks

Your baby is about 15 inches long and weighs about 2-3 pounds. Your baby's bones are getting harder. You may feel your baby kick and move more now.

32 Weeks

Your baby is about 18 inches long and weighs about 5 pounds. Your baby can open its eyes. Your baby may turn around in your uterus (womb) and stay in the new position for the rest of your pregnancy.

36 Weeks

Your baby is about 19 inches long, weighs about 6 pounds, and is gaining about a 1/2 pound each week. At 40 weeks your baby will be "full term" (will have gone through the full length of pregnancy). Your baby could come any time between 37 to 42 weeks. Few babies are born on their "due date".

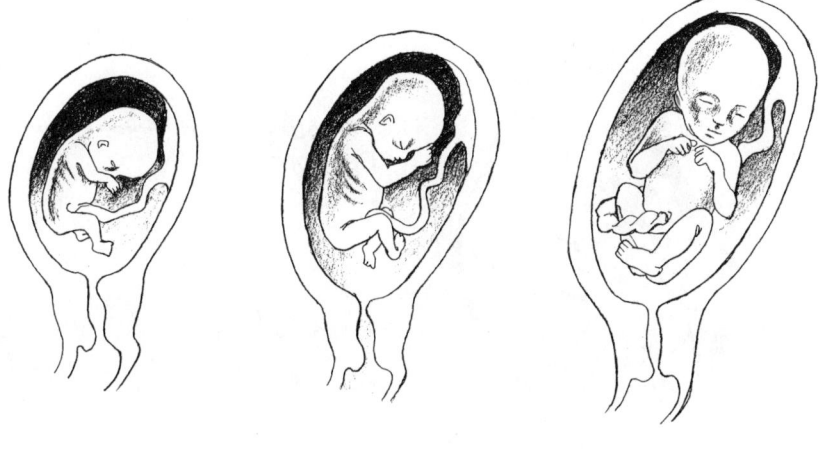

8 Weeks	12 Weeks	16 Weeks
Fetus is 1 inch long, weighs less than 1 ounce.	Fetus is 3 to 4 inches long, weighs about 1 ounce.	Fetus is 6 to 8 inches long, weighs about 6 ounces.

Figure 11.1.a. Fetal Growth and Development.

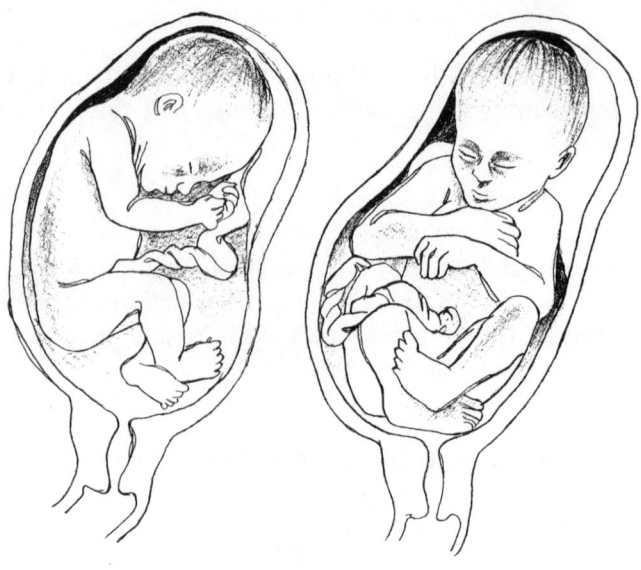

20 Weeks
Fetus is 8 to 12 inches long, weighs 1/2 to 1 pound.

24 Weeks
Fetus is about 14 inches long, weighs 1 to 1½ pounds.

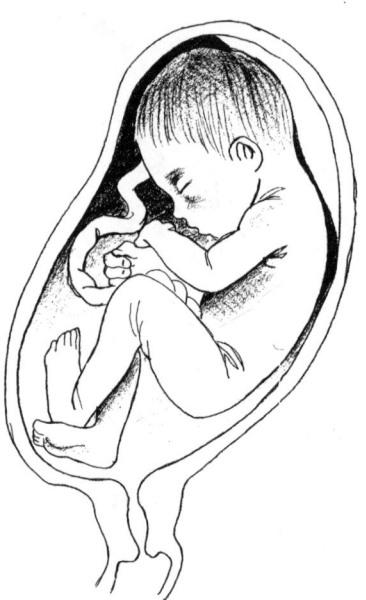

Figure 11.1.b. Fetal Growth and Development

Fetal Growth and Development

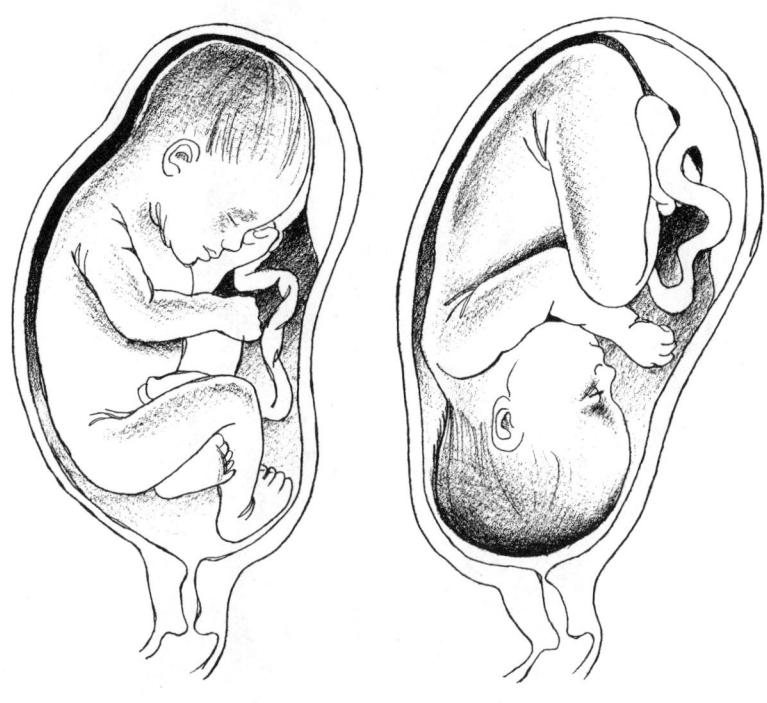

32 Weeks
Fetus is about 18 inches long, weighs about 5 pounds.

36 Weeks
Fetus is about 19 inches long, weighs about 6 pounds.

Figure 11.1.c. Fetal Growth and Development

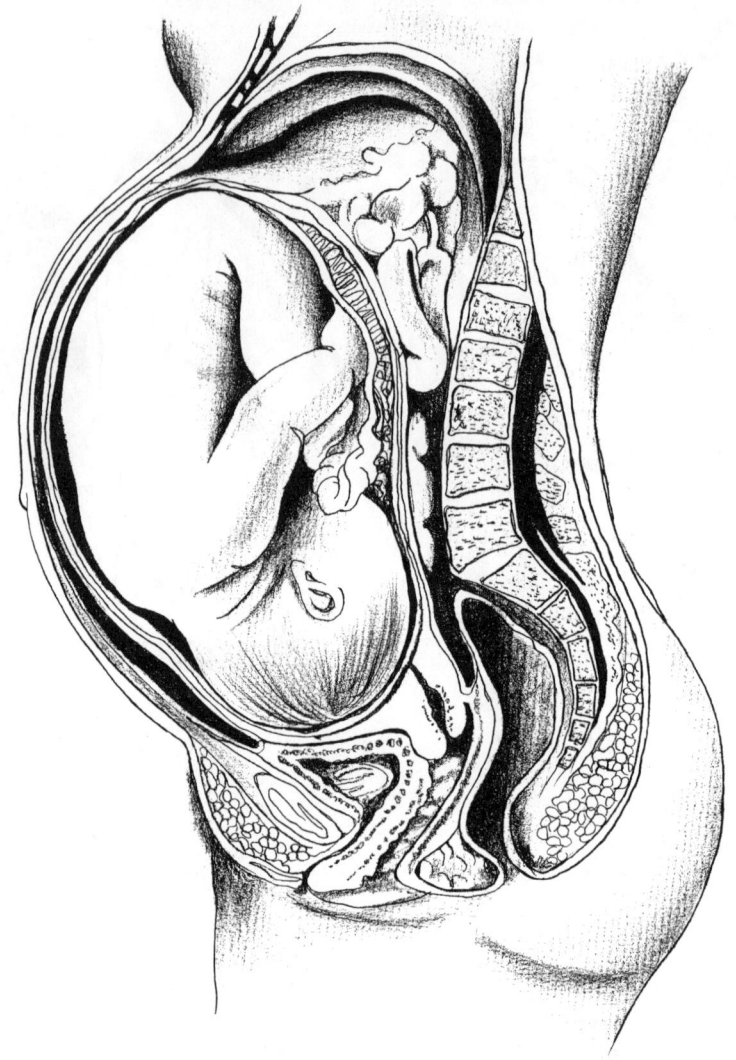

40 Weeks

At term (when fully grown), baby will be about 20 inches long and weigh 7 to 8 pounds.

Figure 11.1.d. Fetal Growth and Development.

Chapter 12

Cautions about Drugs and Their Impact on the Developing Fetus

Chapter Contents

Section 12.1—Drugs and Pregnancy:
 Often the Two Don't Mix 136
Section 12.2—Prescription and Over-the-Counter
 Medications 141
Section 12.3—Tobacco and Pregnancy 148
Section 12.4—Caffeine and Pregnancy 149
Section 12.5—Alcohol and Pregnancy 151
Section 12.6—Illegal Drugs and Pregnancy 157

Section 12.1

Drugs and Pregnancy: Often the Two Don't Mix

Excerpt from DHSS Publication No. (FDA) 90-3174, 1989
by Evelyn Zamula

In the summer of 1986, a group of scientists gathered in Boston to discuss—and to commemorate an event that ruined lives, tore families apart, and left thousands of women with unbearable feelings of anguish and guilt. The occasion was the 25th anniversary of the recognition that the drug thalidomide was a potent producer of birth defects.

One of the speakers at the conference was a young Canadian scientist who had first-hand knowledge of the effects of the drug. Because his mother took the sedative during her pregnancy, he was born with no feet and was missing fingers on both hands. He once asked his parents a disturbing question: If prenatal diagnosis had been available at the time of his birth and could have detected his malformations in the womb, would they have chosen abortion? They answered, "yes," that based on doctors' opinions at that time, they would have aborted. But now they were glad they hadn't because, besides their love for him and pride in his accomplishments, they had gained an empathy with those less fortunate than he.

If that was a bright note in the thalidomide epidemic, there were few others. Although U.S. babies were almost entirely spared thalidomide's devastating effects—FDA drug reviewer Frances O. Kelsey, M.D., did not approve the manufacturer's application to market the drug here—in some countries deformed children were abandoned by their families to be raised in institutions, and it is believed that some were even left to die. About 40 percent of the nearly 6,000 known cases of thalidomide children—born between 1956 and 1963—have already died.

Cautions about Drugs and Their Impact

Birth Defects Long Connected to Drugs

The unusual deformities caused by thalidomide generated worldwide publicity and focused attention on the fact that certain drugs taken at a critical time in pregnancy had the potential for damaging the unborn baby.

Before thalidomide, most birth defects were thought to be genetic, even though observers in the long-ago past had noticed the connection between drug-taking and birth abnormalities. Some of these ancient men of medicine were also aware that though drugs were most dangerous in the early months of pregnancy, the fetus could be affected later, too.

The Greek physician Hippocrates wrote almost 2,500 years ago that for the safety of the fetus, drugs should be administered to pregnant women only from the fourth to the seventh months. In the second century A.D., the Greek physician Soranus of Ephesus warned women not to take drugs at any time during pregnancy, but especially during the first trimester. In particular, he maintained that when drugs taken to cause abortion did not produce the desired result, "let no one assume that the fetus has not been injured at all. For it has been harmed: It is weakened, becomes retarded in growth, less well nourished, and in general, more easily injured and susceptible to harmful agents; it becomes misshapen and of ignoble soul ." (For an interesting fictional account of just such a case, read Robertson Davies' *What's Bred in the Bone.*)

According to the March of Dimes Foundation, each year more than a quarter of a million U.S. babies—or about 1 out of every 14—are born with birth defects. About one-third of the abnormalities are life-threatening, making birth defects—including low birth weight—the leading cause of infant mortality. A half million more potential lives are lost through miscarriage and stillbirth, usually because of faulty fetal development. About 1.2 million infants, children and adults are hospitalized each year for treatment of birth defects. Birth defects contribute to the death of more than 60,000 Americans of all ages annually.

The causes of birth defects are unknown in about 65 percent to 70 percent of the cases; about 20 percent of the defects are genetic, or inherited. (Infections account for 2 percent to 3 percent of congenital malformations, maternal health problems for 1 percent to 2 percent, and chromosomal aberrations for 3 percent to 5 percent.) It is estimated that 2 percent to 3 percent of birth defects are due to chemicals or drugs although it is suspected that the percentage may be higher since many women can't recall all the drugs they took during pregnancy. American women take an average of four prescription or over-the-counter drugs during pregnancy, plus vitamin and mineral supplements.

The effects a drug has on an embryo or fetus (the unborn baby is called an embryo up to eight weeks after conception and a fetus from then until birth) depend mainly on whether a drug has the ability to produce abnormalities, how much of it is taken, and at what point in the pregnancy it is taken.

A drug taken by an expectant mother enters her bloodstream and in most instances passes through the placenta to her unborn child. The drug then passes back through the placenta into the mother's circulatory system and is eventually eliminated. The placenta's normal function is to supply oxygen and nutrients to the fetus and to remove its waste products.

FDA receives more than 50,000 written reports of adverse drug reactions each year from drug companies and health-care providers. Information about the patient the suspect drug and the reaction and its consequences is entered into a computerized data base. FDA scientists use the data to spot patterns of adverse reactions that may call for regulatory action such as occurred with the acne drug Accutane. Reports of birth defects in children born to women who used the drug while they were pregnant led to strengthened label warnings against its use during pregnancy.

Timing Is Important

If a teratogenic (ter-ah-to-JEN-ik) drug—a chemical that can produce birth deformities—is taken in the earliest part of pregnancy (from conception until about 20 days), it will either cause the death of the embryo and subsequent miscarriage, or not affect it at all.

The possibility of harm to normal embryonic development is greatest from the third to eighth weeks, when the organs are forming. In the third week, the brain, heart and blood vessels start to develop and the spine begins to form; the arms and legs appear as tiny buds. By the fourth week, the heart starts to beat, even though the embryo is only a quarter-inch long. At five weeks, the first signs of hands and feet appear. At eight weeks, the arms and legs are separated into upper arm and forearm, thigh and lower leg; the two halves of the hard palate (roof of the mouth) unite.

From then on, the fetus grows and its systems mature. Teratogenic drugs taken after this period usually don't cause major structural defects, but they can affect growth and organ function. Particularly

Cautions about Drugs and Their Impact

vulnerable is the unborn baby's nervous system, which continues to develop throughout pregnancy and in infancy. For example, the antibiotic streptomycin taken at even late stages in pregnancy may cause hearing damage in the baby. Other systems can also be affected. Tetracycline, another antibiotic, taken during the second or third trimester, when the fetus' teeth begin to calcify, will cause permanent staining of the baby teeth.

In some cases, drugs can have delayed effects. Diethylstilbestrol (DES), a synthetic estrogen widely prescribed in the 1940s to prevent miscarriage and other problems, came to be seen as a time bomb in the children of some of the 4 million to 6 million women who took it during pregnancy. Hundreds of young women who had been exposed to this drug as fetuses developed vaginal cancer after puberty. And a greater incidence of reproductive system abnormalities, such as undescended testes, also occurred in male offspring.

FDA requires that every new drug that may be used by women of childbearing potential be tested in pregnant laboratory animals before it can be marketed. (Because any untested drug presents a risk of harm to the fetus, pregnant women cannot participate in the human drug studies that are also required for pre-market approval.) But animal testing alone is by no means foolproof; drugs in animals cannot be guaranteed to act the same way in humans. Drugs that cause birth defects in animals may not cause them in people. Conversely, a drug that may be harmful to the unborn baby may not affect animals, or may not affect them to the same degree. For example, humans are 100 times more sensitive to thalidomide than are rats, and 50 times more sensitive than are rabbits. If a drug causes defects in a wide variety of animal species, however, it's almost certain that it will cause them in people, too.

Post-Market Surveillance

After an approved drug is marketed, FDA continues to gather information about adverse effects from a number of sources. Drug manufacturers are required to report to the agency any adverse drug reactions they learn of; doctors do so voluntarily. The U.S. Centers for Disease Control collects reports from hospitals; and large monitoring studies both here and abroad—such as the Finnish Register of Congenital Malformations—gather and analyze information on birth defects. From this data, epidemiologists (scientists who study disease frequency and distribution) can detect a pattern between use of a certain drug and birth defects.

To date, this system has worked so well since its inception that nothing on the scale of the thalidomide tragedy has occurred in the United States, even though potent teratogens do exist. Isotretinoin (Accutane), for example, is an extremely effective treatment for severe cystic acne, but a known teratogen as well. Women are warned not to take the drug if they are pregnant or intend to become pregnant while undergoing treatment. They run a risk of spontaneous abortion and have at least a 25 percent chance of bearing a baby with birth defects, including outer ear malformations, heart and central nervous system abnormalities, and cleft palate.

Since its approval in 1982, Accutane has been labeled in pregnancy category X, meaning it should not be used during pregnancy. (FDA classifies prescription drugs in five pregnancy categories—A, B, C, D and X—based on teratogenic risk. Drugs in category A appear to be least harmful, while those in category X have risks that clearly outweigh the benefits.) Because FDA, CDC, and the manufacturer continued to receive reports of birth defects, warnings against using Accutane in pregnancy were considerably strengthened in 1988. Patients are now required to have a negative pregnancy test before starting therapy and are given a leaflet that contains a drawing of a baby with the birth deformities associated with Accutane.

Cautions about Drugs and Their Impact

Section 12.2

Prescription and Over-the-Counter Medications

FDA Consumer, October 1988 by Judith Willis and excerpts from DHSS Publication No. (FDA) 90-3174, 1989 by Evelyn Zamula and NIH Publication No. 95-3929, 1995

Accutane Warning

Some likened the decision asked of FDA to that required of the biblical Solomon when two women seemed to have equal claim to being mother of the same child.

The issue before FDA, however, was not one of parentage, but whether a drug that has the ability to clear a very severe and disfiguring form of acne should be taken off the market because it also carries a high risk of causing a deformed baby or miscarriage if taken by a pregnant woman.

The name of the drug is Accutane (generically called isotretinoin). The issues surrounding it could serve as a basis for a course in medical ethics. Summarized, these issues are:

- A relative of vitamin A, Accutane was known to cause birth defects in animals and suspected of causing them in humans even before it was approved by FDA in 1983. Although the labeling has always forbidden use of the drug during pregnancy, such use has nevertheless occurred. Marketing experience with the drug indicates that Accutane causes birth defects in about one out of every four exposed fetuses.

- The condition for which the drug was approved, severe recalcitrant cystic acne unresponsive to other therapy, is much more common in males than in females. Yet 40 percent of the prescriptions are written for women, virtually all of whom are of childbearing age. The primary reason given for this is that women seek treatment for this condition more often than men.

- Accutane is the only drug that can clear this severe and disfiguring form of acne. Other drugs approved to treat the same condition must be taken for extended periods and, when stopped, the condition usually reappears. But with Accutane, most patients need to take the drug for only a few months. When the drug is discontinued, the acne usually does not return.

- Birth defects continued to occur despite repeated revisions of the labeling, letters to physicians from the manufacturer, Hoffmann-La Roche, and articles in the *FDA Drug Bulletin* (a publication sent to more than 1 million health professionals) that the drug should not be used by women of childbearing age unless they were using an effective form of contraception. Miscarriages (technically called spontaneous abortions when occurring in the first three months of pregnancy) also continued to occur at a rate substantially higher than in the general population. In addition, there has been an increased rate of elective abortion among women taking Accutane, apparently resulting from the wish to avoid giving birth to a deformed child.

To publicly consider these issues, FDA convened a meeting of its Dermatologic Drugs Advisory Committee, a panel of experts from outside the agency. Highly knowledgeable and respected scientists lined up on both sides of the issue. Representatives from the federal Centers for Disease Control (part of the Public Health Service) and the American Academy of Pediatrics recommended that the drug be withdrawn from the market. Consumer advocates proposed severe restrictions. Spokespersons from the American Academy of Dermatology, representing skin specialists (who write 90 percent of all Accutane prescriptions), emphasized its therapeutic value and the physical and psychological scarring, along with the social ostracism, that patients with severe cystic acne often endure. They recommended continued marketing with a number of restrictions.

Proponents of keeping the drug on the market showed slides of patients with disfiguring acne, not only on the face but also on the shoulders, arms, back, and chest.

Proponents of severely restricting or totally banning the drug showed slides of babies with the birth defect syndrome known to be associated with the drug: misshapen head, lack of ears or ears placed

Cautions about Drugs and Their Impact

low next to a too-small jaw, and cleft palate. They also described the defects of the brain and heart and explained that the drug does the most damage to the fetus in the early weeks of pregnancy, often before a woman realizes she is pregnant.

How was FDA to choose between protecting the unborn and healing patients with a disfiguring physical problem?

Should the agency allow a drug to remain on the market that continued to be a cause of birth defects despite warnings that it not be used in women who were pregnant or who might become pregnant?

On the other hand, could FDA ethically remove from the market a drug that had the capacity to clear up a disfiguring condition when no other marketed drug was as effective?

Fortunately, FDA had a solution available to it that was not available to Solomon: compromise.

Taking into account advice from consumer and professional organizations, the agency and Hoffmann-La Roche have been hammering out further restrictions and unprecedented labeling warnings in the expectation that these will insure the appropriate use of the drug and, thus, the elimination of birth defects associated with its use.

One aspect of this plan is the inclusion, in the patient information labeling, of a drawing of a baby with the syndrome of deformities associated with Accutane use. The drawing is meant as an attention-getter and as a deterrent to women who might otherwise take lightly the warning not to take the drug unless they are using an effective form of contraception.

The patient labeling will also state that there is at least a one in four chance that a woman who becomes pregnant while taking Accutane will give birth to a deformed baby. The patient consent form, which the woman and her physician must sign, will include a discussion of the potential for birth defects. To prevent starting the drug when a pregnancy has begun but is not yet recognized, the patient leaflet will instruct the woman that the drug should be started only on the second or third day after the start of a normal menstrual period. A phone number will be given for women to call if they think they may be pregnant and want additional information.

The "don't use in pregnancy" symbol (a pregnant woman within a bisected circle, the international symbol for "not" or "don't") will be displayed both on each page of the patient leaflet and on each panel of the new blister-pack packaging. The blister pack will include a tear-off prepaid postcard addressed to Hoffmann-La Roche on which the patient can inform the company of her name, phone number, and address, and grant permission to the company to contact her for follow-up studies to determine whether women taking Accutane are continuing to become pregnant.

The physician labeling, which will also display the "don't use in pregnancy" symbol, will be extensively revised to more strongly emphasize the risk of birth defects. The print size for the boxed pregnancy contraindication will be doubled. The boxed warning will forbid Accutane's use in women of childbearing age unless all of the following conditions are met:

- The patient has severe, disfiguring cystic acne that does not respond to other therapies.

- She is reliable in understanding and carrying out instructions.

- She is capable of complying with mandatory contraceptive measures.

- She has received both verbal and written warnings of the hazards of pregnancy, the risks of contraceptive failure, and has acknowledged these in writing.

- Within two weeks before starting the drug, the patient has had a negative pregnancy test, performed in a physician's office or by a licensed laboratory.

The physician labeling will also contain instructions that Accutane should be prescribed only by physicians, such as dermatologists, who have special competence in the diagnosis and treatment of severe, recalcitrant cystic acne, and who understand the risk of birth defects.

In addition to the labeling changes, Hoffmann-La Roche has agreed to extensive professional educational and follow-up efforts. The firm will report to FDA all cases in which a woman using Accutane becomes pregnant, whether or not a birth defect or other adverse reaction occurs. It also will undertake research into the reasons why, despite warnings, pregnancies have occurred in the past. Data concerning the use of the drug, including information about age and sex of patients, will be supplied to FDA quarterly. The company is also designing studies using lower doses of the drug, and using higher doses for a shorter period.

In conjunction with the labeling changes, the American Academy of Dermatology has developed guidelines for the appropriate use of Accutane.

Cautions about Drugs and Their Impact

This program is a bold example of what can be accomplished when a manufacturer, professional organizations, and FDA cooperate in finding ways to minimize the risks of a drug while preserving its availability to those who can greatly benefit from it. Only time will tell whether the responsible use of Accutane will make the decision to keep it on the market with increased warnings and restrictions a decision worthy of the wisdom of Solomon.

Vitamin A and Birth Defects

It is no secret that high doses of vitamin A may cause birth defects when taken by a pregnant woman. Although data on its effects in humans are sparse, studies in animals have conclusively shown it to be a teratogen—a cause of birth defects.

It was, therefore, no surprise when Accutane, a synthetic derivative of vitamin A, caused human birth defects. From the time the drug first went on the market, it was placed in "Pregnancy Category X," meaning that it should not be used in pregnant women or in those likely to become pregnant. Originally this categorization was based on animal studies, but it took only a few months on the market for it to become evident that it was a potent teratogen in humans as well.

On the heels of the problems with Accutane, concern has arisen about two other drugs that also are vitamin A derivatives: Retin-A (tretinoin), a topical cream and lotion used to treat acne and recently ballyhooed in the press for easing wrinkles, and Tegison (etretinate), an oral medication for the treatment of severe psoriasis unresponsive to other treatments.

Because Retin-A is a topical product and not absorbed a great deal into the body, all evidence to date seems to be reassuring that there is not an increased danger of birth defects to the fetuses of women who may become pregnant while using it. The drug is in Pregnancy Category B, which means that it should be used in pregnancy only when clearly needed.

Tegison, however, is another story. A more potent teratogen than even Accutane, like Accutane it is in Pregnancy Category X. Its teratogenic effect may persist longer than Accutane's; Tegison's labeling warns that it is not known exactly how long this effect lasts after a woman stops taking the drug. Therefore, the labeling requires that a woman taking Tegison use an effective form of contraception one month before starting, during, and for an indefinite period after stopping therapy. Possibly because people suffering from psoriasis are usually older than those with acne (use of Tegison in women of childbearing age is only 5 percent that of Accutane's use in that group), there have been no reports of birth defects associated with Tegison's use in this country since it was approved in late 1986. However, a report from Brazil of a baby born with a syndrome of birth defects similar to that seen with Accutane serves as a warning. In that particular case, that baby was conceived 11 months after the mother stopped taking Tegison.

Regarding vitamin A itself, data from animal studies clearly show it to be a teratogen whose effect, similar to Tegison's, persists for some time after use is discontinued. But it is not yet known at what dosage level it becomes a threat to the developing human fetus. For one thing, because it can be purchased over the counter as a dietary supplement, the extent of its use by pregnant women is unknown, and data on its effects are hard to come by. Further, because it is known to cause birth defects in animals, as do Accutane and Tegison, controlled trials in pregnant women would be unethical. FDA scientists are presently trying to collect more data on vitamin A. But until more definitive studies are completed, women who are pregnant or planning to become pregnant would be wise to avoid taking supplements with more than a total of 8,000 International Units of vitamin A per day. There is no known benefit to anyone, including pregnant women, in taking more than this amounts but there are potential dangers.

Medicines and Pregnancy

Women who must take known teratogens to treat a chronic underlying physical condition present a difficult case for their doctors. Drugs such as anti-convulsants used to treat epilepsy, antibiotics for tuberculosis, oral anticoagulants to prevent blood clots, anti-cancer drugs, drugs to treat an overactive thyroid, and lithium for manic depression are some substances that cannot always be avoided completely. Doctors must advise women taking these drugs—before they become pregnant—of the risk to the unborn baby and how that risk can be reduced. In some cases, it may be possible to withhold the drugs, if only for the first trimester.

For the best outcome, a little prevention is worth a pound of cure. Women who are pregnant or who think they may be pregnant should let their doctors know about their condition when drugs are being prescribed for them. They should take no over-the-counter (OTC) drugs (or prescription drugs left over from another illness) without consulting their doctors. OTC drugs, which look harmless sitting between the candy and housewares departments in drugstores, may not

Cautions about Drugs and Their Impact

be harmless. Even a drug as commonly used as aspirin can prolong labor and alter bleeding and clotting time if taken in the last three months of pregnancy. Many OTC labels warn: *As with any drug, if you are pregnant or nursing a baby, seek the advice of a health professional before using this product.* It's worth paying attention to those words.

It's often true that the critical period for the development of most organs in the unborn baby is over by the time a woman is sure she is pregnant. Nevertheless, it is comforting to know that even women who have taken a known teratogen during the first trimester have given birth to healthy babies free from deformities. Probably a majority of fetuses whose mothers took thalidomide—one of the most potent teratogens known—resisted the effects of the drug. (A recent British survey reported that babies born to women who had thalidomide-caused birth defects are having normal babies, which was expected.) Timing of exposure to a drug is crucial, of course, but some experts think that other factors yet unknown—though perhaps genetic—appear to determine a fetus' vulnerability to a drug's effects.

For the safest pregnancy, the most sensible course is not to drink or smoke, and to take drugs only if necessary and only on the doctors advice.

In general, during pregnancy, all medications (including psychotherapeutic medications) should be avoided where possible, and other methods of treatment should be tried.

A woman who is taking a psychotherapeutic medication and plans to become pregnant should discuss her plans with her doctor; if she discovers that she is pregnant, she should contact her doctor immediately. During early pregnancy, there is a possible risk of birth defects with some of these medications, and for this reason:

1. Lithium is not recommended during the first 3 months of pregnancy.
2. Benzodiazepines are not recommended during the first 3 months of pregnancy.

The decision to use a psychotherapeutic medication should be made only after a careful discussion with the doctor concerning the risks and benefits to the woman and her baby.

Small amounts of medication pass into the breast milk; this is a consideration for mothers who are planning to breast-feed.

A woman who is taking birth-control pills should be sure that her doctor is aware of this. The estrogen in these pills may alter the breakdown of medications by the body, for example increasing side effects of some anti-anxiety medications and/or reducing their efficacy to relieve symptoms of anxiety. For more detailed information, talk to your doctor or mental health professional, consult your local public library, or write to the pharmaceutical company that produces the medication or the U.S. Food and Drug Administration, 5600 Fishers Lane, Rockville, MD 20857.

Section 12.3

Caffeine and Pregnancy

Excerpt from FDA Consumer, November 1990 by Lisa Iannucci

Caffeine—a stimulant found in colas coffee, tea, soft candies, chocolate, cocoa, and over-the-counter and prescription drugs—has been a controversial topic in pregnancy nutrition for more than a decade. A 1980 study by FDA found that caffeine, when fed to pregnant rats, caused birth defects and delayed skeletal development in their offspring. At that time, although the human implications were unknown, FDA advised pregnant women to eliminate caffeine from their diets.

Since then, more studies have been done to determine the effects of caffeine on the fetus. A study of women in Costa Rica, where coffee consumption is high, showed a significantly lower birth weight for infants and a lower concentration of iron in mothers who were coffee drinkers. This report indicated that maternal coffee intake may also contribute to maternal and infant anemia.

Consumed in large quantities, caffeine can cause irritability, nervousness and insomnia. In addition to crossing the placenta and affecting the fetus, it is also a diuretic, dehydrating the mother's body of valuable water. After the baby is born, caffeine can also be transmitted through breast milk.

As mentioned, caffeine is an ingredient in some over-the-counter (OTC) and prescription drugs. Before taking any drugs, a pregnant woman should consult her physician.

Cautions about Drugs and Their Impact

Section 12.4

Tobacco and Pregnancy

Excerpts from DHSS Publication No. (FDA) 90-3174, 1989 and from DHSS Homepage, Smoking and Pregnancy Data by Sandra Smith, April 1992

Among the warnings on packages of cigarettes is a statement that smoking may complicate pregnancy. Still, of the approximately 32 percent of women who smoke cigarettes before pregnancy, 25 percent continue to smoke while pregnant. While no specific malformations are connected with smoking, birth weight of babies born to smokers averages a half pound less than that of babies of nonsmokers. Low-birth-weight babies are 40 times more likely to die in infancy than those of normal weight. It is thought that nicotine, which constricts blood vessels, may reduce placental blood flow, and thus the amounts of nutrients and oxygen to the unborn baby. The March of Dimes states that some research has shown that chest breathing motion in an unborn baby temporarily decreases sharply after its mother has smoked only two cigarettes. Smoking may also increase the risk of miscarriage, stillbirth and death in newborns.

In 1989, 20 percent of mothers smoked during pregnancy, according to an NCHS report, the first to analyze data from the new certificates. Most at risk were older mothers and those who smoked the most: Women who smoked 1.5 to two packs of cigarettes per day were about one-third more likely to have a low-birth-weight infant than those who smoked half a pack—and 2.5 times as likely as nonsmokers.

In releasing the report, DHHS Secretary Louis W. Sullivan, M.D., said, "Our efforts to improve the health of mothers and babies just took a big leap forward. For the first time, we have information on maternal medical and life-style risk factors for the more than 4 million births annually in the United States. We can identify mothers at risk and practices that put them in harm's way."

Also at risk to have low-birth-weight infants were the more than one in five mothers who gained less than 22 to 27 pounds, the weight gain recommendation in effect in 1989. Their infants were two to four times as likely to be low birth weight. Low birth weight was also associated with complications during labor and delivery and abnormal conditions in the newborn such as respiratory distress syndrome, a leading cause of infant deaths.

James Mason, M.D., assistant secretary for health and head of the Public Health Service, said, "This analysis of the smoking risk, as well as other facts and figures still to come, will help as we carry out our Healthy Start programs in high-infant-mortality areas." Mason has been visiting communities to work with them as they develop new efforts to combat infant mortality.

"And most importantly," he said, "teen-age mothers 18 and 19 years of age have the highest smoking rates of any age group—almost one-fourth are smokers." Young teens—those under 15—however, had the lowest rate of cigarette smoking.

Overall, black mothers were less likely to smoke than their white counterparts (17 percent compared to 20 percent), and those who did smoke, smoked fewer cigarettes. The rate of cigarette smoking was also relatively low, at 8 percent, among Hispanic mothers.

Education affects tobacco use. The proportion of smokers generally declined with advanced educational attainment: The highest rate was 35 percent for women with less than high school education, and the lowest was for college graduates, 5 percent.

Section 12.5

Alcohol and Pregnancy

Excerpts from DHSS Publication No's 93-2011, 1993 and 90-3174, 1990
by Evelyn Zamula and *Morbidity and Mortality Weekly*,
April 1995

One drug—alcohol—is so commonly used that some people don't even think of it as a drug. But many experts consider it the most common teratogen in humans. Since more women and teenage girls than ever are drinking now—about 60 percent—and about a quarter of them drink heavily, this has ominous public health implications.

Abuse of alcohol is a significant societal problem in the United States; approximately 18 million Americans are chronic consumers of alcohol. Current estimates indicate that between 8 and 11 percent of women of childbearing age are either problem drinkers or alcoholics. Alcohol abuse exists within all socioeconomic levels of society. Review of drinking habits during pregnancy should form an essential part of perinatal history taking.

No safe level of alcohol consumption during pregnancy has been determined. Alcohol exposure *in utero* may result in a spectrum of abnormalities of fetal growth and development. Maternal consumption of 2 to 3 ounces of alcohol daily, often in association with "binge drinking," is frequently associated with fetal alcohol syndrome (FAS). Lesser intake of alcohol may produce subcombinations of signs of FAS; these lesser signs have been called fetal alcohol effects (FAE).

The effects of alcohol abuse during pregnancy can be summarized as follows:

Adverse Pregnancy Outcome, including an increased risk of spontaneous abortion.

FAS. The worldwide incidence of FAS is 1-3 births per 1,000 live births. To make the diagnosis of FAS, one abnormality from each of the following categories must be present:

- Prenatal or postnatal growth retardation; failure to thrive (weight, length, and/or head circumference less than the 10th percentile).

- Central nervous system dysfunction, including intellectual, neurologic, and behavioral deficits manifested as mild to moderate mental retardation, hypotonia (poor muscle tone), irritability in infancy, and later hyperactivity in childhood. Mental abnormality occurs in 85 percent of FAS children, and although IQ scores vary, affected children rarely show normal mental ability.

- Facial dysmorphology (structural abnormalities) including at least two of three characteristics: 1) Microcephaly (head circumference less than the 10th percentile). 2) Microphthalmia (abnormal smallness of the eye) or short palpebral fissures, ptosis (dropping eyelid), strabismus (imbalance of the eye muscles), or epicanthal folds (folds of the skin of the upper eyelid over the eye). 3) Poorly developed philtrum, thin upper lip (vermilion border), short upturned nose, or flattening or absence of the maxilla (upper jaw).

FAE. Lesser degree of effect.

One to three out of every 1,000 newborns, or about 5,000 babies per year, are born with fetal alcohol syndrome (FAS). (A syndrome is a set of symptoms or characteristics that occur together with reasonable consistency.) The syndrome was first described in France in 1967 by a physician who noticed that children of alcoholic mothers shared such distinct characteristics that a diagnosis of maternal alcoholism could be made by just looking at them.

In 1970, in the United States, a young pediatric resident at the University of Washington Health Sciences Center in Seattle had a similar experience. In reviewing newborns' medical records, she noticed that four babies of alcoholic mothers had abnormally low birth weights. Further search revealed seven more cases. When the 11 children were brought together to the Health Sciences Center for examination, researchers in the birth defects unit were struck by their resemblance to each other. Their heads were abnormally small, and they all had small narrow eyes, drooping eyelids, short upturned noses, and wide upper lips in which the normal center groove was reduced or missing. All were small for their age and all were mentally retarded.

Cautions about Drugs and Their Impact

Since FAS children do not usually improve in intelligence even when placed in foster homes, the damage points to alcohol rather than the family environment, which is usually poor. As many as 20 studies in various western countries indicate that FAS surpasses Down's syndrome and spina bifida (a birth defect in which part of the vertebral column is missing) as a cause of mental retardation. FAS children may also have defects of the heart and genital and urinary organs and may have poor coordination, short attention span, and behavioral problems.

Women who drink the equivalent of three ounces of pure alcohol daily—six average mixed drinks or six cans of beer— frequently give birth to babies with the full range of FAS defects. They are also more likely to miscarry or have stillborn children or children who die in early infancy. Those who drink less but still heavily (more than two drinks a day, according to the U.S. Surgeon General) may give birth to babies who have some, but not all fetal alcohol effects. A new study points out that even two or three drinks a week may trigger spontaneous abortion. Since no one knows at which point in the pregnancy alcohol does the greatest damage or what amount can be consumed safely, pregnant women should drink no alcoholic beverages.

Medical Withdrawal from Alcohol

It should be assumed that pregnant women who consume over 8 ounces of [absolute] alcohol (1 pint of liquor) daily have developed tolerance. However, tolerance may develop at lower levels of consumption in some women and in women using multiple drugs.

The sudden cessation of drinking can result in withdrawal symptoms, some of which may be threatening to the mother and the fetus. It is imperative that medical withdrawal of an alcohol-dependent, pregnant woman be conducted in an inpatient setting and under medical supervision that includes collaboration with an obstetrician. These conditions will ensure

- Close observation and monitoring of maternal alcohol withdrawal status
- Continual monitoring of fetal well-being

Symptoms of Alcohol Withdrawal

Early symptoms of alcohol withdrawal generally appear 6 to 48 hours after drinking has stopped but can occur up to 10 days after the last drink. Withdrawal symptoms may include:

- Restlessness
- Tachycardia
- Irritability
- Hypertension
- Anorexia
- Insomnia
- Nausea
- Nightmares
- Vomiting
- Impaired concentration
- Sweating
- Impaired memory
- Tremor
- Elevated vital signs

More severe symptoms of alcohol withdrawal may include:

- Increased tremulousness
- Increased agitation
- Increased sweating
- Delirium (with confusion, disorientation, impaired memory and judgment)
- Hallucinations (auditory, visual, or tactile)
- Delusions (usually paranoid)
- Grand mal seizures

Note: Withdrawal symptoms do not necessarily progress from mild to severe. In some individuals, a grand mal seizure may be the first sign of withdrawal. Seizures usually occur 12 to 24 hours after cessation or reduction of drinking. One-third of all patients who have seizures develop delirium tremens.

Most programs choose to treat the pregnant, alcohol-dependent woman with short-acting barbiturates or benzodiazepines. Chlordiazepoxide (Librium) and other benzodiazepines, such as diazepam (Valium) and barbiturates (Phenobarbital, Seconal), are valuable for symptomatic treatment during medical withdrawal from alcohol. They are also potentially teratogenic. Some clinicians, therefore, recommend avoiding their use if at all possible. The risks versus the possible benefits of their use need to be assessed.

Disulfiram (Antabuse) is contraindicated during pregnancy. Its use has been associated with clubfoot, VACTERL syndrome (a pattern of congenital anomalies), and phocomelia of the lower extremities. The woman who conceives while taking this drug should receive counseling before deciding to continue the pregnancy.

Maternal and Fetal Effects of Alcohol

Alcohol use during pregnancy may be associated with a variety of serious health consequences for the woman, the fetus, and the subsequent infant.

Possible maternal complications of excessive alcohol consumption:

- Nutritional deficiencies
- Pancreatitis
- Alcoholic ketoacidosis
- Precipitate labor
- Alcoholic hepatitis
- Deficient milk ejection
- Cirrhosis

Possible effects on the fetus:

- Fetal Alcohol Syndrome (FAS)—prenatal/postnatal growth retardation; central nervous system deficits including developmental delay and neurological/intellectual impairments; facial feature anomalies, including microcephaly

- Fetal Alcohol Effects (FAE)—cardiac abnormalities; neonatal irritability and hypotonia; hyperactivity; genitourinary abnormalities; skeletal and muscular abnormalities; ocular problems; hemangiomas

- No effect

Trends in Fetal Alcohol Syndrome—United States, 1979-1993

Based on data from the national Birth Defects Monitoring Program (BDMP), the rate of reported cases of FAS identified among newborns in the United States during 1979-1992 increased approximately fourfold. This text updates data characterizing the occurrence of FAS through 1993, the latest complete year of data reporting for BDMP.

In 1993, FAS was reported in 126 of 188,905 newborns [rate: 6.7 per 10,000].

Overall, during 1979-1993, FAS was reported in 2032 of 9,434,560 newborns (overall rate: 2.2 per 10,000 births). The rate for 1993 was more than sixfold higher than that for 1979 (1.0 per 10,000 births).

Thus, although the cause of FAS-alcohol consumption during pregnancy is preventable, the findings in this report suggest an increasing frequency of this problem. This increase may reflect a true increase in the number of infants with FAS—the most severe expression of in utero alcohol damage to the fetus—or an increase in the awareness and diagnosis by primary-care clinicians of FAS in newborns.

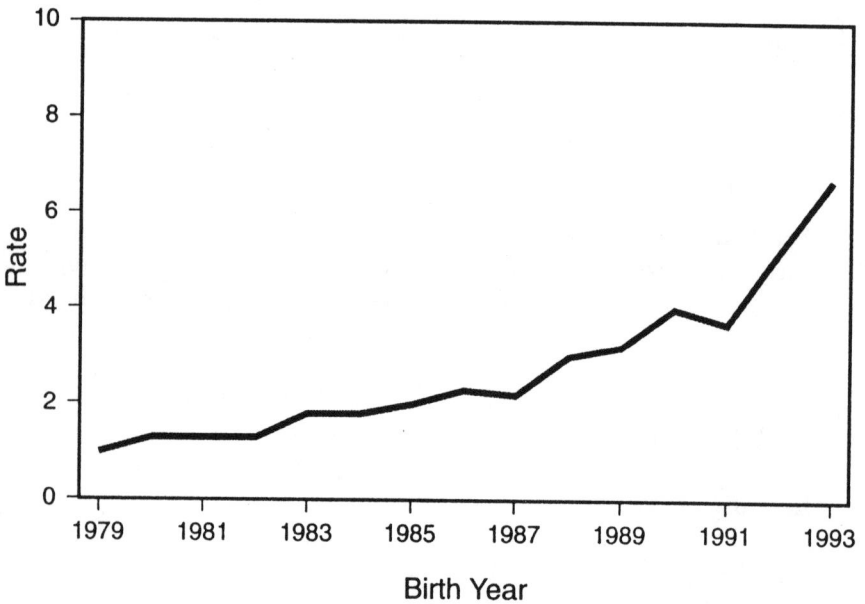

*Per 10,000 births.
†*International Classification of Diseases, Ninth Revision, Clinical Modification*, code 760.71.

Figure 12.1. *Reported rate of fetal alcohol syndrome, by birth year—Birth Defects Monitoring Program, United States, 1979-1993*

Cautions about Drugs and Their Impact

Section 12.6

Illegal Drugs and Pregnancy

Excerpts from DHSS Publication No's (FDA) 93-1998, 1993, 93-2011, 1993 and 90-3174, 1990 by Evelyn Zamula. National Institute on Drug Abuse (NIDA) publication, Capsules, C-89-04, June 1989 and *Research Resources Reporter*, February 1992 by Jane Collins.

Introduction

Paula Crews, a licensed clinical social worker associated with Sharp Memorial Hospital in San Diego, Calif., works with new mothers and their babies. "About 2 percent of the pregnant women in this area are abusing drugs," she says, "which isn't bad compared to some big city hospitals where it's as high as 30 percent or more."

"Cocaine, 'crystal' [methamphetamine], and heroin are the most popular, in that order, and marijuana is used in conjunction with all of them. Many drug abusers haven't had any prenatal care and walk in off the street to deliver. Some of them are high or drunk during labor and delivery. I feel sorry for their babies. The minute the umbilical cord is cut, the baby is on its own. It must clear that drug out of its system. The most pitiful cases are the poor heroin babies, who have classic withdrawal symptoms after they're born. They have feeding problems, sneeze, are irritable, and sometimes have seizures. That's a terrible way to start life."

But the baby's problems are just beginning. "Cocaine users don't have much appetite and are malnourished," continues Crews, "so their babies have low birth weight. These mothers are so skinny that they hardly look pregnant even at term. Some don't make it to term, because cocaine users are at high risk for premature delivery. As far as birth defects go, we don't notice any more overt structural abnormalities among cocaine-exposed babies than usual, but they can sustain neurological damage, which is not apparent at birth, but which we pick up later in infancy and childhood. I've been told that some babies exposed to cocaine late in pregnancy have strokes in utero [in the womb] that can lead to retardation. When we do see malformations, we wouldn't have any idea if a drug is responsible, or which drug is responsible, because many of these women are multiple drug abusers, plus they drink and they smoke, and are often malnourished."

Indeed, increasing numbers of women are abusing drugs during pregnancy and thus endangering the well-being and lives of their children as well as themselves. The spreading abuse of phencyclidine (PCP), cocaine, and its potent form "crack," added to the more well known addictive narcotics such as heroin, has intensified concerns about the implications of maternal drug use for unborn children.

Some harmful effects are generally recognized. Cocaine use, for example, increases risk of hemorrhage and premature delivery, threatening the lives of mother and child. Babies exposed to narcotics in the womb are frequently born addicted, and the misery they suffer from withdrawal makes them difficult to care for, creating special demands on mothers who are often unable to take care of their children adequately. Other effects are less certain. Head size is often smaller in infants exposed to narcotics. While growth erases some of the physical differences, there may be subtle, long-term deficits in mental or neurological functioning in infants exposed to drugs in the womb.

Scientists are just beginning to explore how various drugs may affect the development of physical coordination, language, and emotional interactions. NIDA, through its clinical, epidemiological, and basic research programs, is increasing knowledge of immediate and long-term effects of drug use during pregnancy. NIDA grantees and others are designing and evaluating therapeutic programs to help these mothers and their children overcome the harm caused by drugs.

Scope of the Problem

Evidence of increasing drug use among pregnant women comes from many parts of the country. NIDA estimates that of the women of childbearing age (15-44 years of age), 15 percent are current substance abusers. Approximately 34 million consume alcoholic beverages, more than 18 million are current cigarette smokers, and more than 6 million are current users of an illicit drug, of which 44 percent tried marijuana and 14 percent tried cocaine at least once.

A 1988 survey conducted by the National Association for Perinatal Addiction Research and Education, of 36 hospitals from across the country and representing approximately 155,000 pregnancies annually, found that on average, 11 percent of pregnant women used heroin, methadone, amphetamines, PCP, marijuana, and most commonly,

Cautions about Drugs and Their Impact

cocaine. The researchers estimate that each year, as many as 375,000 infants may be affected by their mother's drug use.

Dr. Barry Zuckerman and his colleagues at Boston University School of Medicine and Boston City Hospital conducted a study of 1,226 women who gave birth at the hospital between 1986 and 1988. Of this group, 27 percent of the women had smoked marijuana and 18 percent used cocaine. They found that marijuana users gave birth to babies who are three ounces lighter and one-fifth of an inch shorter than babies born to women who did not use marijuana, while the cocaine use was associated with still shorter and lighter infants.

Dr. Loretta P. Finnegan, director of the Family Center of Jefferson Medical College of Thomas Jefferson University in Philadelphia reports that in 1985, 7 percent of women at the center were found to have cocaine in their urine, and now urine screens show that 58 percent are using the substance.

Effects on the Pregnant Mother and the Fetus

Until relatively recently, NIDA's research on the effects of maternal drug use on fetal and infant development has focused on narcotics and drugs like methadone that is used in the treatment of narcotic addiction. As the abuse of cocaine, PCP, and other drugs grew, NIDA expanded this research program to non-narcotic drugs. NIDA's research in this area is intended to estimate incidence, prevalence, and patterns of use of illicit drugs among pregnant women, to identify the consequences of maternal drug use on the newborn, to identify the mechanisms underlying organic and behavioral effects resulting from exposure to drugs, and to develop strategies and procedures to prevent, ameliorate, or reverse these toxic effects and their developmental consequences.

A NIDA-supported study by Dr. Ira J. Chasnoff and his colleagues at Northwestern University's Perinatal Center for Chemical Dependence found that women injecting cocaine intravenously during pregnancy immediately experienced complications, including premature separation of the placenta from the womb, which causes hemorrhaging that threatens the lives of both mother and fetus. Another study found that cocaine-addicted women were twice as likely to suffer premature separation of the placenta as women dependent on other drugs and four times as likely as drug-free women to experience this complication. However, this risk is reduced if the pregnant woman discontinues cocaine use early in pregnancy. Isolated cases of birth defects have been associated with cocaine use during pregnancy; however, additional studies are needed to confirm these observations.

Cocaine can also precipitate miscarriage or premature delivery because it raises blood pressure and increases contractions of the uterus. Maternal cocaine use also endangers the fetus directly. Studies show that the drug constricts arteries leading to the womb. This constriction diminishes the amount of blood, and hence oxygen, that reach the fetus. In one extreme case, cocaine apparently caused fetal stroke.

Effects on Infants

Knowledge of drug effects during the early months of life comes largely from studies of children born to women dependent on narcotics. Infants exposed to these drugs in the womb are often born addicted and undergo a characteristic withdrawal sequence called the Neonatal Abstinence Syndrome (NAS). Newborns with NAS show increased sensitivity to noise, irritability, poor coordination, excessive sneezing and yawning, and uncoordinated sucking and swallowing reflexes. If these symptoms persist, they require medication. NIDA-funded researchers are testing carefully controlled doses of phenobarbital, tincture of opium, and other substances to help infants withdraw from narcotics.

Research using ultrasound measurements also raises questions about the rate of brain growth in narcotic-exposed babies. The head circumference tends to be slightly smaller, although this difference soon disappears. By the time infants are six months old, there is little difference between drug-exposed babies and others in brain measurement. But concerns remain, since prenatal harm to these areas of the brain could affect mental functioning, such as memory, in later childhood. Some researchers find, moreover, that certain differences between drug-exposed and other infants persist, adding to concerns about long-term effects.

Other findings include increased risk for Sudden Infant Death Syndrome in which incidence among cocaine exposed infants in the Chicago study was 17 percent as compared to 1.6 percent in the general population and four percent in infants of mothers maintained on methadone. Assessment at four months of age indicate that the cocaine-exposed infants are at considerable risk for motor dysfunction. Data on 30 full-term cocaine-exposed infants and 50 full-term non-drug exposed infants indicate a significant difference in mean total risk scores with 72 percent of the control group infants in the "no risk" category, while 43 percent of the cocaine-exposed infants, were designated "high risk" for motor developmental dysfunction. The infants will be followed to three years of age.

Cautions about Drugs and Their Impact

Long-Term Effects

The epidemic of drug abuse among pregnant women is recent enough that investigators are only now having the opportunity to follow groups of children over several years and thus generalize about more far-reaching effects. Some of the preliminary findings are encouraging. Children at age two to five born to methadone-maintained women seem comparable in intelligence to youngsters of drug-free mothers. However, despite scoring in the normal range for overall intelligence, these children seem to run increased risk of learning disabilities and delayed motor, speech, and language development.

Effective drug intervention programs for drug-dependent mothers and their children may be essential to promoting the youngster's emotional and intellectual well-being. Dr. Judy Howard at the University of California, Los Angeles, is assessing the benefits of a program using a pediatrician, a public health nurse, and a social worker to contact homes regularly to offer information, advice, and referrals to medical and other services. In addition, an infant development specialist works with the children on development skills while a specialist helps mothers and foster parents become sensitive to the child's state of well-being.

The increasing use of drugs by women of childbearing age, the greater numbers of children being born to drug-abusing women, and the environment in which these infants are reared all lend added urgency to conduct additional research in these critical areas.

Guidelines for Pregnant Substance-Abusing Women

Overview

Traditionally, alcohol and other drug treatment programs served adult males, and few women received the treatment they needed. The scarcity of treatment services for women continues today. It is imperative that programs include services designed specifically for women, particularly pregnant women.

Profile of the Women Being Served

Reliable national estimates of the prevalence of drug use by pregnant women are not available. Several factors limit the accuracy and usefulness of current estimates, including differences in the populations studied, the lack of representativeness of samples used, and differences in the methods employed to determine drug use. Results of specific studies, such as those reported below, illustrate to some degree the nature and extent of the problem.

- Data from one study of 36 hospitals, mainly in urban areas, were extrapolated to arrive at an estimate of 375,000 infants exposed in utero to illegal drugs each year, or 11 percent of all births.

- A study conducted in Pinellas County, Florida, of urine samples from more than 700 women enrolling in prenatal care during a 1-month period in 1989 found little difference in the prevalence of drug and alcohol use between women seen at public clinics (16.3 percent) and those seen at private offices (13.1 percent), as well as similar rates of substance abuse among white women (15.4 percent) and black women (14.1 percent).

- A study based on a review of medical records in eight hospitals in Philadelphia in 1989 found that 16.3 percent of women had used cocaine while pregnant.

- A study that assessed drug use, utilizing urine samples obtained at admission for delivery in all seven hospitals in Rhode Island, showed that 3 percent of women used marijuana.

To meet the need for estimates of the prevalence of drug use by pregnant women that are generalizable to the Nation, the National Institute on Drug Abuse has recently sponsored a national, hospital-based study known as the National Pregnancy and Health Survey. Until these and other data become available, service providers should be alert to patterns of alcohol and other drug use occurring locally among women of all socioeconomic and ethnic groups. Those with clinical experience in treating substance-using women have found that the therapeutic needs of women, especially those with children, are markedly different from the needs of men. Substance-using women come from every ethnic and socioeconomic group and have a multitude of needs. Moreover, a substantial portion of the women who seek publicly supported treatment for their addictions share a core group of problems that reflect problems of the communities in which they live. Unless these core problems are addressed, women will be unable to take full advantage of the therapeutic process. Many women who seek treatment for their drug problems through publicly funded programs share the following characteristics:

Cautions about Drugs and Their Impact

- Function as single parents and receive little or no financial support from the birth fathers.
- Lack employment skills and education and are unemployed or underemployed.
- Live in unstable or unsafe environments, including households where others use alcohol and other drugs. Many women are at risk of being homeless and some are homeless.
- Lack transportation and face extreme difficulty getting to and from a variety of appointments, including treatment.
- Lack child care and baby-sitting options and are unable to enroll in treatment.
- Experience special therapeutic needs, including problems with codependency, incest, abuse, victimization, sexuality, and relationships involving significant others.
- Experience special medical needs, including gynecological problems.

Access to Services

Pregnant, substance-using women may access health care services from a variety of sites, including emergency rooms, pregnancy testing sites, clinics treating sexually transmitted diseases, community health centers, and clinics of the Special Supplemental Food Program for Women, Infants, and Children (WIC). Occasionally, alcohol and other drug treatment program staff are the first to notice that a woman is pregnant. Regardless of where she accesses care, appropriate referrals for prenatal care should be provided, and she should be assisted to follow through on these referrals.

Access to care must be simplified for a woman when she enters the system. She should receive whatever support is needed—whether it is financial assistance, help in setting up appointments, or transportation and child care services. Whenever possible, a case manager should schedule a specific prenatal appointment for the woman and initiate other needed services. In addition, a psychiatric assessment should be done to identify cases of alcohol and other drug use and psychiatric illness.

It may be difficult to convince a pregnant, substance-using woman to seek prenatal care. The concept of preventive health care, as opposed to emergency-necessitated health care, may be a foreign concept to her. More importantly, she may have a basic distrust or dislike of the health care system in general, and doctors in particular. Her feelings of fear and guilt, and possible negative past experiences, may cause her to expect poor treatment. Sometimes she provokes a hostile interchange with health care professionals.

Women need to receive health care services in an environment that is nonjudgmental, nonpunitive, nurturing, and culturally and linguistically sensitive. It is essential for all members of the health care team, from the clerical staff to the physicians, to recognize the importance of providing prenatal, postnatal, and pediatric services in a caring way. Staff must avoid comments designed to make the patient feel guilty or ashamed, such as the use of pejorative words like "wino" or "junkie." Each health care visit is an opportunity to provide positive reinforcement to the substance-using patient.

Continuum of Care

The pregnant, substance-using woman requires a continuum of care that includes a broad range of support services provided over an extended period of time. This continuum of care should reflect the complexity of her multiple roles as a person in recovery, parent, partner, and frequently, single head of a household. Ideally, support services should be provided as long as the woman and her family need and can benefit from them, potentially until her last child reaches adulthood. In reality, support services may be available for a period of a few months to several years.

The case management function is essential for the recovery and well-being of the substance-using woman and her family. Virtually any agency can provide case management services, although the lead agency typically assigns an appropriate staff person to this role, such as a social worker or nurse. The case manager assists the patient in accessing services, and monitors her participation and progress in using health care, alcohol and other drug treatment, and other social services.

The multiple services coordinated by the case manager are generally provided by a variety of agencies. Many of these services are initiated during or even prior to pregnancy and should continue after delivery for as long as they are appropriate. The consortium of service providers may change over time, depending on the family's individual circumstances and resources.

The case manager should be aware that differences in philosophies may exist between health and social service agencies and the alcohol and other drug treatment field. Behaviors that health and social service agencies view as helping and supportive are often viewed as codependent behaviors by the treatment field. As agencies work together on behalf of

Case Management

Case management is a vital function that helps to ensure that patients receive and appropriately utilize a variety of services necessary for their improved functioning. Case management should be initiated prenatally and continue throughout the postpartum period for all substance-using women. Services should be provided and maintained as appropriate for the individual woman and her family. The case manager should support and guide the patient to address issues concerning her recovery from alcohol and other drug abuse, develop psychosocial and parenting skills, and meet her survival needs. Key case management functions include:

- A review and assessment
- An individual care plan
- Discussion of the plan with the patient
- Referrals to other agencies, groups, or institutions
- Monitoring of the patient's progress
- Ongoing case management support
- A review of the patient's individual care plan

Comprehensive Service Delivery

The delivery of comprehensive services to substance-using women and their families should continue postpartum. The greatest success is achieved by and for these women when a continuum of care is available to address their special needs as women, mothers, spouses, and heads of households. The following services are often needed:

- Health care services
- Drug treatment services
- Survival-related services
- Psychosocial services
- Parenting and family services

Medical Stabilization and Withdrawal

The initial stabilization as well as the medical withdrawal of pregnant women from their drug(s) of abuse are recognized means of reducing the acute illness associated with the use of drugs. The initial stabilization of the patient should be accomplished within 10 days of first contact or earlier if medically necessary.

During the period of stabilization, caregivers need to monitor the mother and fetus for adverse signs of drug withdrawal, establish a basis for ongoing drug treatment and recovery, and initiate a relationship between the mother and available supportive services within the community. The lead agency is generally responsible for assigning an appropriate staff person to undertake case management functions. The role of the case manager is to monitor and promote completion of this initial phase.

Opioid Stabilization

The following approaches are used to manage the pregnant, opioid-addicted woman. The first approach is methadone maintenance combined with psychosocial counseling. This is a well-documented approach to improve outcomes for both the woman and her fetus.

The second approach is slow medical withdrawal with methadone. The safety of this second approach has not been documented.

Opioid Withdrawal Signs and Symptoms

Mild withdrawal signs and symptoms include:

- Generalized anxiety
- Opioid craving
- Restlessness
- Slight aching of muscles, joints, and bones
- Lower back pain

Mild to moderate withdrawal signs and symptoms include:

- Tension
- Yen sleep (mild insomnia)
- Mydriasis (pupils dilated)
- Lethargy
- Diaphoresis (increased perspiration)

Moderate withdrawal signs and symptoms include:

- Chills alternating with flushing and diaphoresis (sweating) Nausea and/or stomach cramps
- Rhinorrhea (runny nose)

Cautions about Drugs and Their Impact

- Moderate aching of muscles, joints, and bones
- Lower back pain
- Anorexia
- Nausea and/or stomach cramps
- Yawning
- Lacrimation (tearing)
- Goose flesh (earlier if client is in a cold, drafty room)
- Elevated pulse and blood pressure

Moderate to severe withdrawal signs and symptoms include:

- Diarrhea
- Tachycardia (pulse over 100 BPM)
- Vomiting
- Increased respiratory rate and depth
- Tremors

Severe withdrawal signs and symptoms include:

- Doubling over with stomach cramps
- Kicking movements
- Elevated temperature (usually low grade, less than 100°F)

NOTE: Withdrawal signs and symptoms differ in their order of appearance from one individual to another. Some individuals may not exhibit certain withdrawal signs and symptoms. Signs may also include uterine irritability, increased fetal activity, or rarely, hypotension.

Symptoms of Opioid Withdrawal Syndrome

Despite its dramatic appearance, the opioid withdrawal syndrome is rarely life-threatening or permanently disabling to an adult. However, there is good evidence that the fetus may be more susceptible to withdrawal symptoms than the mother. In the mother, the initial signs of opioid withdrawal progress to increasingly painful physical symptoms. In addition to these signs, patients show compelling psychological cravings for drugs, as well as drug-seeking behavior.

Methadone substitution is the standard treatment for heroin addiction. Methadone treatment alternatives consist of (1) high-dose blockage; (2) low-dose maintenance; and (3) medical withdrawal.

Medical withdrawal of the opioid-dependent woman is not recommended in pregnancy because of the increased risk to the fetus of intrauterine death. Methadone maintenance is the treatment of choice.

In addition to methadone maintenance, a comprehensive approach is needed that will provide the patient with counseling and other services.

The administration of methadone, combined with any opioid agonist/antagonist such as pentazocine (Talwin), will precipitate withdrawal. Any pregnant woman receiving methadone should be advised against taking opioid agonist/antagonists under all circumstances.

Neonatal abstinence syndrome (NAS) may or may not be related to maternal dose of methadone; NAS may also be related to fetal gestational age and infant weight. However, studies in both pregnant women and other adults have shown that larger doses of methadone result in a decreased use of other drugs.

Maternal and Fetal Effects of Opioids

These effects may be the result of concomitant maternal lifestyle factors rather than the direct result of drug use.

Possible effects on the pregnancy:

- Toxemia
- Intrauterine growth retardation
- Miscarriage
- Premature rupture of membranes
- Infections
- Breech presentation (abnormal presentation due to premature delivery)
- Preterm labor
- No effect

Possible effects on the mother:

- Poor nourishment, with vitamin deficiencies, iron deficiency anemia, and folic acid deficiency anemia
- Medical complications from frequent use of dirty needles (abscesses, ulcers, thrombophlebitis, bacterial endocarditis, hepatitis, and urinary tract infection)
- Sexually transmitted diseases (gonorrhea, chlamydia, syphilis, herpes, and HIV infection)
- Hypertensive disorder
- No effect

Cautions about Drugs and Their Impact

Possible effects on the fetus and newborn infant:

- Low birth weight
- Prematurity
- Neonatal abstinence syndrome
- Stillbirth
- Sudden infant death syndrome
- No effect

Guidelines for Methadone Maintenance

Methadone maintenance is strongly encouraged for all pregnant, opioid-dependent women. It provides the following advantages:

- Reduces illegal opioid use as well as use of other drugs
- Helps to remove the opioid-dependent woman from the drug-seeking environment and eliminates the necessary illegal behavior
- Prevents fluctuations of the maternal drug level that may occur throughout the day
- Improves maternal nutrition, increasing the weight of the newborn
- Improves the woman's ability to participate in prenatal care and other rehabilitation efforts
- Enhances the woman's ability to prepare for the birth of the infant and begin homemaking
- Reduces obstetrical complications

There are no specific guidelines established for methadone dosages for pregnant women. In general, the clinical trend is toward use of an individually determined, most effective dose that is adequate to prevent withdrawal symptoms. The following guidelines have been used for pregnant and nonpregnant substance users:

- The high-dose methadone blockage dosage is between 50 and 150 mg per day.

- The low-dosage methadone maintenance dosage is less than 60 mg per day.

    Based on current and emerging research, the National Institute on Drug Abuse (NIDA) suggests that maintenance doses below 60 mg are not effective and hence not appropriate. Arbitrary low-dose policies for pregnant and nonpregnant patients is often associated with increased drug use as well as reduced program retention. Based on current informed consensus, the most prudent course is to rely on individually determined methadone dosing that is measured by the absence of subjective and objective abstinence symptoms and the reduction of drug hunger.

An increased methadone dosage may be needed in later stages of pregnancy to prevent withdrawal. (The greater plasma volume and renal blood flow of pregnancy can contribute to a reduced level of methadone in the blood. As a result, the woman's maintenance dose may be insufficient to prevent cravings.) Either administer methadone twice a day to give a more even blood level throughout the day or raise the single daily dose.

Guidelines for Medical Withdrawal from Methadone

Medical withdrawal of the pregnant, opioid-dependent woman from methadone is not indicated or recommended. Few women will have the motivation or the psychosocial supports to accomplish and maintain total abstinence. The goal, therefore, is to achieve the best therapeutic dose possible with which the woman feels comfortable. The neonatal abstinence syndrome can be treated with minimal complications.

Despite the above caution, at times, medical withdrawal may need to be considered due to logistical or geographic barriers. In these cases, the decision to undertake such a program must be a joint decision between the obstetrician, the woman, and her counselor, with the understanding that few women will be appropriate candidates for this approach.

The woman should understand that she must prove she is a candidate for medical withdrawal by complying with prenatal and therapy appointments and supplying clean urines. If at any time the woman is unable to comply with these requirements, no further decrease in dosage of methadone should be ordered.

Timing of withdrawal. There are no research data that suggest withdrawal in one trimester is worse than in others. Some clinical practitioners indicate concerns regarding methadone withdrawal prior to 14 weeks or after 32 weeks. These concerns are based on the theoretical possibility of an increased incidence of spontaneous abortion and premature labor. Other clinicians believe that withdrawal can be performed in all trimesters.

Patients should be allowed to discontinue withdrawal at any time, for any reason, without feelings of guilt. They should then be placed into a methadone maintenance program at a therapeutically sound dose. Clinicians need to be particularly aware that a decrease in methadone dosage could precipitate a relapse to drug use. Patients in continuous treatment who return to illegal drug use should be placed back on methadone. Methadone is preferable to the use of illegal street drugs.

Withdrawal schedule. Medical withdrawal from methadone is usually done in decrements of 2 to 2½ mg every 7 to 10 days. This procedure should only be done in conjunction with an obstetrician who can monitor the effects on the fetus. Intrauterine demise (death of the fetus in utero) has been documented as a complication of medical withdrawal even when done under optimal conditions, such as hospitalization and close fetal monitoring.

Note: At the time of publication, there was no protocol for medical withdrawal from methadone that had been evaluated in an appropriate number of women with suitable scientific and medical rigor.

Opioid Withdrawal Using Clonidine

The long-term effects of the use of clonidine in pregnancy are still unknown. Although clonidine hydrochloride has been used safely and effectively for rapid medical withdrawal in the management of opioid withdrawal in nonpregnant, opioid-dependent individuals, there are no data concerning its safety in pregnancy. Further research in this area needs to be performed before this technique can be recommended as a standard of care for pregnant women.

Cocaine Withdrawal

There are no well-documented studies regarding the safety or efficacy of using drugs to medically withdraw pregnant, cocaine-using women. The evidence is extremely limited for all methods of medical withdrawal. Inpatient treatment is the ideal whenever possible, although these facilities may not always be available. Medical withdrawal is just the first step in the continuum of care for pregnant, cocaine-dependent women. Referral to ongoing alcohol and other drug treatment and relapse prevention services is essential.

Symptoms of Cocaine Withdrawal

Withdrawal from cocaine dependence is characterized by depression, anxiety, and lethargy, which begin to resolve after approximately

1 week. Less common are signs of a paranoid psychosis during withdrawal from chronic use of high doses of cocaine. In cocaine withdrawal, medication is rarely needed for the serious sequelae that are associated with alcohol, barbiturate, and opioid withdrawal.

Maternal and Fetal/Infant Effects of Cocaine

Possible effects of maternal cocaine use during pregnancy:

- Intrauterine growth retardation (IUGR)
- Abruptio placentae
- Premature labor
- Spontaneous abortion
- No effect

Possible effects on the fetus and newborn infant that have been reported:

- Increased congenital anomalies
- Mild neurodysfunction
- Transient electroencephalogram abnormalities
- Cerebral infarction and seizures
- Vascular disruption syndrome
- Sudden infant death syndrome
- Smaller head circumference
- No effect

Guidelines for Withdrawal From Cocaine: Treatment Options

There are no data about the effectiveness of the following guidelines in pregnancy. In those guidelines that substitute other drugs, many of the drugs are problematic to the newborn and some have not been confirmed to be safe. Some centers do not generally use antidepressants for cocaine withdrawal depression. However, other programs prescribe antidepressants for the first 5 days to try to reduce the high dropout rate that occurs during this period. Sedatives and/or antidepressants may cause excessive drowsiness in a cocaine-dependent woman.

Cocaine-dependent women who require sedatives and/or antidepressants for any significant length of time often have an endogenous depressive disorder. Psychiatric consultation is usually indicated.

Cautions about Drugs and Their Impact

Dosing Strategy

To withdraw a pregnant woman dependent on cocaine, the following are options.

- *No medications.* Pregnant patients who are withdrawing from cocaine should not be medicated except in cases of extreme agitation and by individual order of the health care provider.

- *Anxiolytics.* If medication is needed, low doses of diazepam (Valium) or chlordiazepoxide (Librium) (25 mg by mouth, 4 times a day, x 6 doses) may be used.

- *Antidepressants.* A typical withdrawal guideline for cocaine-dependent women uses doxepin (Sinequan) or desipramine (Norpramin). For example,
    Days 1-2: Doxepin 25 mg (one tablet) by mouth 2
        times a day, 50 mg maximum.
    Days 3-5: Doxepin 25 mg (one tablet) by mouth 2
        times a day, then discontinue.
Further therapy should be determined by the treating physician after an initial period of observation.
    No drug therapy is usually indicated after the first 5 days.

- *Barbiturates.* For cocaine withdrawal symptoms:
    Days 1-2: Phenobarbital 30 to 60 mg every 4 hours
        as needed.
    Days 3-4: Phenobarbital 30 to 60 mg every 6 hours
        as needed.

- *Bromocriptine.* Bromocriptine, a drug used to treat menstrual abnormalities and infertility in women, has provided striking and consistent relief from cocaine craving among inpatients. Research indicates that cocaine, when used by the first-time user, seems to stimulate dopamine and also blocks the reuptake of dopamine, which produces the cocaine high. The brains of regular users of cocaine cannot make dopamine as quickly as the cocaine demands; the result is an eventual depletion that creates the crashing and craving effects. The use of bromocriptine in pregnancy is not recommended because of the lack of proven efficacy and unknown effects, both short and long term, on the fetus.

- *Acupuncture.* Acupuncture has been used in the treatment of cocaine addiction. Traditional use of acupuncture for other disorders has usually been contraindicated in pregnancy. At the time of publication, the National Institute on Drug Abuse has not concluded its evaluation of the efficacy of this treatment.

Sedative-Hypnotic Medical Withdrawal

Inpatient medical withdrawal from barbiturates, benzodiazepines, and other sedative-hypnotic drugs is recommended because continual monitoring of the mother and the fetus is required. Drug doses must be tapered so that mother and fetus arrive at a drug-free state without experiencing an uncontrolled withdrawal.

Barbiturates and benzodiazepines are the most commonly abused sedative-hypnotics. There are marked similarities between the withdrawal syndromes seen with both of these drugs. Patients abruptly withdrawn from large doses of benzodiazepines may sustain withdrawal symptoms that closely resemble those associated with barbiturate physical dependence. Because of these similarities, only the barbiturate abstinence syndrome is presented in this guideline.

Symptoms of Barbiturate Abstinence Syndrome

The barbiturate abstinence syndrome begins 6 to 24 hours after the last dose, and symptoms are generally more severe with the short-acting barbiturates. Signs and symptoms of barbiturate abstinence include:

- Tremulousness
- Diaphoresis
- Anxiety
- Postural hypotension
- Insomnia
- Grand mal convulsions (between days 3 and 7)
- Agitation
- Anorexia
- Delirium
- Nausea and vomiting
- Tendon hyperreflexia

If untreated, withdrawal symptoms can progress to hyperpyrexia, electrolyte abnormalities, cardiovascular collapse, and death.

Cautions about Drugs and Their Impact

Management of Withdrawal

Management of withdrawal in patients who may or may not be pregnant can include:

- Substitution of a long-acting agent (phenobarbital, diazepam, clonazepam), and subsequent withdrawal of this agent

- Slow withdrawal of the addicting agent

Risk categories for severe withdrawal:

- Low risk: Sporadic use of a drug or use for relief of cocaine-induced anxiety or insomnia.

- Moderate risk: Daily use of a drug for at least 2 to 4 months at a therapeutic level; concomitant alcohol abuse at low doses; history of mild withdrawal symptoms.

- High risk: Prolonged daily use of a drug at higher than therapeutic doses; higher use of alcohol; history of serious withdrawal symptoms.

- Highest risk: Previous withdrawal seizures or a history of a seizure disorder that is exacerbated by sedative-hypnotic withdrawal.

Some considerations for withdrawal from sedative-hypnotic drugs during pregnancy:

- Severe withdrawal from barbiturates can produce status epilepticus and maternal and fetal respiratory arrest. Immediate obstetrical intervention and hospitalization are warranted.

- Use of dilantin and other anticonvulsants have been considered for a patient with a history of withdrawal seizures. However, these drugs have been associated with congenital anomalies. Therefore, their use in pregnancy must be based on an assessment of the risks versus the benefits. Although there are concerns of teratogenicity regarding benzodiazepines and barbiturates, these appear to have a lower risk versus benefit ratio.

Mental Health Considerations

Mental disorders in pregnant, substance-using women often go undetected by health care providers and alcohol and other drug treatment staff. It is essential that a dual diagnosis be made, when appropriate, and addressed in subsequent treatment planning. The complex combination of pregnancy, addiction, and mental illness requires a carefully coordinated approach. The following general guidelines can be useful in assessing the mental health of pregnant, substance-using women.

Mental Health Assessment

Distinguish between drug-induced psychiatric symptoms and a major mental disorder. Symptoms such as anxiety, agitation, and paranoia can be manifestations of a state of drug intoxication or of the withdrawal syndrome itself and at times require no medications. Ongoing psychosocial support may help minimize many of these symptoms.

On the other hand, confirmed mental illness may necessitate the continuation of medications, such as antidepressants or antipsychotics, which have been previously effective in treating the underlying disorder. It is mandatory that a diagnosis of mental illness be ruled out before such medication is stopped. It must be remembered that evidence is inconclusive regarding the safe use of any psychotropic medication in pregnant women. A thorough assessment of the risks versus the benefits must be made prior to administering these medications.

Establish any previous history of psychiatric illness before developing the medical withdrawal treatment plan. Efforts should be made to contact previous therapists, treating agencies, and mental health facilities for this crucial information.

Establish communication early in treatment with mental health personnel involved in the patient's care. These individuals often can provide important history, help build an alliance with the patient, support discharge planning, and provide assistance in the event of an acute management crisis.

Individualize medical withdrawal plans for each patient. Carefully review standard guidelines and amend them if there are significant psychiatric problems to be treated.

Set up arrangements to involve mental health personnel, where appropriate, in establishing diagnoses and in developing the treatment plan.

Continue prescribed medications and provide appropriate followup for patients who enter alcohol and other drug treatment programs with well-documented, diagnosed psychiatric illnesses that require psychopharmacologic medication. Continue any prescribed medications, such as methadone and chlordiazepoxide, except as advised by the patient's health and mental health care providers. Patients should be supported in this decision by treatment programs. Some support groups may inappropriately encourage women to abandon all medications.

Do not avoid seeking therapy for the patient because of the complex combination of pregnancy, addiction, and psychiatric problems. Careful planning and staff coordination are usually effective in treatment.

Use well-validated psychiatric assessment scales in the diagnosis and followup of individual patients.

Consider issues of codependency, adult children of alcoholics/other addictions, and deep trauma from childhood in the evaluation of patients.

Guidelines for Medical Withdrawal

Orders for medication should be individualized to minimize the types and doses prescribed. Psychotropic drugs may need to be prescribed throughout medical withdrawal. The use of psychotropic drugs must be considered on a case-by-case basis, taking into consideration their effects on the mother and fetus, particularly with respect to interactions with methadone and possible congenital abnormalities. Behavioral management techniques should be developed to minimize the need for these medications. Providing adequate staff, structure, limits, and support are important treatment methods.

Other Issues

Agitation and oppositional or impulsive behavior can be manifestations of cognitive impairments, such as attention deficit disorder, limited intelligence, mild retardation, or psychotic illness. Patients with these behaviors can appear to have difficulty comprehending or complying with treatment expectations. Awareness of these deficits can help staff manage these problems and adapt treatment methods to minimize or avoid unnecessary confrontations.

Neurologic Abnormalities in Infants of Substance-Abusing Mothers

Apparently healthy infants of substance-abusing mothers have elevated blood levels of the neurotransmitter norepinephrine, according to California neonatologists and pediatricians. The researchers suggest that the high norepinephrine levels may be responsible for some of the neurologic abnormalities in these infants.

Dr. Sally L. Davidson Ward, assistant professor of pediatrics at the University of Southern California (USC) School of Medicine and Childrens Hospital of Los Angeles, and her colleagues found almost twice as much norepinephrine in the blood of substance-exposed babies as in infants of mothers who did not use any substances of abuse. In contrast, no differences were detected in the blood levels of epinephrine and dopamine, two related neurotransmitters, Dr. Ward says.

With associates at USC, the Los Angeles County/USC Medical Center, and the Martin Luther King Hospital in Los Angeles, Dr. Ward studied 15 healthy babies and 22 otherwise healthy offspring of substance-abusing women. All of these mothers had used cocaine and a variety of other drugs during pregnancy but, according to Dr. Ward, "cocaine was the common denominator."

"The cocaine-exposed babies had no chemical evidence of cocaine in their bodies yet they cried uncontrollably and appeared jittery and were almost continuously in motion," Dr. Ward says. Unlike control babies they were small and had low birthweights despite being term babies. Another characteristic—excessive muscle tone, or hypertonicity—produced abnormal stiffness in their upper bodies. "Together with a high level of physical activity, this upper-body stiffness often causes the babies to injure themselves as they move about in their cribs. When they become agitated, cocaine-exposed babies tremble and shake," Dr. Ward says, "and the movements can abrade their skin. Even bedclothes can hurt them."

Blood specimens were obtained from the infants when they were 1 to 4 months old, "at least 1 month after exposure to cocaine," Dr. Ward notes. The blood samples were analyzed for epinephrine, norepinephrine, and dopamine differences that might be associated with cocaine or cocaine withdrawal. In addition, the receptors by which those neurotransmitters attach to lymphocytes and blood platelets were also measured. Ideally the neurotransmitter receptors should have been measured in the brain, but that is of course not possible to do in live persons. Other investigators have reported, however, that the receptor concentration on blood cells reflects the concentration in the brain, according to Dr. Ward.

Although the scientists found norepinephrine at nearly twice its normal level in the blood of cocaine-exposed infants, they found no significant differences in the number of receptors in the two groups of babies. "This seems a paradox," Dr. Ward says. "With an increase in the amount of norepinephrine circulating in these cocaine-exposed babies one would expect to see a homeostatic decrease in the number of norepinephrine receptors. The number of receptors ordinarily declines when the neurochemicals saturate the nerve endings; conversely, receptor number rises when the neurochemical level decreases.

"But we did not find that. The number of norepinephrine receptors was the same in the blood of high-norepinephrine, cocaine-exposed babies as it was in the control infants." Dr. Ward adds that she and her associates think they may be detecting an increased sensitivity of the entire system of neurotransmitter-receptor interactions. "Of course we are measuring neurochemical evidence from the peripheral nervous system, not the actual receptors in the brain that have been measured by other investigators in animals exposed to cocaine," she says.

Neurologic abnormalities may occur even when cocaine use stops after the first trimester, according to Dr. Ward. Cocaine damage to the fetus is attributed in part to the vasoconstrictive effect of norepinephrine and directly to cocaine itself; cocaine narrows maternal and fetal blood vessels that carry oxygen-rich blood to the fetal brain and developing internal organs. Dopamine and probably norepinephrine are also thought to inhibit breathing, Dr. Ward says. "It's not fully understood, but we think that breathing problems may place cocaine-exposed infants at a relatively high risk of sudden infant death syndrome (SIDS)," she adds.

Dr. Ward says that babies exposed to opiates—notably heroin and methadone—during fetal life are also at risk of SIDS; they display some of the same symptoms these babies have, but for a shorter time. For cocaine-exposed babies the problems persist at least through the first year of life.

"The hypertonicity we see in these babies is there long after the cocaine itself is gone. Why are these babies still troubled, why are the effects there after the cocaine is long gone? These are the questions we are trying to answer," she says.

"Of course, the ideal medicine for these babies is preventive medicine," says Dr. Ward. "The statistics are alarming. There are close to a half-million cocaine-exposed babies born in the United States each year." She notes that more than 4 percent of pregnant women aged 12 to 34 years used cocaine during pregnancy, according to the 1990 Household Survey of the National Institute on Drug Abuse. Dr. Ward believes the best approach to the problem is drug rehabilitation in nonjudgmental settings for cocaine-addicted women before they begin a pregnancy.

Additional Reading

1. Ward, S. L. D., Schuetz, S., Wachsman, L., et al., Elevated plasma norepinephrine levels in infants of substance-abusing mothers. *American Journal of Diseases of Children* 145:45-48, 1991.
2. Dixon, S. D., Effects of transplacental exposure to cocaine and methamphetamine on the neonate. *Western Journal of Medicine* 150:436-442, 1989.
3. Woods, J. R., Plessinger, M. A., and Clark, K. E., Effects of cocaine use on uterine blood flow and fetal oxygenation. *Journal of the American Medical Association* 257:957-961, 1987.
4. Chasnoff, I. J., Burns, W. J., Schnoll, S. H., and Burns, K. A. Cocaine use in pregnancy. *New England Journal of Medicine* 313:666-669, 1985.

Medical Management of The Drug-Exposed Infant

Medical management of the drug-exposed infant has emerged in recent years as a major challenge to health care professionals. This section presents the TIP [Treatment Improvement Protocol] consensus panel's recommendations and guidelines for diagnosis of in utero drug exposure, medical assessment of the neonate, effects of exposure to different types of drugs, guidelines for appropriate treatment, promotion of positive parent-infant interaction, and discharge criteria and instructions. As a foundation for its guidelines in these specific areas, the consensus panel recommends the following:

Surveillance. Clinicians should be aware of shifting local trends due to user preferences and street market availability of particular

Cautions about Drugs and Their Impact

drugs within the community. Networking with local emergency and trauma services, drug treatment providers, social service agencies, and the criminal justice system provides neonatal caregivers with an opportunity for community surveillance. However, each nursery also should monitor the changing patterns of drug exposure in its newborn population. Further, the quality of data on drug abuse patterns obtained from maternal histories or anonymous toxicology screens should be continually monitored.

Preconception. Ideally, obstetricians, family practitioners, midwives, family planning clinicians, and other clinicians providing health care to women of childbearing age should provide counseling regarding abstinence from alcohol and other drugs prior to and during pregnancy.

Reducing Barriers to Access. Federal, State, and local agencies should reduce barriers to the use of family planning services and increase access to early prenatal care and other health services, including drug rehabilitation.

Interdisciplinary Treatment. Interdisciplinary intervention for the mother and her offspring (and the father, when possible) should be available at all points of access to care. Professionals involved in this care should include obstetricians, neonatologists, pediatricians, nurses, nutritionists, mental health professionals, social workers, substance abuse counselors, and child development specialists, at a minimum.

Staying Abreast of New Information. The medical literature is replete with research and anecdotal observations on the effects of drugs and alcohol on the infant. Long-term studies of exposure to opiates are sparse, and few systematic studies of long-term alcohol effects are available. Recent research has documented the possible long-term effect of maternal marijuana use on the infant. Longitudinal followup investigations on the effects of *in utero* cocaine exposure are in progress.

Attempts to assess the effects of drug exposure on newborns are confounded by numerous medical and environmental variables. However, acknowledging these limitations, the TIP consensus panel offers these guidelines to the medical management of drug-exposed infants. *In utero* exposure to opiates (heroin and methadone) and cocaine is emphasized. Many of the suggested approaches are also applicable to infants exposed prenatally to other drugs, including alcohol. It is very important to remember that alcohol use frequently coexists with other forms of substance abuse.

Diagnosis of In Utero Drug Exposure

Maternal Substance Use History

A maternal AOD [Alcohol and Other Drug] use interview should be conducted at the earliest point of access into the health care system. (If possible, information about paternal substance use should also be obtained by interviewing the father or questioning the mother.) Despite concerted efforts by health care professionals to promote prenatal care, the mother may not have received such care and the delivery hospitalization may be the only opportunity to elicit information on the nature and extent of the infant's *in utero* exposure to drugs and alcohol. The mother's concern for her infant's health may encourage valid responses; conversely, fear of legal reprisals or loss of custody of the infant may cause the mother to deny drug use.

Treatment Planning

Treatment planning for mothers and involvement of representatives from all participating agencies should include referral to an appropriate AOD abuse treatment program and continued involvement with medical and psychosocial agencies. Adequate arrangements should be made to ensure that the mother can get to the treatment facility, which may, in certain instances, require the provision of transportation for the mother to the location. An indepth treatment plan should be developed for the infant through multidisciplinary efforts of doctors, nurses, social workers, and others. The mother and father should be given the opportunity and urged to take part in treatment planning. If assessment reveals that the infant may be at risk for future harm due to the mother's potential for abuse or neglect, a report should be made to the child protective services agency so that further evaluation can occur. At a minimum, the treatment team must develop a clear followup plan for the infant upon discharge from the hospital, and must arrange for careful monitoring of compliance with the plan.

Cautions about Drugs and Their Impact

Toxicology Screening of Mothers and Infants

Maternal AOD use history should be complemented by toxicology screening of the mother and/or infant at the time of delivery only in certain situations (when a complete drug history cannot be obtained and the mother is manifesting symptoms of possible addiction and withdrawal and when the infant is showing withdrawal signs.)

Legal and Ethical Considerations

The diagnosis of infants with in utero drug exposure has significant legal and ethical ramifications. [For a discussion of these issues, refer to the complete copy of *Improving Treatment for Drug-Exposed Infants*, DHHS Publication No. (SMA) 92-1022 available from the Substance Abuse and Mental Health Services Administration's Center for Substance Abuse Treatment.]

Medical Assessment of the Drug-Exposed Neonate

Physical Examination

A thorough physical examination of the neonate should include accurate assessment of weight, length, and head circumference and a standardized assessment of gestational age. Special attention should be paid to signs of intrauterine growth retardation, microcephaly or decreased head circumference, prematurity, congenital infection, and major and minor congenital malformations. Various tools and scoring systems can be used to chart and compare the infant's neuromuscular and physical maturity and size to normal ranges for infants (Ballard et al., 1977; Ballard et al., 1979; Brazelton, 1984; Lubchenco et al., 1966).

Screening for Congenital Infection

Drug-exposed infants are at increased risk of acquiring infections transmitted from mothers whose lifestyles include unsafe sexual practices or intravenous drug abuse. Assessment of the mother for sexually transmitted diseases and human immunodeficiency virus (HIV) should be incorporated into the prenatal care setting and delivery hospitalization.

In Utero *Exposure To Opiates Effects And Treatment*

Effects of In Utero *Heroin Exposure*

The effects of heroin on the neonate as follows:

Low Birth Weight. The low birth weight is due primarily to symmetric intrauterine growth retardation. Low birth weight may also be due to prematurity. In either case, low birth weight results in the slowing of both body and head growth.

Meconium Aspiration. Meconium aspiration may be caused by hypoxia in association with antepartum or intrapartum passage of meconium secondary to fetal stress.

Neonatal Abstinence Syndrome (Withdrawal). Neonatal abstinence syndrome occurs in about 60 to 80 percent of heroin-exposed infants. Its onset is usually within 72 hours of birth, with possible mortality if the syndrome is severe and untreated. The syndrome involves several body systems. Central nervous system (CNS) signs of abstinence include irritability, hypertonia, hyperreflexia, abnormal suck, and poor feeding. Skin abrasions may result from general hyperactivity. Seizures are seen in 1 to 3 percent of heroin-exposed infants. Gastrointestinal signs include diarrhea and vomiting. Respiratory signs include tachypnea, hyperpnea, and respiratory alkalosis. Autonomic signs include sneezing, yawning, lacrimation, sweating, and hyperpyrexia. If the infant is hypermetabolic, the postnatal weight loss may be excessive and subsequent weight gain suboptimal unless higher caloric intake is provided. In cases demonstrating signs suggestive of the abstinence syndrome, other diagnoses should also receive the clinician's full attention. For example, sepsis, metabolic disorders, and CNS hemorrhage or ischemia should be considered in making the differential diagnosis.

Premature infants seem to manifest fewer overt symptoms of opiate abstinence syndrome. These differences may be due to the developmental immaturity of the preterm CNS, which might ameliorate the clinical appearance of abstinence symptoms, or to variations in total drug exposure due to a shortened gestation.

Delayed Effects. Delayed effects include subacute withdrawal with symptoms such as restlessness, agitation, irritability, and poor socialization that may persist for 4 to 6 months.

Cautions about Drugs and Their Impact

Sudden Infant Death Syndrome (SIDS). Epidemiologic studies suggest an association between SIDS and interuterine exposure to opiates (including methadone), but somewhat weaker links between SIDS and cocaine exposure.

Effects of mother's behavior. Adverse effects may be due to the life circumstances and behavior of the mother who uses heroin. Lack of prenatal care, poor nutrition, medical problems and the abuse of other drugs pose significant risk to the mother and the fetus. In addition, heroin use can cause sexual disinhibition, which increases the possibility of the mother's engaging in behaviors that place her at high risk for contracting HIV, such as sharing needles. Or the addicted mother may engage in sex for drugs with partners infected with HIV and other sexually transmitted diseases (STDs).

Effects of In Utero *Methadone Exposure*

Maternal methadone maintenance is a valuable treatment modality when administered under medical supervision. Although methadone poses some threat to the fetus, it is important to contrast the benefits of methadone in pregnancy with the risks associated with the continuing use of heroin. For this reason, methadone maintenance is often recommended for pregnant opioid-dependent women.

Benefits of methadone maintenance during pregnancy:

- Assists women in staying heroin free
- Leads to more consistent prenatal care
- Lessens possibility of fetal death
- Lessens decreased fetal growth and improves growth of newborn
- Reduces risk of HIV infection
- Enables the woman to breastfeed her infant

Risks of In Utero *Methadone Exposure*

Despite the significant advantages of methadone to an opioid-dependent pregnant woman, dangers to the fetus and to the newborn still exist, as described below.

Low Birth Weight. *In utero* exposure to methadone may lead to low birth weight caused by symmetric fetal growth retardation involving fetal weight, length, and head circumference. There is a lack of consensus on the appropriate methadone dosage schedule during pregnancy. Some studies indicate that a higher dose in the first trimester leads to a more optimal birth weight. Thus, a higher dosing schedule during this period may be considered.

Neonatal Methadone Abstinence Syndrome. Although the neonatal methadone abstinence syndrome is similar to that of heroin, it is typically more severe. Whether severity is related to maternal dosage is controversial. Late withdrawal can occur at 2 to 3 weeks of age, and subacute withdrawal can persist until 6 months of age. These phenomena may be related to variations in the metabolism of methadone due to placental transfer or neonatal metabolism. Methadone is also known to accumulate in CNS tissue.

Seizures. Seizures attributed to withdrawal will be seen in some drug-exposed infants. For example, in one study of 301 neonates passively addicted to narcotics, 18 had seizures attributed to withdrawal. Some studies have shown that infants exposed to methadone may have an increased incidence of seizures. Others in the field believe that it is actually the use of diazepam and phenobarbital that increases the incidence of seizures in methadone-exposed babies. The latter recommend the use of paregoric.

Thrombocytosis. At 4 to 10 weeks, methadone-exposed neonates are at risk to develop thrombocytosis, which may persist for 6 to 10 months. [Thrombocytosis is an abnormal increase in the number of blood platelets.]

Hyperthyroid State. Elevation of T_3 and T_4 during the first week of life has been documented.

SIDS. When controlled for other high-risk variables, the rate of SIDS among opiate-exposed infants is about 3-4 times higher than in the general population. The increased rate of SIDS is less impressive for cocaine-exposed infants.

Treatment Protocol for Opiate-Exposed Infants

Neonates exposed *in utero* to opiates should be examined systematically for signs of neonatal abstinence syndrome to assess the need for intervention.

Paregoric has been found to decrease seizure activity, increase sucking coordination, and decrease the incidence of explosive stools.

Phenobarbital is also a commonly used agent, and may be especially helpful in cases of polydrug abuse. Other specific agents have been considered in the treatment of neonatal abstinence syndrome, but experience with morphine, methadone, chlorpromazine, and rauwolfia is much too limited to support their use. Diazepam has been used to treat neonatal abstinence, but this agent controls seizures poorly and may lead to respiratory depression in the neonate.

Naloxone is sometimes given to newborns to reverse the perinatally acquired effects of analgesics administered to the mother during labor and delivery. Naloxone is contraindicated in opiate-exposed infants with respiratory depression due to its potential for precipitating a severe narcotic withdrawal. Naloxone is not specifically contraindicated for infants born to cocaine-using mothers, but providers should be aware that such mothers may be polydrug abusers who have also used opiates and that in this circumstance, naloxone may precipitate narcotic withdrawal in the infant.

Modification of the infant's environment—by placing the infant in a dimly-lit, quiet room; swaddling him or her; and using a non-oscillating waterbed if available—may be useful. However, this environmental modification does not eliminate the need for close observation of the infant. Drug-exposed infants in a prone or lateral position are generally comforted best. But caretakers should note an ongoing debate over prone versus supine positioning as possible factors in SIDS.

In Utero *Exposure To Cocaine: Effects And Treatment*

Effects of Cocaine Exposure on the Neonate

The abuse of cocaine became an alarming problem during the last decade. It is estimated that up to 8 million Americans use cocaine regularly and 30 to 40 percent of cocaine addicts are women. Cocaine use by pregnant women has multiple adverse influences on the mother's health, pregnancy outcome, and the well-being of the infants.

As with heroin addiction, adverse effects may be due to the life circumstances and behavior of the mother as well as to the pharmacologic properties of cocaine itself.

Lack of prenatal care, poor nutrition, medical problems, and abuse of other drugs and alcohol pose significant risk to the mother and the fetus. In addition, cocaine use increases the possibility of the mother's engaging in behaviors such as unprotected sex that place her at risk for contracting HIV.

The pharmacologic action of cocaine inhibits uptake of norepinephrine in the synaptic cleft, thus leading to vasoconstriction, hypertension, and tachycardia. In animal models, cocaine increases uterine vascular resistance and decreases uterine blood flow with resulting fetal hypoxemia.

Therefore, cocaine may play an etiologic role in causation of *abruptio placentae*, premature labor, intrauterine growth retardation, and fetal vascular disruption. Cocaine exposure causes a direct neurotoxicity manifested by neurobehavioral disturbances that are usually less striking than those associated with opiate abstinence syndrome.

These neurobehavioral disturbances may be transient, and usually do not require treatment. An encephalopathic syndrome—including irritability, tremulousness, lethargy, somnolence, labile state, decreased habituation, and visual tracking difficulties—has been described in cocaine-exposed newborn infants by many investigators. In addition to clinical signs of cocaine-induced neurotoxicity, transient encephalographic abnormalities can be demonstrated in this population of infants. Besides clinical and encephalographic abnormalities, echoencephalographic abnormalities are found in some cocaine-exposed infants. Lesions varying from ischemic injury with cavitation to intraventricular hemorrhage and ventricular dilation are observed in 8-14 percent of the study population. Cerebral infarctions have also been described in other reports. In some infants, physiologic dysfunction is indicated by alterations in vital signs including tachycardia and hypertension, and cardiac arrhythmias. The risk of sudden infant death syndrome in this population of infants may be increased, but large epidemiologic studies are needed in order to differentiate between effects of cocaine and other factors, such as low socioeconomic status, polydrug abuse, and smoking.

Long-term effects of intrauterine cocaine exposure, as well as polydrug exposure, are described in anecdotal reports, and include attention deficits, flat apathetic moods, decreased fantasy play, and other observations. However, long-term followup studies of cocaine-exposed children are scarce at present.

Subtle neurobehavioral aberrations may persist beyond the neonatal period. Cocaine may produce long term neurodysfunction, which is now being described anecdotally among the first cohort of babies exposed to crack *in utero* as they enter nursery school. The biologic vulnerability of infants exposed to crack *in utero* is modulated by the environment. The poor psychosocial, nutritional, medical, and socioeconomic status of the mother can all contribute to long-term

Cautions about Drugs and Their Impact

neurodysfunctional sequelae in the infant. Additional risk factors—including intrauterine growth retardation, CNS pathology, prolonged hospitalization, and lack of intellectual nurturing—must be taken into consideration in evaluation of long-term neurobehavioral outcome of cocaine-exposed infants.

Possible Complications of Maternal and Neonatal Effects of Cocaine Use that May Occur in Pregnancy

Maternal Complications:

- Poor nutritional status
- Increased risk for infections
- Hypertension/tachycardia/arrhythmias/myocardial infarctions
- Central nervous system hemorrhage
- Depression and low self-esteem
- Increased tendency to engage in risk behaviors for HIV

Pregnancy, Labor and Delivery Complications:

- Spontaneous abortion
- Poor weight gain
- Abruptio placentae
- Fetal demise
- Precipitous delivery

Neonatal Complications:

- Intrauterine growth retardation
- Microencephaly or reduced head circumference
- Prematurity
- Congenital malformations/vascular disruption
- Congenital infections
- Cardiovascular dysfunction/arrhythmias
- Feeding difficulties/necrotizing enterocolitis
- Central nervous system hemorrhagic-ischemic lesions
- Neurobehavioral dysfunction
- Seizure activity
- Sudden infant death syndrome (SIDS)
- Increased possibility of HIV involvement

Treatment for Cocaine Exposed Neonates

Treatment for the neonate demands an appropriate nursery environment, comprehensive assessments, pharmacologic intervention, and clinical diagnostic studies.

Optimal Nursery Environment. Such an environment features sound primary nursing care, gentle handling by as few care takers as possible, and an avoidance of stimuli such as light and noise that will irritate the baby. To facilitate and promote optimal infant growth and development, nursery personnel should carefully monitor feeds, initiate strategies to facilitate intake for those infants experiencing feeding difficulties, observe for feeding intolerance or necrotizing enterocolitis, provide opportunities to interact with parents and environment as the infant is able to tolerate them, and provide primary nursing to facilitate parent-infant interactions.

Brazelton Neonatal Behavioral Assessment Scale. Use of the Brazelton Neonatal Behavioral Assessment Scale (Brazelton, 1984) is encouraged. This scale has been used extensively to evaluate newborn behavior such as habituation and responsivity to stimuli (faces, voices, light, bell, rattle, etc.); state (sleeping, alertness); characteristics of changes in state (irritability, inconsolability); and neurological and motor development. Although clinical expertise is demanded to administer the Brazelton Scale, programs will find it useful in evaluating infants exposed to drugs.

Neonatal Neurotoxicity Assessment. While asymptomatic infants do not need to be systematically assessed for neonatal neurotoxicity, consideration should be given to developing scoring criteria for those infants who are symptomatic. In the presence of significant withdrawal symptoms, other etiologies, including polydrug and alcohol exposure and metabolic problems, should be explored.

Pharmacotherapy. If irritability persists in an infant, a short course of phenobarbital is recommended.

Central Nervous System Imaging. Cranial sonograms are not routinely recommended, but recent literature is suggestive of CNS abnormalities, including hemorrhagic ischemic lesions in some drug-exposed infants. As yet, evidence is insufficient to support a mandate for cranial sonograms in all cocaine-exposed infants. However, special

Cautions about Drugs and Their Impact

consideration should be given to specific neuroimaging of cocaine-exposed preterm infants, infants whose head circumference falls below the 10th percentile on standardized fetal growth curves, and infants with abnormal neurologic signs, neurobehavioral dysfunction, or seizure activity.

Assessment for Congenital Malformations/Vascular Disruptions. Clinicians should have a heightened awareness of the possibility of uncommon but significant congenital malformations or vascular disruptions reported in cocaine-exposed neonates. Systems that may be affected include the genitourinary tract, cardiovascular system (congenital heart malformations), gastrointestinal tract, and skeletal system. Echocardiography and abdominal ultrasound are not currently recommended as routine assessments in cocaine-exposed infants, but should be performed based on clinical indications.

Sudden Infant Death Syndrome. As indicated earlier, SIDS is a multifactorial problem, and opiate exposure is known to increase the neonate's risk of SIDS. There is some controversy over the incidence of SIDS in cocaine-exposed infants, but crack cocaine does appear to raise the risk slightly over controls. Data also suggest that cocaine-exposed infants may exhibit respiratory dysfunction. There are no indications that apnea monitoring decreases the incidence of SIDS. Routine home apnea monitoring for drug-exposed infants is therefore not recommended.

Promoting Positive Mother-Infant Interaction

Hospitals can promote positive interaction between parents and infants by adopting liberal visiting policies and mother-infant interaction time for newborn nurseries. Two other areas of concern are breastfeeding and instruction of mothers in handling drug-exposed infants.

Breastfeeding Drug-Exposed Infants

Breastfeeding is a key area of concern, especially among substance-using women. The advantages of breastfeeding are many, and are well documented. Benefits include the fact that breastfeeding strengthens the bond between the mother and the infant—an advantage that is of vital importance. Despite the instances described below, when breastfeeding is contraindicated, the decision on the part of service providers to advise women against breastfeeding should not be made without careful thought and training, taking into account the particular circumstances of the individual woman. Service providers must often become active breastfeeding advocates, encouraging the mother to breastfeed despite initial resistance to do so and educating her on breastfeeding's advantages to both herself and the newborn.

Nonetheless, there are instances when breastfeeding of drug-exposed infants is contraindicated. Since most drugs are secreted in breast milk, it has often been the practice to advise drug-using mothers not to breastfeed. Women who have been actively using drugs through the pregnancy and after the delivery have been discouraged from breastfeeding because of a number of factors including possible drug toxicity from diverse agents in varying levels, including the risk of exposure to drugs used intravenously, and the mother's medical and nutritional problems associated with continued drug use. Cocaine readily passes into breast milk and may lead to neonatal neurotoxicity, including irritability, tremors, brisk reflexes, mood lability, and even seizures. In addition, breastfeeding is contraindicated if the mother is HIV positive. (It should be noted, however, that the HIV status of the mother may not be known to the care provider or the mother.)

Despite these warnings, the well-known advantages of breastfeeding have led to a reconsideration of breastfeeding in selected substance-using women. There are two kinds of situations, highlighted below, in which care providers might wish to recommend that substance-using women breastfeed their babies: when the woman is on methadone or abstinent.

- In many instances, women who are methadone-maintained should be encouraged to breastfeed, particularly if the woman is known to be HIV-negative and free of other drug use. The fact that breastfeeding is not contraindicated among methadone-maintained patients is an advantage to methadone that is sometimes underemphasized, yet is of crucial importance.

- The recovering user of other substances (including cocaine), who has complied with rehabilitation and been documented to be AOD-free for a suitable period of time before delivery, may be able to breastfeed the infant, provided she continues to abstain from AODs and consents to frequent, random toxicology screens.

In sum, the recommendation regarding whether a substance-using woman should breastfeed her newborn should be made on

Cautions about Drugs and Their Impact

an individual basis, taking a variety of factors into account. Service providers should receive ongoing training on the issue to keep up with the latest developments in the field.

Instructions in Infant Handling

Parents and other providers of primary care should be taught:

- To assess the baby, interpret his or her cues for more or less interaction, and synchronize one's behavior with that of the infant.

- To organize care and handling so that the baby is not bombarded by multiple stimuli that overwhelm her or his limited ability to habituate.

- To utilize graduated interventions in quieting the fussy, irritable baby.

- To appreciate the infant's unique competencies: The baby's ability to see, hear, and interact with the environment.

Discharging the Drug-Exposed Infant from the Hospital

It is often quite difficult to follow an AOD-using mother and her newborn after release from the hospital, and thus it is vital that the infant and the mother not be discharged too early. According to the Newborn Assessment Score, most babies (96 percent) are symptom-free of withdrawal seizures by the third or fourth day after birth and might otherwise be ready to be discharged from the hospital. However, a small but significant percentage of babies present with withdrawal seizures within 7 to 10 days after birth. For this reason, it is important to closely monitor the drug-exposed infant to determine if he or she needs to remain in the hospital after 4 days. Other medical, social, or environmental issues may further prolong the need for hospitalization.

Discharge Criteria

The infant's discharge should occur after the following criteria are met:

- The infant is taking oral feeds and gaining weight satisfactorily.

- The infant is physiologically stable (has normal vital signs including blood pressure).

- The infant is showing neurobehavioral recovery (can reach full alert state, responds to social stimuli, and can be consoled with appropriate measures).

- All necessary assessments have been completed, since adherence to followup schedules cannot be ensured.

Discharge Instructions

- The parent(s) or alternate primary care provider should receive anticipatory guidance (oral and written) regarding late and subacute withdrawal, seizures, behavioral interventions, and medications (side effects, route of administration, dose, etc.).

- A home evaluation should be performed on all drug-exposed infants or those with multiple risks by a public health nurse or a protective social service worker within 7 days of discharge, when feasible.

- A follow-up appointment for pediatric care should be scheduled within 2 to 4 weeks.

- Mothers and fathers who are not already enrolled in drug abuse treatment and need to be should be referred to an accessible and suitable treatment program prior to the infant's discharge.

- Facilitation of mother's postpartum gynecologic care and family planning should be incorporated into discharge planning of the infant.

- To promote quality improvement, discharge planning instructions should be documented in medical records, and a discharge summary of the hospital course should be given to parents or alternate primary caregiver.

Followup and Aftercare of Drug-Exposed Infants

Drug-exposed infants should not be viewed as a homogeneous group but as individual at-risk infants presenting with a broad spectrum of possible effects, ranging from healthy term newborns with no apparent effects to high-risk births with significant effects. Living in a drug-abusing family is, in itself, a significant risk factor, regardless of prenatal exposure. Maternal drug use (and paternal drug

Cautions about Drugs and Their Impact

use as well) represents a health, biological, and psychosocial risk to the developing fetus and a social risk to the young child. The primary focus of the addicted woman is characteristically on her drug of choice, not on her child. A child whose mother abuses drugs often lives in a chaotic environment. Prenatal drug exposure and suboptimal home environments are highly correlated. In combination, they have a synergistic and devastating effect on the child's health and development.

Because the infant exists as part of a mother-child dyad, effective treatment must occur within the context of that relationship, as the mother often serves as the gatekeeper for the child's access to services. Knowledge of other siblings, extended family, the father, friends, neighbors, and other caregivers is also crucial to treatment. Followup and aftercare services should also be based on a multicultural and multilinguistic model that takes into account the cultural backgrounds of the mother, the father, and the extended family, as well as the service providers. Staff should reflect the different cultural and racial backgrounds of the communities being served. When appropriate, bilingual staff should be hired or other provisions made so that the inability to speak English is not a barrier to care. In sum, to be effective, treatment must occur within the cultural context of the mother and father, the extended family, and the community.

Knowledge of specific drug exposure is necessary for the appropriate medical management and treatment during the newborn period; the type of pharmacotherapy used in treating neonatal abstinence varies according to the specific drugs or combinations of drugs used by the mother. But followup and aftercare should not be based on a deficit model that assumes and screens for specific abnormalities caused by specific drugs. Rather, followup and aftercare should be based on a multirisk model that takes into account not only the prenatal drug exposure but also the medical status of the mother and the caregiving environment of the infant.

All health care and other service providers should consider the possibility that a number of environmental factors may contribute to specific deficits that have been attributed to drug exposure, as outlined below.

Experience with drug-using mothers and their children has demonstrated that drug exposure is only one of a number of risk factors that may affect the lives of the mothers and children. Other risk factors include:

- Chronic poverty
- Poor nutrition

- Inadequate or no prenatal health care
- Sexually transmitted diseases, including HIV exposure
- Domestic violence
- Child abuse or neglect
- AOD abuse within the family (including the father and the extended family)
- Homelessness, transient or inadequate living arrangements, or substandard housing
- Unemployment
- History of incarceration
- Low educational achievement
- Poor parenting skills
- Discrimination based on race, gender, or culture.

The lack of sufficient training among providers also affects the quality of the followup care given to drug-exposed infants and families. To counter the drug-exposed child's early disadvantages, service providers must be prepared to intervene early, often, and from many perspectives. Above all, health care and other service providers should not adopt the attitude that all drug-exposed infants are doomed to an unhappy, unhealthy life. Many, if not most, can eventually lead productive lives, given adequate intervention, education, and treatment services. The following recommendations address interventions for infants and toddlers, the transition to the preschool period, and training for child-oriented professionals. In general, many services require pediatric supervision by a specially trained physician.

Early Interventions for Infants

Components

Because of their distinctive needs, drug-exposed infants should receive more than the standard medical followup. Such followup should preferably be carried out under the supervision of a specially trained pediatrician. Followup interventions include but are not limited to:

- Nutrition (especially if inadequate sucking reflex is evident)
- Psychomotor assessment and monitoring of development
- Vision and hearing screening
- Speech and language assessments and therapy
- Emotional development assessments and therapy

Cautions about Drugs and Their Impact

- Play therapy
- Early educational needs assessments
- Physical therapy
- Immunization

Referrals

All health care and other service providers, including physicians, should stay abreast of available community services for drug-exposed infants and their families. Administrators should develop clear procedures to ensure that referrals are made to the appropriate resources. (For example, procedures might clarify whose responsibility it is to make referrals, such as case managers or social workers.)

Examples of routine health care referrals for drug-exposed infants and their families should include referrals to Federal programs such as:

- Early Periodic Screening, Diagnosis and Testing Program
- Maternal and child health services
- Community health centers
- Healthy Start Program.

Although federally supported, these programs vary from State to State and city to city. In addition, regulations and resources associated with these programs may be subject to change each fiscal year. It is important for programs and individual providers serving this population to be aware of these Federal and State resources and to utilize them. Developing and maintaining contact with a public agency (such as the local maternal and child health office, usually housed under the jurisdiction's public health department) can facilitate the process of keeping abreast of programs and resources appropriate for AOD-using mothers and infants.

In addition, in order to provide appropriate referral and followup services to drug-exposed infants and their families, providers and administrators should develop personal contacts among: physicians, social workers, alcohol and other drug counselors, speech and language specialists, early childhood educators, child development specialists, community volunteers, child protective services staff, and others. The new Substance Abuse Block Grant regulations require programs receiving block grant funds set aside for pregnant women and women with dependent children to provide a comprehensive range of services to women and their children, either directly or through linkages with community-based organizations. Thus, contacts with appropriate personnel in these AOD treatment programs should help other agencies with the provision of appropriate referrals.

The appropriateness of certain referrals will vary with the income of the mother, among other factors. For instance, referrals for mothers below the poverty level will usually differ from referrals for mothers who are in a middle-income bracket.

Outcomes

Intervention strategies for drug-exposed infants should promote the following outcomes:

- Self-regulation: the ability to regulate activity, attention, and affect.
- Secure relationships with mother and other significant caregivers.
- Developmentally appropriate progress in motor, cognitive, and speech and language skills.

Delivery System

The Federal early intervention system, mandated under the Individuals with Disabilities Education Act (IDEA), should be used when ever possible to deliver these family-focused services to both infant and mother. (IDEA was formerly known as P.L. 99457, The Education of the Handicapped Act Amendments of 1986. In 1990, the title of the Act was changed, and some changes were made as well in the content of the law. For instance, greater emphasis is now placed on the transition component from toddlers to children aged 3 to 5. The numbers of the law were also dropped when referring to the Act, since the numbers change each time the law is reauthorized. In 1992, the Act is authorized under P.L. 101476.)

IDEA, which focuses on disabled and "at-risk" children aged 6 and younger and their families, establishes two new Federal programs. One (Part H) addresses disabled and at-risk infants and toddlers from birth to 3 years of age; the other program (Part B) addresses disabled children aged 3 to 5. The law provides States with Federal funds to plan and implement early intervention services for children, aimed primarily at coordination. Each State must designate a single lead agency, assisted by a 25-member interagency council. Close coordination among health, social services, and educational agencies is required. The State must establish a public awareness program, a system to locate eligible children, procedural safeguards, data collection, and a State definition

Cautions about Drugs and Their Impact

of developmental delay. Because designated Federal dollars are for coordination, States must develop strategies for funding direct services. The local school system can be contacted for help in identifying the lead agency responsible for coordination of Part H (infants to toddlers) as well as Part B (children aged 3 to 5) of IDEA.

Eligible children must include those who experience developmental delays as well as children with diagnosed physical or mental conditions, such as Down's syndrome or spina bifida, which are likely to cause delays. States also have the option of including children who are medically or environmentally at risk of substantial delay. Thus, States can, but are not required to, include all children born to mothers who have used drugs *in utero*. However, if an infant is developmentally delayed as a result of this drug exposure, the infant must be included in the program.

The Act also requires an Individualized Family Service Plan (IFSP), which must be developed by a multidisciplinary team and reviewed at least once every 6 months. The following section on the service plan describes what the IFSP must include.

Despite the significance of IDEA, there is a concern that many early intervention programs are designed for infants with more obvious impairments and do not address the more subtle and shared needs of drug-exposed infants and their parents. New models of service delivery and curriculum development must be created to meet the needs of these multirisk infants within the mainstream of early childhood education. Intervention strategies can also be delivered through:

- Home visits (by early intervention programs or home health services)
- Parent-child services delivered within an integrated treatment program of drug treatment and pediatric care
- Parent-child groups that are center- or community-based.

Service Plan

The intensity and format of interventions should be based on the needs of the individual child and family, using a format such as the Individual Family Service Plan (IFSP), developed through early intervention programs. The IFSP must include statements regarding:

- The child's present developmental status and
- The family's strengths and needs.

Major outcomes expected to be achieved for both the child and the family are:

- Timelines for measuring progress
- Specific early intervention services (including health care services) necessary to meet the distinctive needs of the child and the family
- Projected startup dates and the expected duration of service provision
- Name of the case manager
- Steps for transition from early intervention into the preschool program.

However, there is a concern among some in the field that the utility of the required IFSP is questionable and problematic.

Additional Casefinding

When an infant receives early intervention services, providers should explore the possibility that siblings may also have been exposed to drugs *in utero*, have been living in a home affected by drug use, and have unidentified or unaddressed service needs.

Supportive Services

Quality child care should be provided for the infant and siblings when the mother or the mother-infant dyad are in treatment. Likewise, transportation services for mothers and their children should be provided to facilitate treatment and other community services.

Schedule

Followup and aftercare services should be regularly scheduled.

Recommendations for Universal Hepatitis B Immunization

Hepatitis B immunization is now universally recommended. In order of priority, the following groups should be immunized: high-risk children and all infants, adolescents living in high-risk areas, and all adolescents. A summary of recommendations follow.

All pregnant women should receive routine serologic screening for HBsAg. All newborn infants should be immunized with the HBV vaccine.

Cautions about Drugs and Their Impact

Infants born to women who are HBsAg-negative should be administered the first dose prior to discharge from the hospital. The second dose should be administered at 1 to 2 months of age. The third dose should be administered at 6 to 18 months of age. Those infants not receiving a dose of vaccine at birth should be administered three doses by 18 months of age. The minimal interval between the first two doses is 1 month. The minimal interval between the second and third dose is 2 months, although 4 months or more may be preferable. An alternative scheduling at months 1, 4, and between months 6 and 18 is acceptable—provided the infant's mother is HBsAg-negative—but is not a preferred schedule.

Infants born to HBsAg-positive women must be immunized at or shortly following birth, and should receive one dose of HBIG as soon as possible after birth. The second vaccine dose should be administered at 1 month, and the third dose at 6 months. Their serologic status should be checked at 9 months of age.

Infants born to women whose HBsAg status is unknown at the time of delivery should be immunized at birth with the dose of vaccine recommended for infants born to HBsAg-positive mothers. In order to determine the subsequent management of the infant, including the need to administer HBIG, the mother should be screened for HBsAg as soon as possible.

Older children, adolescents, and adults who are at increased risk of HBV infection should be immunized with HBV vaccine. The routine immunization of all adolescents against HBV should be encouraged and implemented when feasible.

Interventions for Toddlers

Early Childhood Programs

For toddlers who have been receiving early intervention services and whose behavior and development are within normal limits, interventions would include quality, developmentally based early childhood programs like Head Start (modified for younger children with appropriate staffing and curriculum), preschool programs, and parent-child groups.

Quality early childhood programs offer children and their parents the opportunity to be exposed to other adults who have different approaches to childrearing, to try out new activities and learning experiences within a supportive environment, to participate as part of a group, to interact with peers, to receive feedback from others about their behavior, and to experience success and a sense of accomplishment. Children at risk for school failure because of their drug exposure or drug-using home environment can master these critical tasks within an integrated early childhood program.

Individual Therapy

Some children may not have received early intervention, or may still need individual therapy. Interventions, including speech and language services and physical and play therapy should be based on individual profiles of abilities and weaknesses. Low child:teacher ratios (1:1 being optimal) are recommended to allow for quality programming and an individualized focus.

Self-Regulation

Early childhood marks the beginning of self-regulation. Specific strategies to support self-regulation include:

- An orderly, consistent, child-appropriate environment.
- Predictable routines and consistent schedules.
- Clear expectations and rules.
- Clear patterns for transitions (such as a daily routine, warning signals, and signals to move to next activity).
- Offering choices to children.
- Praising a child's efforts, not just successes, each day.
- Using anticipatory guidance to avoid difficult situations.
- Explaining how a child's actions affect others.

Relationships

Strategies to support secure relationships with ongoing caregivers include:

- Individual attention, encouragement of mutual respect, and celebration of each person to build healthy self-esteem.
- Activities that foster self-esteem in both mother and child.
- Labeling of feelings, so the child can learn to identify and express a range of emotions.
- Clear boundaries within adult-child relationships.

Cautions about Drugs and Their Impact

Transition to the Preschool Period

Transition from the toddler to preschool period should involve careful planning and preparation with the mother and child to ensure compliance with the new program. Early intervention and developmentally based parent-child and early childhood programs should continue to provide services within a family-centered model, and should feature low child to teacher ratios of 4:1 for multirisk children. In addition, class size should remain small, with no more than eight children and two teachers per classroom. Lower ratios and small class size ensure that the children receive the individualized attention critical to their educational development.

To deal adequately with the complex problems of multirisk children in a school setting:

- Needed therapeutic services should be provided: speech and language services; physical therapy; occupational therapy; play therapy.

- Teachers should be provided with training to: understand addiction issues in general; understand women's addiction issues and family systems; understand cultural and racial factors in the family's background; recognize behavioral cues in individual children to promote the child's self-regulation; provide a consistent, predictable, well-structured environment to promote the child's self-regulation; plan for transitions to promote the child's self-regulation; address issues relating to addiction, abuse, and violence.

Quality Assurance Checklist

To ensure the quality of followup and aftercare services to the drug exposed child, the hospital AOD abuse treatment program should provide the following services:

- Qualified staff and inservice education programs.
- Interdisciplinary staff that includes AOD treatment providers.
- Appropriate AOD treatment services for the mother as well as the father.
- Significant involvement of mother and child dyad; if the father is present, he should be involved.

- Child to staff ratio not exceeding 3:1 up to 3 years of age in the early intervention program.
- Transportation.
- Regular medical exams according to schedule.
- Up-to-date immunizations.
- Weekly monitoring visits during first 3 months, and monthly visits up to 18 months; visits should be conducted by the organization responsible for case management.
- Availability of visiting nurses.
- Regular reports to and from social services.
- Ongoing relationship with child protective services.
- Long-term retention of mothers in the program.
- Mechanism for peer review.

Training for Child Oriented Professionals

Health professionals often lack training and experience working with substance-abusing women, addicted families, prenatal drug exposure, and effective intervention strategies. Educators and health care providers must understand addiction, family functioning, and be able to communicate effectively with families.

Child-oriented professionals need specific training and supervision in: taking AOD histories; addiction models and issues for women; family systems—especially regarding the addicted family; prenatal drug exposure (medical, developmental, and behavioral outcomes); child development; family-focused interventions; parent-child interactions; intervention strategies for mothers and children (and fathers); HIV and its relationship to AOD abuse; treatment and referral strategies; and the impact of culture and ethnicity on service delivery.

All professionals working with addicted people and their children must have access to regular clinical supervision. Clinical supervision provides information, support, and stress management.

This chapter contains excerpts from DHHS Pub. No. (SMA) 93-2011: *Improving Treatment for Drug-Exposed Infants*. To receive a copy of the complete report write: Substance Abuse and Mental Health Services Administration, Center for Substance Abuse Treatment—Publications, Rockwall II Building, 10th Floor, 5600 Fishers Lake, Rockville, MD 20852-9949.

Chapter 13

Infectious Organisms and Fetal Development

Chapter Contents

Section 13.1—Sexually Transmitted Diseases and
 Your Baby 206
Section 13.2—Toxoplasmosis 212
Section 13.3—Group B Streptococcal Infections 221
Section 13.4—Listeriosis During Pregnancy 225

Section 13.1

Protect Yourself and Your Baby from Sexually Transmitted Disease

Reprinted with permission for the American Social Health Association, a nonprofit organization dedicated to stopping STDs and their harmful consequences.

How do STDs cause special problems for women?

- Some STD infections show no signs. Often a woman does not know she has an STD because the infection is hidden inside her body.

- Some STDs cause lasting damage to the female reproductive organs. This might keep a woman from having babies when she wants to.

Can STDs hurt babies?

Yes. A pregnant woman who has an STD can pass the disease to her baby. Thousands of infants die or suffer birth defects each year because of STD infections they get from their mother during pregnancy or birth.

What about AIDS?

AIDS is caused by a virus. People who have the AIDS virus (also known as HIV, human immunodeficiency virus) may seem to be healthy for months or years after getting the virus. But they can spread the virus to others without knowing it. Later they might become very sick and develop AIDS.

A woman could get pregnant without knowing she carries the AIDS virus. If she does, she could pass the virus to her baby. It may also be possible to pass this virus through breast milk.

People who have had any STD are more likely to get the AIDS virus than people who have not had an STD.

Infectious Organisms and Fetal Development

What should I do if I'm planning to get pregnant?

- See your doctor or health clinic for a check-up and get tested for STDs. Most STDs can be cured.

- Get tested. Even if the STD cannot be cured, your doctor can treat your symptoms and can take steps to protect your baby. There is no cure for AIDS, but a test can help you and the doctor to manage your care and the care of your baby.

Can STDs keep me from having children?

Yes. STDs such as gonorrhea and chlamydia often cause damage that makes it hard or impossible for a woman to get pregnant.

These STDs can lead to pelvic inflammatory disease (PID), which often causes severe pain in the abdomen. PID can scar the tubes that carry the egg to the uterus. If these tubes are blocked by scars, the egg cannot grow properly. Women with scarred tubes often have a tubal or ectopic pregnancy. During an ectopic pregnancy, the egg will grow outside the uterus. This condition can cause death and requires immediate surgery.

How can I avoid getting an STD?

Your risk for getting an STD increases with the number of sexual partners you have. You can avoid all STDs if you don't have sexual contact with anyone and don't share drug needles. But *you can greatly decrease your risk if you have only one partner (this person must not have sex with anyone but you and must not have an STD) and if you use condoms (rubbers).*

If you are not sure that your partner is free from STDs, use condoms during any sexual contact. Make sure the condom is used from start to finish during vaginal sex, oral sex, or anal sex. Other products will provide protection for many sexual practices, and the National STD Hotline (1-800-227-8922) can answer questions about this.

Use spermicides with a condom. Spermicides alone can't be trusted to prevent disease, but they can give protection in case a condom breaks. Spermicides are available in a foam or a cream and must cover the entire vagina. Follow the directions on the package, and do not use spermicides for oral sex. Spermicides may not protect against STDs when used for anal sex.

Get checked. If you have sex with more than one person, see a doctor or health clinic often. Doctors can test for hidden STDs like chlamydia. Since some STDs are linked to the risk of cervical cancer, get a Pap smear often, too.

How do drug needles spread STDs?

Even a small amount of blood can carry many viruses. Many cases of AIDS are spread when a person is injected with needles or syringes that have been used by a person with the AIDS virus. Hepatitis and some other diseases also are spread this way. If you must use or lend needles, make sure they are cleaned in bleach. In clinics and doctors' offices in the United States, needles are never used twice.

Gonorrhea

How Women Suffer. Symptoms are often unseen. But without treatment, gonorrhea can keep you from having babies and can cause arthritis.

How Babies Suffer. Eye infection that could lead to blindness. Since babies get gonorrhea during birth, treatment during pregnancy will protect your baby.

Special Considerations. Gonorrhea and chlamydia can cause pelvic inflammatory disease (PID) in women. PID can scar the tubes that carry the egg to the uterus, and this can make it hard to have children. PID can also lead to ectopic pregnancy, and this can threaten your life.

Chlamydia

How Women Suffer. Chlamydia Symptoms are often unseen. But without treatment, chlamydia can keep you from having babies.

How Babies Suffer. Eye infection or pneumonia. Since babies get chlamydia when born, treatment during pregnancy will protect your baby.

Special Considerations. Chlamydia and gonorrhea symptoms are similar, but the drugs that cure gonorrhea will not cure chlamydia.

Infectious Organisms and Fetal Development

Genital Herpes

How Women Suffer. Genital Herpes Symptoms are often unseen, but a person with genital herpes may develop very painful blisters or bumps near or inside the vagina or rectum. There is no cure for herpes, and the symptoms can return again and again.

How Babies Suffer. May cause very painful blisters on the skin. May damage the eyes, the brain, and other internal organs. Can lead to retardation. While herpes is rare in babies, about one in six babies who get it will not survive. Since babies most often get herpes at delivery, there are ways to protect your baby from herpes if you know you have it.

Special Considerations. If you think you or your partner could have herpes, be sure to tell your doctor or health clinic. A doctor can tell if you need a cesarean section delivery to protect the baby. More than half of babies born with herpes come from mothers who don't know about their own herpes infection.

Drug treatment will control herpes outbreaks, but this treatment may not be safe during pregnancy. Even after birth, keep your baby from touching your herpes sores. Do not let people who have herpes sores on the lip kiss your baby.

Syphilis

How Women Suffer. Usually a painless sore appears near or inside the vagina, the mouth or rectum. Often the sore, rash, or growth is not seen. These sores may appear to heal by themselves, but the disease is still in the body.

How Babies Suffer. Eye damage, dental and bone deformities, blindness, brain damage, death. Symptoms might appear at birth or months or years later. Early treatment will protect your baby.

Special Considerations. Infection might lead to miscarriage. Without treatment, the disease stays in the body for years and can cause severe damage or death. It can be cured at any time with antibiotics, but some damage may be permanent.

AIDS

How Women Suffer. AIDS HIV, the AIDS virus, usually leads to AIDS. AIDS makes it difficult for the body to fight disease, and often leads to death.

How Babies Suffer. Many babies whose mothers have the AIDS virus will get it from their mothers and develop AIDS during early childhood. Treatment during pregnancy can help protect your baby. Babies can get the AIDS virus before birth, during birth, or possibly through breast milk.

Special Considerations. A woman may have the virus but not have symptoms. There is no cure yet, but treatment can keep you healthier. Testing will help you prevent the spread of the AIDS virus to your baby or others. People with the AIDS virus should consult their doctor about the risks of pregnancy. The virus usually causes no symptoms, but blood tests can find it.

STD Warning Signs

You can get an STD whether you're pregnant or not. If you have any of these symptoms, see your doctor:

- excess discharge or unusual smell from the vagina
- irritation, discomfort, itching, swelling, soreness, or pain in or around the vagina or rectum
- genital sores, blisters, rashes, bumps, or growths (even if they don't hurt)
- painful urination
- swollen glands in the groin
- abdominal pain, especially during sex
- bleeding from the vagina when you're not having a period.

Signs often appear where you are infected. If you have oral sex, you could show symptoms in the mouth.

If you have an STD, you may also have these symptoms:

- swelling, soreness, or redness in the throat
- fever, chills, and aches
- sores or white patches inside the mouth.

If you think you have an STD:

- See a doctor or health clinic right away. It is important for your doctor to know if you have an STD or if you are pregnant. If you have an STD, make sure your sexual partner is tested and treated.

Infectious Organisms and Fetal Development

- Follow the doctor's instructions carefully. If the doctor prescribes medicine, take all of it. The infection can still cause problems even if the symptoms go away.

- Don't have sex until you and your partner are completely cured. Until you're well, you can give the disease to your partner.

Sex and Disease

One out of every 20 Americans will get a Sexually Transmitted Disease (STD) this year.
One out of five already has one.
These diseases will cause serious health problems for women.
But you can protect yourself... and your baby.
You can get a sexually transmitted disease (STD) if you have sexual contact with someone who has an STD. This includes vaginal, anal, and oral sex. These diseases are spread by both men and women.
STDs are caused by germs that live on the skin or in body fluids like semen, vaginal secretions, or blood. These germs can enter a person's body through the vagina, the mouth, the anus, an open sore, or a cut. Some germs like those that cause herpes or genital warts, can even infect a person through the skin of the genitals or anywhere on the body.
Many kinds of STDs can seriously damage your health if you don't get treatment. Some STDs, like AIDS, can kill you or your baby.

Where can I get more information about STDs?

Check the following sources for additional information:

- your doctor
- your local health department or free STD clinic
- the National STD Hotline at 1-800-227-8922, toll-free. The hotline is open from 8 A.M. to 11 P.M., (Eastern time) Monday through Friday.
- Call the National AIDS Hotline (1-800-342-AIDS) any day, 24 hours a day.

This brochure is published by the American Social Health Association (ASHA). ASHA is a private, nonprofit organization dedicated to stopping all STDs and their harmful consequences to individuals, families, and communities. ASHA produces educational materials on sexual health; operates national hotlines for STDs, AIDS, and herpes; advocates for strong public health programs to prevent the spread of STDs; and funds research to find better treatments.

For more information on our programs or other materials, please write to us at the address below.

American Social Health Association
P.O. Box 13827
Research Triangle Park, NC 27709
Phone: (919) 361-8422

Section 13.2

Toxoplasmosis and Pregnancy

National Institute of Allergy and Infectious Diseases publication, July 1992.

Why be Concerned about Toxoplasmosis?

Although up to 50 percent of the U.S. adult population has been infected with the parasite that causes toxoplasmosis, most people have no clue that their bodies are home to the parasite. However, for the baby of a woman who acquires the infection during pregnancy, the disease can cause stillbirth, neurologic problems, and blindness. And in immune-deficiency patients, the illness can be life-threatening.

The main sources of infection for people are cat feces and raw or poorly cooked meat. Without realizing it, people touch these materials and then carry the microscopic parasites from their hands to their mouths. Simple precautions can reduce the risk of contact during pregnancy:

- Avoid kitty-litter boxes (cat droppings also contaminate soil and sandboxes).
- Cook meat thoroughly.
- Wash hands regularly, especially after touching raw meat.

Infectious Organisms and Fetal Development

Background

Toxoplasmosis is a parasitic disease that is found throughout the world. It is caused by a single-celled organism, a protozoan, called *Toxoplasma gondii*. This parasite was first discovered more than 80 years ago in a small African rodent, the gondi, from which it derives its name. It has since been found that any warm-blooded animal, and many reptiles, can be infected with the parasite.

Symptoms

In a newly acquired infection in otherwise healthy persons, the disease usually runs a mild, self-limited course, with few or no symptoms. Among people who do have signs of infection (about 10 percent of the cases), the symptoms resemble those of infectious mononucleosis, where patients typically experience swollen glands and fatigue. The other common symptoms are malaise, muscle pain, a fluctuating low fever, rash, headache, and sore throat. Eye inflammation, with blurred vision, occurs in about one percent of persons with acquired infection. In rare instances, the lungs, heart, brain, and liver may be affected.

Generally, the symptoms appear a week or two after infection and then subside gradually over a period of two weeks to several months. The parasite itself goes into a dormant state, although it never leaves the body.

The parasite, however, can become active again if the immune system is suppressed—for example, by drugs given to treat cancer or to prevent rejection of transplanted organs. Reactivated toxoplasmosis in patients with acquired immunodeficiency syndrome (AIDS) can be fatal.

Toxoplasmosis in Pregnancy and the Newborn

An estimated 10 to 20 percent of women of childbearing age in the United States have been infected with *T. gondii* and, therefore, harbor the organism in their bodies. If these women become pregnant, there is no threat to the fetus because the parasite is dormant in the mother's body. But if the woman contracts the parasite for the first time while she is pregnant, the fetus may also become infected. The disease can severely damage an unborn child while being mild or symptomless in the mother.

If a pregnant woman becomes infected during her first trimester of pregnancy, there is only a small chance that the fetus will become infected, but if it does, it is probable that the consequences to the fetus will be severe. Spontaneous abortion, stillbirth, or delivery of a premature or full-term infant with congenital disease may result.

Symptoms at Birth

Generalized illness or significant damage to the central nervous system and eyes is apparent at birth in about 30 percent of infants born with toxoplasmosis. Among the first symptoms apparent at birth are hydrocephalus (fluid in the skull) and neurologic symptoms such as convulsions and seizures.

The number of babies born with toxoplasmosis has not been determined. Some estimates are as high as one per 1,000 live births, while other studies indicate an infection rate of only one per 10,000.

Late-Developing Symptoms

In cases where a woman first becomes infected with *T. gondii* during her third trimester of pregnancy, the chances that the infant will be infected are greatly increased. Although such infants appear to be normal at birth, they may develop severe symptoms later in life, including blindness, epilepsy, and mental retardation. Increasingly, there are reports of eye damage that does not become evident until the person reaches adulthood or late maturity.

Diagnosis

The primary method for diagnosing toxoplasmosis is a blood test that detects Toxoplasma antibodies, proteins our bodies produce to defend against the parasite. A positive test result indicates only that the patient has been infected with the parasite at some point in the past. Determining whether it is a newly acquired infection—which is crucial if a woman is pregnant—may require a combination of tests that must be carefully interpreted. At present, researchers are working to making the tests more accurate.

Pre-Pregnancy Screening

Ideally, every woman who might become pregnant should undergo systematic toxoplasmosis screening—starting before she becomes pregnant. However, until more is known about the number of babies affected, the cost effectiveness of this approach is not clear. A woman who tests positive before pregnancy can be reasonably sure

Infectious Organisms and Fetal Development

that she has already been exposed to the parasite, that she has developed protective antibodies, and that there is little, if any, risk to the fetus.

Testing During Pregnancy

In cases where a newly pregnant patient develops symptoms suggestive of toxoplasmosis, her doctor will start screening for potential infection as early as possible, beginning in the first trimester, with follow-up testing in the second and the third trimesters. If any of the tests comes out positive, the woman is retested three weeks later. Generally, a significant rise in antibody level in the second testing confirms the diagnosis of recently acquired infection.

Testing the Fetus

When the tests indicate that the fetus is at risk, the doctor may request a prenatal ultrasound examination to detect possible physical abnormalities in the fetus. In a new diagnostic technique, samples of amniotic fluid or umbilical blood, which are drawn through the uterine wall with a syringe, can be cultured to detect *Toxoplasma* antibodies. If fetal infection is confirmed, the patient and her doctor can discuss medical options.

Treatment

Most individuals with toxoplasmosis do not require treatment. However, pregnant women who acquire their infection during gestation, infected newborns, and immune-deficient patients with new or reactivated infection should undergo therapy. Of the women who become infected during pregnancy—and do not receive treatment—50 percent will give birth to infected infants.

The standard treatment in the United States is a combination of pyrimethamine (an antimalarial drug) with sulfadiazine or triplesulfa drugs. The drugs kill the active form of the parasite but have no effect on the dormant stage. The need for treatment depends on the severity and duration of symptoms, evidence of serious damage to vital organs, any underlying medical problems, and whether or not the patient is pregnant. People taking these drugs must be monitored regularly because the side effects can include toxicity due to bone marrow depression. Treatment with a drug called folinic acid is used in adults to reverse these effects.

In Pregnancy

Treatment of toxoplasmosis acquired during pregnancy decreases but does not eliminate the chance of a congenitally infected infant. Unfortunately, little can be done to reverse any damage already done to the fetus. In cases where the patient chooses to begin drug therapy, sulfa drugs alone are the treatment of choice because pyrimethamine can cause birth defects.

In the Newborn

If the mother has been diagnosed as having toxoplasmosis during pregnancy and has received treatment, the baby is usually begun on treatment at birth, whether the infection is symptomatic or not. The drugs are given for as long as a year, and if started early in infancy, can significantly reduce the chance of serious complications later in life. In infants born with severe toxoplasmosis, further damage may be prevented by adding corticosteroids to the pyrimethamine/sulfa drug regimen.

Transmission

Emptying kitty-litter boxes and handling raw meat without washing the hands immediately afterward are two of the most common ways people become infected. Unknowingly, people carry the parasites from their hands to their mouth and ingest them. Eating raw or undercooked meat is also risky. The parasites have been found in pork, mutton, and beef. In addition, infection may be transmitted through blood transfusions, organ transplants, and laboratory accidents.

Role of the Cat

Only cats are known to shed *Toxoplasma* organisms in their feces. This is why the common household cat plays a major role in human Toxoplasma infections.

Like other animals that harbor the toxoplasmosis parasite in their tissues and organs, the cat shows no sign of infection. If a cat eats infected birds or rodents, the parasites multiply within the cat's intestine. The cat excretes the parasites for 10 days or longer in the form of microscopic egg-like capsules known as oocysts. Generally, once a cat has been infected and has excreted oocysts, it will not shed oocysts if it becomes infected again. Thus, it can transmit the parasite only around the time of its first infection.

Infectious Organisms and Fetal Development

The oocysts mature two to four days after being expelled in cat feces. When mature, each oocyst contains infectious organisms known as sporozoites, which can remain infective for months in moist soil. Similarly, a litter box used by an infected cat is a significant reservoir of oocysts.

How People are Exposed

When a person accidentally ingests mature oocysts, the sporozoites are released in the intestine. The parasites penetrate the intestinal wall, spread throughout the body in the bloodstream, and multiply within the host's cells. Eventually, the body's immune defenses cause the parasite to transform into cysts, which usually remain dormant in the tissues for the rest of the person's life.

Transmission to the Fetus

If a woman is first exposed to the parasite during her pregnancy, the parasite can be transmitted to the fetus. The ingested parasite travels through the woman's intestinal tract, where it enters the bloodstream and reaches the fetus through the placenta.

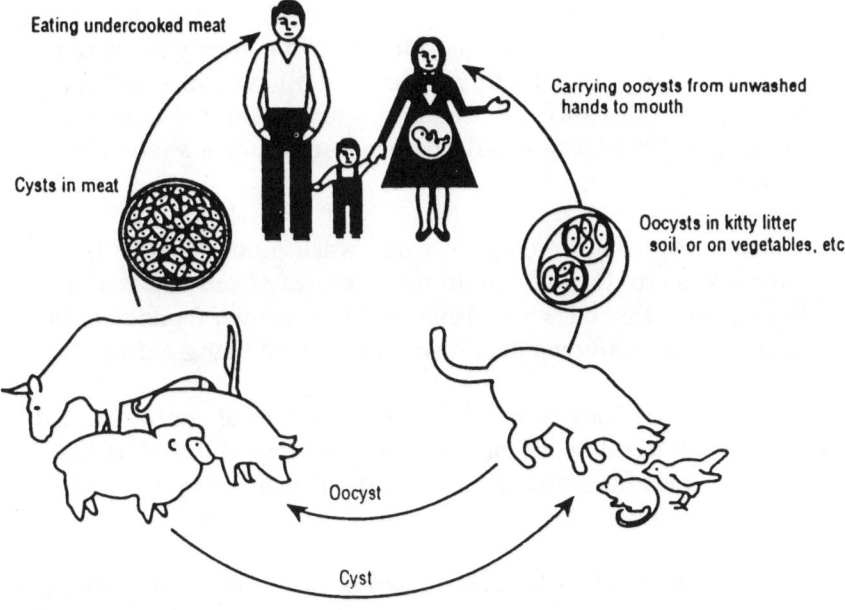

Figure 13.1. Toxoplasmosis Transmission to People

Prevention

Fortunately, there are several preventive measures one can take to avoid toxoplasmosis. Naturally, many of these center around the cat.

- A cat can be maintained free of infection by feeding it only well-cooked meat or commercial cat food. It should also be kept indoors and not allowed to hunt mice and birds. These strict precautions are especially important if a woman is planning to become or is already pregnant. The pregnant woman should avoid close contact with the animal throughout her pregnancy.

    Testing the cat is not recommended because the results may be misleading. Positive results could mean that the cat has been infected, has shed oocysts, will probably not shed oocysts again, and is therefore not a threat to a pregnant woman. Negative results could mean that the cat was never infected, was so recently infected that antibodies have not yet appeared, or was infected in the past but for some reason did not develop antibodies.

- Someone other than the expectant mother should be responsible for regularly changing the kitty litter. This should be done daily, since excreted organisms are not infectious when passed but become infective within two to four days. The empty litter pan should be filled with boiling water and allowed to stand for a least five minutes. If the pregnant woman must change the litter, disposable gloves should be used and hands washed immediately afterward.

- Similar care should be taken when working in gardens that cats have access to. Hands should be kept away from the face and thoroughly washed when finished. Homegrown foods should also be thoroughly washed or cooked before being eaten.

- Children's sandboxes may be a prime source of contaminated cat feces. When not in use, keep the sandbox covered. If the sandbox does become contaminated with cat feces, discard all sand and replace it.

- Prevent flies and cockroaches from getting into food since these insects are capable of carrying infectious oocysts from cat feces to food.

Infectious Organisms and Fetal Development

- All meat should be well cooked—especially pork, mutton, and lamb, which should be cooked at 151 F (66 C) or higher.

- Finally, hands should be washed after touching uncooked meat.

Research

Much of what is known about the link between cats and toxoplasmosis derives from work supported by the National Institute of Allergy and Infectious Diseases (NIAID). NIAID continues to fund a broad spectrum of research on toxoplasmosis.

Improving Diagnostic Tests

The chemical make-up of the parasite is being analyzed, and methods of detecting very small amounts of these chemicals are being developed. The end result may be more sensitive and rapid tests for diagnosis of congenital and acquired toxoplasmosis.

Testing New Drugs

NIAID-supported scientists are developing better methods of treatment and prevention of *Toxoplasma* infections. Studies of the antibiotic spiramycin are being extended to test its effectiveness in congenital toxoplasmosis. Preliminary results suggest that highly specific monoclonal antibodies, made in the laboratory, may have a protective effect. Perhaps with further testing, these antibodies may one day be used to prevent human toxoplasmosis.

Finding Who gets Toxoplasmosis

Other NIAID-supported research includes studies to ascertain whether certain people are at greater risk for the disease or if there is a genetic tendency to develop it. They are also studying children born with asymptomatic *Toxoplasma* infections, to see how many will develop complications later in life. To assess the need for widespread pre-pregnancy screening, the U.S. Public Health Service is currently doing studies to get a clearer estimate of the number of pregnancies affected by toxoplasmosis.

Investigating What Happens during Pregnancy

Other NIAID-supported scientists are studying various aspects of human toxoplasmosis. Of particular interest is the way the immune system responds to *Toxoplasma* during pregnancy. Scientists are investigating the relationship between the immune response, the transmission of the parasite to the fetus, and spontaneous abortion.

Understanding Immune-Deficiency

NIAID grantees are studying *Toxoplasma* infections in persons whose immune systems are not working properly because of other medical problems. Specifically, the researchers are studying the signs of infection, how the deficient immune system responds, and better ways of diagnosing the infection, which is often fatal in immuno-suppressed people.

Past and Present Goals of Biomedical Research

Earlier research solved the mysteries of what caused toxoplasmosis and how the parasite was transmitted. Current research holds the promise of finding more effective ways to diagnose and treat persons with this potentially handicapping, and sometimes fatal, disease.

Section 13.3

Group B Streptococcal Infections

Homepage of the National Center for Infectious Diseases, January 1996

Group B streptococcus (GBS) is a type of bacterium that causes illness in newborn babies, pregnant women, the elderly, and adults with other illnesses, such as diabetes or cancer. GBS is the most common cause of life-threatening infections in newborns.

How common is GBS disease?

GBS is the most common cause of sepsis (blood infection) and meningitis (infection of the fluid and lining surrounding the brain) in newborns. GBS is a frequent cause of newborn pneumonia and is more common than other, better known, newborn problems such as rubella, congenital syphilis, and spina bifida.

Approximately 8,000 babies in the United States get GBS disease each year; 5%-15% of these babies die. Babies that survive, particularly those who have meningitis, may have long-term problems, such as hearing or vision loss or learning disabilities.

In pregnant women, GBS can cause urinary tract infections, womb infections (amnionitis, endometritis), and stillbirth. Among men and among women who are not pregnant, the most common diseases caused by GBS are blood infections, skin or soft tissue infections, and pneumonia. Approximately 20% of men and nonpregnant women with GBS disease die of the disease.

Does everyone who has GBS get sick?

Many people carry GBS in their bodies but do not become ill. These people are considered to be "colonized." Adults can be colonized in the bowel, genital tract, urinary tract, throat, or respiratory tract. Fifteen percent to 40% of pregnant women are colonized with GBS in the rectum or vagina. A fetus may become colonized with GBS on the skin if the mother is colonized with GBS in the rectum or vagina; colonization occurs before or during birth.

How does GBS disease affect newborns?

Approximately 1%-2% of babies who are colonized with GBS develop signs and symptoms of GBS disease. Three-fourths of the cases of GBS disease among newborns occur in the first week of life ("early-onset disease"), and most of these cases are apparent a few hours after birth. Sepsis, pneumonia, and meningitis are the most common problems. Premature babies are more susceptible to GBS infection than full-term babies, but most (75%) babies who get GBS disease are full term.

GBS disease may also develop in infants 1 week to several months after birth ("late-onset disease"). Meningitis is more common with late-onset GBS disease. Only about half of late-onset GBS disease among newborns comes from a mother who is colonized with GBS; the source of infection for others with late-onset GBS disease is unknown.

How is GBS disease diagnosed and treated?

GBS disease is diagnosed when the bacterium is grown from usually sterile body fluids, such as blood or spinal fluid. Cultures take a few days to complete. GBS infections in both newborns and adults are usually treated with antibiotics (e.g., penicillin or ampicillin) given through a vein.

Can pregnant women be checked for GBS?

GBS colonization can be detected during pregnancy or just before delivery by a vaginal and rectal swab for special culture or rapid screening. Rapid screening tests are not as good at detecting the bacteria but can be completed in 30 minutes to a few hours. Physicians who culture for GBS colonization during prenatal visits should do so late in pregnancy because cultures collected before 25 weeks' gestation do not predict whether a mother will be colonized with GBS at delivery. Authorities suggest that cultures be done at 35-37 weeks' gestation, by swabbing both the vagina and rectum.

A positive culture result means that the mother is colonized with GBS—not that she or her baby will definitely become ill. Colonized women should not be given oral antibiotics before labor because

Infectious Organisms and Fetal Development

antibiotic treatment at this time does not prevent GBS disease in newborns. Whether a woman is colonized with GBS becomes important at the time of labor and delivery—when antibiotics are effective in preventing GBS disease.

Can GBS disease among newborns be prevented?

Most GBS disease in newborns can be prevented by giving certain pregnant women antibiotics through the vein during labor. Any pregnant woman who previously had a baby with GBS disease or who has a urinary tract infection caused by GBS should receive antibiotics during labor. Pregnant women colonized with GBS should be offered antibiotics at the time of labor or membrane rupture. Colonized women at highest risk are those with any of the following conditions:

- fever during labor
- rupture of membranes 18 hours or more before delivery
- labor or rupture of membranes before 37 weeks ("preterm").

Because women who are colonized with GBS but do not develop any of the above complications have a relatively low risk of delivering an infant with GBS disease, the decision to take antibiotics during labor should balance risks and benefits. Penicillin is very effective at preventing GBS disease in the newborn and is generally safe. A colonized woman with none of the conditions above has the following risks:

- a 1 in 200 chance of delivering a baby with GBS disease if no antibiotics are given.

- a 1 in 10 chance, or lower, of experiencing a mild allergic reaction to penicillin (such as rash).

- a 1 in 10,000 chance of developing a severe allergic reaction—anaphylaxis—to penicillin.

Anaphylaxis requires emergency treatment and can be life-threatening.

If a prenatal culture for GBS was not done or the results are not available, physicians may give antibiotics to women with one or more of the risk conditions listed above.

What research is being done on prevention of GBS disease?

Unfortunately, some babies still get GBS disease in spite of testing and antibiotic treatment. Vaccines to prevent GBS disease are being developed. In the future, women who are vaccinated may make antibodies that cross the placenta and protect the baby during birth and early infancy.

Who is at higher risk for GBS disease?

Pregnant women with the following conditions are at higher risk of having a baby with GBS disease:

- previous baby with GBS disease
- urinary tract infection due to GBS
- GBS colonization late in pregnancy
- fever during labor
- rupture of membranes 18 hours or more before delivery
- labor or rupture of membranes before 37 weeks ("preterm").

Adults with illnesses that suppress the immune system, such as diabetes or cancer, are at higher risk of getting GBS disease.

For more information, contact:

Childhood and Respiratory Diseases Branch
Division of Bacterial and Mycotic Diseases
National Center for Infectious Diseases
Centers for Disease Control and Prevention
MS C-09
1600 Clifton Rd NE
Atlanta, GA 30333

Section 13.4

Listeriosis During Pregnancy

DHSS Publication No. (FDA) 92-22556S, 1992

For your baby's sake, avoid soft cheeses (such as Mexican-style, feta, Brie, Camembert, and Roquefort).

Is there anything in soft cheese that could hurt me or the baby I'm carrying?

Yes. Sometimes soft cheeses, such as Mexican-style queso blanco, queso fresco, queso de hoja, queso de crema, and asadero, become contaminated with bacteria called *Listeria*. These bacteria can cause an illness called listeriosis. If you're pregnant and get this disease, the baby you're carrying could die.

Public health experts say you should not eat Mexican-style or other types of soft cheeses like feta (sometimes called goat cheese), Brie, Camembert, and blue-veined cheeses (such as Roquefort) while you are pregnant.

I've never heard of Listeria. Please tell me more.

Food poisoning from Listeria is not nearly as common as it is from other microorganisms. But Listeria is much more dangerous than other bacteria to unborn babies. In 1985, an outbreak of the illness in Los Angeles caused 19 stillbirths and 10 newborn deaths. Many of those stillbirths and deaths were babies of Hispanic women. The outbreak in Los Angeles was linked to eating Mexican-style soft cheese that was contaminated with Listeria.

Is listeriosis dangerous only if I'm pregnant?

No. In addition to pregnant women, other persons can become very ill with listeriosis. These include:

- the elderly
- transplant recipients
- people receiving anti-cancer drug therapy
- people who have tested positive for the human immunodeficiency virus (which causes AIDS).

How would I know if I have listeriosis?

Listeriosis usually shows up from seven days to six weeks after eating the contaminated food. But if the food is heavily contaminated, you could start to feel sick in as little as two to four days. Symptoms include fever, headache, nausea, and vomiting.

Pregnant women may get mild, flu-like symptoms of chills and fever. If you have these symptoms, tell your doctor right away.

The real danger is if the infection spreads to the baby itself. If it does, you could start premature labor. Unborn or newborn babies could develop a serious Listeria infection. Studies show that 25 percent of those babies die from the disease.

Why are Hispanic women particularly at risk for this illness?

Soft cheese, preferred over other cheeses in Latin American kitchens, is traditionally part of Hispanic diets and is used in many dishes. However, because of its high moisture content, soft cheese can easily become contaminated with Listeria if it is not carefully manufactured and properly handled.

Some dishes call for soft cheese. Is there a substitute I can safely use?

Yes. Cottage cheese can be used in place of Mexican-style soft cheese in most dishes. Hard cheeses, such as cheddar and other yellow cheeses, are also less likely to be contaminated with Listeria. If a hard cheese is made from unpasteurized milk, it must be aged at a processing plant for at least 60 days. The aging process kills harmful bacteria These cheeses must be clearly marked "aged 60 (or more) days."

How can I tell if a food is contaminated with Listeria?

You can't. The food will not smell or taste bad, nor does it look spoiled. The bacteria are invisible to the naked eye and, unlike other

Infectious Organisms and Fetal Development

common food bacteria, they continue to grow during refrigeration. Since you can't see, smell or taste Listeria, it's best not to eat Mexican-style soft cheese while you're pregnant.

What makes Listeria different from other bacteria?

Listeria are "tough bugs" because they can live in conditions that would kill most other bacteria. Although Listeria can grow in the refrigerator at temperatures below 40 degrees Fahrenheit, the bacteria are killed with thorough cooking (until the cheese is bubbling).

Can I keep from getting listeriosis by not eating soft cheese?

This will help, but there are other precautions you need to take. The bacteria that cause listeriosis are sometimes in raw or undercooked poultry and meat as well, and in raw and smoked seafood.

Because *Listeria* is naturally found in the soil—like other bacteria—it can also be on the vegetables you buy in markets, and in delicatessen foods. Although the risk of getting listeriosis from these two sources is low, pregnant women may choose to avoid food from delicatessen counters, thoroughly reheat cold cuts before eating them, and wash fruits and vegetables well. And, of course, they should eat meat, poultry or seafood only if it is thoroughly cooked.

What can I do to protect myself from food poisoning?

These food safety rules apply to everyone:

- Buy only pasteurized dairy products, as indicated on the label, and hard cheeses marked "aged 60 days" (or longer) if unpasteurized milk is used to make them.

- After you've handled or cut raw meat, poultry or seafood, wash your hands, the cutting board, counter, knives, and any other utensil you've used with hot soapy water before you use them again to prepare any other food.

- Thoroughly cook all meat, poultry and seafood, especially shellfish.

- Cover and store leftover cooked food in the refrigerator as soon as possible.

- Reheat all leftovers until they are steaming hot.

- Thoroughly wash raw fruits and vegetables with tap water.

- Follow label instructions on products that must be refrigerated or that have a "use by" date.

- Keep the inside of the refrigerator and the counter tops clean.

Part Four

Labor and Delivery

Chapter 14

Stages of Labor and Delivery

Labor Starts

What Happens

The way labor begins and progresses is different for each pregnancy. Sometimes you may not know that you are in the early stages of labor, but feel as though you have gas, heartburn, indigestion or backache. The woman may have some or all of the following symptoms as labor begins. These are the main signs that labor has started.

- Bloody mucous comes out of the vagina.

- Irregular contractions (pains or tightening) which become regular. These most often begin in your lower back and move through to the lower front of your abdomen (stomach).

- Bag of waters breaks—fluid may gush or trickle out from the vagina. This is painless.

Guidelines for the Expectant Mother

Unless you and your health care giver have made other plans, call right away when your "water breaks" or when your contractions are regular and about 5 minutes apart or last more than 30 seconds each.

Association of Asian/Pacific Community Health Organizations, 1988 and excerpts from DHSS Publication No. HRSA-MCHB-92-4-A, November 1994 and document From NIH Homepage, NIH-NICHD study, Sept 1995

- If your bag of waters breaks or if you have heavy red vaginal bleeding or clots, call your health care provider. Be ready to go to the hospital.

- Notify the person who will accompany you to the hospital.

- Time contractions (the number of minutes from the beginning of one contraction to the beginning of the next contraction).

- If contractions start during the day, continue with light activities.

- If contractions start during the night, try to rest.

Induction of Labor

Sometimes you may receive medication to start labor. This is done instead of waiting for labor to start on its own and is called induction of labor.

Before labor is induced, an amniocentesis may be done to show that the baby is ready to be born.

Labor can be induced by giving a medicine called Pitocin through an IV. Sometimes your doctor may try to start your labor by putting some gel into your birth canal. Your doctor will decide which way is best for you and your baby.

Induction of labor may be necessary because of:

- your medical condition

- a change in your baby's condition

- the possibility of infection.

First Stage of Labor

What Happens

- Entrance to the uterus starts to open up (dilate).

- Contractions occur closer together and become stronger.

- Backache may occur.

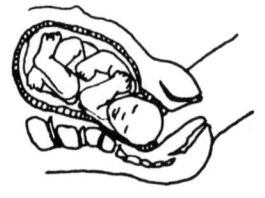

Figure 14.1. First Stage. Beginning of Labor: Entrance of uterus begins to open.

Stages of Labor and Delivery

Guidelines for the Expectant Mother

- Continue timing contractions.
- Go to hospital at the time you and your health care provider have discussed.
- Relax as much as possible. Use breathing techniques to help relax, avoid tensing muscles and reduce pain.
- Make yourself as comfortable as possible. If possible, try different positions. Walk, sit, lean forward, stand, lie back propped up with pillows, lie on side. Do not lie flat on your back—it reduces blood flow to baby.
- Try to urinate every hour.
- Avoid heavy meals.

Guidelines for the Support Person

- Help time contractions.
- Help make the mother comfortable. You can offer juice, cool damp towel, lip balm, ice chips, hot water bottle, help in taking a warm shower or bath.
- Offer to massage the expectant mother's back.
- Suggest different positions for the mother to try.
- Encourage appropriate breathing and relaxation techniques.

Transition in Labor

What Happens

- The opening of the uterus opens the last 2-3 cm to 10 cm (4 inches) and baby moves further down.
- Contractions become very intense—long, strong, and close together. About 12-20 contractions per hour. For most women the most difficult part of labor.

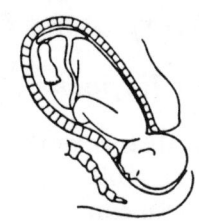

Figure 14.2. Transition. Entrance of uterus fully opens.

- May have severe low backache, nausea, vomiting, trembling, chills, or sweating.
- Mother is typically less responsive, more restless and more irritable.
- Mother may become overwhelmed or feel she's losing control.

Guidelines for the Expectant Mother

- Focus on doing the breathing and relaxation techniques.
- Relax muscles as much as possible.
- Remember you're almost ready to push the baby out.
- Do not push until told it is okay to do so. Pushing too soon can slow the labor.

Guidelines for the Support Person

- Provide lots and lots of support and comfort.
- Check for muscle tension and encourage mother to relax whole body.
- Offer massage, warm blankets, cool towel.
- Firmly hold shaking arms or legs.
- Help mother focus on appropriate breathing. It may help to have her look at you and follow your breathing.

Second Stage: Pushing and Delivery of the Baby.

What Happens

- Entrance of the uterus fully opened and mother pushes the baby down the birth canal.
- Contractions very strong but less frequent than before.

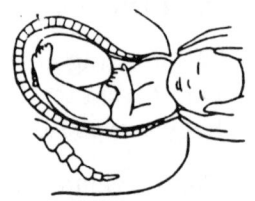

Figure 14.3. Second Stage of Labor

Stages of Labor and Delivery

- As the baby moves down the birth canal, burning and stretching sensations are felt.
- Health practitioner may perform a cut around the birth canal to prevent tearing as the baby comes out.
- The baby is born!

Guidelines for the Expectant Mother

- Follow the health practitioner's instructions for pushing and not pushing.
- May try different positions for pushing (squatting, propped up, lying on side)
- Use appropriate breathing techniques to control pushing.
- Relax muscles in bottom area.
- Rest between contractions.

Guidelines for the Support Person

- Stay with the mother.
- Help her into effective positions for pushing.
- Encourage appropriate breathing for pushing and not pushing.
- Encourage and support the mother!
- Watch the baby being born!

Third Stage: Delivery of Afterbirth.

What Happens

- Contractions continue to free the afterbirth (placenta) from the uterus. May or may not be painful.
- After-birth is expelled from uterus.
- Stitching is done if a cut (episiotomy) was performed at birth.

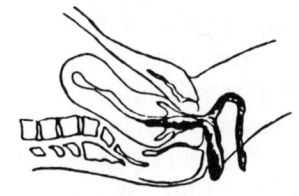

Figure 14.4. Third Stage of Labor

Guidelines for the Expectant Mother

- Push if instructed to do so.
- Hold your new baby. You can put your baby to your breast.
- Use breathing techniques if contractions are painful.
- Massage uterus to reduce bleeding.

Guidelines for the Support Person

- Get to know the baby!
- Praise mother for job well done.

Actively Managed Labor and Delivery

A team of researchers supported by the National Institute of Child Health and Human Development (NICHD) has found that a highly regarded "active management" approach to labor and delivery yielded mixed results for U.S. women. The extensive clinical trial was the largest, most intensive effort yet to test the new approach.

On one hand, the researchers discovered several benefits of the approach: it decreased the average length of labor, reduced by three fold the percentage of women experiencing labor lasting longer than 12 hours, and also cut back the likelihood of maternal fever, an indication of uterine infection.

On the other hand, the method did not reduce the rate of cesarean delivery—something its proponents eagerly hoped it would.

The study appeared as the lead article in the September 21 issue of the *New England Journal of Medicine*. The research team was led by Fredric D. Frigoletto, Jr., MD, from the Departments of Obstetrics and Gynecology at Brigham and Women's Hospital in Boston and Harvard Medical School in Boston when the study was conducted, and now at Massachusetts General Hospital in Boston. In addition to financial support from the NICHD, the investigators also received funding from Brigham and Women's Hospital and the Harvard Community Health Foundation.

In recent years, concern has been voiced that the cesarean rate may be too high, as cesarean delivery carries an increased risk of maternal and infant illness and death. In the report Healthy People 2000: National Health Promotion and Disease Prevention Objectives, the U.S. Department of Health and Human Services recommended that

Stages of Labor and Delivery

the cesarean rate be reduced to no more than 15 deliveries per 100 births. Approximately 24 percent of all births now are by cesarean section.

The active management approach to labor was pioneered by physicians at the National Maternity Hospital in Dublin, Ireland, the authors explained in the article. This active approach involves strict criteria for diagnosing labor, intervention with a labor-inducing drug in the event of weak uterine contractions, and ensuring that hospital staff never leave a woman unattended during labor. Because the rate of cesarean delivery at the National Maternity Hospital has remained consistently lower than in most of the industrialized world, many practitioners of obstetrics have employed it to try to reduce cesarean rates at their facilities. Several smaller studies have also found that the approach reduced cesarean rates.

A total of 1915 women delivering their first baby participated in the U.S. study. Of these, 1009 were assigned to the active management group, and the remaining 906 were assigned to the usual care group before the 30th week of pregnancy. Women in the usual care group were observed in the hospital labor and delivery unit, which was staffed with one nurse for every two patients, until a late stage of labor, when a single nurse provided care to each patient.

Unlike the active management group, the physicians in the usual care group did not adhere to a standardized protocol for administering or stopping oxytocin, the drug used for initiating or intensifying labor. Women in the active management group were seen by nurse midwives throughout the course of their labor.

Fetal monitoring was used for both groups of women, and all the women had similar access to pain relieving methods.

All of the women received prenatal care from their own health care providers. Women in the active management group took classes that explained the active management method. Women in the usual care group received payments to allow them to take childbirth education classes they chose for themselves.

Cesarean rates did not differ significantly—10.9 percent for the active management group, versus 11.5 percent in the usual care group.

Although the results are not what was hoped for regarding cesarean section rates, the trial did identify several advantages of the active management method, said Donald McNellis, MD, a project officer with NICHD's Pregnancy and Perinatology Branch. For example, the median duration of labor was 6.2 hours in the active management group, versus 8.9 hours in the usual care group. Furthermore, the percentage of women experiencing labor lasting longer than 12 hours was 3 times higher in the usual care group than in the active management group—26 percent versus 9 percent.

The active management group also was significantly less likely to experience maternal fever during delivery. Such fevers indicate a possible infection of the uterine lining. These infections may jeopardize a fetus' life and place him or her at greater risk of neonatal infections.

The researchers found that the active management group and the usual care group experienced similar cesarean section rates in the first stage of labor. Moreover, these rates were similar to cesarean section rates in Ireland.

For the second stage of labor, the cesarean section rate was again similar for both the active management and usual care groups. However, the rates for both of these groups were much higher than typically seen in the Irish studies, suggesting that some unexplained difference may exist between obstetrical practices in America and Ireland.

This difference suggests the need for a careful assessment of practices for the management of the second stage of labor in North America, the investigators wrote.

Unlike previous studies, the current study excluded women with conditions predisposing them to higher cesarean rates, such as hypertension and diabetes.

Chapter 15

Pre-Term Labor

Chapter Contents

Section 15.1—Management of Pre-Term Labor 240
Section 15.2—Cervix Length a Predictor of
 Pre-Term Labor 245
Section 15.3—Common Vaginal Condition Increases
 Risk of Preterm Delivery and Low Birth
 Weight 247
Section 15.4—Treatment of Pre-Term Labor with
 Corticosteroids 250
Section 15.5—Pre-Term Babies 262

Section 15.1

Management of Pre-Term Labor

From FDA Consumer, March 1992 by Deborah Bash and AHCPR Publication No. 92-0064, August 1992.

Introduction

Preterm delivery occurs in 7-10 percent of all pregnancies and is a major cause of infant mortality and morbidity. In addition, preterm births are associated with more than $2 billion in health care costs annually. Preterm infants account for the majority of all neonatal deaths. Immature infants may have numerous complications including respiratory distress syndrome (RDS), intraventricular hemorrhage (IVH), necrotizing enterocolitis (NEC), bronchopulmonary dysplasia (BPD), sepsis, patent ductus arteriosus (PDA), and retinopathy of prematurity. RDS is often the most acute problem of the very immature infant and, along with IVH, accounts for a significant proportion of neonatal deaths. Although most premature infants survive without major sequelae, some require rehospitalization and special services.

A woman who has a medical condition complicating pregnancy may be more likely to have an early labor and delivery. Smoking, poor nutritional habits, drug and alcohol abuse, and other poor health practices during pregnancy also increase the risk of early delivery and birth of stillborn or sick infants. Early in pregnancy, health professionals try to identify women who are at risk for pre-term labor and delivery so they can be monitored more frequently for early signs of the problem.

The usual length of a pregnancy is 38 to 40 weeks after the first day of the last menstrual period. Premature or pre-term labor is defined as labor occurring after 20 weeks and before 37 completed weeks of pregnancy. Although there is no firm data, estimates on the incidence of preterm delivery suggest that 6 to 10 percent of all births in the United States occur between the 20th and the 37th week of pregnancy.

According to Robert K. Creasy, M.D., chairman of the department of obstetrics, gynecology, and reproductive sciences at the University

Pre-Term Labor

of Texas Science Center at Houston, prematurity accounts for over 50 percent of the neurologically handicapped children in this country and is the greatest single cause of newborn illness and death.

Unfortunately, it is difficult to predict which women are at risk for pre-term labor. Since pre-term labor can occur in all age groups and within all social settings, researchers continue to explore what lifestyles and risk factors are common to women who experience pre-term labor.

Sometimes women mistake a certain type of contraction for labor. As early as six weeks into all pregnancies, the uterus, which is a large muscle, begins to contract rhythmically. These contractions (called Braxton Hicks contractions) are usually irregular and painless, and, because they usually do not cause the cervix to dilate, they do not threaten the pregnancy.

Braxton Hicks contractions that tend to increase in frequency and intensity toward the end of the pregnancy may be misinterpreted as contractions of labor and are sometimes referred to as "false labor" contractions. Women are not usually aware of cervical dilatation, the stretching and opening of the entrance to the uterus, and cervical dilatation can only be measured by a health practitioner during a pelvic examination.

Trish Mooney of Takoma Park, Md., has had two high-risk pregnancies. During the first one, however, she didn't recognize the symptoms. Her son Isaiah was born after only 34 weeks' gestation, weighing 5 pounds, 8 ounces. During her second pregnancy, her contractions were recognized and, due also to her history of previous pre-term birth, she was put on bed rest. She also developed gestational diabetes. She was closely monitored and last May, after a full-term pregnancy, gave birth to her daughter Leslie, who weighed in at 8 pounds, 4 ounces.

What to Do

A pregnant woman experiencing contractions, either painful or painless, anytime during pregnancy, that occur more than four times an hour or are less than 15 minutes apart should report this activity to her physician or midwife, and be prepared to answer the following questions:

- When did the discomfort start?

- What is the type and frequency of the contractions?

- What were you doing when the symptoms began?

- Do you have any other signs or symptoms such as:
  1. menstrual-like cramps that may come and go
  2. abdominal cramps with or without diarrhea
  3. backache that is dull and may radiate around toward the abdomen
  4. vaginal discharge increase or a noticeable change in color
  5. pelvic pressure that is constant or intermittent.

While waiting for her provider to return her call, the woman should:

- lie down with her feet elevated

- drink two or three glasses of water or juice.

These two activities sometimes cause contractions to subside. If symptoms do not lessen within one hour and the woman is not able to get in touch with her healthcare provider, she should go to the nearest hospital for further evaluation.

Home Monitoring

Home monitoring of the mother-to-be who has signs of pre-term labor may be ordered by her health-care provider, especially if she must be on bed rest for a significant time (often 20 weeks or more). Home care, although quite expensive itself, may help reduce costs and continue to provide a safe and satisfactory means of monitoring the pregnancy. Some insurance companies cover the cost of home care visits and some aspects of home monitoring equipment. Not all insurance companies cover home uterine activity monitoring.

In the fall of 1990, FDA approved for marketing the Genesis Home Uterine Activity Monitoring System to monitor uterine activity in women past their 24th week of pregnancy who have histories of previous pre-term births. The purpose of such monitoring is the early detection of uterine activity, which can cause cervical dilatation and pre-term labor.

Wearing an elastic belt around her waist, the expectant mother places the transducer attached to the belt on her abdomen. The transducer is a small, flat, pressure-sensitive recorder that looks like a "compact" or a small "beeper" and detects uterine contractions. A computer program transfers the data reporting the uterine activity over the telephone lines to communication centers such as the obstetrician's office, the home health service office, or a hospital relay station. Some women complain of skin irritation from the belt and the transducer because the belt is worn for two hours a day, usually one hour in the morning and one hour in the evening.

However, while the use of home uterine monitoring devices may result in detection of preterm labor at an earlier stage of cervical dilation, it has not been established that use of this technology results in a reduction in the incidence of preterm birth, nor that it is superior to patient education coupled with frequent provider-initiated contact with patients.

Drug Treatment

Pregnant women at risk for premature labor are often placed on medications that can stop contractions and give the fetus more time in the uterus. Such medications are called tocolytic agents. The word is derived from the Greek words *tokos,* meaning birth, and *lysis,* meaning dissolution.

The following fictionalized example, based on several real-life examples, explains the benefits of tocolytics.

Robin believes her 6-month-old daughter is alive and well today because of the tocolytic drug treatment Robin received in her 22nd week of pregnancy. Hospitalized for painful uterine contractions, Robin received tocolytic medication intravenously. After one week, she was sent home on strict bed rest, oral medication to prevent contractions, and a regimen of careful monitoring.

The only tocolytic medication approved by FDA for use in pre-term labor is Yutopar (ritodrine hydrochloride). Yutopar can be prescribed if labor begins between 20 and 36 weeks gestation and if the fetus weighs between 500 and 2,499 grams (1 to 5 pounds). The initial dose of Yutopar is usually given intravenously. Once the best dose for the patient is found, she may receive the medication by oral or intramuscular route. The amount and frequency of subsequent dosages depend on the woman's response to the initial therapy.

Yutopar should not be used in women who have cardiovascular disease, pregnancy-induced high blood pressure, intra/uterine infection, vaginal bleeding, or uncontrolled diabetes. Nor should it be used if the woman is in active labor or has a history of repeated miscarriages due to an incompetent cervix, or if the fetal membranes have ruptured.

Side effects include: heart palpitations, excessively rapid heartbeat, tremors, anxiety, headaches, vomiting, and fever.

Low blood sugar, bowel problems, and a low level of calcium in the blood have been reported in infants of mothers who were given tocolytics such as Yutopar. The labeling instructs physicians to carefully weigh the risks and benefits of administering the drug to women who are more than 32 weeks pregnant because of its possible effect on the fetus.

An electrocardiogram is recommended before starting Yutopar therapy. Before and often during tocolytic therapy, the patient may be monitored for serial blood glucose and blood electrolyte levels.

When a woman in pre-term labor also has diabetes or heart disease, she may be placed on magnesium sulfate to reduce uterine activity. Magnesium sulfate is approved for magnesium deficiency states but not specifically for use in pre-term labor. However, because there is extensive literature and clinical data on this use, some physicians prescribe it. The most uncomfortable side effect of magnesium sulfate is a feeling of warmth and flushing when the drug is first administered. Women must also be carefully monitored for respiratory or cardiac complications during the therapy.

Terbutaline sulfate, a drug approved for asthma and other lung disorders, has been used by some physicians to treat pre-term labor. However, it has not been approved by FDA for this use, nor has the agency been asked to review an application for marketing terbutaline sulfate for treating pre-term labor. The labeling for terbutaline sulfate was revised in 1988 by the drug's manufacturer to specify that it is not approved for treatment of pre-term labor.

Health professionals hope that proper use of home monitoring will lead to more appropriate and effective use of tocolytics.

Home Health-Care Services

Many communities have home healthcare services specializing in pregnancy. Nurses from these services provide specialized care for pregnant patients at home, including evaluation of:

- weight
- urine
- blood pressure
- blood glucose levels
- bed rest compliance
- psychological status
- uterine contractions

- fetal heart tones using a fetoscope, a stethoscope—like instrument. Home services also provide medication therapy as prescribed by a physician.

Pre-term birth is a serious medical conditions that cause parents-to-be much concern and worry. High costs of hospitalization and the rate of illness and death in newborns are factors in the increased use of home monitoring for women who have high-risk pregnancies. Educating expectant mothers to get early prenatal care, eat nutritionally sound diets, stop smoking, practice stress reduction, and detect signs of pre-term labor can go a long way towards lowering the incidence of infant mortality and illness.

Section 15.2

Cervix Length a Predictor of Premature Labor

NIH Home Page, February 1996 by Robert Bock

Researchers funded by the National Institute of Child Health and Human Development (NICHD) have identified a significant risk factor for premature birth, which, in turn, is a major cause of infant mortality.

Specifically, a pregnant woman who has been determined by ultrasound to have a short cervix during pregnancy is more likely to give birth prematurely than is a woman with a longer cervix, according to a study by the NICHD's Maternal Fetal Medicine Network. Established in 1986, the Maternal-Fetal Medicine Units Network was formed to permit more effective evaluation of existing and new prenatal and perinatal health treatments through clinical trials.

The study, the largest of its kind to date, appears in the February 29 issue of the *New England Journal of Medicine*. The finding provides a relatively easy method for evaluating the chances of a woman giving birth prematurely, the authors wrote. In addition, it may prove particularly useful for selecting women who are candidates for clinical trials of cerclage, the surgical practice of preventing early labor by placing a single suture through the cervix. Premature birth is a major public health problem. Roughly 11 percent of U.S. infants are born prematurely (before the 36th week of pregnancy, according to the National Center for Health Statistics. Of these infants, 4.7 percent will die in infancy, accounting for 58.6 percent of all infant deaths. A method for identifying and preventing premature labor would significantly reduce the infant mortality rate.

"The length of the cervix is directly correlated with the duration of pregnancy: the shorter the cervix, the greater the likelihood of preterm delivery," they wrote.

For the study, the researchers made use of transvaginal ultrasonography, in which the ultrasound probe is placed at the vaginal opening. This method was used to evaluate 2915 women recruited nation wide from the 10 centers of NICHD's Maternal and Fetal Medicine Units, at approximately the 24th week of pregnancy. The women were again scheduled to undergo the transvaginal ultrasound examination at the 28th week, but because some either gave birth, withdrew from the study, or failed to appear for the examination at the scheduled interval, only 2531 actually did so.

The cervix length of each woman was recorded and ranked serially. Based on the length of the cervix each woman was assigned to a particular grouping called a percentile. After the women had all given birth, the researchers calculated their risks of giving birth prematurely, based on the women's ultrasound readings at the time of each evaluation.

Women whose cervical length was above the 75 percentile were the least likely to give birth prematurely. Using these women as a reference point, the researchers calculated the relative risk of giving birth prematurely for the women in the remaining percentiles. "Relative risk" refers to the chances of women giving birth prematurely, as compared to women above a certain percentile. For example, women below the 75 percentile at 24 weeks had a relative risk of 1.98, meaning they were almost twice as likely as the women above the 75 percentile to give birth prematurely.

The researchers conceded that a shortened cervix may not be a predictor of early labor, but due instead to uterine contractions. Such contractions, which shorten the cervix, could have resulted from the beginnings of labor. The NICHD-supported researchers discounted this possibility, however, as the women enrolled in the study gave no other indications of beginning labor at the time they were examined. Although previous studies have suggested a link between cervical length and prematurity, the current study is the largest of its kind to do so.

Section 15.3

Common Vaginal Condition Increases Risk of Preterm Delivery and Low Birth Weight

From NIH Homepage, December 1995

A common vaginal condition known as bacterial vaginosis (BV) significantly increases a woman's risk of the premature delivery of a low-birth-weight infant, according to research funded by the National Institute of Child Health and Human Development (NICHD) and the National Institute of Allergy and Infectious Diseases (NIAID).

Pregnant women who were diagnosed with BV during the second trimester were 40 percent more likely to give birth to a premature infant with low birth weight (i.e., an infant born before 37 weeks' gestation and weighing less than 5 pounds) than were women who did not have the vaginal infection. This increased risk remained after adjusting for other variables, including smoking, race, previous delivery of a low-birth-weight infant, previous pregnancy loss, number of previous live births, maternal age, antibiotic use, and other vaginal infections. The research, part of a larger NICHD/NIAID clinical study called the Vaginal Infections and Prematurity (VIP) Study, will appear in the December 28 issue of the New England Journal of Medicine.

"Preterm delivery and low-birth-weight delivery remain two of the most difficult unsolved problems in our country," said principal investigator Dr. Sharon Hillier, now at the University of Pittsburgh/Magee Women's Hospital. "If we find that treating this very common vaginal condition can prevent preterm birth, this would be a really important step in preventing the long-term sequelae that some preterm, low-birth-weight infants face."

BV is caused by an imbalance among the bacteria that are normally found in the vagina. In healthy women, the predominant strain of bacteria found is Lactobacillus. With BV, increased numbers of anaerobic organisms are found, including Gardnerella vaginalis, Mycoplasma hominis, and bacteroides. Although these bacteria are also found in healthy women, they signal an abnormality when they outnumber the normal Lactobacillus flora.

Previously called Gardnerella vaginitis or nonspecific vaginitis, BV is the most common vaginal infection in reproductive-aged women. It is also one of the most common vaginal infections in pregnancy, affecting from 12 to 22 percent of pregnant women.

While BV has been linked to preterm birth before, this study is the first large enough in size to document the association between the infection and the premature delivery of a low-birth-weight infant after controlling for other variables, such as smoking and obstetrical history.

Research Study

Between 1984 and 1989, the VIP research team enrolled 10,397 pregnant women from seven medical centers in five cities into this cohort study. None of the women had known medical risk factors for preterm delivery.

At 23-26 weeks of gestation, all women were screened for BV using laboratory staining for bacterial strains associated with BV. Since vaginal pH tends to be less acidic with BV, pH testing was also used to determine if infection was present.

The women were then followed until delivery to identify birth outcome involving prematurity and low birth weight. Of 504 women who delivered premature, low-birth-weight infants, 20 percent had been diagnosed with BV. Further statistical analysis indicated that women with BV were 40 percent more likely than women without the condition to have such a birth. At highest risk were women with two particular strains of bacteria, Mycoplasma hominis and bacteroides.

In addition to BV, the primary risk factors for preterm delivery of a low-birth-weight infant were smoking, which increased the risk of preterm delivery by about 40 percent; having already had a preterm infant, which increased the risk about six fold; and being of African American race, which increased the risk by about 40 percent. Women with a history of bladder infections or antibiotic use prior to the study were also more likely to have a premature, low-birth-weight infant.

Although BV is more common among women with new or multiple sexual partners, the organisms that cause it have been isolated in young women who are not sexually active. The use of intrauterine devices has been linked to an increased risk of becoming infected.

The main symptom associated with BV is an abnormal vaginal discharge with a characteristic "fishy" odor. As many as 50 percent of

Pre-Term Labor

women, however, have no symptoms at all, and are only diagnosed after microscopic examination of a sample of vaginal discharge under a microscope. The infection can be treated with antibiotics. "Pregnant women who have genital symptoms should be screened for this and treated appropriately if they're found to have bacterial vaginosis," Dr. Hillier said.

The mechanisms underlying the increased risk of prematurity and low birth weight associated with BV are unclear. The investigators theorize that, in addition to causing an infection in the vagina, BV may cause an infection in the uterus, which somehow triggers preterm birth.

Although premature delivery and low birth weight are major contributors to perinatal mortality, there is no effective way to prevent them at this time. The findings from this study, however, may be the first step toward a prevention strategy that would involve screening and treatment of high-risk women.

Already, a related study by Hauth, et al, has demonstrated that antibiotic treatment is an effective way to reduce the risk of premature delivery among women with BV and other noninfectious risk factors for preterm birth. In this study, also appearing in the December 28 New England Journal of Medicine, investigators at the University of Alabama at Birmingham found that they were able to reduce the rate of premature delivery in such women by treating them with the antibiotics metronidazole and erythromycin.

Currently, the NICHD's Maternal/Fetal Medicine Unit Network is conducting a large clinical trial involving approximately 1,900 pregnant women to determine whether metronidazole alone will reduce the risk of preterm delivery in low-risk women with asymptomatic bacterial vaginosis.

Section 15.4

Treatment of Preterm Labor with Corticosteroids

NIH Consensus Statement, Volume 12, Number 2, 1994.

Corticosteroid treatment of pregnant women delivering prematurely was first introduced in 1972 to enhance fetal lung maturity. A recent meta-analysis concluded that corticosteroid administration prior to anticipated preterm delivery is associated with a large reduction in the incidence of early neonatal death, RDS, IVH, and NEC.

Despite evidence of beneficial effects from both experimental models and randomized controlled trials in humans, a minority of women delivering prematurely receive antenatal corticosteroid treatment. In reports from approximately 500 perinatal centers, only 12-18 percent of women who deliver preterm infants of 501-1,500 grams birthweight are treated with antenatal corticosteroids. Clinicians are not treating many patients who might benefit because of concerns about the efficacy of corticosteroids and the potential complications of treatment in certain conditions. Use of this therapy is further impeded by lack of access to prenatal care and to appropriate delivery services.

To address these issues, the National Institute of Child Health and Human Development, together with the Office of Medical Applications of Research of the National Institutes of Health, convened a Consensus Development Conference on the Effect of Corticosteroids for Fetal Maturation on Perinatal Outcomes. The conference was cosponsored by the National Heart, Lung, and Blood Institute and the National Institute of Nursing Research. After a year of study and preparation concluding with 1 1/2 days presentations by experts in the relevant fields and discussion from the audience, an independent consensus panel composed of representatives from the medical and related scientific disciplines, as well as representatives from the public, considered the evidence and formulated a consensus statement in response to the following key questions:

- For what conditions and purposes are antenatal corticosteroids used, and what is the scientific basis for that use?

- What are the short-term and long-term benefits of antenatal corticosteroid treatment?

- What are the short-term and long-term adverse effects for the infant and mother?

- What is the influence of the type of corticosteroid, dosage, timing and circumstances of administration, and associated therapy on treatment outcome?

- What are the economic consequences of this treatment?

- What are the recommendations for use of antenatal corticosteroids?

- What research is needed to guide clinical care?

For what conditions and purposes are antenatal corticosteroids used, and what is the scientific basis for that use?

Animal studies conducted in the 1950's and 1960's showed that the pituitary adrenal system affected differentiation of the intestine and lung. Later studies found physiologic surges in corticosteroids just before term or preterm delivery, and a relationship between fetal cortisol levels at delivery and lung maturity. Since then, randomized controlled trials in women have confirmed the maturational effects of corticosteroids on fetal organ systems such as the cardiovascular, respiratory, nervous, and gastrointestinal systems. As a result, antenatal corticosteroids are now administered for the purpose of hastening maturation of the preterm infant's organs and tissues, thus reducing morbidity and mortality related to prematurity.

The clinical conditions under which antenatal corticosteroid administration has been investigated are those associated with threatened or inevitable preterm delivery. These include:

1. Preterm labor, which accounts for 30-50 percent of all preterm deliveries

2. Preterm premature rupture of membranes, which accounts for 20-50 percent of all preterm deliveries

3. Preeclampsia, which is associated with 10-25 percent of preterm deliveries

4. Other conditions, such as diabetes mellitus, third-trimester bleeding, fetal distress, or isoimmunization necessitating preterm delivery, which account for up to 10 percent of preterm deliveries. The use of antenatal corticosteroid therapy has been studied in relatively few pregnancies less than 24 weeks' or greater than 34 weeks' gestation.

Additional issues that have been investigated include duration of the "treatment window," the gender and race of the fetus, the relationship of gestational age to the risks and benefits of treatment, and the use of antenatal corticosteroids along with other treatments, such as postnatal pulmonary surfactant and tocolytic administration.

Scientific Basis

Studies of antenatal corticosteroid treatment were evaluated with the grading system developed by the Canadian Task Force on the Periodic Health Examination and adapted by the U.S. Preventive Services Task Force (Figure 15.1).

The ratings reflect both the quality of evidence and the strength of the recommendations that can be based on that evidence. For most of these conditions or outcomes, at least some data were available from randomized controlled trials. For some outcomes, such as RDS, data were extensive. For other maternal conditions or neonatal outcomes, though derived from randomized controlled trials, data were limited. Hence, for some conditions or outcomes, although grade I evidence was available, this evidence was judged insufficient to allow a recommendation concerning the use of corticosteroids.

Quality of Evidence.

- I—Evidence obtained from at least one properly designed randomized controlled trial.

- II-1—Evidence obtained from well-designed controlled trials without randomization.

- II-2—Evidence obtained from well-designed cohort or case-control analytic studies, preferably from more than one center or research group.

Pre-Term Labor

- II-3—Evidence obtained from multiple time series with or without the intervention. Dramatic results in uncontrolled experiments (such as the results of the introduction of penicillin treatment in the 1940's) could also be regarded as this type of evidence.

- III—Opinions of respected authorities, based on clinical experience, descriptive studies, or reports of expert committees.

Strength of Recommendation Regarding Corticosteroid Administration.

- A—There is good evidence to support use.

- B—There is fair evidence to support use.

- C—There is inadequate evidence to argue for or against use.

- D—There is fair evidence to avoid use.

- E—There is good evidence to avoid use.

	Quality of evidence for benefit	Strength of recommendation
Interval from treatment to delivery		
<24 hours	I	B
24 hours to 7 days	I	A
>7 days	I	C
Gestational age		
Delivery age 24–28 weeks	I	A
Delivery at 29–34 weeks	I	A
Delivery at >34 weeks	I	C
Preterm premature rupture of membranes	I	B
Neonatal outcomes		
Mortality	I	A
Respiratory distress syndrome	I	A
Intraventricular hemorrhage	I	A

Figure 15.1. Evidence of efficacy of corticosteroids and strength of recommendation according to delivery interval, gestational age, status of membranes, and neonatal outcome. See text for explanation of symbols.

What are the short-term and long-term benefits of antenatal corticosteroid treatment?

Short-Term Benefits for the Infant

Antenatal corticosteroid therapy in the preterm fetus in many randomized controlled trials has reduced neonatal mortality and the incidence of RDS. A meta-analysis based on 15 such trials showed a reduction in the incidence of RDS with a typical odds ratio of 0.5 (95% CI = 0.4-0.6) and a reduction of neonatal mortality with a typical odds ratio of 0.6 (95% CI = 0.5-0.8). These data are not only statistically significant but also clinically compelling. In subgroup analysis, these benefits were confirmed regardless of the infant's gender or race.

One recent randomized controlled trial showed a significant reduction in IVH with antenatal corticosteroid treatment. Secondary outcome variables reported in the meta-analysis of randomized controlled trials also showed a significant reduction in the incidence of IVH with an odds ratio of 0.5 (95% Cl = 0.3-0.9). This reduction in IVH is supported by the results of the observational database, information prospectively collected in five registries involving more than 30,000 low birthweight infants. Since IVH is an important contributor to mortality and serious long-term neuro-developmental disability, this reduction is a major benefit.

Improved circulatory stability and reduced requirements for oxygen and ventilatory support were additional benefits identified in randomized controlled trials. Data are conflicting for NEC and PDA. The meta-analysis of the randomized controlled trials revealed a reduction of the incidence of NEC however; this finding was not corroborated by the observational database. Conversely, the incidence of PDA was not found to be reduced in the meta-analysis but was significantly reduced in the observational database.

Long-Term Benefits for the Infant

Several studies have followed infants from the randomized trials for as long as 12 years. The increased survival of treated infants has not resulted in the appearance of adverse long-term effects.

What are the short-term and long-term adverse effects for the infant and mother?

Short-Term Adverse Effects for the Infant

Short-term adverse effects of antenatal corticosteroid administration of greatest concern in the neonate include infection and adrenal suppression. The evidence presented to date shows no increase in infection in treated infants, no clinically important adrenal suppression, and rapid return of adrenal function when antenatal corticosteroids are discontinued.

Some animal studies have suggested that antenatal corticosteroid treatment might promote maladaptive responses to hypoxia. Other animal studies have shown that corticosteroids in doses similar to those used in humans antenatally provide protection against hypoxic-ischemic brain injury. More data are needed from human studies in this area of research.

Long-Term Adverse Effects for the Infant

Studies initiated in the 1970's, which followed the development of children treated antenatally with corticosteroids up to the age of 12 years, showed no adverse outcomes in the areas of motor skills, language, cognition, memory, concentration, or scholastic achievement. The possibility of adverse, long-term neurodevelopmental outcomes has been suggested by studies of corticosteroid administration in animals. These studies were conducted using doses approximately 10 times the doses used in human clinical trials. There does not seem to be an increased risk in children of long-term neurodevelopmental impairment, as reflected in any greater prevalence of learning, behavioral, motor, or sensory disturbances. Long-term effects of antenatal corticosteroids on growth and the onset of puberty are not fully known.

Short-Term and Long-Term Adverse Maternal Effects

Maternal pulmonary edema can occur when antenatal corticosteroids are used in combination with tocolytic agents. This complication is more commonly associated with maternal infection, fluid overload, and multiple gestation. Pulmonary edema has not been reported when antenatal corticosteroids are used alone.

The risk of maternal infection may be increased when corticosteroids are used in preterm premature rupture of membranes (PPROM); however, the degree of this effect, if any, is unclear. Furthermore, there is no evidence that antenatal corticosteroid treatment interferes with the ability to diagnose maternal infection. When corticosteroids are administered to pregnant diabetic women, diabetic control may become more difficult and insulin may have to be adjusted accordingly. Screening for gestational diabetes may similarly be affected. In serious maternal medical conditions that necessitate premature delivery, the delay necessary to demonstrate maximal corticosteroid effects for the fetus may worsen the maternal medical status. A subgroup analysis in the first randomized trial suggested that antenatal corticosteroid administration might predispose to fetal death in hypertensive women. Subsequent trials failed to demonstrate this effect. No long-term maternal adverse effects have been reported.

What is the influence of the type of corticosteroid, dosage, timing and circumstances of administration, and associated therapy on treatment outcome?

Type of Corticosteroid

Dexamethasone and betamethasone are the preferred corticosteroids for antenatal therapy. These two compounds are identical in biological activity and readily cross the placenta in their biologically active forms. They are devoid of mineralocorticoid activity, relatively weak in immunosuppressive activity, and exert longer duration of action than cortisol and methylprednisolone. They also are the most extensively studied antenatal corticosteroids for accelerating fetal maturation.

Dose

Treatment of two doses of 12 mg of betamethasone given intramuscularly 24 hours apart or four doses of 6 mg of dexamethasone given intramuscularly 12 hours apart has been shown to be effective. Although these regimens were arbitrarily selected, they have subsequently been shown to deliver concentrations to the fetus that are comparable to physiologic stress levels of cortisol occurring after birth in untreated premature infants who develop RDS.

These regimens result in an estimated 75 percent occupancy of available corticosteroid receptors, which should provide a near maximal induction of antenatal corticosteroid receptor-mediated response in fetal target tissues. Higher or more frequent doses do not increase the benefits of antenatal corticosteroid therapy and may increase the likelihood of adverse effects.

Timing

Strong evidence exists for neonatal benefits from a complete course of antenatal corticosteroids starting at 24 hours and lasting up to 7 days after treatment. Evidence suggests a reduction in mortality, RDS, and IVH, even with treatment initiated less than 24 hours prior to delivery. Both clinical and *in vitro* evidence suggest that the corticosteroid biological effects persist up to 7 days following initial treatment.

Data are inadequate to establish the clinical benefit beyond 7 days after antenatal corticosteroid therapy. The potential benefits or risks of repeated administration after 7 days are unknown. *In vitro* experiments in human fetal lung explants show that inducible biochemical effects have dissipated by 7 days, although structural changes persist.

Circumstances of Administration

Gestational Age. For infants born at 29-34 weeks' gestation, treatment with antenatal corticosteroids clearly reduces the incidence of RDS and overall mortality. Although antenatal corticosteroids do not clearly decrease the incidence of RDS in infants born at 24-28 weeks' gestation, they reduce its severity. More important, antenatal corticosteroids clearly reduce mortality and the incidence of IVH in this age group. All fetuses between 24 and 34 weeks' gestation threatened with premature delivery are candidates for treatment with antenatal corticosteroids.

In infants born beyond 34 weeks' gestation, the risk of neonatal mortality, RDS, and IVH is low. The evidence for significant improvement in outcomes in these infants with antenatal corticosteroid use is limited. Use of corticosteroids in mothers expected to deliver at greater than 34 weeks is, therefore, not recommended unless there is evidence of pulmonary immaturity.

Race and Sex. There is no convincing evidence from any of the clinical trials that either gender or race of the fetus affects the response to therapy with antenatal corticosteroids.

Preterm Premature Rupture of Membranes. The use of antenatal corticosteroids to reduce infant morbidity in the presence of PPROM remains controversial. Antenatal corticosteroids reduced the risk of RDS in PPROM in randomized controlled trials, although the magnitude of the reduction was not as great as when the membranes were intact. Strong evidence from observational studies suggests that, even in the presence of PPROM, the incidence of neonatal mortality and IVH is reduced when antenatal corticosteroids are used. Although the risk of neonatal infection associated with antenatal corticosteroid use in the face of PPROM may be increased, the magnitude of the increase is small. Because of the effectiveness of antenatal corticosteroids in reducing mortality and IVH in fetuses of less than 30-32 weeks' gestation, antenatal corticosteroid use is appropriate in the absence of chorioamnionitis

Other Conditions. Data are insufficient to assess the effectiveness of antenatal corticosteroid use in certain maternal high-risk conditions such as hypertension and diabetes. In the absence of evidence of adverse effects, it may be reasonable to treat these women as one would others with threatened premature delivery. Similarly, in the presence of high-risk fetal conditions, such as multiple gestation, intrauterine growth retardation, and hydrops, it is reasonable to treat these patients as one would others with threatened premature delivery.

Associated Therapies

Surfactant. Antenatal administration of corticosteroids acts additively with postnatal administration of surfactant to reduce mortality, RDS, and IVH. Furthermore, surfactant replacement appears to have little or no impact on the incidence of IVH or PDA. For these reasons the decision to use antenatal corticosteroids should not be altered by availability of surfactant replacement therapy.

Thyrotropin-Releasing Hormone. Thyroid hormones accelerate fetal lung maturation in animal studies. However, T3 and T4 do not cross the placenta. This problem has been circumvented by maternal administration of thyrotropin-releasing hormone (TRH). The combination of TRH plus antenatal corticosteroids was more effective than corticosteroids alone in two randomized studies. Women who received both drugs had infants with fewer adverse outcomes, fewer days on the ventilator, and a lower incidence of BPD. The use of TRH to accelerate fetal pulmonary maturation currently is experimental, and randomized studies are in progress.

Beta-Mimetic Tocolytics. Beta-mimetic agents such as ritodrine and terbutaline are frequently administered in an attempt to arrest preterm labor. Women receiving tocolytic therapy are candidates for antenatal corticosteroids to accelerate fetal maturation in the face of threatened premature delivery. Several studies have examined the outcomes of infants born prematurely to mothers who received both ritodrine and dexamethasone or betamethasone. Although there are flaws in the design of each of

Pre-Term Labor

these studies, they all showed a significant decrease in incidence of RDS. In addition, one study demonstrated a decrease in ventilator dependency and incidence of PDA. There is evidence that beta-mimetic agents may be associated with increased risk of IVH. However, the use of antenatal corticosteroids may reduce this risk.

What are the economic consequences of this treatment?

Neonatal intensive care is expensive but is more cost-effective in terms of years of life gained than many other accepted medical interventions. Because the costs of caring for infants with RDS are so high, interventions that may reduce its incidence, such as antenatal corticosteroids or prophylactic surfactant, have the potential of producing large cost savings, in addition to improving health.

The net economic consequences include the costs of initial treatment, changes in treatment made to allow the corticosteroids to work, the costs of any harmful side effects of treatment, the savings resulting from reduced length of stay and intensity of treatment, and the long-term costs of the burden of chronic diseases in surviving infants. Because the direct costs of corticosteroid treatment are so low and differential extra long-term burden has not been well quantified, net cost estimates were derived from the balance of costs of the health outcomes of initial treatment. Costs of infant care are relatively low for both uncomplicated preterm infants and early neonatal deaths. For any proposed clinical situation, costs are decreased to the extent that corticosteroids reduce illness in survivors and increased for infants that would have died quickly without them. Data on costs from randomized trials are scant, but length of stay was reduced by about one-third in corticosteroid-treated infants in the four trials for which these data were collected. To estimate costs or savings from increased use, data on efficacy from all corticosteroid trials can be applied to data on current costs of caring for infants with and without disease. The resulting calculated base-case cost savings were more than $3,000 per treated neonate. Of the 4,100,000 babies born in the United States each year, 106,000 weigh less than 2,000 grams at birth. Currently, 15 percent of these babies are treated with corticosteroids. If this were increased to 60 percent, as observed in some hospitals, a conservative estimate of the annual savings in health care costs would be $157 million from the initial hospitalization alone.

What are the recommendations for use of antenatal corticosteroids?

- The benefits of antenatal administration of corticosteroids to fetuses at risk of preterm delivery vastly outweigh the potential risks. These benefits include not only a reduction in the risk of RDS but also a substantial reduction in mortality and IVH.

- All fetuses between 24 and 34 weeks' gestation at risk of preterm delivery should be considered candidates for antenatal treatment with corticosteroids.

- The decision to use antenatal corticosteroids should not be altered by fetal race or gender or by the availability of surfactant replacement therapy.

- Patients eligible for therapy with tocolytics should also be eligible for treatment with antenatal corticosteroids.

- Treatment consists of two doses of 12 mg of betamethasone given intramuscularly 24 hours apart or four doses of 6 mg of dexamethasone given intramuscularly 12 hours apart. Optimal benefit begins 24 hours after initiation of therapy and lasts 7 days.

- Because treatment with corticosteroids for less than 24 hours is still associated with significant reductions in neonatal mortality, RDS, and IVH, antenatal corticosteroids should be given unless immediate delivery is anticipated.

- In PPROM at less than 30-32 weeks' gestation in the absence of clinical chorioamnionitis, antenatal corticosteroid use is recommended because of the high risk of IVH at these early gestational ages.

- In complicated pregnancies where delivery prior to 34 weeks' gestation is likely, antenatal corticosteroid use is recommended unless there is evidence that corticosteroids will have an adverse effect on the mother or delivery is imminent.

What research is needed to guide clinical care?

Areas of animal and human research that need to be addressed include the following:

- The short-term and long-term benefits and risks of repeating administration of antenatal corticosteroids 7 days after the initial course.

- Long-term effect of antenatal corticosteroids on cognitive, behavioral, psychological, and physical development of the neonate.

- Effects of antenatal corticosteroids on organ maturation.

- Effects of antenatal corticosteroids on hypoxic-ischemic insults.

- Effects of antenatal corticosteroids on neonatal hemodynamic stability.

- Mechanism of antenatal corticosteroid induction of cell and organ maturation at the molecular level.

- The interaction of antenatal corticosteroids with other therapies administered during the perinatal period (e.g., the effect of corticosteroids and tocolytics on the incidence of IVH).

- Development of alternative therapies to antenatal corticosteroids for fetal maturation.

- Systematic study of the diffusion of these scientifically based recommendations into clinical practice.

Conclusion

Antenatal corticosteroid therapy for fetal maturation reduces mortality, respiratory distress syndrome, and intraventricular hemorrhage in preterm infants. These benefits extend to a broad range of gestational ages (24-34 weeks) and are not limited by gender or race. Although the beneficial effects of corticosteroids are greatest more than 24 hours after beginning treatment, treatment less than 24 hours in duration also improves outcomes. The benefits of antenatal corticosteroids are additive to those derived from surfactant therapy.

In the presence of preterm premature rupture of the membranes, antenatal corticosteroid therapy reduces the frequency of respiratory distress syndrome, intraventricular hemorrhage, and neonatal death, although to a lesser extent than with intact membranes. Whether this therapy increases either neonatal or maternal infection is unclear. However, the risk of death from prematurity is greater than the risk from infection.

Data from trials with followup of children up to 12 years indicate that antenatal corticosteroid therapy does not adversely affect physical growth or psychomotor development.

Antenatal corticosteroid therapy is indicated for women at risk of premature delivery with few exceptions and will result in a substantial decrease in neonatal morbidity and mortality, as well as substantial savings in health care costs. The use of antenatal corticosteroids for fetal maturation is a rare example of a technology that yields substantial cost savings in addition to improving health.

Section 15.5

Pre-Term Babies

FDA Consumer, April 1992

When Benjamin McClatchey was born almost three months premature on July 27, 1990, he weighed only 2 pounds, 13 ounces, and his underdeveloped lungs struggled for every breath.

Benjamin's parents, Steve and Trillis McClatchey of Lafayette, Ind., got only a glimpse of their son before doctors whisked him off to another hospital an hour away. They called Trillis McClatchey at 5 o'clock the next morning for her permission to give Benjamin a pulmonary surfactant, a new lifesaving drug, to help him breathe.

"[They] told us it worked best if given in the first six hours of life," McClatchey remembers. "I said, 'He was born at 11:10 last night—you have 10 minutes!'

"The doctor laughed. He said 'Everything's going to be fine.'"

Benjamin received the drug and is indeed fine today. But at birth he developed respiratory distress syndrome, or RDS, a life-threatening lung condition that strikes about 65,000 infants each year. RDS has become more treatable in recent years because of surfactant and new ventilators recently approved by FDA.

RDS is common among the approximately 380,000 premature infants born in the United States each year. About 3,000 infants died of RDS in 1988, making it the fourth most common cause of all infant deaths.

RDS is also called hyaline membrane disease. In 1963, a baby boy born to the then-President and Mrs. John F. Kennedy died of the condition.

But neonatal medicine has improved since then, reducing deaths from RDS steadily over the last 15 years. Preliminary statistics indicate they may have fallen even further—more than 30 percent between 1987 and 1990. FDA's recent approval of several new ventilators and two kinds of surfactant to treat RDS has contributed to premature infants' chances or survival.

Lubricating Lungs

Short for "surface-active agent," a pulmonary surfactant is perhaps the most beneficial new treatment RDS patients like Benjamin can receive. FDA has approved two kinds of surfactant, the first in July 1990 and second a year later.

A pulmonary surfactant is a foamy liquid produced naturally in human and animal lungs. It reduces the surface tension between the wet lung tissue and dry air to keep the tiny air sacs in the lungs, called alveoli, from collapsing between breaths.

Without lung surfactant, every breath requires tremendous force, like blowing up a new balloon.

Because surfactant production is one of the last processes a fetus develops in the womb, preterm infants often don't have it. Commercially prepared surfactants replace the missing natural lung surfactant until the infant can produce his or her own a few days after birth.

"Surfactant has made a dramatic difference in the survival of very-low-birthweight infants," says Dr. K. N. Siva Subramanian, the chief of the Division of Neonatology at Georgetown University Hospital in Washington D.C.

Georgetown has been using a surfactant in clinical trials for more than three years, and doctors say babies who get it require less intensive medical care and less time on ventilators because of it.

The first FDA-approved surfactant was Exosurf Pediatric, a synthetic compound made by Burroughs Wellcome Co. of Research Triangle Park, N.C. The second approved surfactant, Survanta, is a compound made from cow lungs. It was developed in Japan and is distributed by Ross Laboratories of Columbus, Ohio.

Both drugs are passed down the infants' lungs through a ventilator tube. They can be given as "rescue" treatments to babies who have already developed RDS, or "prophylactic" (preventive) treatments to infants at risk of developing RDS.

In either case, studies show that surfactant reduces RDS deaths by about half. They also shorten the time infants need to be on ventilators.

Pulmonary surfactant has been a life-saver to children born unexpectedly early. It has also given hope to parents who know their unborn children are at high risk for prematurity.

For example, in 1990, Leslie and Matthew Carter of Carmel, Ind., chose to have their children at the Indiana University Medical Center in part because they knew the hospital had surfactant.

Leslie Carter was carrying quadruplets, and she knew she would probably deliver early as is often the case with multiple births. Surfactants were not approved for general use at the time, but the Indiana hospital had one through an FDA treatment program that allows lifesaving drugs to be used in certain hospitals before they receive approval.

"We were aware of the drug called surfactant," Leslie Carter remembers, "and we were really glad to be in a hospital where they could use that."

Katelin, Katherine, Abigail, and Elizabeth Carter were born nearly 10 weeks early on Jan. 30, 1990 weighing less than 3 pounds each. They all developed respiratory distress syndrome, were treated with surfactant, and placed on ventilators. At first their progress was slow, but after 2 months in the hospital, all were home and doing well.

"We've been very fortunate," their mother says. "They're really healthy."

The Indiana University Medical Center has participated in clinical trials of both approved pulmonary surfactants for about four years, according to associate professor of pediatrics William A. Engle, M.D., who treated the Carter quadruplets and Benjamin McClatchey.

He says his colleagues have used both kinds with promising results.

"I think the major benefits of surfactant is that it reduces the risks associated with respiratory distress syndrome," Engle says, "and we know that about 50 percent of the babies less than 1,500 grams (3.3 pounds) will have severe hyaline membrane disease."

Bellows for Baby

A surfactant is no miracle cure for respiratory distress syndrome, however. Like Benjamin McClatchey and the Carter quadruplets, infants born too early may still spend months hooked to ventilators to help them breathe.

The newest kind of respirator for newborns is called a "high-frequency ventilator," which works very differently from the older, conventional ventilators.

Conventional ventilators have been used on infants for years and are largely responsible for the drastic drop in infant deaths from RDS throughout the 1970s. The high-frequency concept, a modification of conventional ventilation, was first described in 1959 but wasn't tested on infants until the early 1980s or approved by FDA until 1987.

Conventional ventilators force air down an infants lungs with pressures high enough to expand them, sometimes damaging the delicate airways in the process.

A high-frequency ventilator, however, supplies oxygen to the baby through tiny, rapid puffs of air that barely move the lungs. It creates a vibrating column of air in the lungs without forcing them to expand in the traditional manner.

While a conventional ventilator "breathes" only about 14 times per minute, a high-frequency ventilator puffs at least 150 times per minute.

It's still not scientifically proven, however, whether high-frequency ventilators are better in the long run then the older machines for all premature infants. Doctors use them mostly when conventional ventilation isn't successful.

Since 1987, FDA has approved for use on infants three high-frequency ventilators made by Bunnell Inc. of Salt Lake City, Utah, Infrasonics Inc. of San Diego, Calif., and SensorMedics Corp. of Yorba Linda, Calif.

Despite the benefits of both surfactants and high-frequency ventilators, problems remain.

Neither the surfactant drugs nor the high-frequency ventilator seem to reduce the incidence of a chronic lung condition stemming from long-term ventilator use called bronchopulmonary dysplasia, or BPD.

"That's kind of disappointing," says Dorothy Gail, PhD., chief of the Cell and Developmental Biology Branch at the National Heart, Lung, and Blood Institute.

"Surfactant's great for RDS, but as far as the chronic lung diseases go, it's not what everyone had hoped."

Benjamin McClatchey, for example, developed BPD. He still requires oxygen fed to his nose from a portable tank at home.

Babies on high-frequency ventilators develop other common side effects found with conventional ventilation, such as high blood pressure, a rise in heart rate, brain hemorrhaging, and a condition called pneumothorax, in which air blows out the side of the lungs and in to the chest cavity.

"High-frequency ventilation is just not natural, so the body perceives it as something different and reacts to it," says Jim Dillard, a review scientist at FDA. "Over time, more light will be shed on the overall survival improvements with high-frequency ventilators, if any."

At Indiana University's Riley Hospital for Children, where Benjamin and the Carter quadruplets were treated, doctors use high-frequency ventilators in the severest cases.

Two of the Carters' daughters developed more serious lung problems, and one of them, Abigail, was placed on a Bunnell high-frequency ventilator. The other Katelin, had similar problems but was placed on a conventional ventilator.

"Abigail's lungs healed a lot better and she did a lot better than Katelin did. And their problems were very, very similar," Caret says. "We felt the [high-frequency ventilator] really helped."

"I think it's been moderately successful," says Engle, of the Riley Hospital program. "Babies that would have had less than a 20 percent chance of survival [on conventional ventilation] now have a 50 to 60 percent chance."

Looking for Tomorrow's Cures

In the future, scientists hope to provide even better chances for premature infants like Benjamin and the Carter quadruplets.

In October 1991, a scientist from the Scripps Research Institute in La Jolla, Calif., described in the journal *Science* a new kind of surfactant he manufactured with synthetic human proteins. He said the synthetic human surfactant, if successful in humans, could be more like human surfactant than those presently on the market. It has not been tested in humans to show effectiveness and safety, however, one requirement for FDA approval.

According to the National Heart, Lung, and Blood Institute, scientists are examining human surfactant in a number of studies, researching its basic genetic makeup and how it is produced and used by lungs.

Pre-Term Labor

In clinical settings, doctors are still testing for the best possible dose and time to give a surfactant to newborns, as well as ways to use the drug to treat adult lung disorders.

For many premature children, new technologies have already eased their untimely transitions from the womb to the world.

The Carter quadruplets, for example, are still not as physically mature as other 2-year-olds, but in other ways they have developed normally. "They're doing just wonderfully," their mother says.

Benjamin McClatchey also is doing well. Now nearly 2 years old, he talks as well as any child his age, even though he, too, is catching up to his peers physically.

"I don't let that get me down," says his mother. "He spent a total of seven months in the hospital out of his first 10 months of life, and a baby can't develop in a hospital bed.

"But he's made a lot of progress since we've had him home. He's doing just great."

—by Rebecca Williams

Chapter 16

Medical Care During Labor and Delivery

Chapter Contents

Section 16.1—Pain Relief Options 270
Section 16.2—Epidural 272
Section 16.3—Use of Forceps 273
Section 16.4—Episiotomy 275
Section 16.5—Electronic Fetal Monitoring During Labor 277

Section 16.1

Pain Relief Options

Excerpt from FDA Consumer, December 1992 by Dori Stehlin

Almost every pregnant woman wonders how her labor is going to be. Will it be long and difficult? Will it be so short she'll barely make it to the hospital? And what about the pain?

"There are some women who come in and they're 9 centimeters dilated [dilation is complete at 10 centimeters, when the baby is usually ready to come out], and they say, 'I'm not really sure if I'm in labor,' " says Marion McCartney, a certified nurse-midwife in Bethesda, Md.

No pain; just a little discomfort and then the baby slides out. Wouldn't that be great?

McCartney says it happens. She also says that there are some women who, from the beginning, are in terrible agony. "Those are the extremes," says McCartney. "All the rest of us sort of fall in the middle. You can deal with the early part of labor and you can deal with the middle part of labor and then from 7 to 10 centimeters it really is terrible."

How does a woman deal with the terrible part? For a low-risk woman—one without any medical problems such as diabetes or high blood pressure—the way she copes frequently depends on the philosophy of the person giving her medical care.

Should a woman in labor receive painkillers and anesthetics? While some natural childbirth proponents believe that women who are knowledgeable about and well-prepared for labor will be able to handle the pain without drugs, some medical professionals can't imagine why any woman would want to deal with "unnecessary" pain.

Yet there is a middle ground.

"Labor and delivery should not be an ego trip," says Phill Price, M.D. "It's not about how much pain a woman can endure. It is about producing a healthy baby with a happy mother who is not traumatized for the rest of her life."

That said, Price, who has a private obstetrics practice in Washington, D.C., and reviews new drug applications for the Food and Drug Administration, is quick to point out that drugs are not the only answer. First he encourages his patients experiencing labor pains to walk and to breathe in patterns learned in prepared childbirth class. At the hospital where he delivers babies, there's even a Jacuzzi whirlpool bath that some women find eases the pain.

"The key to having a baby is the ability to relax between the pains," he says. "If you can do it with breathing, fine. If you can do it with a Jacuzzi, fine. But it's easier said than done."

He explains that while many women may think they're relaxing between contractions, "they're actually waiting for that next pain to come. With drugs, a woman may actually go to sleep during the minute or two between contractions."

The drugs that can reduce the pain are either narcotics such as Demerol or non-narcotics such as Nubain. The drugs should be administered only when a woman is between 3 centimeters and 8 centimeters dilated.

"The timing is most important," he says. The drugs may cause breathing problems for the baby if it is born with the drug in its system. Demerol should not be given within two hours of birth and Nubain not within one hour.

The Personal Touch

Perhaps the most important thing to remember is that one 'normal' labor may be very different from the next, says Price. "Things should be individualized," he says. "All deliveries are not the same."

Barbara Good, a certified nurse-midwife who delivers babies at the Columbia Hospital for Women, agrees. "Women are very individual in their responses to pain," she says. "If a woman says, 'I've had it and I'm really ready for [an epidural],' I'm not going to say no. I share the information and I let her choose. It's her birth. I want her to be happy with the experience.

Section 16.2

Epidural

Excerpt from FDA Consumer, December 1992 by Dori Stehlin

If analgesics don't provide enough relief, epidurals may be the next step. Epidurals are anesthetic drugs that cause a loss of pain sensation in the lower half of the body by blocking the pain messages the nerves around the spine normally send to the brain. Injected into the lower back, the amount of numbness depends on the amount of the drug used.

Because administration of an epidural requires the skills of an anesthesiologist, nurse-midwives who, like McCartney, deliver at birth centers instead of hospitals must transfer their patients to a hospital if an epidural is necessary.

Anesthesiologist Murray Malin, M.D., who practices at the Columbia Hospital for Women in Washington, D.C., feels the benefits of epidurals far outweigh the risks, especially if the medication is given continuously through a pump. Not used routinely as little as five years ago, a pump allows a much lower concentration of the drug than would be necessary if the drug were given in intermittent doses.

When a pump isn't used, a higher dose of the drug becomes necessary to ensure enough pain relief as the medication's effects wear off, and this could result in a drop in the mother's blood pressure. That, in turn, could cause fetal distress. While those risks aren't eliminated with the use of a pump, they are substantially reduced. However, other risks still exist.

"Epidurals are a double-edged sword," says Price. "They help to relieve pain. They also have a tendency to arrest labor. Worst of all, epidurals take away the bearing down reflex [necessary to push the baby out]."

Those disadvantages—slowing the labor and not being able to push—outweigh the benefits, according to McCartney.

If labor slows down, the woman may be given Pitocin (oxytocin), a synthetic hormone, to speed things up. But contractions resulting from

Medical Care During Labor and Delivery

Pitocin are usually stronger than naturally occurring ones and may cause some fetal distress.

"The safest way to have babies is not to have any medication," she says. "Only if there is a problem—a terribly long labor, the woman is exhausted—should you start to intervene. You shouldn't intervene in a process that's going very well. Save those good anesthesias for people that really, really need them."

Section 16.3

Use of Forceps

Excerpt from FDA Consumer, December 1992 by Dori Stehlin

A forceps is a surgical instrument that looks like two large spoons or salad tongs. A medical device, it is regulated by FDA. The doctor inserts the forceps into the birth canal, places the "spoons" around the baby's head, and, with each contraction, moves the baby down, and eventually out of, the birth canal.

Another medical device, the vacuum extractor, may be used in place of forceps. The extractor consists of a soft plastic or rubber cap held in place on the baby's head by suction from a vacuum pump.

Medical reasons for forceps delivery include a slow or irregular fetal heartbeat, failure of the baby's head to rotate into the proper position, or failure of the mother to push because of fatigue or an epidural.

Outlet forceps delivery—when the head is visible at the vaginal opening—involves the least risk. A study by Michael K. Yancey, M.D., and colleagues at the Madigan Army Medical Center, Tacoma, Wash., reported in the October 1991 issue of *Obstetrics and Gynecology,* found that an outlet forceps delivery in an uncomplicated labor causes no immediate harm to the baby. (The study did not address the possibility of any long-term effects.) However, the study did find these mothers had increased incidence of cuts and tears in the perineum (the area between the anus and the vagina) compared to women whose babies were delivered without forceps.

The risk level of outlet forceps delivery increases as the doctor moves the forceps higher into the birth canal.

"Difficult forceps deliveries involving a lot of rotation of the baby's head or pulling it down from high up in the birth canal are done quite infrequently in most parts of this country," says Wayne R. Cohen, M.D., vice chairman of the department of obstetrics and gynecology at the Albert Einstein College of Medicine in New York City. "The basic principle is that the more difficult the forceps delivery, the greater the risk."

The risks from a difficult forceps delivery range from minor injuries to the baby's head, such as bruises and indentations—both temporary—to serious problems, including skull fracture, eye injury, facial paralysis, and brain damage. Forceps may also cause damage to the mother's bladder or urethra (the tube that carries urine from the bladder to the outside of the body).

If the baby must be delivered right away, says Cohen, a Caesarean section (surgical delivery of the baby through an incision in the abdominal and uterine walls) involves less risk to both mother and baby and is therefore usually preferable to a difficult forceps delivery.

Besides helping a baby in distress, another reason for using forceps often cited by obstetricians is to shorten the second stage of labor and, in turn, reduce the risk of damage to the pelvic floor and tissues supporting the bladder and rectum that might occur with prolonged pushing. (The second stage of labor begins when the cervix is fully dilated and ends with the baby's birth. It can last for more than two hours, especially during a first labor.) But according to Yancey's study, routine use of forceps "does not significantly shorten the second stage of labor."

"No one wants to put forceps on babies unless there's a medical reason for doing it," says Price. That's why he tells his patients that he will let the epidural wear off so they can feel and push the baby out themselves.

McCartney advocates that women be allowed to keep pushing as long as fetal heart tones are good and progress is being made.

Cohen agrees. "Intervening with forceps during the second stage offers no advantage to the fetus as long as the fetal condition is good."

Section 16.4

Episiotomy

Excerpt from FDA Consumer, December 1992 by Dori Stehlin

Another intervention, one of the most common surgical procedures performed in North America, is episiotomy, the cutting of the perineum. The rationale behind routine episiotomy—that cutting is safer for the mother than the tearing that sometimes occurs during delivery—has been increasingly questioned in recent years.

The two types of episiotomies are:

- *Midline* — cut straight down from the vagina in the direction of the rectum. Considered to be more comfortable afterward and easier to repair.

- *Mediolateral* — perineum is cut diagonally to one side. Will prevent a tear from continuing on to the rectum, but is more difficult to repair and takes longer to heal than midline.

The American College of Obstetricians and Gynecologists recommends that doctors perform episiotomies if the baby is large, the woman's perineum is short, or to make room for a forceps delivery.

In addition, while an episiotomy can speed delivery by only a few minutes, even that amount of time can be critical if the baby is in distress.

But what about performing episiotomy just as a measure to prevent tearing?

The common philosophy is that a straight cut will be less painful and heal quicker than a jagged tear. But according to a study in the July 1, 1992, *Online Journal of Current Clinical Trials,* there was no difference in pain levels or recovery time between women who had an episiotomy and women who had spontaneous tissue tears.

The theory that an episiotomy prevents severe, out-of-control tears that reach the rectum was also refuted in that study. Doctors who restricted the use of episiotomies to cases of fetal distress or forceps delivery had a severe tear rate of 4.9 percent. The other group of doctors, who performed episiotomies on all patients, had a severe tear rate of 23 percent.

Even without the severe tear, any woman who gets an episiotomy gets a second-degree laceration, which means underlying tissue is involved. (Third-degree lacerations extend to the rectal sphincter (muscle) and fourth-degree go into the rectum.)

However, many women don't tear at all while giving birth or only tear the skin (first-degree laceration). First-degree tears may not require any stitches.

Another argument often cited to support performing episiotomies is that without the incision, the pressure on both the perineum and the baby's head could cause long-term damage to the mother's pelvic floor or to the baby's brain.

There are no strong studies to support or refute that hypothesis, according to Stephen B. Thacker, M.D., a researcher with the national Centers for Disease Control.

Preventing tears is possible in some cases, but it requires extra effort from both the mother and the person delivering the baby.

Delivery position is one important factor in preventing tears. McCartney recommends upright positions such as sitting, squatting or kneeling because in these positions "the pelvic area, including the perineum, is relaxed, and pushing with gravity is easier."

Finally, the care-giver needs to encourage the mother not to push the baby out too fast. McCartney always tells her mothers, "I want you to push this baby out one hair at a time so you don't tear."

Medical Care During Labor and Delivery

Section 16.5

Electronic Fetal Monitoring During Labor

Excerpt from FDA Consumer, December 1992 by Dori Stehlin and Online Publication of the U.S. Preventative Services Task Force, Feb 1997 by Carolyn DiGuiseppi

The unborn baby's heart rate is an important indicator of how things are going. The heartbeat can be monitored by a care-giver with a special stethoscope called a fetoscope or by an electronic fetal monitor.

Electronic fetal monitors, which are FDA-approved medical devices, measure the baby's heart rate continuously in one of two ways: externally or internally. With external monitors, two belts are placed around the mother's abdomen. One belt uses ultrasound to monitor the baby's heartbeat while the other measures the length of contractions. Internal monitors measure the baby's heart rate through an electrode attached to the baby's scalp.

Both types of monitors usually require the mother to stay in bed so the belts or electrodes stay in place.

Although measuring and recording every heartbeat sounds ideal, not everyone thinks the technology is an advantage.

"When I started delivering babies in 1971," says FDA's Phill Price, M.D., "physicians really believed that electronic fetal monitoring would be a tool that would tell us if a baby was going to be in trouble. But the last 8 to 10 years have told us that electronic fetal monitoring has not done a lot to actually improve the overall care of mothers or babies."

The theory behind the continuous monitoring is that the care-giver could note a change in the baby's heart rate immediately and take immediate action to prevent any harm to the baby. That action, almost always, is a Caesarean section.

The harm doctors are most concerned about is oxygen starvation, which can lead to conditions such as cerebral palsy.

However, in the last 25 years the incidence of cerebral palsy has remained the same—3 per 1,000 whether the patient was monitored or not, says Price.

Some babies are going to have problems, and in all likelihood those problems occurred during the nine months of pregnancy, he explains. "To think that because 1 waited 5 or 10 or 15 minutes before doing a C-section the baby will come up with cerebral palsy is ludicrous," he says. "If you have a nurse who listens every 15 minutes in the first stage of labor and every five minutes in the second stage, you can get the same outcome."

"If I'm physically present, I can be pretty sure if things are fine or if things are starting to go wrong," says Barbara Good, a certified nurse-midwife in Takoma Park, Md.

But Wayne Cohen, M.D., of the Albert Einstein College of Medicine in New York City, says he has serious doubts about replacing electronic monitors with "old-fashioned" intermittent listening to the heart rate, because a monitor can pick up very uncommon patterns that might be missed by the intermittent method. While he agrees with Price that some of those uncommon patterns may indicate brain damage that occurred before labor even began, "I don't think our knowledge is sophisticated enough yet to be able to be say when we see a very abnormal pattern that no benefit can be accrued by delivering as quickly as possible."

Recommendation

Routine electronic fetal monitoring for low-risk women in labor is not recommended. There is insufficient evidence to recommend for or against intrapartum electronic fetal monitoring for high-risk pregnant women.

Burden of Suffering

Intrapartum fetal asphyxia is an important cause of stillbirth and neonatal death. In the U.S. in 1993, an estimated 700 infant deaths (17.3/100,000 live births) were attributed to intrauterine hypoxia and birth asphyxia. Some neonates with intrauterine hypoxia require resuscitation and other aggressive medical interventions for such complications as acidosis and seizures. Asphyxia has also been implicated as a cause of cerebral palsy, although most cases of cerebral palsy occur in persons without evidence of birth asphyxia or other intrapartum events. Most fetuses tolerate intrauterine hypoxia during labor and are delivered without complications, but assessments suggesting fetal distress are associated with an increased likelihood of cesarean delivery (63% compared to 23% for all births). The exact

Medical Care During Labor and Delivery

incidence of fetal distress is uncertain; a rate of 42.9/1,000 live births was reported from 1991 U.S. birth certificate data, with the highest rates in infants born to mothers under age 20 or over age 40, and in blacks.

Accuracy of Fetal Monitoring

The principal screening technique for fetal distress and hypoxia during labor is the measurement of fetal heart rate. Abnormal decelerations in fetal heart rate and decreased beat-to-beat variability during uterine contractions are considered to be suggestive of fetal distress. The detection of these patterns during monitoring by auscultation or during electronic monitoring (cardiotocography) increases the likelihood that the fetus is in distress, but the patterns are not diagnostic. In addition, normal or equivocal heart rate patterns do not exclude the diagnosis of fetal distress. Precise information on the frequency of false-negative and false-positive results is lacking, however, due in large part to the absence of an accepted definition of fetal distress. For many years, acidosis and hypoxemia as determined by fetal scalp blood pH were used for this purpose in research and clinical practice, but it is now clear that neither finding is diagnostic of fetal distress.

Electronic fetal heart rate monitoring can detect at least some cases of fetal distress, and it is often used for routine monitoring of women in labor. In 1991, the reported rate of electronic fetal monitoring in the U.S. was 755/1,000 live births. The published performance characteristics of this technology, derived largely from research at major academic centers, may overestimate the accuracy that can be expected when this test is performed for routine screening in typical community settings. Two factors in particular that may limit the accuracy and reliability achievable in actual practice are the method used to measure fetal heart activity and the variability associated with cardiotocogram interpretations.

Measurement of Fetal Heart Rate

The measurement of fetal heart activity is performed most accurately by attaching an electrode directly to the fetal scalp, an invasive procedure requiring amniotomy and associated with occasional complications. This has been the technique used in most clinical trials of electronic fetal monitoring.

Other noninvasive techniques of monitoring fetal heart rate, which include external Doppler ultrasound and periodic auscultation of heart sounds by clinicians, are more appropriate for widespread screening but provide less precise data than the direct electrocardiogram using a fetal scalp electrode. In studies comparing external ultrasound with the direct electrocardiogram, about 20-25% of tracings differed by at least 5 beats per minute.

A second factor influencing the reliability of widespread fetal heart rate monitoring is inconsistency in interpreting results. Several studies have documented significant intra- and interobserver variation in assessing cardiotocograms even when tracings are read by experts in electronic fetal monitoring. It would be expected that routine performance of electronic monitoring in the community setting with interpretations by less experienced clinicians would generate a higher proportion of inaccurate results and potentially unnecessary interventions than has been observed in the published work of major research centers.

Effectiveness of Early Detection

A potentially more important issue is whether electronic evidence of fetal distress during labor results in benefit to either the fetus or mother. Observational studies in the 1960s and 1970s suggested that electronic fetal monitoring during labor reduced the risk of intrapartum stillbirth, neonatal death, and developmental disability, but methodologic problems in these largely retrospective studies left the issue unsettled. Ten randomized controlled trials and four meta-analyses of electronic fetal monitoring have since been published, all of which compared electronic monitoring, with or without fetal scalp blood sampling, to active clinical monitoring including intermittent auscultation by trained personnel.

Three trials in low-risk women, the largest of which involved nearly 13,000 patients, compared continuous electronic monitoring to intermittent auscultation; where described, auscultation was performed at least every 15 minutes during the first stage of labor and between each contraction during the second stage. Two trials included scalp blood sampling. These trials found no significant differences between the study groups in intrapartum or perinatal deaths, maternal or neonatal morbidity, Apgar scores, umbilical cord blood gases, the need for assisted ventilation, or admission to the special care nursery. The results of one of these trials may have been biased by the method of randomization, however, which resulted in a large disparity in the distribution of primigravidae between the study groups. Similarly, no differences in clinical outcomes were reported in a subgroup analysis of low-risk women enrolled in a prospective study of nearly 35,000 pregnancies in which routine monitoring was compared with selective monitoring of high-risk pregnancies. A controlled trial that assigned intervention by week of admission also reported no effect of electronic fetal monitoring on low Apgar scores, admissions to special care nurseries, or neonatal infection. A trial from Greece carried out in predominantly low-risk pregnant women found no differences in most neonatal outcome measures, but reported a significant reduction in perinatal mortality rates (2.6 compared to 13/1,000 total births). This study may not be generalizable to the U.S., however, given higher perinatal mortality and substantially lower cesarean delivery rates (about 10%) than are typical in the U.S. In addition, the method of randomization and the large disparity in numbers between study and control group (746 vs. 682 women) raise the possibility of biased randomization.

Fetal Monitoring in High-Risk Pregnancy

The potential benefits of electronic fetal monitoring during labor have also been examined in high-risk pregnancies. Four clinical trials in developed countries found that electronic fetal heart rate monitoring in high-risk pregnancies, with or without scalp blood sampling, was of limited benefit when compared with intermittent auscultation during labor. Neonatal death, Apgar scores, cord blood gases, and neonatal nursery morbidity were unchanged in three of the trials, all of which performed intermittent auscultation systematically in control women: every 15 minutes in the first stage of labor and every 5 minutes in the second stage. The fourth trial found that continuous monitoring was associated with improved umbilical cord blood gases and neurologic symptoms and signs, and decreased need for intensive care. This study has been criticized, however, because monitoring techniques in the control group were poorly described and one physician withdrew his patients from the control group after the trial began.

Meta-analyses that included all but the two most recently published randomized controlled trials reported no effect of electronic fetal monitoring on low Apgar scores, admissions to special care nurseries, or neonatal infection. With electronic fetal monitoring combined with scalp blood sampling, the relative risk of intrapartum death was 0.81 (95% confidence interval, 0.22 to 2.98) and of perinatal death was 0.98 (95% confidence interval, 0.58 to 1.64) when compared to intermittent auscultation. Relative risk of perinatal mortality when electronic fetal monitoring without blood sampling was used was 1.94 (95% confidence interval, 0.2 to 18.62). A meta-analysis of all trials from developed countries also reported no significant effect on overall perinatal mortality (typical odds ratio 0.87; 95% confidence interval, 0.57 to 1.33). The confidence intervals around these point estimates of the risk of perinatal death are wide, indicating that sample size is insufficient to exclude the possibility of clinically important increases or declines in mortality. One meta-analysis reported a significant reduction in perinatal mortality due to fetal hypoxia, but the method for attributing deaths to hypoxia was not standardized. The results appeared to be strongly influenced by the inclusion of one trial with questionable randomization methods and generalizability to the U.S.

Although most outcome measures in these studies were not influenced by electronic fetal monitoring, there is evidence that it reduces the incidence of neonatal seizures. This was suggested in early research and confirmed in the Dublin trial of low-risk women. This study reported a statistically significant reduction in the rate of neonatal seizures when continuous intrapartum fetal monitoring was compared with intermittent auscultation. Secondary analysis suggested that the reduced risk was limited to labors that were prolonged or induced or augmented with oxytocin. In a meta-analysis of the controlled trials that included scalp blood sampling as an adjunct, the odds of neonatal seizures were reduced by about one half with electronic monitoring. A separate meta-analysis found no effect of electronic monitoring on neonatal seizures when no scalp blood sampling was performed, raising the possibility that the benefit may have been due to the blood sampling rather than the electronic monitoring. What also remains unclear is the extent to which infants benefit from the prevention of neonatal seizures by monitoring. Seizures have been viewed by many as a poor prognostic indicator; in the Dublin trial, death occurred in 23% of the babies who experienced seizures, and autopsy confirmed that at least two thirds of these deaths were due to asphyxia during labor. There are few prospective data on whether the prevention of neonatal seizures reduces the risk of neonatal death or long-term neurologic sequelae. The neonatal seizures prevented by electronic monitoring may not be those associated with long-term impairment. At 4-year follow-up of survivors after seizures in the Dublin trial, the total number and rate with cerebral palsy (n = 3, and 0.5/1,000 enrolled subjects) were identical in the monitored and control groups.

None of the three trials reporting longer term follow-up found that electronic fetal monitoring improved neurologic or developmental outcomes. A follow-up study of the growth and development at 9 months of age of infants involved in the second Denver trial failed to show any long-term benefits of electronic fetal monitoring; the direction of the effect on mental and psychomotor development scores suggested increased risk in the monitored group. In the Dublin trial, the overall rates of cerebral palsy at 4-year follow-up were 1.8/1,000 in the electronically monitored group and 1.5/1,000 in the auscultation group. Eighteen-month follow-up in a trial in high-risk women revealed little difference in mean mental or psychomotor development scores on the Bayley Scales, but cerebral palsy and low mental development scores were both significantly more common in the electronically monitored group. Cerebral palsy was associated with an increased duration of abnormal fetal heart rate patterns and time to delivery after diagnosis of such patterns in the electronically monitored group. Meta-analyses combining these three studies confirm little benefit from monitoring on adverse neurologic outcomes.

Benefits Versus Risks

Any potential benefit of intrapartum monitoring must be weighed against the potential risks associated both with diagnostic procedures and operative interventions for fetal distress. The insertion of fetal scalp electrodes, for example, is generally a safe procedure, but it may occasionally cause umbilical cord prolapse or infection due to early amniotomy; electrode or pressure catheter trauma to the eye, fetal vessels, umbilical cord, or placenta; and scalp infections with Herpes hominis type 2 or group B streptococcus. Concerns have also been raised about the potential for enhancing transmission of human immunodeficiency virus (HIV) infection by the use of scalp electrodes. Meta-analysis of randomized controlled trials indicates no increased risk of neonatal infection from electronic fetal monitoring compared to intermittent auscultation. Perhaps the most important complication of intrapartum electronic fetal monitoring is the increased performance of cesarean delivery, an operation associated with maternal and neonatal morbidity and a small but measurable operative mortality. Fetal distress is a common indication for cesarean delivery, and all trials showed a higher cesarean delivery rate in the electronically monitored group. The randomized controlled trials from the 1970s reported that cesarean delivery was performed significantly more frequently in association with electronic fetal monitoring. In recent years, an effort has been made to lower the frequency of cesarean delivery, and four of five trials carried out in developed countries in the 1980s or 1990s reported no significant increase in the overall cesarean delivery rate with electronic fetal monitoring. A fifth trial, comparing routine to selective electronic monitoring, reported a very small increase that was statistically but not clinically significant.

On the other hand, operative vaginal (e.g., forceps) deliveries were significantly increased in the newer trials, suggesting an inverse relationship between cesarean and operative vaginal delivery.

The meta-analyses previously cited reported a 1.3- to 2.7-fold increased likelihood of cesarean delivery and a 2-to 4.1-fold increased likelihood of cesarean delivery for fetal distress with continuous electronic fetal monitoring, with lower rates in the meta-analysis of studies that used scalp blood sampling. The likelihood of any operative delivery was increased by about 30% with electronic fetal monitoring. The meta-analyses also reported higher rates of both maternal infection and general anesthesia with electronic monitoring, presumably secondary to the higher rates of operative delivery. Electronic monitoring may also have adverse psychological effects. In a comparison of subsamples from the randomized groups in one trial, women who had electronic fetal monitoring reported an increased likelihood of feeling "too restricted" during labor and were also more likely to report feeling left alone, although the latter difference was of only borderline significance. On the other hand, in a subsample from a different trial, there were no differences between women in the two groups in their assessment of their monitoring experience, medical or nursing support, or the labor or delivery experience.

Recommendations of Other Groups

The American College of Obstetricians and Gynecologists states that all patients in labor need some form of fetal monitoring, with more intensified monitoring indicated in high-risk pregnancies; the choice of technique (electronic fetal monitoring or intermittent auscultation) is based on various factors, including the resources available. The Canadian Task Force on the Periodic Health Examination advises against routine electronic fetal monitoring in normal pregnancies but found poor evidence regarding the inclusion or exclusion of its routine use in high-risk pregnancies.

Discussion

Electronic fetal monitoring has become an accepted standard of care in many settings in the U.S. for the management of labor. Birth certificate data suggest that this technology was used in about three fourths of all live births in 1991; in certain academic centers the rate may be as high as 86-100%. As discussed above, there are important questions regarding the definition of fetal distress, as well as about the accuracy and reliability of electronic fetal monitoring in discriminating accurately between pregnancies with and without this disorder. It is also unclear whether the use of this technology results in significantly improved outcome for the baby when compared to active clinical monitoring. Adequately conducted trials generalizable to obstetric care in the U.S. have not reported a reduction in perinatal mortality, although sample sizes are not adequate to exclude a benefit.

Evidence does support a reduced risk of neonatal seizures, but the benefit was mainly seen in women with complicated labors (i.e., induced, augmented with oxytocin, or prolonged), and it is not clear that there are long-term adverse effects associated with the types of seizures prevented. Follow-up of study subjects at 9 months to 4 years of age has not revealed any long-term neurologic benefits from electronic monitoring. If anything, effect estimates suggest an increased risk of cerebral palsy and low developmental scores in electronically monitored infants, possibly due to false reassurance and consequent delayed intervention.

In addition to the maternal risks associated with electronic fetal monitoring, including increased rates of cesarean or operative vaginal (e.g., forceps) delivery, general anesthesia and maternal infection, and the possible increased risk of adverse neonatal neurologic outcome, increased use of this technology is associated with increased costs of labor care. The widespread use of electronic fetal monitoring in low-risk pregnancies in the face of uncertain benefits, and certain maternal risks and costs, has been attributed to concerns about litigation.

It has been estimated that nearly 40% of all obstetric malpractice losses are due to fetal monitoring problems, and this may be a major motivating factor behind the widespread use of electronic fetal monitoring during labor.

Clinical Intervention

Routine electronic fetal monitoring is not recommended for low-risk women in labor when adequate clinical monitoring including intermittent auscultation by trained staff is available. There is insufficient evidence to recommend for or against electronic fetal monitoring over intermittent auscultation for high-risk pregnancies.

For pregnant women with complicated labor (i.e., induced, prolonged, or oxytocin augmented), recommendations for electronic monitoring plus scalp blood sampling may be made on the basis of evidence for a reduced risk of neonatal seizures, although the long-term neurologic benefit to the neonate is unclear and must be weighed against the increased risk to the mother and neonate of operative delivery, general anesthesia, and maternal infection, and a possible increased risk of adverse neurologic outcome in the infant. There is currently no evidence available to evaluate electronic fetal monitoring in comparison to no monitoring.

References

National Center for Health Statistics. Annual summary of births, marriages, divorces, and deaths: United States,1993. Monthly vital statistics report; vol 42, no 13. Hyattsville, MD:Public Health Service, 1994.

Freeman JM, Nelson KB. Intrapartum asphyxia and cerebral palsy. Pediatrics 1988; 82:240-249.

Nelson KB, Ellenberg JH. Antecedents of cerebral palsy. Multivariate analysis of risk. N Engl J Med 1986; 315:81-86.

Shy KK, Larson EB, Luthy DA. Evaluating a new technology: the effectiveness of electronic fetal heart rate monitoring. Ann Rev Public Health 1987; 8:165-190.

Goodlin RC, Haesslein HC. When is it fetal distress? Am J Obstet Gynecol 1977; 128:440-445.

Taffel SM. Cesarean delivery in the United States,1990. National Center for Health Statistics. Vital Health Statistics, Series 21, no. 51. Washington, DC:Government Printing Office, 1994. (Publication no. DHHS (PHS) 94-1929.)

National Center for Health Statistics. Advance report of maternal and infant health data from the birth certificate, 1991. Monthly vital statistics report; vol 42, no 11. Hyattsville, MD: Public Health Service, 1994.

Prentice A, Lind T. Fetal heart rate monitoring during labour: too frequent intervention, too little benefit? Lancet 1987; 2:1375-1377.

American College of Obstetricians and Gynecologists Committee on Obstetric Practice. Fetal distress and birth asphyxia. Committee Opinion no. 137. Washington, DC: American College of Obstetricians and Gyecologists, 1994.

Pritchard JA, MacDonald PC, Gant NF. Williams obstetrics, 17th ed. Norwalk, CT: Appleton-Century-Crofts, 1985: 281-293.

Perkins RP. Perinatal observations in a high-risk population managed without intrapartum fetal pH studies. Am J Obstet Gynecol 1984; 149:327-334.

Clark SL, Paul RH. Intrapartum fetal surveillance: the role of fetal scalp blood sampling. Am J Obstet Gynecol 1985; 153:717-720.

Suidan JS, Young BK, Hochberg HM, et al. Observations on perinatal heart rate monitoring. II. Quantitative unreliability of Doppler fetal heart rate variability. J Reprod Med 1985; 30:519-522.

Boehm FH, Fields LM, Hutchison JM, et al. The indirectly obtained fetal heart rate: comparison of first-and second-generation electronic fetal monitors. Am J Obstet Gynecol 1986; 155:10-14.

Cohen AB, Klapholz H, Thompson MS. Electronic fetal monitoring and clinical practice: a survey of obstetric opinion. Med Decis Making 1982; 2:79-95.

Beaulieu MD, Fabia J, Leduc B, et al. The reproducibility of intrapartum cardiotocogram assessments. Can Med Assoc J 1982; 127:214-216.

Nielsen PV, Stigsby B, Nickelsen C, et al. Intra-and inter-observer variability in the assessment of intrapartum cardiotocograms. Acta Obstet Gynecol Scand 1987; 66:421-424.

Kelso IM, Parsons RJ, Lawrence GF, et al. An assessment of continuous fetal heart rate monitoring in labor: a randomized trial. Am J Obstet Gynecol 1978; 131:526-531.

Wood C, Renou P, Oats J, et al. A controlled trial of fetal heart rate monitoring in a low-risk obstetric population. Am J Obstet Gynecol 1981; 141:527-534.

MacDonald D, Grant A, Sheridan-Pereira M, et al. The Dublin randomized controlled trial of intrapartum fetal heart rate monitoring. Am J Obstet Gynecol 1985; 152:524-539.

Leveno KJ, Cunningham FG, Nelson S, et al. A prospective comparison of selective and universal electronic fetal monitoring in 34,995 pregnancies. N Engl J Med 1986; 315:615-619.

Neilson JP. Liberal vs. restrictive use of EFM in labour (low-risk labours). In: Enkin MW, Keirse MJNC, Renfrew MJ, Neilson JP, eds. Pregnancy and childbirth module. Cochrane database of systematic reviews:review no. 03886, 12 May 1994, "Cochrane Updates on Disk." Oxford:Update Software, 1994, Disk Issue 1.

Neldam S, Osler M, Hansen PK, et al. Intrapartum fetal heart rate monitoring in a combined low-and high-risk population: a controlled clinical trial. Eur J Obstet Gynecol Reprod Biol 1986; 23:1-11.

Vintzileos AM, Antsaklis A, Varvarigos I, et al. A randomized trial of intrapartum fetal heart rate monitoring versus intermittent auscultation. Obstet Gynecol 1993; 81:899-907.

Renou P, Chang A, Anderson I, et al. Controlled trial of fetal intensive care. Am J Obstet Gynecol 1976; 126:470-476.

Haverkamp AD, Thompson HE, McFee JG, et al. The evaluation of continuous fetal heart rate monitoring in high-risk pregnancy. Am J Obstet Gynecol 1976; 125:310-317.

Haverkamp AD, Orleans M, Langendoerfer S, et al. A controlled trial of the differential effects of intrapartum fetal monitoring. Am J Obstet Gynecol 1979; 134:399-409.

Luthy DA, Shy KK, van Belle G, et al. A randomized trial of electronic fetal monitoring in preterm labor. Obstet Gynecol 1987; 69:687-695.

Thacker SB. The efficacy of intrapartum electronic fetal monitoring. Am J Obstet Gynecol 1987; 156:24-30.

Mahomed K, Nyoni R, Mulambo T, et al. Randomised controlled trial of intrapartum fetal heart rate monitoring. BMJ 1994; 308:497-500.

Neilson JP. EFM + scalp sampling vs. intermittent auscultation in labour. In: Enkin MW, Keirse MJNC, Renfrew MJ, Neilson JP, eds. Pregnancy and childbirth module. Cochrane database of systematic reviews:review no. 03297, 4 May 1994, "Cochrane Updates on Disk." Oxford: Update Software, 1994, Disk Issue 1.

Neilson JP. EFM alone vs. intermittent auscultation in labour. In: Enkin MW, Keirse MJNC, Renfrew MJ, Neilson JP, eds. Pregnancy and childbirth module. Cochrane database of systematic reviews:review no. 03298, 4 May 1994, "Cochrane Updates on Disk." Oxford: Update Software, 1994, Disk Issue 1.

Neilson JP. EFM vs. intermittent auscultation in labour. In: Enkin MW, Keirse MJNC, Renfrew MJ, Neilson JP, eds. Pregnancy and childbirth module. Cochrane database of systematic reviews:review no. 03884, 4 May 1994, "Cochrane Updates on Disk." Oxford: Update Software, 1994, Disk Issue 1.

Vintzileos AM, Nochimson DJ, Guzman ER, et al. Intrapartum electronic fetal heart rate monitoring versus intermittent auscultation: a meta-analysis. Obstet Gynecol 1995; 85:149-155.

Chalmers I. Randomized controlled trials of intrapartum monitoring. In: Thalhammer O, Baumgarten KV, Pollak A, eds. Perinatal Medicine. Stuttgart: Georg Thieme, 1979: 260-265.

Grant A, O'Brien N, Joy M-T, et al. Cerebral palsy among children born during the Dublin randomised trial of intrapartum monitoring. Lancet 1989; ii:1233-1236.

Langendoerfer S, Haverkamp AD, Murphy J, et al. Pediatric follow-up of a randomized controlled trial of intrapartum fetal monitoring techniques. J Pediatr 1980; 97:103-107.

Shy KK, Luthy DA, Bennett FC, et al. Effects of electronic fetal-heart-rate monitoring, as compared with periodic auscultation, on the neurologic development of premature infants. N Engl J Med 1990; 322:588-593.

American College of Obstetricians and Gynecologists. Human immunodeficiency virus infections. Technical Bulletin no. 169. Washington, DC: American College of Obstetricians and Gynecologists, 1992.

American Academy of Pediatrics and American College of Obstetricians and Gynecologists. Guidelines for perinatal care. 3rd ed. Elk Grove Village, IL: American Academy of Pediatrics, 1992.

Pearson J, Rees G. Technique of caesarean section. In: Chalmers I, Enkin M, Keirse MJNC, eds. Effective care in pregnancy and childbirth, volume 2: childbirth. Oxford: Oxford University Press, 1989: 1234-1269.

Garcia J, Corry M, MacDonald D, et al. Mothers' views of continuous electronic fetal heart monitoring and intermittent auscultation in a randomised controlled trial. Birth 1985; 12:79-85.

Killien MG, Shy K. A randomized trial of electronic fetal monitoring in preterm labor: mothers' views. Birth 1989; 16:7-12.

American College of Obstetricians and Gynecologists. Intrapartum fetal heart rate monitoring. Technical Bulletin no. 132. Washington, DC: American College of Obstetricians and Gynecologists, 1989.

Canadian Task Force on the Periodic Health Examination. Canadian guide to clinical preventive health care. Ottawa: Canada Communication Group, 1994: 158-165.

Cunningham AS. Electronic fetal monitoring in labour. J R Soc Med 1987; 80:783.

Frigoletto FD Jr, Nadel AS. Electronic fetal heart rate monitoring: why the dilemma? Clin Obstet Gynecol 1988; 31:179-183.

Chapter 17

Cesarean Childbirth

Cesarean childbirth, an operation to deliver a baby through an incision in the abdomen, can be traced back through history to Egypt in 3000 B.C. The procedures's name comes from a set of Roman laws, *Lex Caesare,* which in 715 B.C. mandated surgical removal of an unborn fetus upon death of the mother.

Until recent decades the operation usually had been used as a last resort because of a high rate of maternal complications and death. But with the availability of antibiotics to fight infection and the development of modern surgical techniques, the once high maternal mortality rate has dropped dramatically. As a result, the cesarean childbirth rate has increased dramatically. From 1970 to 1980, the number of cesareans in the U.S. more than tripled, increasing from 5 percent of all births to 16.5 percent. In some localities the rate is much higher.

This startling increase has become a matter of national concern. In the fall of 1980, the National Institute of Child Health and Human Development convened a panel to gather information and develop a draft report on the subject. This report formed the basis for a three-day conference held to examine the issues related to cesarean childbirth, reach general agreement and make recommendations to guide practicing physicians. This "consensus development" panel, made up of leading scientists, practicing physicians and consumers, produced a 540 page final report.

NIH document entitled Facts about Cesarean Childbirth, 1982

Basically, the panel concluded that the rising cesarean birth rate can be stopped and perhaps reversed, without sacrificing continued improvements in the quality and success of pregnancy care.

What is cesarean childbirth?

A major operation, each cesarean actually involves a series of separate incisions in the mother. The skin, underlying muscles and abdomen are opened first and then the uterus is opened allowing removal of the infant.

There are two main types of cesarean operations, each named according to the location and direction of the uterine incision:

- cervical—a transverse (horizontal) or vertical incision in the lower uterus, and

- classical—a vertical incision in the main body of the uterus.

Today, the *low transverse* cervical incision is used almost exclusively. It has the lowest incidence of hemorrhage during surgery as well as the least chance of rupturing in later pregnancies. Sometimes, because of fetal size (very large or very small) or position problems (breech or transverse), a *low vertical* cesarean may be performed.

In the *classical* operation, a vertical incision allows a greater opening and is used for fetal size or position problems and in some emergency situations. This approach involves more bleeding in surgery and a higher risk of abdominal infection. Although any uterine incision

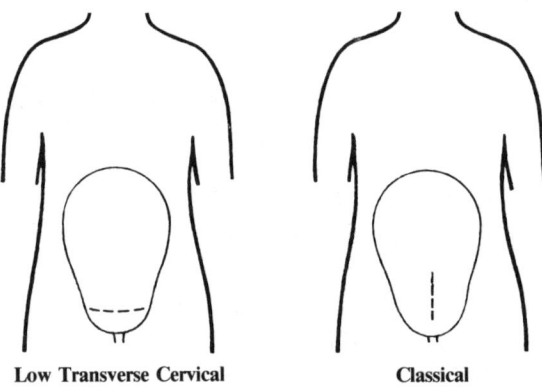

Figure 17.1. Types of Cesarean Incisions

may rupture during a subsequent labor, the classical is more likely to do so and more likely to result in death for the mother and fetus than a cervical incision.

Why have cesarean rates increased?

Many factors account for rising cesarean birth rates. By the 1960's, increasing emphasis was being placed on the health of the fetus. With declining birth rates and couples having fewer children, even greater attention was given to improving the outcome of pregnancy, and infant survival in general. The nation's infant mortality rate began to be seen as an international yardstick on the quality of health care.

At the same time, advances in medical care combined to make maternal death from cesarean childbirth a rare occurrence. The safer the procedure became, the easier it was to decide to perform the operation. As a safe alternative to normal delivery, the cesarean became a practical way to try to improve the outcome of difficult pregnancies.

Studies suggesting the benefit of cesarean birth in dealing with various pregnancy complications also led to more cesareans. Obstetricians came to favor surgery in pregnancies with difficult deliveries that formerly would have required the use of forceps. The diagnosis of "dystocia," a catch-all term meaning difficult labor, was made more frequently and handled more often with the cesarean operation. Fetal distress during labor—a condition often resulting in a cesarean—was more apt to be detected with the introduction of electronic fetal monitoring. Increasingly, physicians used the cesarean method to deliver infants in the breech position prior to birth, adding still further to the rising cesarean rate.

Another important contributing factor was the rising number of repeat cesareans. As the number of women having their first cesarean increased, the long-held tenet "once a cesarean, always a cesarean" led to a rapid increase in the number of repeat cesarean births.

What is the current medical thinking about repeat cesarean deliveries?

Having had a prior cesarean delivery is one of the two major reasons women have the operation today. (The other is the diagnosis of dystocia.) The consensus development panel found that the rate of repeat cesareans is likely to increase further if present trends continue. Currently more than 98 percent of women in the U.S. who have had a cesarean undergo a repeat cesarean for subsequent pregnancies.

This practice was begun in the late 1900's to avoid the risk of uterine scar rupture and hemorrhage during labor. At that time the classical cesarean incision was most widely used and the cesarean birth rate was extremely low.

Physicians now know that the classical, low vertical and "inverted T" incisions have a higher rate of rupture than the low transverse incision now in general use. The low transverse cervical cesarean also has been shown to result in fewer cases of lasting health disorders or death among mothers and infants. Today, many women who had earlier low transverse cesareans safely delivery subsequent children vaginally.

In studying the issue, the consensus panel found that the risk of maternal death in a repeat cesarean is two times that of a vaginal delivery. In addition, the maternal mortality rate for repeat cesareans has not fallen since 1970. The group concluded that the practice of routine repeat cesarean birth is open to question, and that labor and vaginal delivery after a previous low transverse cervical cesarean birth are of low risk to the mother and child in properly selected cases.

The panel recommended that:

- In hospitals with appropriate facilities, services and staff for prompt emergency cesarean birth, some women who have had a previous low transverse cervical cesarean may safely be allowed a trial of labor and vaginal delivery.

- The present practice of repeat cesareans should continue for patients who have had previous cesareans with classical, inverted T or low vertical incisions, or for whom there is no record or the type of incision.

- In hospitals without appropriate facilities, services and staff, the risk of labor for women having had a previous cesarean may exceed the risk to mother and infant from a properly timed, elective repeat cesarean birth. To allow patients to make an informed decision, they should be told in advance about the limits of the institution's capabilities and the availability of other institutions offering this service.

- More adequate information should be compiled on the risks and benefits of trying labor in patients with previous low transverse cervical incisions.

- Institutions offering labor trials following low transverse cesareans should develop guidelines for managing those labors.

Cesarean Childbirth

- Patient education on initial and repeat cesarean birth should continue throughout pregnancy as an important part of patient participation in making decisions about the delivery.

What if the baby is in the breech position prior to birth?

There is a continuing trend to use the cesarean method to deliver a "breech baby"—a fetus positioned in the womb to be born in some way other than the normal head first manner. Nationally, the proportion of breech positioned infants delivered by cesarean rose from about 12 percent in 1970 to 60 percent in 1978.

Breech positioning involves higher risks for the mother and child, regardless of whether the delivery is vaginal or cesarean. Cesareans are being selected more often in these cases to try to improve the outcome in the face of the increased risks. But the consensus group found scientific data in this area generally inadequate to make firm conclusions about the desirability of one approach over the other.

Most clinical reviews suggest that the cesarean may involve less risk for the premature breech infant, but this may not be true for term breech babies. Several studies indicate that vaginal delivery of the uncomplicated term breech infant is preferable because an elective cesarean birth involves risk of significant complications for the mother and little or no decrease in the risk of infant death.

Deciding which method of delivery to use in these situations involves considering many factors. These include maternal pelvic size, size of the fetus, the type of breech position and the experience of the physician with vaginal breech delivery.

In general, the consensus panel concluded that the cesarean presents a lower risk to the infant than a vaginal delivery when a breech fetus is 8 pounds or larger, when a fetus is in a complete or footling breech position or when a fetus is breech with marked hyperextension of the head.

The group recommended that vaginal delivery of term breech babies should remain an acceptable choice when the following conditions exist:

- anticipated fetal weight of less than 8 pounds;
- normal pelvic dimensions and structure in the mother;
- frank breech positioning without hyperextended head; and
- delivery by a physician experienced in vaginal breech delivery.

What is the most common, single reason for performing a cesarean?

Dystocia is a catch-all medical term covering a broad range of problems which can complicate labor. The consensus group found that this diagnosis was the largest contributor to the overall rise in the cesarean rate, accounting for 30 percent of all cesareans.

Included under the dystocia, or difficult labor, diagnosis are the following three basic types of problems which may impede labor:

- abnormalities of the mother's birth canal, such as a small pelvis;

- abnormalities in the position of the fetus, including breech position or large fetal size; and

- abnormalities in the forces of labor, including infrequent or weak uterine contractions.

The first two categories are well-defined areas. The physician usually recognizes size or position problems early; guidelines for appropriate obstetrical action are available; and the effects of the various approaches for mother and infant are reasonably well known.

The consensus panel agreed that the last category—forces of labor—is most in need of scrutiny and offers an opportunity for moderating the cesarean rate. Generally, this diagnosis occurs with low-risk infants of normal weight and size. Studies have not shown that infants in this group are better off with either cesarean or vaginal deliveries, although the maternal mortality rate for dystocia in 1978 was 41.9 deaths per 100,000 cesarean births compared with 11.1 deaths per 100,000 vaginal births.

The panel concluded that in handling a difficult or slowly progressing labor without fetal distress, a physician should consider various options before performing a cesarean. These include having the patient rest or walk around, sedating the patient or stimulating labor with a drug called oxytocin.

The panel recommended that because the diagnosis of dystocia is poorly defined and so prominent in increasing the cesarean rate, practice review boards in hospitals should include dystocia cases when conducting reviews. The panel also stressed the need for more research on the factors affecting the progress of labor.

Cesarean Childbirth

Has the use of electronic fetal monitoring led to more cesareans?

Another diagnosis accounting for the rise in cesarean birth rates is fetal distress. Occurring during labor, this problem can result in various complications, the most serious being fetal brain damage because of oxygen deprivation.

The use of electronic fetal monitoring techniques has led to an increase in the diagnosis of fetal distress but not necessarily to the increase in cesarean deliveries, according to the consensus panel.

Because current data are insufficient on the possible risks or benefits of handling this condition with either cesarean or vaginal deliveries, the panel recommended studies to gather information on the outcomes of births involving fetal distress and development of new techniques to improve the accuracy of the diagnosis. These steps, the panel said, may be expected to improve fetal outcome and lower cesarean birth rates.

Are there other medical conditions which would necessitate a cesarean?

Because of a need for early delivery, certain medical problems in either the mother or fetus can lead to cesarean birth. Examples include maternal diabetes, pregnancy induced hypertension, vaginal herpes infection, and erythroblastosis fetalis, a blood disease related to the Rh factor in the mother. This entire group, however, contributes only a small part of the cesarean birth rate increases.

The consensus panel said that in some of these situations vaginal birth would be a safe alternative if a more effective method of stimulating labor before term was available. The panel recommended research to develop such methods.

What are the benefits of the cesarean method?

There are certain times when conditions in the mother or infant make cesarean delivery the method of first choice. By providing an alternate route of delivery, the procedure offers great benefit in situations when a vaginal delivery carries a high risk of complications and death.

A cesarean is usually used when an expectant mother has diabetes mellitus. Such women have a high risk of having stillborns late in pregnancy. In these cases, a slightly early cesarean helps prevent this occurrence.

The cesarean can also be a lifesaving procedure when the following conditions are present:

- Placenta previa—when the placenta blocks the infant from being born.

- Abruptio placentae—when the placenta prematurely separates from the uterine wall and hemorrhage occurs.

- Obstructed labor—which can occur with a fetus in the shoulder breech, or any other abnormal position.

- Ruptured uterus.

- Presence of weak uterine scars from previous surgery or cesarean.

- Fetus too large for the mother's birth canal.

- Rapid toxemia—a condition in which high blood pressure can lead to convulsions in late pregnancy.

- Vaginal herpes infection—which could infect an infant being born vaginally, and lead to its eventual death.

- Pelvic tumors—which obstruct the birth canal and weaken the uterine wall.

- Absence of effective uterine contractions after labor has begun.

- Prolapse of the umbilical cord—when the cord is pushed out ahead of the infant, compressing the cord and cutting off blood flow.

What are the maternal risks in cesarean childbirth?

The risks of any medical procedure are determined by examining the related mortality statistics showing death rates and morbidity figures showing complications, injuries or disorders linked to the event. These vary from hospital to hospital and from locale to locale.

Cesarean Childbirth

Although maternal death during childbirth is extremely uncommon, national figures show cesarean birth carries up to four times the risk of death compared to a vaginal delivery. The maternal mortality rate for vaginal delivery in 1978 was about 10 deaths per 100,000 births. For cesareans, the rate was about 41 deaths per 100,000 births. (In some cases, maternal deaths indicated in these figures were caused by illness rather than the surgery.)

The morbidity rates associated with cesarean births are higher than with vaginal delivery. Because major surgery is involved, the chance of infection and complication is greater. The most common are endometritis (an inflammation of tissue lining the uterus) and urinary tract or incision infections.

Does cesarean childbirth require special anesthesia?

The use of anesthesia during childbirth is unique because it requires attention to the infant about to be born as well as the mother. Although rare, anesthesia-related maternal deaths continue to occur. Most, however, are potentially avoidable.

There are three major anesthetic techniques for cesarean birth. Spinal anesthesia is widely used, although the use of lumbar epidural anesthesia is increasing. Both are considered "regional" anesthesia because they deaden pain in only part of the body without putting the patient to sleep. General anesthesia, which renders the patient unconscious, is often used in an emergency situation and with women who object to the spinal or epidural approach.

The consensus panel recommended that the types of anesthesia available should be discussed among the patient, obstetrician and anesthesiologist. Each approach has advantages and disadvantages. If possible, the report recommends, the patient should have the option of receiving regional instead of general anesthesia.

Are there risks to the infant?

Infants delivered with elective cesarean surgery, especially if it is performed before the onset of labor, appear to have a greater risk of respiratory distress syndrome (RDS). This condition, in which the infant's lungs are not fully mature, may result if an error is made in estimating the age of the developing fetus. Under these circumstances, an infant—who otherwise would have been healthy if allowed to develop fully—encounters the problems of prematurity when removed too soon by cesarean. These include RDS and other lung disorders, feeding problems and various complications which in some cases require a long hospital stay.

Measures and techniques to assess the maturity of the fetus and the degree of lung development are readily available in the United States. The consensus report stressed the need for improving physician and patient education about the safe and effective use of these techniques in planning for elective cesarean delivery. Respiratory distress is unlikely to be a problem, regardless of the type of delivery, if the infant is born at or near term.

What are the psychological effects of cesarean childbirth?

Other factors must be taken into consideration when weighing the prospects of a cesarean. Although there has been only limited research on the psychological effects on parents following a cesarean birth, it is clear that surgery is an increased psychological and physical burden compared to vaginal delivery. In limited follow-up studies of infants, there has been no evidence of an adverse psychologic effect on infants born by cesarean.

In some hospitals, family-centered maternity care has been extended to cesarean deliveries. The presence of the father in the operating room and the closer contact between the mother and newborn in this approach appear to improve the cesarean process.

The consensus panel recommended strengthening the information exchange and education of prospective parents about the overall cesarean experience. They urged hospitals to allow fathers in the operating room when possible and to avoid routinely separating the newborn from its parents immediately following delivery.

For More Information

Single free copies of the following publications are available by writing to

NICHD
P.O. Box 2911
Washington, D.C. 20040.

- Cesarean Childbirth is the 540-page final report of the consensus development task force. The report contains evidence gathered by the panel, as well as findings and recommendations. Ask for NIH Publication No. 82-2067.

Cesarean Childbirth

- "Cesarean Childbirth Consensus Statement" is a ten-page summary of the questions examined at the three-day Consensus Development Conference held September 22-24, 1980. The summary contains the specific findings and recommendations of the panel.'

Part Five

Postpartum and Perinatal Care

Chapter 18

Postpartum Concerns

Chapter Contents

Section 18.1—Taking Care of Yourself After
 the Baby is Born 306
Section 18.2—Childbirth and Bladder Control 313
Section 18.3—Postpartum Depression 317
Section 18.4—Planning Your Family 320

Section 18.1

Taking Care of Yourself After the Baby is Born

Reprinted by permission of Group Health Cooperative of Puget Sound, copyright, 1996. *Disclaimer of Warranties:* This publication was developed by Group Health for use in communicating with our enrollees. Group Health specifically disclaims any warranties, implied or expressed, including the warranty of merchantability and the warranty of fitness for a particular purpose.

In the Hospital

Security in the Hospital

All hospital personnel wear name badges (identification or ID badges), some with photos. Do not allow your baby to leave your room with anyone not wearing an ID badge. If an unfamiliar person wants to take your baby, or if you have any concerns about the person's identity, turn on the nurse call-light.

You and your baby will also have identification bands with matching numbers. Notify your nurse immediately if you notice your or your baby's ID band is missing.

Try to Limit Visitors

Everyone will want to see your new baby. That can tire you out quickly. We suggest that you limit the number of visitors at the hospital. Your time in the hospital is short and you'll need to rest and get to know your baby. Partners may come and go at any time. Other visitors should come during visiting hours. Also, try to limit your visitors at home during the first few weeks so you don't get overtired.

Your Changing Body

Weight

You will lose about 12 pounds with the birth of your baby and delivery of the "afterbirth." You'll lose an additional four to five pounds

Postpartum Concerns

in the next week as you lose the extra fluid you've accumulated during the pregnancy. (You may notice that you pass a lot of urine and sweat a lot.) You'll continue to lose weight gradually. Many women will be close to their pre-pregnancy weight by six weeks after the birth. If you breastfeed, it may take you a little longer to return to your pre-pregnancy weight because of the weight of lactating breasts and because nursing mothers need additional nutrients.

Vaginal discharge

For several weeks after the birth, you will have vaginal discharge of blood and tissue left from pregnancy. For the first 3-5 days, it is bloody and red with some clots. It gradually becomes lighter, pinkish and then brownish in color. By about the 10th day, it is pale cream in color. This lasts for 2-6 weeks. Use sanitary napkins, not tampons, to absorb the flow.

Afterpains

"Afterpains" are contractions of the uterus, similar to menstrual cramps, which occur as the uterus regains its original size. They often occur during breastfeeding but usually disappear after the first week. "Afterpains" are often unnoticeable after the first baby. They become more noticeable with each birth.

Menstrual periods

If you formula-feed your baby, you may start menstruating 6-8 weeks after birth. If you are breastfeeding, your periods may not start for several months. However, since ovulation (release of an egg) often occurs before your periods start, you can get pregnant even if you have not started menstruation. Be sure to use birth control if you do not want to get pregnant right away.

Skin changes

Stretch marks will fade but they do not disappear completely. Any increase in skin pigmentation and hair growth that occurred during pregnancy will slowly go away.

Constipation

Constipation is fairly common during the first few days after delivery. You can help prevent constipation by drinking plenty of fluids and eating high fiber foods, such as raw vegetables, fresh fruit, and whole grain breads and cereals. If you have stitches, pressing a clean pad on the stitches may make you feel more comfortable during a bowel movement.

How to prevent lower back pain

- Avoid lifting anything heavier than your baby for the first few weeks.

- Bend your knees when lifting your baby.

- Avoid twisting movements.

- Follow the pregnancy guidelines for getting up and lying down (found in Chapter 7); be sure your lower back is supported when you are sitting down.

- Perform exercises for strengthening your abdominal muscles. When the abdominal muscles are weak, the back has less support and is more likely to be strained.

When to Call your Healthcare Provider

If:

- You have chills or a temperature of 100.4 degrees or more that lasts longer than four hours.

- You feel pain while urinating.

- Your abdomen feels tender, your vaginal discharge is foul-smelling or contains large clots (the size of a golfball or bigger), or you have bright red bleeding that doesn't go away with rest.

- You notice a red, warm, swollen area in your leg, or pain in your calf when you step down.

- One or both breasts have a red, warm, or swollen area that feels tender, and you have chills or fever.

Sexual Activity

The many postpartum physical and emotional changes can also affect a couple's sexual relationship and desire. You can have intercourse

Postpartum Concerns

when you feel ready, usually four to six weeks after delivery. Postpartum intercourse may be less exciting at first than intercourse before the baby's birth.

Stitches from an episiotomy or tear can be sensitive during intercourse. You may also feel tense because of new feelings related to motherhood. You may have less vaginal lubrication. The following suggestions may help with these difficulties.

Positions with the woman on top or lying on her side may be more comfortable because they decrease tension on the perineum. K-Y jelly is an effective lubricant. Touch and massage can help both partners relax. Remember that you'll need time to recover from pregnancy and birth. You may both be preoccupied with the baby and short of sleep. Your breasts may be tender and if you are breastfeeding, you may leak milk when sexually aroused. It may take a few weeks before you feel comfortable with one another and sexually satisfied. You'll need patience, humor, optimism, and sharing of feelings. Remember to use birth control to avoid getting pregnant sooner than you wish.

How to Get Some Sleep

Getting enough sleep is a problem for all new parents. Newborns sleep about 16 hours a day but they sleep on a different schedule than adults. A newborn's sleep cycle is about 45-50 minutes. Just like adults, they may stir without fully waking during each sleep cycle. New parents often assume their baby is hungry when the baby stirs. Giving your baby time to settle back to sleep allows for better rest for both parents and the baby. A two-week-old baby will only sleep for 3 or 4 hours before waking up to be fed. By four months, some babies may sleep up to 8 hours. What you do now, and during the first months of your baby's life, will help everyone sleep better. Here are some tips to promote good sleep habits:

- Keep the sleep area quiet and cool.

- Turn TV and radios down or off.

- Have a consistent place and time for sleep—especially nighttime.

- Have relaxing bedtime routines—singing, hugs, kisses. Follow your routine every night. Your baby will learn that being in bed means going to sleep.

- Do not change a sleeping baby after feeding, most babies can tolerate wet diapers for 1-2 hours. They may wake up and be fitful if changed when they are asleep.
- For yourself (and older children), try low-fat, high carbohydrate snacks or warm milk before bedtime.
- Limit your caffeine to 1-2 cups in the morning only.
- Get out daily for a walk—fresh air and exercise will help both mom and baby to sleep.

By using these tips, you can help your baby learn good sleep habits. In the meantime, sleep when the baby sleeps. You may also want to read some books, such as *Crying Baby, Sleepless Nights* by Sandy Jones (1992).

Getting Back in Shape

Exercise will help you recover your pre-pregnancy shape and strength. After birth, two areas of your body need special attention—your pelvic floor and your abdominal area. The following exercises tone and strengthen both areas. These exercises can usually be started as early as a few hours after the baby's birth. If you've had a cesarean birth, you should start more gradually. Ask your healthcare provider when it is safe for you to start exercising.

Walking

Most healthcare providers recommend that you get out of bed and walk within 6-8 hours after the birth, even a cesarean birth. Walking promotes circulation and improves bladder and bowel tone. This helps prevent bladder infections and constipation. Walking helps the vaginal discharge and strengthens the abdominal muscles.

Kegel Exercises for the Pelvic Floor Muscles

The Kegel exercise will help your vagina regain its muscle tone and shape, prevent leaking of urine when coughing, laughing, or sneezing, and lessen hemorrhoid problems.

What to do:

1. Tighten the muscles around the vagina and rectum (as if to stop urinating midstream) and hold for a count of three. (Keep your abdomen and buttocks relaxed.)

Postpartum Concerns

2. Relax and tighten them again.
3. Repeat tightening and relaxing 10 times.
4. Over the next few days, hold the muscles for longer periods, until you can hold for a slow count of five.

At first you may not be able to do this exercise for ten repetitions or hold your muscles tight for as long as 3-5 seconds. Do them for as long as you can and practice every day, 5-10 times a day.

Another way you can check the tone and strength of the muscles, after the vaginal discharge has faded, is to place one finger in the vagina and tighten the muscles around your finger.

Follow-Up Care

Your healthcare provider will tell you when to come to your postpartum checkup. Be sure to ask your healthcare provider about:

- When it is safe for you to have intercourse and about birth control.
- Breastfeeding and breast care.
- Exercises.
- Any special precautions.

Your Baby's Healthcare

Ask your baby's healthcare provider about infant care and other things such as:

- When to bring your baby for his or her first checkup. (The first visit to your baby's healthcare provider should be no later than at 7-10 days of age.)

- Immunization schedule.

- What to do if your baby cries excessively.

Write down other questions you want to ask.

Learning to Be a Parent

During this time of change, remember that neither women nor men are born with an automatic ability to be a parent. Parenting is not an instinctive skill. At times you may feel overwhelmed and helpless. Most new parents have positive and negative feelings about their changing roles and their child. Don't worry if you have mixed feelings at first. In time things will get easier. Although you will be a parent for the rest of your life, the time with an infant is short—but intense.

In Brief (Excerpt from DHSS publication No. HRSA-MCHB-92-4-A, 1994)

- You should go to your health care giver about 2-6 weeks after your baby is born. Make an appointment for this "postpartum" visit as soon as possible. If you have questions or problems before then, call your health care provider.

- Ask your health care giver if you are protected against rubella. If not, get a shot to protect you before you leave the hospital.

- Ask your health care giver about family planning. You can get pregnant again even if you are breastfeeding. Your body is not ready for another healthy pregnancy right now.

- Call your care giver right away if you have any of these postpartum warning signs:
  1. Heavy, bright red bleeding or large clots
  2. Fever over 100 degrees F
  3. Painful cramps
  4. Hard, painful lumps in your breasts
  5. Increased pain in episiotomy (stitches)
  6. Pain when you empty your bladder
  7. Feeling that you might harm yourself or your baby

- Many new mothers feel depressed, cry easily, or are just very tired. These feelings are often due to lack of sleep; it doesn't mean you don't love your baby. If you have some of these feelings, you may want to talk to your family, a friend, or another mother about it. If you need help to cope with your feelings, call your health care giver.

- Breastfeeding is best for your baby. It is good for you too. It will help get your uterus (womb) back in shape. Almost all mothers breastfeed easily. Some need advice or help. Call your childbirth educator, nutritionist, or the La Leche League (1-800 LA LECHE) if you have problems or questions.

Postpartum Concerns

- Eat a variety of healthful foods and drink 6 to 8 glasses of water and other liquids each day, just as you did while you were pregnant. You need food for energy and to pass on to your baby if you are breastfeeding. Avoid alcohol, cigarettes, and drugs. They are not healthy for you and can harm your baby if passed through your breast milk.

- Try to sleep when your baby sleeps. If you feel under stress, take a break. Put your baby in the crib and take a shower or bath or call a friend. Ask a family member or a friend to watch the baby while you go for a short walk. If you feel as though you are under too much stress, call your health care giver and ask where you can get help. Taking good care of yourself and your baby is most important now.

- Spend some special time with your other children.

Section 18.2

Childbirth and Bladder Control

NIH publication No. 97-4189, 1997

Do pregnancy and childbirth affect bladder control?

Yes. But don't panic. If you lose bladder control after childbirth, the problem often goes away by itself. Your muscles may just need time to recover.

When do you need medical help?

If you still have a problem after 6 weeks, talk to your doctor. Without treatment, lost bladder control can become a long-term problem. Accidental leaking can also signal that something else is wrong in your body.

Bladder control problems do not always show up right after childbirth. Some women do not begin to have problems until later, often in their 40's.

You and your health care team must first find out why you have lost bladder control. Then you can discuss treatment.

After treatment, most women regain or improve their bladder control. Regaining control helps you enjoy a healthier and happier life.

Can you prevent bladder problems?

Yes. Women who exercise certain pelvic muscles have fewer bladder problems later on. These muscles are called pelvic floor muscles. If you plan to have a baby, talk to your doctor. Ask if you should do pelvic floor exercises.

Exercises after childbirth also help prevent bladder problems in middle age. Ask your health care team how to do pelvic exercises.

How does bladder control work?

Your bladder is a muscle shaped like a balloon. While the bladder stores urine, the bladder muscle relaxes. When you go to the bathroom, the bladder muscle tightens to squeeze urine out of the bladder. More muscles help with bladder control. Two sphincter muscles surround the tube that carries urine from your bladder down to an opening in front of the vagina. The tube is called the urethra. Urine leaves your body through this tube. The sphincters keep the urethra closed by squeezing like rubber bands. Pelvic floor muscles under the bladder also help keep the urethra closed.

When the bladder is full, nerves in your bladder signal the brain. That's when you get the urge to go to the bathroom. Once you reach the toilet, your brain sends a message down to the sphincter and pelvic floor muscles. The brain tells them to relax. The brain signal also tells the bladder muscles to tighten up. That squeezes urine out of the bladder.

Strong sphincter (bladder control) muscles prevent urine leakage in pregnancy and after childbirth. You can exercise these muscles to make them strong. Talk to your doctor about learning how to do pelvic floor exercises.

What do pregnancy and childbirth have to do with bladder control?

The added weight and pressure of pregnancy can weaken pelvic floor muscles. Other aspects of pregnancy and childbirth can also cause problems:

- changed position of bladder and urethra
- vaginal delivery
- episiotomy (the cut in the muscle that makes it easier for the baby to come out)
- Damage to bladder control nerves.

Which professionals can help you with bladder control?

Professionals who can help you with bladder control include:

- your primary care doctor
- a gynecologist
- a women's doctor
- a urogynecologist: an expert in women's bladder problems
- a urologist: an expert in bladder problems
- a nurse or nurse practitioner
- a physical therapist.

Points to Remember

- Temporary bladder control problems are common during pregnancy.

- Exercising pelvic floor muscles can help prevent bladder control problems.

- Bladder control problems may show up months to years after childbirth.

- Talk to your health care team if this happens to you.

For More Information

Contact:

National Kidney and Urologic Diseases Information Clearinghouse
3 Information Way
Bethesda, MD 20892-3580
E-mail: nkudic@aerie.com

The National Kidney and Urologic Diseases Information Clearinghouse is a service of the National Institute of Diabetes and Digestive and Kidney Diseases, of the National Institutes of Health, under the U.S. Public Health Service. Established in 1987, the clearinghouse provides information about diseases of the kidneys and urologic system to people with these disorders and to their families, health care professionals, and the public. The clearinghouse answers inquiries; develops, reviews, and distributes publications; and works closely with professional and patient organizations and government agencies to coordinate resources about kidney and urologic diseases.

Section 18.3

Postpartum Depression

Excerpt reprinted with permission from Group Health Cooperative, 1996 and excerpt, marked [ ], from NIH Publication No. 93-0551

After childbirth, you may feel emotional ups and downs. You may feel happy, proud, and excited one day and sad, lonely, or depressed the next day. You may be unable to sleep, lack energy, cry easily, feel irritable, overwhelmed, and anxious. You may worry about all sorts of things. These feelings are common among new moms—about eighty women out of one hundred experience "baby blues." These feelings can come and go, but they usually go away in two weeks. They are caused by hormonal changes and the fact that you are very tired. Here are some things you can do to help you cope with "baby blues":

- Try to get as much rest as possible. Rest whenever your baby is asleep. Don't worry if your house is not as neat as it used to be sleep is more important to you right now than a neat house. Let others, especially your partner, help you with household chores and the baby. Your partner can help change the diapers, dress the baby, give the baby a bath, or gently rock the baby to sleep at night.

- Talk with your partner, friends, and other new moms about your feelings.

- Take time for yourself. Ask someone you trust to baby-sit so you can get away and do something you enjoy.

- Keep visits from relatives and friends short—unless they come to help you out.

A few women may get more than just "blue." They feel very depressed and unable to bring themselves out of it. Postpartum depression can start as late as two to four weeks after childbirth. Symptoms include headaches, numbness, chest pains, despair, inability to cope, sense of powerlessness, lack of concentration, loss of interest in sex, thoughts of suicide, panic attacks, hostility, new fears or phobias, nightmares, hallucinations, or no feelings for the baby. If you have any of these symptoms, you need to get professional help. Call your healthcare provider or Group Health Mental Health Services. If you don't get help, your depression can get worse and affect your health as well as your relationship with your baby and your partner.

Your partner's feelings

The baby's father or your partner may also have moments when he feels sad and anxious. Your partner may feel "left out" because of all the attention you are giving to the baby. Pregnancy and the birth of the baby can be a strain on any relationship. Both you and your partner will need loving care and support. Remember to:

- Talk with your partner and let him know he is still very important to you.
- Spend time alone together.
- Share your feelings about being new parents.
- Be affectionate and good to each other.

Classification of Postpartum Mood Disorders

[Postpartum mood symptoms are divided into three categories based on severity:

1. Blues
2. Psychosis
3. Depression

Postpartum blues are brief episodes (1 to 4 days) of unstable mood/tearfulness that normally occur in 50 to 80 percent of women within 1 to 5 days of delivery. Treatment consists of reassurance and time to resolve this normal postpartum response.

Postpartum psychoses can be divided in to depressed and manic types. Patients with the depressed type show more psychotic, disorientated, agitated, and emotionally unstable features, as well as more psychomotor retardation, than do non-postpartum matched depressed

Postpartum Concerns

controls. Most of these cases are associated with signs of organic impairment. Features of the manic type are similar to features of a classic mania. The incidence of postpartum psychosis is low (0.5 to 2.0 per 1,000 deliveries), as shown in eight studies. Many early cases were mistaken for toxic/infectious states.

The symptoms of postpartum psychosis develop rapidly (Over 24 to 72 hours), typically beginning 2 to 3 days after delivery. The period of risk for developing postpartum psychosis is within the first month following delivery. For acute postpartum psychosis, the prognosis is generally good. However, many patients have previously had or subsequently develop a bipolar disorder. The risk of postpartum psychosis is higher for those with episodes at prior deliveries. The recurrence rate is from 33 to 51 percent.

Non-psychotic postpartum depressions (major or minor depressive disorders) have also been identified. These conditions may occur from 2 weeks to 12 months postpartum, but typically occur within 6 months. The prevalence of non-psychotic depressions is 10 to 15 percent within the first 3 to 6 months after childbirth, which is somewhat higher than are the rates (5 to 7 percent) in non-childbearing matched controls. However, the risk for non-psychotic postpartum depression is higher for persons with a psychiatric history.

No randomized controlled treatment trials for any of the postpartum mood conditions are available. Logic and clinical experience suggest that prophylactic lithium be given as soon as possible after delivery to prevent a postpartum precipitation in patients with a history of bipolar disorder. Likewise, given the high likelihood of recurrence, other previously effective psychotropic medications should be considered in those with a history of psychotic postpartum mood episodes immediately after giving birth.]

Section 18.4

Planning Your Family

Excerpts from FDA Consumer, April 1997 and DHSS Publication No. HRSA-MCHB-92-4-A, 1994

Before You Become Pregnant Again

Think about your own health first. Take care of yourself before you get pregnant again. Make sure that you and your family are ready for another baby.

Another baby will change your life in many ways. More babies add new responsibilities as well as new joys. Mothers and fathers both need to be ready to be good parents to another baby. Family planning services are available. For information, call your local health department.

Look at Your Health

If you have a health problem (such as diabetes or high blood pressure), try to get it under control before you become pregnant. Then you and your health care givers can work together to avoid problems and have a healthy pregnancy. If you are healthy, it is still a good idea to talk with your care giver before you become pregnant about:

- If you should keep taking any prescribed drugs
- If you should be immunized against rubella (get a German measles shot). Do not get pregnant for 3 months following this shot.
- If you should think about genetic testing (to detect problems you could pass on to your baby).
- If the time is right for you to try to become pregnant. Wait several months after you stop taking oral contraceptives (the "pill") or if you have just had a miscarriage.
- If you should change your diet or gain or lose weight.
- If there are other lifestyle changes you should make before you become pregnant (such as quitting smoking and drinking alcohol).

Contraceptive Choices

The Food and Drug Administration has approved a number of birth control methods, ranging from over-the-counter male and female condoms and vaginal spermicides to doctor-prescribed birth control pills, diaphragms, intrauterine devices (IUD's), injected hormones, and hormonal implants. Other contraceptive options include fertility awareness and voluntary surgical sterilization.

"On the whole, the contraceptive choices that Americans have are very safe and effective," says Dennis Barbour, president of the Association of Reproductive Health Professionals, "but a method that is very good for one women may be lousy for another."

The choice of birth control depends on factors such as a person's health, frequency of sexual activity, number of partners, and desire to have children in the future. Effectiveness rates, based on statistical estimates, are another key consideration. FDA is developing a more consumer-friendly table to be added to the labeling of all contraceptive drugs and devices.

Barrier Methods

Male Condom. The male condom is a sheath placed over the erect penis before penetration, preventing pregnancy by blocking the passage of sperm.

A condom can be used only once. Some have spermicide added, usually nonoxynol-9 in the United States, to kill sperm. Spermicide has not been scientifically shown to provide additional contraceptive protection over the condom alone. Because they act as a mechanical barrier, condoms prevent direct vaginal contact with semen, infectious genital secretions, and genital lesions and discharges.

Most condoms are made from latex rubber, while a small percentage are made from lamb intestines (sometimes called "lambskin" condoms). Condoms made from polyurethane have been marketed in the United States since 1994.

Except for abstinence, latex condoms are the most effective method for reducing the risk of infection from the viruses that cause AIDS, other HIV-related illnesses, and other STD's.

Some condoms are prelubricated. These lubricants don't provide more birth control or STD protection. Non oil-based lubricants, such as water or K-Y jelly can be used with latex or lambskin condoms, but oil-based lubricants, such as petroleum jelly (Vaseline), lotions, or massage or baby oil, should not be used because they can weaken the material.

Female Condom. The Reality Female Condom, approved by FDA in April 1993, consists of a lubricated polyurethane sheath shaped similarly to the male condom. The closed end, which has a flexible ring, is inserted into the vagina, while the open end remains outside, partially covering the labia.

The female condom, like the male condom is available without a prescription and is intended for one-time use. It should not be used together with a male condom because they may not both stay in place.

Diaphragm. Available by prescription only and sized by a health professional to achieve a proper fit, the diaphragm has a dual mechanism to prevent pregnancy. A dome-shaped rubber disk with a flexible ring covers the cervix so sperm can't reach the uterus, while a spermicide applied to the diaphragm before insertion kills sperm.

The diaphragm protect for six hours. For intercourse after the six-hour period, or for repeated intercourse within this period, fresh spermicide should be placed in the vagina with the diaphragm still in place. The diaphragm should be left in place for at least six hours after the last intercourse but not for longer than a total of 24 hours because of the risk of toxic shock syndrome (TSS), a rare but potentially fatal infection. Symptoms of TSS include sudden fever, stomach upset, sunburn-like rash, and a drop in blood pressure.

Cervical Cap. The cap is a soft rubber cup with a round rim, sized by a health professional to fit snugly around the cervix. It is available by prescription only and, like the diaphragm, is used with spermicide.

It protects for 48 hours and for multiple acts of intercourse within this time. Wearing it for more than 48 hours is not recommended because of the risk, though low, of TSS. Also, with prolonged use of two or more days, the cap may cause an unpleasant vaginal odor or discharge in some women.

Sponge. The vaginal contraceptive sponge has not been available since the sole manufacturer, Whitehall Laboratories of Madison, N.J., voluntarily stopped selling it in 1995. It remains an approved product and could be marketed again.

The sponge, a donut-shaped polyurethane device containing the spermicide nonoxynol-9, is inserted in to the vagina to cover the cervix. A woven polyester loop is designed to ease removal.

The sponge protects for up to 24 hours and for multiple acts of intercourse within this time. It should be left in place for at least six hours after intercourse but should be removed no more than 30 hours after insertion because of the risk, though low, of TSS.

Vaginal Spermicides Alone

Vaginal spermicides are available in foam, cream, jelly, film, suppository, or tablet forms. All types contain a sperm killing chemical.

Studies have not produced definitive data on the efficacy of spermicides alone, but according to the authors of *Contraceptive Technology*, a leading resource for contraceptive information, the failure rate for typical users may be 21 percent per year.

Package instructions must be carefully followed because some spermicide products require the couple to wait 10 minutes or more after inserting the spermicide before having sex. One dose of spermicide is usually effective for one hour. For repeated intercourse, additional spermicide must be applied. And after intercourse, the spermicide has to remain in place for at least six to eight hours to ensure that all sperm are killed. The women should not douche or rinse the vagina during this time.

Hormonal Methods

Combined Oral Contraceptives. Typically called "the pill", combined oral contraceptives have been on the market for more than 35 years and are the most popular form of reversible birth control in the United States. This form of birth control suppresses ovulation (the monthly release of an egg from the ovaries) by the combined action of the hormones estrogen and progestin.

If a women remembers to take the pill every day as directed, she has an extremely low chance of becoming pregnant in a year. But the pill's effectiveness may be reduced if the women is taking some medications, such as certain antibiotics.

Beside preventing pregnancy, the pill offers additional benefits. As stated in the labeling, the pill can make periods more regular. It also has a protective effect against pelvic inflammatory disease, an infection of the fallopian tubes or uterus that is a major cause of infertility in women, and against ovarian and endometrial cancers.

The decision whether to take the pill should be made in consultation with a health professional. Birth control pills are safe for most women—safer even than delivering a baby—but they carry some risks.

Current low-dose pills have fewer risks associated with them than earlier versions. But women who smoke—especially those over 35—and women with certain medical conditions, such as a history of blood clots or breast or endometrial cancer, may be advised against taking the pill. The pill may contribute to cardiovascular disease, including high blood pressure, blood clots, and blockage of the arteries.

One of the biggest questions has been whether the pill increases the risk of breast cancer in past and current pill users. An international study published in the September 1996 journal *Contraception* concluded that women's risk of breast cancer 10 years after going off birth control pills was no higher than that of women who had never used the pill. During pill use and for the first 10 years after stopping the pill, women's risk of breast cancer was only slightly higher in pill users than non-pill users.

Side effects of the pill, which often subside after a few months' use, include nausea, headache, breast tenderness, weight gain, irregular bleeding, and depression.

Doctor's sometimes prescribe higher doses of combined oral contraceptives for use as "morning after" pills to be taken within 72 hours of unprotected intercourse to prevent the possibly fertilized egg from reaching the uterus. In a Feb. 25, 1997, *Federal Register* notice, FDA stated its conclusion that, on the basis of current scientific evidence, certain oral contraceptives are safe and effective for this use.

Mini-pills. Although taken daily like combined oral contraceptives, mini-pills contain only progestin and no estrogen. They work by reducing and thickening cervical mucus to prevent sperm from reaching egg. They also keep the uterine lining from thickening, which prevents a fertilized egg from implanting in the uterus. These pills are generally less effective than combined oral contraceptives.

Mini-pills can decrease menstrual bleeding and cramps, as well as the risk of endometrial and ovarian cancer and pelvic inflammatory disease. Because they contain no estrogen, mini-pills don't present the risk of blood clots associated with estrogen in combined pills. They are a good option for women who can't take estrogen because they are breastfeeding or because estrogen-containing products cause them to have severe headaches or high blood pressure.

Side-effects of mini-pills include menstrual cycle changes, weight gain, and breast tenderness.

Injectable Progestins. Depo-Provera, approved by FDA in 1992, is injected by a health professional into the buttocks or arm muscle every 3 months. Depo-Provera prevents pregnancy in three ways:

Postpartum Concerns

It inhibits ovulation, changes the cervical mucus to help prevent sperm from reaching the egg, and changes the uterine lining to prevent the fertilized egg from implanting in the uterus. The progestin injection is extremely effective in preventing pregnancy, in large part because it requires little effort for the women to comply: She simply has to get an injection by a doctor once every three months.

The benefits are similar to those of the mini-pill and another progestin-only contraceptive, Norplant. Side effects are also similar and can include irregular or missed periods, weight gain, and breast tenderness.

Implantable Progestins. Norplant, approved by FDA in 1990, and the newer Norplant 2, approved in 1996, are the third type of progestin-only contraceptive. Made up of matchstick-sized rubber rods, this contraceptive is surgically implanted under the skin of the upper arm, where it steadily releases the contraceptive steroid levonorgestrel.

The six-rod Norplant provides protection for up to five years (or until it is removed), while the two-rod Norplant 2 protects for up to three years. Norplant failures are rare, but are higher with increased body weight.

Some women may experience inflammatory or infection at the site of the implant. Other side effects include menstrual changes, weight gain, and breast tenderness.

Intrauterine Devices

An IUD is a T-shaped device inserted into the uterus by a healthcare professional. Two types of IUD are available in the United States: the Paragard CopperT 380A and the Progestasert Progesterone T. The Paragard IUD can remain in place for 10 years, while the Progestasert IUD must be replaced every year.

It's not entirely clear how IUD's prevent pregnancy. They seem to prevent sperm and eggs from meeting by either immobilizing the sperm on their way to the fallopian tubes or changing the uterus lining so the fertilized egg cannot implant in it.

IUD's have one of the lowest failure rates of any contraceptive method. "In the population for which the IUD is appropriate—for those in a mutually monogamous, stable relationship who aren't at high risk of infection—the IUD is a very safe and effective method of contraception," says Lisa Rarick, M.D., director of FDA's division of reproductive and urologic drug products.

The IUD's image suffered when the Dalkon Shield IUD was taken off the market in 1975. This IUD was associated with a high incidence of pelvic infections and infertility, and some deaths. Today, serious complications from IUD's are rare, although IUD users may be at increased risk of developing pelvic inflammatory disease. Other side effects can include perforation of the uterus, abnormal bleeding, and cramps. Complications occur most often during and immediately after insertion.

Traditional Methods

Fertility Awareness. Also known as natural family planning or periodic abstinence, fertility awareness entails not having sexual intercourse on the days of a woman's menstrual cycle when she could become pregnant or using a barrier method of birth control on those days.

Because a sperm may live in the female's reproductive tract for up to seven days and the egg remains fertile for about 24 hours, a women can get pregnant within a substantial window of time—from seven days before ovulation to three days after. Methods to approximate when a women is fertile are usually based on the menstrual cycle, changes in cervical mucus, or changes in body temperature.

"Natural family planning can work," Rarick says, "but it takes an extremely motivated couple to use the method effectively."

Withdrawal. In this method, also called *coitus interruptus,* the man withdraws his penis from the vagina before ejaculation. Fertilization is prevented because the sperm do not enter the vagina.

Effectiveness depends on the male's ability to withdraw before ejaculation. Also, withdrawal doesn't provide protection from STD's including HIV. Infectious diseases can be transmitted by direct contact with surface lesions and pre-ejaculatory fluid.

Surgical Sterilization

Surgical sterilization is a contraceptive option intended for people who don't want children in the future. It is considered permanent because reversal requires major surgery that is often unsuccessful.

Female Sterilization. Female sterilization blocks the fallopian tubes so the egg can't travel to the uterus. Sterilization is done by various surgical techniques performed under general anesthesia.

Postpartum Concerns

Complications from these operations are rare and can include infection, hemorrhage, and problems related to the use of general anesthesia.

Male Sterilization. This procedure, called a vasectomy, involves sealing, tying or cutting a man's vas deferens, which otherwise would carry the sperm from the testicle to the penis.

Vasectomy involves a quick operation, usually under 30 minutes, with possible minor post-surgical complications, such as bleeding or infection.

Research continues on effective contraceptives that minimize side effects. One important research focus, according to FDA's Rarick, is the development of birth control methods that are both spermicidal and microbicidal to prevent not only pregnancy but also transmission of HIV and other STD's.

Type	Male Condom	Female Condom	Diaphragm with Spermicide	Cervical Cap with Spermicide	Sponge with Spermicide (not currently marketed)	Spermicides Alone
Estimated Effectiveness	88%[a]	79%	82%	64–82%[b]	64–82%[b]	79%
Some Risks[d]	Irritation and allergic reactions (less likely with polyurethane)	Irritation and allergic reactions	Irritation and allergic reactions, urinary tract infection	Irritation and allergic reactions, abnormal Pap test	Irritation and allergic reactions, difficulty in removal	Irritation and allergic reactions
Protection from Sexually Transmitted Diseases (STDs)	Except for abstinence, latex condoms are the best protection against STDs, including herpes and AIDS.	May give some STD protection; not as effective as latex condom.	Protects against cervical infection; spermicide may give some protection against chlamydia and gonorrhea; otherwise unknown.	Spermicide may give some protection against chlamydia and gonorrhea; otherwise unknown.	Spermicide may give some protection against chlamydia and gonorrhea; otherwise unknown.	May give some protection against chlamydia and gonorrhea; otherwise unknown.
Convenience	Applied immediately before intercourse; used only once and discarded.	Applied immediately before intercourse; used only once and discarded.	Inserted before intercourse and left in place at least six hours after; can be left in place for 24 hours, with additional spermicide for repeated intercourse.	May be difficult to insert; can remain in place for 48 hours without reapplying spermicide for repeated intercourse.	Inserted before intercourse and protects for 24 hours without additional spermicide; must be left in place for at least six hours after intercourse; must be removed within 30 hours of insertion; used only once and discarded.	Instructions vary; usually applied no more than one hour before intercourse and left in place at least six to eight hours after.
Availability	Nonprescription	Nonprescription	Prescription	Prescription	Nonprescription; not currently marketed.	Nonprescription

Figure 18.1. Birth Control Guide. Efficacy rates in this chart are based on Contraceptive Technology (16th edition, 1994). They are yearly estimates of effectiveness in typical use, which refers to a method's reliability in real life, when people don't always use a method properly. For comparison, about 85 percent of sexually active women using no contraception would be expected to become pregnant in a year. This chart is a summary; it is not intended to be used alone. All product labeling should be followed carefully, and a health-care professional should be consulted for some methods.

Postpartum Concerns

Oral Contraceptives—combined pill	Oral Contraceptives—progestin-only minipill	Injection (Depo-Provera)	Implant (Norplant)	IUD (Intrauterine Device)	Periodic Abstinence	Surgical Sterilization—female or male
Over 99%[c]	Over 99%[c]	Over 99%	Over 99%	98–99%	About 80% (varies, based on method)	Over 99%
Dizziness; nausea; changes in menstruation, mood, and weight; rarely, cardiovascular disease, including high blood pressure, blood clots, heart attack, and strokes	Ectopic pregnancy, irregular bleeding, weight gain, breast tenderness	Irregular bleeding, weight gain, breast tenderness, headaches	Irregular bleeding, weight gain, breast tenderness, headaches, difficulty in removal	Cramps, bleeding, pelvic inflammatory disease, infertility, perforation of uterus	None	Pain, bleeding, infection, other minor postsurgical complications
None, except some protection against pelvic inflammatory disease.	None, except some protection against pelvic inflammatory disease.	None	None	None	None	None
Must be taken on daily schedule, regardless of frequency of intercourse.	Must be taken on daily schedule, regardless of frequency of intercourse.	One injection every three months	Implanted by health-care provider—minor outpatient surgical procedure; effective for up to five years.	After insertion by physician, can remain in place for up to one or 10 years, depending on type.	Requires frequent monitoring of body functions (for example, body temperature for one method).	One-time surgical procedure
Prescription	Prescription	Prescription	Prescription	Prescription	Instructions from health-care provider	Surgery

a. Effectiveness rate for polyurethane condoms has not been established.
b. Less effective for women who have had a baby because the birth process stretches the vagina and cervix, making it more difficult to achieve a proper fit.
c. Based on perfect use, when the woman takes the pill every day as directed.
d. Serious medical risks from contraceptives are rare.

Chapter 19

Breastfeeding

Chapter Contents

Section 19.1 — Breastfeeding Statistics 332
Section 19.2 — Feeding Baby: Nature and Nurture 334
Section 19.3 — Lactation Suppression: Safer Without
  Drugs 341
Section 19.4 — Breastfeeding and the Working Mother 346
Section 19.5 — Potential Health Care Cost of Not
  Breastfeeding 352
Section 19.6 — Recent Advances in Maternal and
  Infant Nutrition 355

Section 19.1

Breastfeeding Statistics

Excerpts from DHSS Publication Numbers HRSA-M-DSEA-96-5, September 1996 and HRSA-MCH-95-1, July 1995.

From 1971 to 1982, the percentage of mothers who began breastfeeding in the hospital increased steadily to a high of 62%, but then gradually declined to 51.5% by 1990. Since 1991, however, there has been an increase for black, Hispanic and white women.

With steeper increases in the rate of breastfeeding for black women, the gap between breastfeeding rates for black and white women narrowed slightly in 1994 but was still nearly twice as high for white women as for black women.

Breastfeeding rates for women of all races decrease substantially between delivery and 5 to 6 months postpartum, the period of breastfeeding recommended as most critical for the infant's health by the Surgeon General of the United States. In 1992, only 23.3% of white women and 9.3% of black women were breastfeeding after 6 months. The 1994 rate at 5 to 6 months postpartum were only 23.9%, 18.9% and 10.3% for white, Hispanic, and black women respectively, representing a decline of 38.4% among whites, 38.9% among Hispanics, and 22.9% among blacks from the rates just after delivery.

Breastfeeding rates are highest among women over 30 years of age, college educated, relatively affluent, women not participating in the Women, Infants, and Children (WIC) dietary supplement program and/or and/or who live in the western United States.

Women least likely to breastfeed were younger than 20, employed full-time, low income (less than $10,000/year), are black, Hispanic and/ or live in the southeastern United States. Also women were less likely to breastfeed their first child.

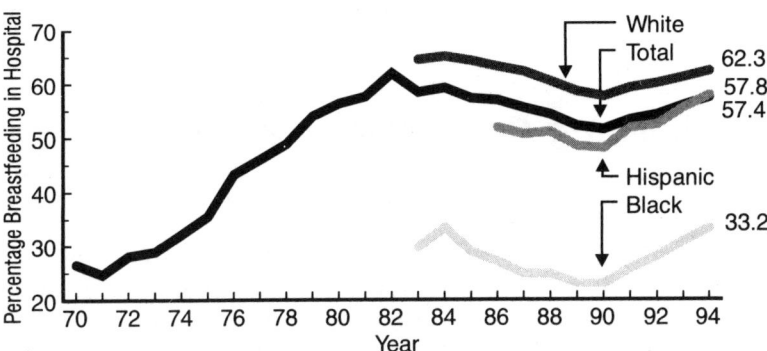

Figure 19.1. Trends in Breastfeeding by Race: 1970-1994. Source (III.6): Abbott Laboratories.

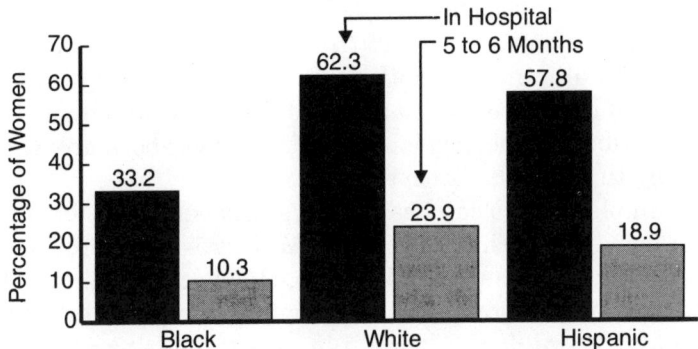

Figure 19.2. Breastfeeding by Rates by Race: 1994. Includes exclusive and supplemented breastfeeding. Source (III.6): Abbott Laboratories.

Section 19.2

Feeding Baby: Nature and Nurture

FDA Consumer, September 1990

Parents of a new baby have a million things to do, but menu-planning isn't one of them. Until a baby is 4 to 6 months old, for breakfast, lunch and dinner—and, of course, the infamous middle-of-the-night feeding—the only items on the menu are either breast milk or infant formula.

Breast Milk Is Best

Usually a manufacturer won't announce that the competition's product is a better choice. But when the competition is breast milk, infant formula manufacturers concede—right on the label—that breast milk is best.

Human breast milk is the ideal nourishment for human babies. Its protein content is particularly suited to a baby's metabolism, and the fat content is more easily absorbed and digested than the fats in cow's milk.

Breast milk also may protect the infant against certain diseases, infections and allergies. A mother's milk contains cells from her immune system and antibodies against diseases to which she has been exposed. Antibodies she develops after the baby is born are also passed to the baby through the breast milk.

For example, if Mom catches the flu, she develops antibodies to that strain of flu virus. Richard Schanler, M.D., associate professor of pediatrics at Baylor College of Medicine, Houston, explains. "The baby will get some protection. [The baby] might not get the flu at all, or the case may be milder . . . than if he or she wasn't breast-fed to begin with."

However, risks of breast milk may outweigh advantages if a nursing mother takes certain medications or abuses drugs. The quality and quantity of the mother's diet may affect the quality and quantity of breast milk.

Breastfeeding

Breast-Feeding Success

"Learn about breast-feeding before the baby is born," says Julie Stock of the La Leche League, an international breast-feeding support and educational organization. "If you know a lot beforehand, you start to build a sense of confidence. Many attempts at breast-feeding fail because of wrong information."

Once the baby is born, breast-feeding as soon as possible after delivery and often is the first of three essential keys for success, says Stock.

The second key is no artificial nipples—that includes pacifiers as well as bottles of water or formula—during the first few weeks. Stock explains that some babies can become very confused by the different feel and the different way of sucking needed with a bottle or pacifier, and they may not be able to switch back to the breast.

Finally, it is important to make sure that the baby "latches on" to the mother's nipple correctly. "If [a mother] has those three things going for her, in general that will eliminate about 90 percent of the common problems that mothers have," says Stock.

The La Leche League has local chapter meetings throughout the country where expectant and new mothers can learn about breast-feeding, nutrition, and other aspects of child care. For the number of your local chapter, call the La Leche League at 1-708-455-7730 or write to La Leche League International, 9616 Minneapolis Ave., P.O. Box 1209, Franklin Park, Ill. 60131-8209.

Second Best

The composition of infant formula is similar to breast milk, but it isn't a perfect match. Further, the exact chemical makeup of breast milk is still unknown.

"We're always discovering things in human milk that are there in small quantities that hadn't been looked at before," says John C. Wallingford, Ph.D., an infant nutrition specialist with FDA's Center for Food Safety and Applied Nutrition. "But [infant formula] is increasingly close to breast milk, especially in the area of fatty acids and lipids."

More than half the calories in breast milk come from fat, and the same is true for today's infant formulas. This may be alarming to many American adults watching their intake of fat and cholesterol, especially when high saturated fats, such as coconut oil are used in formulas. (High saturated fats tend to increase blood cholesterol levels more than other fats or oils.) But the low-fat diet recommended for adults doesn't apply to infants.

"Infants have a very high energy requirement, and they have a restricted volume of food that they can digest," says Wallingford. "The only way to get the energy density of a food up is to increase the amount of fat."

Homemade Isn't Best

Homemade formulas should not be used, says Nick Duy, assistant to the director in FDA's division of regulatory guidance. Homemade formulas based on whole cows' milk don't meet all of an infant's vitamin and mineral needs. In addition, the high protein content of cow's milk makes it difficult for an infant to digest and may put a strain on the baby's immature kidneys. Substituting evaporated milk for whole milk may make the formula easier to digest, but it is still nutritionally inadequate when compared to commercially prepared formula. Use of soy drinks as an infant formula can actually be life-threatening.

Commercially prepared formulas are regulated by the Food and Drug Administration as a food for special dietary use. "Infant formulas are the most heavily regulated food that there is," says Wallingford.

FDA regulations specify exact nutrient level requirements for infant formulas, based on recommendations by the American Academy of Pediatrics Committee on Nutrition. The following must be included in all formulas:

- protein
- fat
- linoleic acid
- vitamin A
- vitamin D
- vitamin E
- vitamin K
- thiamine (vitamin B1)
- riboflavin (vitamin B2)
- vitamin B6
- vitamin B12
- niacin
- folic acid

- pantothenic acid
- vitamin C
- calcium
- phosphorus
- magnesium
- iron
- zinc
- manganese
- copper
- iodine
- sodium
- potassium
- chloride

In addition, formulas not made with cow's milk must include biotin, choline and inositol.

The safety of commercially prepared formula is also enhanced by strict quality control procedures that require manufacturers to analyze each batch of formula for required nutrients, to test representative samples for stability over the shelf life of the product, to code containers to identify the batch, and to make all records available to FDA investigators.

Formula Choices

The most common sources of protein in infant formulas are either cow's milk or soybeans. "For term infants, soy formulas appear to be as nutritionally sound as milk-based formulas, and their use is unlikely to expose infants to nutritional risk," wrote pediatrician Samuel J. Foman in 1987 in the *American Journal of Clinical Nutrition*. Baylor's Schanler agrees, but says that there is some question about whether the minerals in soy-based formulas can be used by the infant's body as well as those from cow's milk formula.

For a healthy, full-term infant, "cow's milk formula would be the first choice," Schanler says. "The only indication that I see for soy formula is for babies with lactose intolerance."

Lactose, also known as milk sugar, is the main carbohydrate in milk. Infants who don't have enough of the enzyme lactase to digest the lactose may suffer from abdominal pain, diarrhea, gas, bloating, or cramps. There is no lactose in soy formula.

Schanler does not think soy formula is a good choice for infants with milk allergies, however. "If there is a real history of [milk] allergy in the family, the baby might be allergic to soy, too," he says. Instead of soy, Schanler recommends special cow's milk formulas known as protein hydrolysates, which won't cause allergic reactions because the proteins are already broken down. "That way the chance of a cross reaction with the soy protein is eliminated," he explains.

Both milk and soy formulas are available in powder, liquid concentrate, or ready-to-feed forms. The choice should depend on "whatever the parents find convenient and can afford," says Schanler.

Whatever form is chosen, proper preparation and refrigeration are essential. Opened cans of ready-to-feed and liquid concentrate must be refrigerated and used within the time specified on the can. Once the powder is mixed with water it should also be refrigerated, if it is not used right away. The exact amounts of water recommended on the label must be used. Under-diluted formula can cause problems for the infant's organs and digestive system. Over-diluted formula will not provide adequate nutrition, and the baby may fail to thrive and grow.

Warming the formula isn't necessary for proper nutrition, says William MacLean, M.D., a pediatrician at infant formula manufacturer Ross Laboratories. "There is nothing magical about having [the formula] warmed up to body temperature," he says. "But if it's cold, some babies may refuse it. It's the baby's preference."

Bottles should not be heated in microwave ovens because the ovens don't heat evenly, MacLean warns. "The drop a mother tests on her wrist could be fine," he says. But, he explains, undetected "hot spots" in the formula could seriously burn the baby.

The best way to warm a bottle of formula is by placing the bottle in a pot of water and heating the pot on the stove, according to Christine Watson, a nurse who specializes in maternal and newborn care at the Shady Grove Adventist Hospital in Gaithersburg, Md. "You can also run hot tap water over the bottle but that isn't very quick," she says.

Vitamin Supplements—Yes or No?

The American Academy of Pediatrics says "the normal breast-fed infant of the well-nourished mother has not been shown conclusively to need any specific vitamin and mineral supplement. Similarly, there is no evidence that supplementation is necessary for the full-term, formula-fed infant and for the properly nourished normal child."

Many physicians recommend supplements, nevertheless—especially for breast-fed infants. "There is definitely some controversy here," says Wallingford.

The controversy on supplements usually revolves around the following:

- **Iron**—Although the amount of iron in breast milk is very low (0.3 milligrams of iron per liter), the infant absorbs almost half. In contrast, while iron-fortified formulas contain 10 to 12 mg per liter, babies absorb only about 4 percent, amounting to about 0.4 mg per liter to 0.5 mg per liter. In either case, those amounts of iron are adequate for the first 4 to 6 months, according to the American Academy of Pediatrics.

  In the past, there was concern that iron-fortified formulas could cause gastrointestinal problems such as colic, constipation, diarrhea, or vomiting. But, based on several studies over the last 10 years, the American Academy of Pediatrics does not believe there is any evidence connecting these problems to iron and recommends that iron-fortified formula be used for all formula-fed infants.

- **Vitamin D**—Insufficient vitamin D can cause rickets, a disease that results in softening and bending of the bones. Although the amounts of vitamin D in breast milk are small, rickets is uncommon in the breast-fed term infant. This may be because, like the iron in breast milk, the vitamin D in breast milk is easily absorbed by the baby.

  Sunlight is important for the formation of vitamin D, but probably as little as a few minutes exposure a day is all the baby needs, says Schanler, and exposure to the whole body isn't necessary—just the arms and face are enough.

- **Fluoride**—No one knows for sure if giving fluoride during the first six months of life will result in fewer cavities. Reflecting the uncertainty surrounding fluoride supplements, the American Academy of Pediatrics recommends starting fluoride supplements shortly after birth in breast-fed infants, but also says that waiting up to six months is acceptable. Because there is no fluoride in infant formula, that twofold recommendation also applies when ready-to-feed formula is used or when the water used for powdered or concentrated formula has less than 0.3 parts per million of fluoride.

Solid Evidence

Sometime between a baby's 4-month and 6-month birthdays solid food can be introduced. Exactly when depends on several factors.

One factor involves the disappearance of the involuntary action called the extrusion reflex. Before this reflex disappears, feeding solids usually involves putting a spoonful in the mouth and scraping most of it off the baby's face as he or she spits it back out.

Also, babies should be able to sit up and turn their heads away. That way, Schanler explains, they can communicate that they're not ready for the next spoonful or just not hungry anymore.

Usually, the first food recommended is a single-grain, iron-fortified infant cereal. Starting with single-grain cereals makes it easier to pinpoint any allergic reactions.

The biggest concern with feeding solids too early is that the solids will replace breast milk or formula in the baby's diet. "Solids vary nutritionally depending on the food," says Schanler. "None of them is as complete as formula or breast milk. You don't want to rob [the baby] of milk."

Feeding babies exclusively with breast milk or formula during the first few months is not only the best thing for the babies' health, it can also be a blessing for busy, overtired parents. Now if only the baby would sleep through the night.

Soy Beverages Not Complete Formulas

A severely malnourished 5-month-old infant was admitted to Arkansas Children's Hospital, Little Rock, Ark., last February with symptoms including heart failure, rickets, vasculitis (blood vessel inflammation), and possible neurological damage. According to the hospital, the baby girl had been fed nothing but Soy Moo since she was 3 days old. Soy Moo is a soy beverage sold in health food stores.

This kind of soy beverage, sometimes improperly called "soy milk," should not be confused with soy-based infant formulas. Unlike true infant formulas, which are nutritionally complete and appropriate for infants, soy beverages are lacking some of the nutrients infants need. Analysis of Soy Moo by the Arkansas Children's Hospital revealed deficiencies in calcium, niacin, and vitamins D, E and C.

Labels on Soy Moo cartons and literature about the drink do not suggest that Soy Moo be used as an infant formula. In addition, an FDA investigation found no evidence that the infant's parents were explicitly told that Soy Moo could be used as a baby's sole nourishment. Nevertheless, Soy Moo's distributor, Health Valley Foods, Irwindale, Calif., has voluntarily stopped distribution until new labels stating "Do Not Use As Infant Formula" can be printed.

FDA learned of a similar incident that occurred last April when a California couple questioned a physician about their 2-month-old daughter's failure to gain weight. The physician discovered that the baby had been exclusively fed Edensoy, another brand of soy beverage. A midwife had recommended Edensoy to the parents, according to the FDA investigator assigned to the case.

In response to this incident, Edensoy's manufacturer, Eden Foods, Clinton, Mich., wrote all its retailers in the United States and Canada to remind them that Edensoy is not an infant formula. In addition, the letter said, "Please make sure that no store personnel suggest or imply that Edensoy or other soy beverages are suitable for use as infant formula."

In an effort to prevent this problem with similar soy beverages, FDA asked all 68 known manufacturers, importers, and private label distributors of these products to include a warning against using the beverages as infant formula. The agency does not, however, have the regulatory authority to require this warning.

— by Dori Stehlin

Section 19.3

Lactation Suppression: Safer without Drugs

FDA Consumer, April 1990

Rosellen Bowen was having a tough time completing her master's thesis. The graduate nursing student was researching whether breast massage would help relieve the pain and discomfort some new mothers experience when they don't breast-feed their babies. But she had trouble finding participants.

During the year she worked on her thesis, over 3,000 babies were born at the University of Rochester Medical School Hospital, where she worked, and the Rochester Community Hospital. But out of the 800 women at these two hospitals who didn't breast-feed their babies, Bowen could only find 46 who said they felt pain when their breasts filled up with milk.

Determining pain is subjective, experts say. But on a 10-point pain scale that Bowen provided for the participants, no mother, at any time, scored pain above a 6.

"She had a lot of trouble completing her thesis with a valid number of patients because [pain] was not a common complaint," says Ruth Lawrence, M.D., a pediatrician who worked with Bowen.

Bowen found that although breast massage did help some new mothers, for most, the long-standing traditional treatment of pain relievers, ice packs, and a well-fitting bra or specially made breast binder was sufficient.

Use of Lactation Suppressants in U.S. (1988)

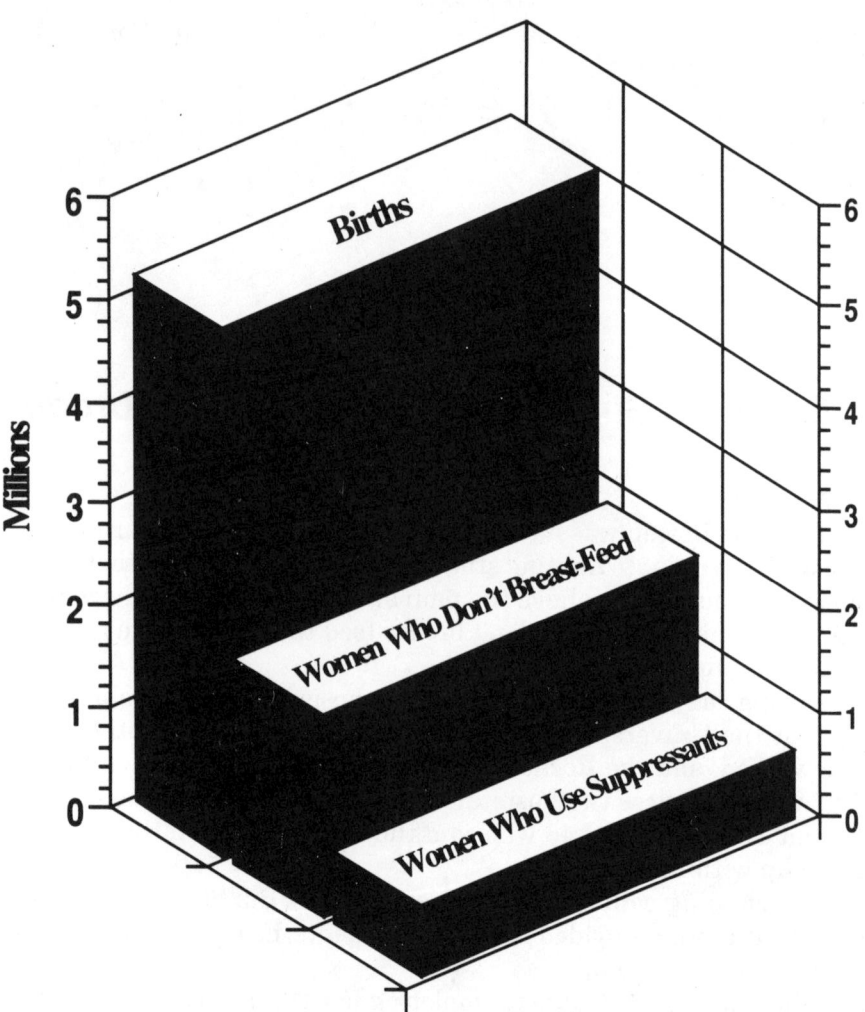

Figure 19.3. In 1982, 5.2 million babies were born in the United States. Of the 2 million mothers who didn't breast-feed their babies, 700,000 took lactation suppressants.

Because other studies have also shown that these traditional treatments provide enough help for the minority of women who do experience pain, and because the drugs used to suppress lactation carry risks, the Food and Drug Administration's Fertility and Maternal Health Drugs Advisory Committee recently recommended that drugs to prevent milk production not be used. Following the committee's recommendation, FDA has asked the manufacturers of these drugs to stop including lactation suppression as an approved use.

The major drug used for suppressing lactation is a non-hormonal substance called bromocriptine. It is also used to treat Parkinson's disease, but because this is a serious disease, the risks associated with the drug's use do not outweigh its benefits. The other lactation-suppressing products all contain the female sex hormone estrogen, alone or in combination with the hormone testosterone.

Sending a Message

Even when a woman knows long before her baby is born that she isn't going to breast-feed, her body needs a few nonbreast-feeding days after the baby is born to get the message.

In the meantime, milk production begins. First, levels of the hormones estrogen and progesterone, which are very high during pregnancy, drop abruptly after birth. This drop signals another hormone, prolactin, to stimulate milk production in the breast. The milk is produced in cells throughout the breast and then travels through the milk ducts to the openings in the nipple. In a mother who breast-feeds, her baby's suckling signals the prolactin to keep the milk coming. But when a woman doesn't breast-feed her baby, the prolactin levels drop, and milk production ceases.

In the few days it takes before lactation stops, the mother's breasts can fill up with milk. For some non-nursing women, this engorgement is uncomfortable, and occasionally even painful.

Lactation suppression drugs prevent engorgement and, in fact, prevent lactation before it begins. The most commonly prescribed drug, bromocriptine, acts by cutting the production of prolactin. In contrast, the sex hormones keep the estrogen at pre-birth levels, tricking the body into thinking it is still pregnant.

Do They Work?

The National Academy of Sciences/National Research Council (NAS/NRC) reviewed the effectiveness of estrogens and androgens such as testosterone as lactation suppressants approximately 20 years ago as part of a review of all drugs approved before the 1962 drug amendments. (The amendments required, for the first time, that drugs must be effective as well as safe.)

NAS/NRC explained that it did not know of any satisfactory evidence that these drugs could effectively prevent lactation. Nevertheless, since the drugs were commonly used for lactation suppression, the panel decided the indication could be continued.

Evidence on the safety of the sex hormones for lactation suppression is also lacking. (Since the safety problems connected with other uses of these hormones had not surfaced in the 1950s, the indication was allowed at that time.) The risk of thromboembolism has been connected with estrogens used as oral contraceptives. But, according to FDA's Diane Wysowski, Ph.D., "there is a paucity of good, definitive data on the acute and long-term effects of sex hormones used for prevention of postpartum breast engorgement. The bottom line is, nobody really knows."

The same uncertainty about safety and effectiveness surrounds bromocriptine. When FDA approved this drug for lactation suppression, clinical trials had not uncovered any serious side effects and the results of several studies showed that the majority of women given the drug did not experience engorgement. However, what was impossible to determine with these studies was whether engorgement was actually prevented. There is no way to predict whether a woman's breasts will become engorged or, if they do, whether the engorgement will cause pain.

In addition, even when bromocriptine seems to work, the drug's success may be short-lived. According to the official labeling, up to 40 percent of the time, rebound engorgement occurs after the two week course of treatment with bromocriptine ends.

According to FDA's division of metabolism and endocrine drug products, bromocriptine has been associated with seizures, strokes, and heart attacks, but the connection has not been firmly established. What has been established are bromocriptine's less severe side effects—nausea, dizziness, and drop in blood pressure.

Benefit vs. Risk

Based on several different studies, FDA estimates that only a very small minority of women given lactation suppressants may possibly benefit from the treatment. For the majority, taking the drug only exposes them to possible side effects. In August 1989, the Health Research Group, a consumer organization, requested action against the use of lactation suppressants. In its response, FDA said that because the drugs are not therapeutically required, any risks are unacceptable.

What about the side effects from doing nothing to stop milk from coming in? "The side effects of letting nature take its course—breast engorgement, leakage, discomfort—are short-lived," says Lisa Rarick, M.D., an obstetrician with FDA's division of metabolism and endocrine drug products. "Doing nothing is 100 percent effective. It's an issue similar to any physiological problem that resolves on its own, like painful [menstrual] periods. When you have an adolescent come to your office and she hasn't had a period yet, you don't just automatically give her a prescription to prevent painful cramps. If somebody comes to you and she has the pain, then you treat her."

Where does that leave women who decide not to breast-feed? First, the symptoms can be treated by other means if they occur. According to the University of Rochester's Lawrence, who has written a book for physicians on all aspects of breast-feeding, nonprescription pain relievers such as acetaminophen "seem to take care of women's discomforts. Only rarely is something [stronger] needed."

Second, except for two estrogen drugs that are only used for lactation suppression, all the other products will still be on the market. FDA does not regulate the practice of medicine. Physicians are free to use approved drugs in any way they feel is medically necessary.

Lawrence adds that the risks of letting lactation end naturally "seem to be close to zero. I think in some respects we've assumed that women would rather be medicated than experience any discomfort at all, and that is probably not true."

—*by Dori Stehlin*

Section 19.4

Breastfeeding and the Working Mother

BEST START-Kentucky,
Lexington-Fayette County Health Department, 1993

As more mothers come back to work soon after their babies are born, they are thinking about how to balance work and breastfeeding. This guide can help you plan for breastfeeding once you go back to work.

Step 1. Explore Your Options During Your Pregnancy

- Learn about your company's maternity leave policies -how long you can be out, with or without pay, after the baby is born. The older the baby is when you return, the less you will need to pump your milk during the day. Learn if you can come back at first on a part-time or flex-time schedule, or if there is a job-sharing plan. This way you don't have to work as many hours at first and can gradually get used to being back.

- See if your company has a policy about breastfeeding babies or expressing breastmilk during the workday:
    1. Flexible time during the day.
    2. A clean, private, and quiet place.
    3. A place to store your breastmilk.

- Talk to other breastfeeding working moms to see what they did. Consider a support group at work.

- Look at your current job and see how breastfeeding can fit in. Look for times in your current schedule that could be used for nursing or pumping, like morning or afternoon breaks and lunchtimes. See if your employer will let you work earlier or later so that you can have longer breaks during the day.

Breastfeeding

- Find a place at work to nurse or express your milk.

    1. If the baby will be in an on-site or nearby child care center, you may be able to go and nurse during the day. Also, your child care provider may be able to bring the baby to you on your breaks.

    2. Use a "do not disturb" sign to help insure privacy.

    3. You will want a place that is quiet, private, clean, and has a comfortable chair. This could be a private office, store-room, women's lounge, health service office, or athletic facility. A nearby sink is very useful. A public restroom or toilet stall is a last choice—they are not usually very clean or comfortable, but are better than nothing.

    4. Some companies with many breastfeeding mothers may have a special place set aside. Ask the Personnel Manager or Health Nurse.

- Plan a way to store your milk. Keep the bottles of milk in the employee refrigerator. Put them in a box or container labeled with your name. This will protect the milk from spilling, getting lost or thrown out. If you work in a food service (restaurant, hotel, bakery, etc.), ask your employer if you can store your breastmilk in the commercial refrigerator. There are no laws against storing breastmilk with other foods. Alternatively, use ice packs with a small cooler, ice chest, or thermos to store breastmilk in your locker or other safe storage place.

- Discuss your ideas and plans with your employer before you have your baby. See how well they fit with your employer's policies. If your employer doesn't have a policy, see if your plan is acceptable given the current work environment. Remind them of the long-term benefits of breastfeeding compared with your short-term needs to keep pumping.

- Some moms find it impossible to arrange a system for nursing or expressing during the day. These moms nurse when they are at home with the baby and have the child care provider give formula during the day.

Step 2. Prepare Yourself During Maternity Leave

- Give yourself time to get to know your baby, yourself, and how breastfeeding works. The more comfortable you feel with breastfeeding, the easier it will be once you return to work.

- Wait for at least 3-4 weeks to give your baby a bottle of breastmilk. By this time, breastfeeding becomes easier. Give a bottle every once in a while so the baby learns how to drink from it. Have someone else besides you give the bottle. An older baby could be given breastmilk directly from a cup. Express your breastmilk every time the baby takes a bottle so you keep up your own supply.

- Nurse in different places so you will feel more comfortable nursing or expressing milk away from home—at work, the child care provider's, etc.

- Keep track of the times your baby usually wants to breastfeed, so that you can try to express milk or nurse about the same times once you've gone back to work. This will help you feel more comfortable and keep you from feeling too full or leaking.

- Find a child care provider who will support your plans for breastfeeding and is near where you work.

- Learn how to express your breastmilk by hand. This can help with your own comfort as your body learns to make milk. Some women are able to express as much milk by hand as they can by using a pump.

- If you use a pump, choose one that is best for your needs:

  1. A large electric pump is most efficient—you can express from both breasts at the same time, taking about 15 minutes. They can be rented from medical equipment suppliers for between $1.00 and $3.00 a day. Some mothers share the use and cost of a pump, making it more affordable.

  2. A battery-operated pump is less expensive and more portable, but not as efficient. They only pump one side at a time (unless you buy two pumps), so they take a little longer to use. They cost between $50 and $75.

3. Manual pumps come in many different designs. The most efficient are the Loyd-B, Medela Manualectric, and Ameda Egnell Mother's Touch. They will only pump one side at a time, and will take about 15 minutes for each side.

- Fresh breastmilk can be refrigerated safely for 48 hours. Breastmilk may be safely frozen for a month in a combination refrigerator/freezer, or up to six months in a deep-freeze. Store milk in the amounts your baby usually takes for a single feeding—try 2-oz amounts for a young baby.

- One week before you return, start to practice. If you haven't started pumping yet, begin expressing milk at the same times you will pump at work. This gives you a chance to learn how to use the pump, how long it will take, and how your body feels. It will also help you build up an extra supply of stored breastmilk. Also, visit your child care provider and leave the baby for some short periods. This lets you, the provider, and the baby get used to each other. Let the provider know your baby's usual feeding times so she can feed then. You may want to make a whole-day trial run a few days before you really go back to work to see how things go.

Step 3. Breastfeeding When You Return to Work

- Try to go back to work mid-week or late in the week. Keep a light schedule if possible, or work shorter hours. This will make you less tired and less worried about being away from your baby.

- Get up a little early so you can nurse the baby (even if you both are still sleepy). Then the baby will be happy while you get ready for the day. Try to nurse again just before you leave home or when dropping the baby off at the child care provider's.

- Express your breastmilk on your "usual" schedule. Have pictures of your baby, a blanket, or toy to remind you about your baby. This can help you relax and make it easier to express milk.

- Store breastmilk in small amounts, 2 to 4 ounces, for a young baby. Label the bottle with the baby's name and the date so the child care provider knows who the milk is for and how fresh it is. Fresh milk should be used within 2 days.

- Wear two-piece outfits to make pumping or nursing easier. If you leak milk, try to express more often, use nursing pads inside your bra, or press gently against your nipples to stop the leak. Wear clothing with a pattern, a sweater, or a jacket to hide leak marks.

- Nurse again when you pick the baby up from day care or when you get home. Relaxing together for the first 30 minutes can refresh you and keep your baby happy while you fix dinner.

- Breastfeed when you're with the baby to keep up your milk supply—mornings, evenings and weekends. Try not to use bottles or formula.

- Drink plenty of fluids like water and juice during the day. Limit caffeine drinks like coffee, tea, or colas to two drinks a day.

- As your baby gets older and starts eating other foods, you may not need to pump as often during the day.

- Give your employers feedback about how it is going. Let them know your satisfaction or dissatisfaction with the system, and encourage them to keep helping you. Tell them how healthy your baby has been.

Other Tips

- Many areas in your life will change when you have a new baby. Learning to breastfeed and work are part of those changes. Once a routine is set up, it will get easier. Don't be too hard on yourself—give yourself and your family time to settle in to your new life.

- Give yourself time to rest. Consider a nap when you get home. Get other family members or friends to make meals, clean house or do laundry. Cut down on your activities and things that do not need to get done. You and your baby are most important—let other people help take care of you.

- If you have questions or problems with breastfeeding after you go back to work, call your local health department, lactation consultant, or La Leche League (1-800-LA-LECHE) for help.

- If you want to learn more, read "Of Cradles and Careers: A Guide to Reshaping Your Job to Include A Baby In Your Life" by

Kaye Lowman or "The Working Woman's Guide to Breastfeeding" by Nancy Dana and Anne Price. They may be available at your local bookstore or library.

The period of time you will be breastfeeding is short compared to your whole working career. The long-term benefits of a healthy and happy child are worth the short-term extra effort for you and your employer.

Resources for Breastfeeding Education, Management and Support

American Academy of Pediatrics (AAP)
141 Northwest Point Road
P.O. Box 927
Elk Grove Village
IL 660009-0927
Contact Mary Claire Walsh (708) 981-7933

American Society of Psychoprophylaxis in Obstetrics, Inc. (ASPO/Lamaze)
1101 Connecticut Avenue, NW, Suite 700
Washington, D.C. 20036
(800) 36-4404

International Lactation Consultant Association
201 Brown Avenue
Evanston, IL 60202
Contact: Jan Barger (708) 260-8874

La Leche League International
9616 Minneapolis Avenue
Franklin Park, IL 60131
(708) 455-7730

National Center for Education in Maternal and Child Health
2000 15th Street North, Suite 701
Arlington, VA 22201
(703) 524-7802

National Healthy Mothers, Healthy Babies Coalition
409 12th Street SW
Washington, DC 20024
(202) 863-2458

Section 19.5

Potential Health Care Costs of Not Breastfeeding

Excerpts from BEST START-Kentucky, Lexington-Fayette County Health Department, 1993

Every time a child is ill, the working parent faces increased stress. This stress can be transferred to the workplace through employees who are absent, distracted, and thus less productive. The Los Angeles Department of Water and Power estimated that it cost $360 each day a $15 per hour employee was off work caring for a sick child.

Breastfeeding is one way in which infants and children can be protected from and strengthened against many common childhood infectious diseases.

The Health Benefits of Breastfeeding

Breastfed children are half as likely to have any illnesses within the first year as formula-fed children, and are 10 times less likely to be hospitalized for any bacterial infection.

Breastmilk has components which coat the digestive tract, making it more difficult for bacteria to grow and spread. It also contains anti-infective agents which help to destroy bacteria and viruses, further protecting the vulnerable baby.

The American Academy of Pediatrics recommends that infants be breastfed a minimum of three months in order to protect the immature systems as they finish growing. Breastfeeding for a longer period is beneficial as the amount of protection is often related to the total length of breastfeeding.

Cow's milk formulas are more difficult for the baby's immature systems to digest, so the baby may be at more risk for food allergies. They do not contain the other protective components of breastmilk, making the baby more susceptible to infection, illness, and chronic diseases.

Breastfeeding

Determining the bottom line on children's illnesses

1. **Diarrhea.** These digestive tract infections result in dehydration and sometimes hospitalization. In the U.S., diarrheal disease kills about 500 infants and children annually, around 200,000 are hospitalized each year, and total treatment costs range from $4 million to $10.3 million. Breastfed infants are 3 to 4 times less likely to have diarrheal diseases than formula-fed infants.

2. **Ear Infections.** By age 3, 1/3 of all children have had more than three episodes of ear infections. In the U.S., ear infections cost more than $1 billion annually in visits to physicians. Breastfed children have a 60% decrease in risk for ear infections compared with formula-fed children.

3. **Allergies.** Food allergies are often triggered by proteins the infant is unable to digest. The infant with a family history of respiratory or food allergies is at higher risk for a severe reaction due to an immature immune system. Breastfed infants and children have a significantly lower risk for food allergies, especially cow's milk and other protein reactions, and are often protected from other respiratory allergies due to immunological factors in breastmilk.

4. **Respiratory Synctial Virus (RSV).** This is an upper and lower respiratory infection that is the widest spread virus in the U.S. It is usually more severe among infants under 6 months, and is often associated with or compounded by influenza, bronchitis, or pneumonia. RSV has a high risk for annual reinfections, and can even lead to death. Breastfed infants have a significant decrease in severity for RSV, with fewer hospitalizations.

5. **Bronchitis/Pneumonia.** These conditions can start as a mild lung infection, often from contact with large numbers of other children. As the infection increases in severity, it can cause high fevers, breathing difficulties, and lead to hospitalization. In the U.S., treatment for such infections cost more than $19 million annually. Breastfed children have an 80% decrease in risk for lower respiratory infections.

6. **Meningitis.** An infection that targets the nervous system, meningitis can be caused by a variety of bacteria and viruses. Different types of meningitis are seasonal and can be of varying degrees, ranging from a severe headache to brain damage and death. Breastfed children have a 4-fold decrease in risk for infections causing meningitis, and a significant decrease in severity when infected.

7. **Baby Bottle Tooth Decay.** Pooling of sweet liquids around the gums and teeth can cause damage or loss of the front teeth. This often happens when the child is put to bed with a bottle of sweet liquid (formula, milk, juice) or sips these liquids constantly from a bottle during the day. Breastfed infants and children are at a very low risk for baby bottle tooth decay because the infant is typically not at the breast long enough for significant pooling to occur.

8. **Diabetes Mellitus.** Genetically susceptible infants and children may become insulin-dependent around age 7 or 8. Nationally, about 120,000 children are affected by Insulin Dependent Diabetes Mellitus (IDDM). However, only 5 or 6 per 1000 genetically susceptible children develop this disease. Current research suggests that the early introduction of inappropriate proteins (especially those found in cow's milk) may trigger the development of IDDM. Children with IDDM are more susceptible to infections than IDDM adults or non-affected children. Breastfed infants and children are at reduced risk for developing IDDM, especially those given only breastmilk for the first several months.

References

Cunningham, in Jelliffe and Jelliffe Advances in International Maternal and Child Health, Oxford: Oxford Univ. Press, vol. 1, 1981.

Duffy, Riepenhoff-Talty, Ogra, et.al, Am J Dis Child 140:1164-68, 1986.

Pullan, Toms, Martin, et.al Br. Med J. 281 (6247):1034-36, 1980.

Section 19.6

Recent Advances in Maternal and Infant Nutrition

Excerpt from *Nutrition: Eating for Good Health*, U.S. Department of Agriculture, Agriculture Information Bulletin 685.

Milk fat provides infants with the essential fatty acids important for the growth of their neurological tissue and cell membranes. It also provides about 50 percent of their energy needs. Scientists need to understand how dietary fat is used to produce human milk, so food recommendations can be formulated for breast-feeding mothers.

Maternal Nutrition and Lactation

Most of the dietary fatty acids consumed by lactating women are (1) converted to energy through oxidation, (2) secreted into milk, or (3) stored in maternal adipose tissues. The Children's Nutrition Research Center has studied what happens to dietary fats in lactating, well-nourished women who consume either a low-fat diet or a high-fat diet. The diets were randomly assigned to 16 women who were nursing their infants.

The results of the study indicate that women on the low-fat diet had a lower concentration of fat in their milk but produced greater amounts of milk. Thus, their daily secretion of milk fat did not change, but their total carbohydrate production increased. The study also indicates that women with more body fat are better able to store dietary lipids and consequently may have difficulty losing weight

In contrast, Otomi Indian women living in rural Mexico who consume a low-fat diet and have low body fat may produce milk that has a low fat content. Lactation was studied in these women because their infants were growing poorly. The Otomi women consume a low-fat, corn-predominant diet. Although their milk production rates were actually 15-20 percent higher than rates reported for well-nourished women, the concentrations of fat and energy in their milk were lower and may have contributed to the poor growth of their infants.

Infant Nutrition

Growth standards for infants from the National Center for Health Statistics (NCHS), Washington, DC, were derived primarily from formula-fed infants studied 20-50 years ago.

Efforts are now under way to revise growth standards for infants. In a study at the Children's Nutrition Research Center, the growth of breast-fed and formula-fed infants was monitored for 9 months. Investigators found that formula-fed infants gained more weight after 3 months than breast-fed infants of the same age.

Until recently, most nutrition studies in infants relied on measurements of weight and length to estimate growth and body composition. Today, however, scientists have new techniques, such as total body

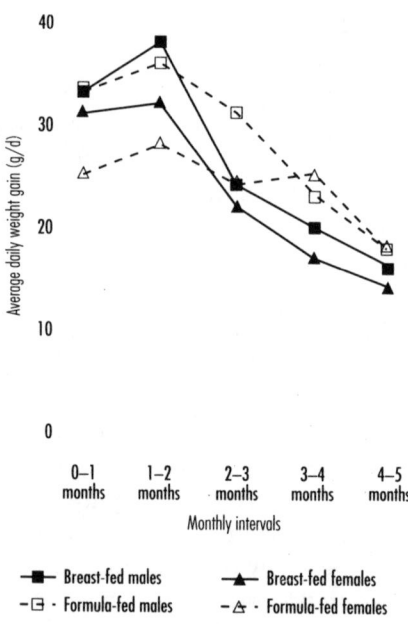

Figure 19.4. Composition of weight gain in breast-fed and formula-fed infants

electrical conductivity, to measure lean and fat body mass. Surprisingly, initial studies suggest that breast-fed infants may have more body fat than formula-fed infants. Other methods make it possible to measure how infants use the nutrients in the food they eat. Using indirect calorimetry and the doubly labeled water ($^2H_2{}^{18}O$) method, investigators have shown that breast-fed infants not only consume fewer calories than formula-fed babies but also expend fewer calories.

Besides differences in how breast-fed and formula-fed infants use calories, there are important differences in their biochemical makeup. Breast-fed infants have higher plasma cholesterol concentrations than formula-fed infants, presumably because of the higher cholesterol content of human milk than formula. The synthesis of cholesterol in breast-fed infants is one-third that of formula-fed infants. Scientists are now trying to determine how cholesterol intake in infancy affects cholesterol levels in adulthood.

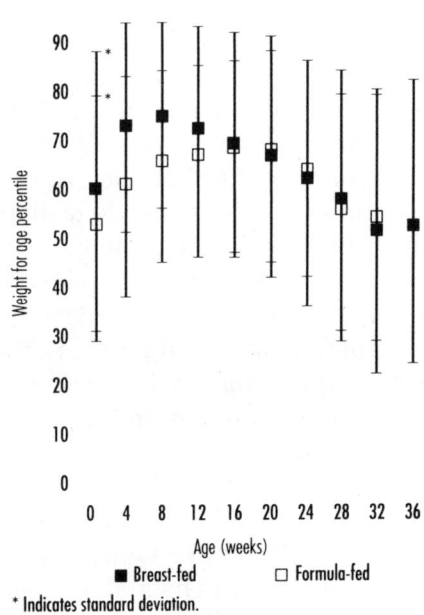

Figure 19.5. Growth of breast-fed and formula-fed infants measured by growth standards of the National Center for Health Statistics (courtesy of J.E. Stuff)

Nutrition of the Preterm Infant

The survival rate of preterm infants has increased dramatically in the last several years; at least 90 percent of infants born prematurely survive. Scientists are studying differences in the composition of human and cow's milk to determine the levels of nutrients most suitable for preterm infants. Feeding human milk to preterm infants appears to be advantageous, because (1) the fat content of human milk is more appropriate than that of cow's milk for infant brain development, and (2) the levels of immunoglobulins in human milk may increase an infant's ability to defend against infection. Human milk, however, is "designed" by nature for full-term infants, whose bones are more fully developed, so investigators at the Children's Nutrition Research Center are studying how much additional calcium and phosphorus must be added to human milk to ensure healthy bone growth in preterm infants.

Studying Postnatal Growth and Development

Some infant nutrition questions must be studied in animals, such as the infant pig, to avoid the possibility of harming human subjects. Scientists at the Children's Nutrition Research Center are studying genetically lean and obese piglets to learn how fat and cholesterol are used in early life. They have found that cholesterol levels in genetically obese piglets continue to rise when their diets contain cholesterol, suggesting that these piglets may not be able to shut down cholesterol synthesis when cholesterol is provided in the diet. Studies have also shown that piglets with low levels of plasma cholesterol grow more slowly than piglets with higher levels. Because infant formula has very little cholesterol compared with human milk, both findings are important in designing human infant formulas, whether for full-term or preterm infants.

Rats are also studied to learn more about human infants. Because they are particularly immature at birth, rats are relevant to studies of preterm infants. Investigators have found that before 10 days of age, the weight gain of rat pups consists almost entirely of protein, with very little increase in body fat. This phenomenon can also be seen in preterm infants. From the studies in rats, scientists have learned that adequate nutrition immediately after birth is very important to ensure normal maturation.

Continuing Research

Nutrient utilization in lactating females and their offspring is being investigated through noninvasive techniques and animal models. We have yet to fully understand how maternal diet and nutritional status affect milk composition and how dietary manipulation of infant weight gain, body composition, and serum cholesterol affects health later in life. Studies to ensure that preterm infants get adequate nutrition will enable normal growth and development and promote optimal cognitive and immune functions. Both short- and long-term effects of infant nutrition on the developing organism are important in defining the nutritional requirements of infants.

Nancy F. Butte
Associate Professor,
USDA-ARS Children's Nutrition Research Center,
Department of Pediatrics,
Baylor College of Medicine,
Houston, TX

Chapter 20

Routine Medical Screening of Newborns

Newborn screening began in the early 1960's with the research interests of Dr. Robert Guthrie and financial support from the Maternal and Child Health Division of the U.S. Children's Bureau at the direction of Mr. Rudolf Hormuth. Since that time, this vital area of preventative medicine has expanded to all states and territories. To date there is no national law regarding screening and each program functions independently.

While hemoglobinopathy screening has been a part of some newborn screening programs for many years, its major expansion occurred after 1987. Programs continue to expand their follow-up efforts and to better understand the complex issues which must be addressed. Similarly, laboratory techniques for identifying various hemoglobin disorders continue to improve in both sensitivity and specificity.

Newborn screening programs exist in all states and territories. There are 9 disorders commonly included in newborn screening programs:

1. Hyperphenylalaninemia (PKU)
2. Hyperthyroidism
3. Galactosemia
4. Maple Syrup Urine Disease
5. Homocystinuria
6. Biotinidase Deficiency

NIH Consensus Development Conference Statement, 1987 and excerpts from the National Newborn Screening Report, 1992

7. Cystic Fibrosis
8. Congenital Adrenal Hyperplasia
9. Hemoglobinopathies

Other tests that may be included are Tyrosinemia and toxoplasmosis.

In 1992, all programs except Delaware and Maryland, North Carolina, and Vermont report that newborn screening was required by statute. In all programs, a legal mandate existed which allowed for the provision of newborn screening. All U.S. newborn screening programs included screening for phenylketonuria and congenital hypothyroidism in 1992.

Earlier hospital discharge (less than 24 hours) of maternity patients continues to increase. For physiologic reasons, the corresponding early collection of specimens increases the risk of missing an infant with one of the tested disorders. It is important for programs and practitioners to monitor the age of the infant at the time of screening so that proper interpretations of results can be made.

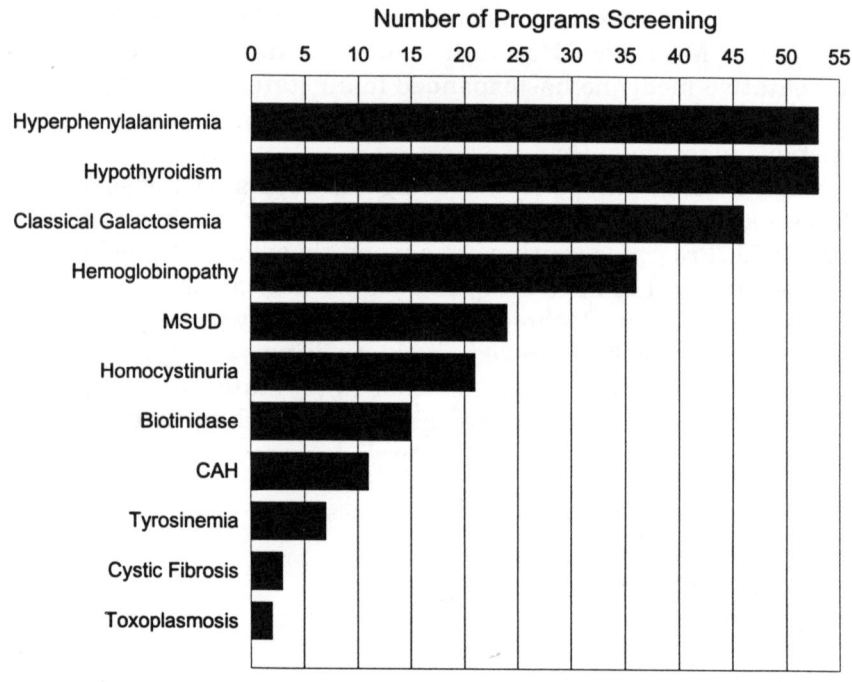

Figure 20.1. Disorders Screened in 1992

Routine Medical Screening of Newborns

Newborn screening is and has been working to prevent death and debilitating conditions. Over 4500 cases of classical PKU are reported with most programs starting PKU screening during the 1960's and over 8800 cases of primary congenital hyperthyroidism are reported with most starting in the early 1980's. In evaluating cost effectiveness of such screening detections, it is important to remember that institutionalization costs for mental retardation which might occur as a consequence of these and other screening disorders is cumulative over the lifetime of the patient.

Newborn Screening for Sickle Cell Disease and Other Hemoglobinopathies

Hemoglobinopathies represent one of the major health problems in the United States and constitute the most common genetic disorders in some populations. Sickle cell diseases (SS, SC, S-beta thalassemia) alone affect about 1/400 American black newborns. These and other hemoglobinopathies are common in persons of African, Mediterranean, Asian, Caribbean, and South and Central American origins as well. Although the technology to screen infants for hemoglobinopathies in the newborn period has been available for many years, widespread adoption of screening has not occurred. Reasons have included lack of a demonstrated improvement in outcome with early diagnosis, uncertainty about whom to test, technical difficulties caused by the high level of fetal hemoglobin in the neonate, and questions about obligations to those identified as carriers.

For at least 20 years, it has been known that children with sickle cell anemia have an increased susceptibility to severe bacterial infection, particularly due to Streptococcus pneumoniae. The risk of major infection with this organism is greatest in the first 3 years of life and can occur as early as 4 months of age. This infection may be the first clinical manifestation of disease and carries a case fatality rate as high as 30 percent. Acute splenic sequestration crisis, another catastrophic event, also contributes to mortality in infancy. Data are now available documenting a reduction of morbidity and mortality through early diagnosis and immediate entry into programs of comprehensive care, including penicillin prophylaxis. Early diagnosis of hemoglobinopathies is facilitated by newborn screening. Screening has the capability of reaching infants who might otherwise be lost to the health care system or delayed in their entry into it. Neonatal testing to identify infants with major sickling diseases allows prompt institution of ongoing care, including the provision of effective prophylaxis.

It is unclear whether presymptomatic interventions offer significant advantage to infants with other hemoglobinopathies (e.g., Hb E-beta thalassemia and homozygous beta and alpha thalassemias). Identification by newborn screening may, however, provide natural history data and/or allow testing of potential interventions.

To examine questions surrounding the issue of neonatal screening and to enhance understanding among scientists, health care providers, and the public at large, the National Heart, Lung, and Blood Institute and the National Institute of Child Health and Human Development of the National Institutes of Health (NIH), the Genetic Disease Services Branch, the Division of Maternal and Child Health, the Bureau of Health Care Delivery and Assistance of the Health Resources and Services Administration, and the NIH Office of Medical Applications of Research convened an NIH Consensus Development Conference on Newborn Screening for Sickle Cell Disease and Other Hemoglobinopathies on April 6-8, 1987. For 1 1/2 days, experts in the field presented their findings, and an audience that included health professionals, parents, patients, and other interested persons discussed the issues. A consensus panel representing the fields of biochemistry, genetics, pediatrics, obstetrics, hematology, public health, nursing, law, epidemiology, and counseling considered the scientific evidence and developed answers to the following questions:

1. Are programs for screening the newborn for sickle cell disease effective in decreasing morbidity and mortality?
2. What are the techniques of screening, and what is their efficacy?
3. What are the major factors to be considered, including benefits and risks, in conducting newborn screening programs?
4. What are the optimal followup and management of infants identified with hemoglobinopathies (disease and carriers)?
5. What future research directions are indicated?

Are programs for screening the newborn for sickle cell disease effective in decreasing morbidity and mortality?

Although the technology to screen infants in the newborn period has been available for the past 15 to 20 years, screening has not received widespread acceptance largely because of the perception that, without effective treatment, early diagnosis would not decrease morbidity and mortality.

There is now indisputable evidence that rates of morbidity and mortality can be significantly reduced by programs that screen newborns for sickle cell disease, if they are linked to comprehensive clinical management systems that include parental education. A recent multicenter randomized trial of oral penicillin prophylaxis in children with sickle cell disease showed an impressive 85 percent reduction in the incidence of infection in the group treated with oral penicillin as compared with the group given placebo. The 13 septic episodes among the 110 patients in the placebo group resulted in 3 deaths compared with no deaths and only 2 septic episodes among the 105 patients treated with prophylactic penicillin. These significant differences between the placebo and penicillin groups were compelling reasons to terminate the study 8 months early, after an average followup of 15 months.

Over the past 20 years, a case fatality rate of 30 percent has been commonly observed among children with sickle cell anemia who develop sepsis. Because babies with sickle cell disease may develop sepsis as young as 4 months of age, early provision of comprehensive care coupled with prophylactic penicillin beginning prior to age 4 months is now recommended. An additional factor possibly contributing to improved survival is the widespread availability of pneumococcal vaccine. These effective interventions fully justify the establishment of newborn screening programs to assure early access to care.

What are the techniques of screening, and what is their efficacy?

The panel recommends centralized laboratories for mass screening programs and for confirmation of diagnosis of sickle cell disease states because of the expertise available and the experience gained from analysis of large numbers of samples.

Effective laboratory procedures exist that are currently being applied in statewide programs for newborn screening for sickle cell disease. The technology for mass screening for hemoglobinopathies is still evolving, especially for the detection of thalassemia states. Electrophoresis at alkaline pH on cellulose acetate followed by further examination of abnormal samples by acid electrophoresis on citrate agar is presently the most popular procedure used for mass screening. Advantages include simplicity, low cost, and standardization. These techniques provide reliable detection of hemoglobins (Hb) S, C, and A even in the presence of large amounts of Hb F. Disadvantages include the need for two different electrophoretic procedures to ensure accurate results and limited resolution of other abnormal hemoglobins. Several large pilot studies have demonstrated low error rates.

However, more data are needed to assess the technical adequacy of each screening procedure with regard to its reproducibility, sensitivity, specificity, and error rates.

Thin layer isoelectric focusing is also currently being employed in many newborn screening programs. This methodology provides better resolution of Hbs A, S, and C from Hb F and detection of many other abnormal hemoglobins by a single procedure. It is, however, more costly, and there has been less experience in its use. High pressure liquid chromatography (HPLC) is a highly sensitive, rapid, and reproducible technique capable of differentiating among many abnormal hemoglobins. This method is currently being evaluated in a few newborn screening programs. Solubility testing procedures are not satisfactory for screening purposes.

The panel concludes that at the present time, cellulose acetate followed by citrate agar electrophoresis is the method of choice for large-scale centralized mass screening. However, isoelectric focusing is a satisfactory alternative and may be the method of choice for some screening programs. Blood collected from heel puncture and dried on filter paper has been the most common method of sample collection for newborn screening programs for inborn errors of metabolism (phenylketonuria, etc.). The use of these same blood samples in neonatal testing for sickle cell disease is advantageous because the system for collection already exists; no duplicate blood sampling is required; and transmittal to centralized laboratories is in place. Disadvantages include susceptibility to sample deterioration and the possibility of contamination by neonatal blood transfusion. Missed sampling is a problem when infants are in special care units or are discharged early.

Alternatively, cord blood samples can be used for neonatal screening. The hemoglobin components within these samples (especially Hb Barts) are more stable, and the problem of contamination by transfusion is avoided. However, cord blood can be contaminated with maternal blood. It is not easily transported and may not be collected during unattended deliveries.

Techniques recommended for newborn screening also can be used for the testing of individuals of any age. Whatever screening method is used, confirmation of abnormal results by analysis of followup blood samples is imperative. Every screening laboratory must participate in a quality-control program that includes proficiency testing. Establishment of a national proficiency testing program should be a high priority, and it should yield predictive values of all test results.

Routine Medical Screening of Newborns

What are the major factors to be considered, including benefits and risks, in conducting newborn screening programs?

In conducting an adequate newborn screening program, the following factors should be considered.

Population To Be Screened. The panel recommends universal screening of all newborns for hemoglobinopathies. Programs that screen only specific high-risk segments of a population tend to miss individuals who are inaccurately registered and to encourage nonscreening because of provider complacency. This panel believes that the health risks to children with sickle cell diseases are so great that major efforts should be made to identify every affected child. Therefore, the panel recommends that most states adopt a policy of screening all newborns. For those states with very few at risk members, targeted screening might be considered. State genetic planning committees and sickle cell advisory committees should provide an appropriate forum for considering the advisability of adopting this exception to the recommended norm.

The Role of Prenatal Screening. The screening for hemoglobinopathies should include both prenatal maternal and neonatal screening as a continuum of health care. Prenatal maternal hemoglobin screening will help to determine maternal obstetrical and neonatal risk and will provide genetic information for the parents, as well as make prenatal diagnosis possible.

Mandating the Provision of Screening Education of Professionals and the Public. Good medical practice dictates that screening be provided for all neonates as a part of ordinary health care. The benefits of screening are so compelling that its provision should not be left to the discretion of individual physicians or health care facilities. State law should require the provision of such services.

Providers should inform pregnant women about the availability and purpose of antenatal and neonatal hemoglobin screening as early as possible in pregnancy. Screening should be presented to the parent as a part of the usual panel of neonatal tests. The parent may refuse any of these tests. If the parent does so, the provider should document this fact.

Implications of the Heterozygous State. A specific protocol portrait followup should be developed by each screening program.

When a neonate with trait is identified, a health care provider must contact the family with the results of the screening and offer family testing and counseling or referral for these services. The health care provider must, however, understand that this information could be disruptive to family well-being because it may raise fears of chronic illness, exposure of nonpaternity, and concern about sickle cell disease in future pregnancies. Therefore, the provider must approach and counsel first and foremost the mother, as the pivotal caretaker. Subsequent decisions regarding testing and counseling of other family members should be done with guidance from the mother, and always with sensitivity and discretion.

Education of Professionals and the Public. The training and continuing education of professional providers of care is of paramount importance and must be regularly included within the curricula of schools of medicine, nursing, social work, and other appropriate professions as well as in continuing postgraduate courses. Such education should provide the student and professional with knowledge of the etiology, pathophysiology, medical management, and psychosocial issues of relevance in assuring the comprehensive care of patients with hemoglobinopathies.

Public education is also critical to an effective neonatal screening program. Focal points should include schools, day care providers, mass media, and appropriate literature. Such education ought to include a clear understanding of the purpose of screening and the nature of sickle cell disease and sickle cell trait.

Risks of Screening. The benefits of sickle cell screening in terms of reduced morbidity and mortality of children with sickle hemoglobinopathies clearly outweigh the risks of screening. Risks include misdiagnosis, stigmatization, diminished self-esteem, and potential discrimination. These risks, however, can be minimized by careful programmatic design and monitoring.

One risk of screening is the anxiety to the family from the discovery of homozygous sickle states. Although this risk is unavoidable, the family can be helped to deal with the problem through sympathetic and sensitive support and careful education regarding appropriate care. Anxiety can also result from the discovery that a child has a heterozygous state. Counselors should emphasize that the condition will have little clinical impact on the child. If retesting of a child to confirm an uncertain test result is required, the retesting should also be handled with sensitivity to parental and child concerns. In all these matters, direct patient contact by providers in an organized program is preferred over indirect methods such as mailed information.

Legal safeguards against discrimination in employment opportunities and insurance eligibility are also necessary, in view of the historical abuses of sickle cell screening. Considerable care should be taken to ensure confidentiality of screening results and to maintain the privacy of the family.

What are the optimal followup and management of infants identified with hemoglobinopathies (disease and carriers)?

Comprehensive specialized care should be the right of every child who is affected by a clinically significant hemoglobinopathy. Economic, social, cultural, or geographic concerns should not limit access to this care but should be taken into account when structuring a followup program. Local factors will dictate how such continuous, consistent, and comprehensive care is best provided. Sickle cell centers with staff and support services to care for the physical and psychosocial needs of sickle cell patients and their families provide a model for comprehensive care. This model, however, may be unattainable in many areas. A multidisciplinary approach and 24-hour availability of care must be a part of all systems. Primary care physicians should educate themselves about sickle cell diseases and about the availability of consultation and support services in their local area. In rural areas, health departments should designate health professionals who can assist in resource identification and network linkage. Consideration should be given to satellite clinics from tertiary centers that use local health care services. All components of the care system must be present in any followup program even though these components may be delivered by a single individual.

Whether the care of a child with sickle cell disease is obtained through a single provider, in a health maintenance organization, by a comprehensive sickle cell clinic, or a hematology clinic, the care must either be a component of a sickle cell network or have ties to such a network. Such followup capabilities should be in place before a screening program is instituted.

Sickle Cell Diseases. In the first few months of the child's life, the screening program should assist the family to identify an appropriate health care provider and to become established with the network before the onset of symptoms.

Components of the ideal network should include the sickle cell experts, genetic counselors, social services, interpreters, and knowledgeable sub-specialists such as neurologists, orthopedists, ophthalmologists, and others. The value of local and national sickle cell organizations in providing supportive counseling, peer groups, tutoring, intra-community referrals, and advocacy cannot be overemphasized. These organizations should be involved in all phases of planning for the institution of neonatal screening for sickle cell disease. The continuity provider must be prepared to:

1. Perform appropriate tests on the patient or the family to make the definitive diagnosis of the type of sickle cell disease.
2. Start penicillin prophylaxis prior to age 4 months and make every effort to assure compliance.
3. Institute routine immunization as well as *Hemophilus influenzae* B vaccine at 18 months and 2 years and *Streptococcus pneumoniae* vaccine at 2 years.
4. Monitor growth and development.
5. Advise optimal nutrition and dietary supplements as needed.
6. Perform periodic physical examinations and whatever laboratory and radiographic tests are indicated.
7. Educate and counsel parents on early identification of symptoms of impending serious complications (e.g., fever, lethargy, pallor, enlarging abdomen).
8. Provide genetic counseling to family.
9. Advise on health care management.
10. Identify peers and peer groups that the patient might relate to in the immediate health provider system or through the sickle cell network.
11. Provide access to blood banking expertise.
12. Provide access to knowledgeable emergency and inpatient pediatric services, preferably in a tertiary care center.
13. Provide supportive counseling to the parents and other family members or make referral to mental health services.

Key professionals include pediatricians, nurses, genetic counselors, social workers, nutritionists, and child developmentalists. If these disciplines are not available as separate individuals, their function can be subsumed by the provider or his or her designee.

Other Hemoglobinopathies. Patients with hemoglobinopathies of questionable or minimal significance (e.g., CC, EE) can be followed in a sickle cell setting at the option of the patient or the provider. Patients with beta thalassemia other than S-beta thalassemia are best followed in thalassemia programs because of their need for intensive, long-term transfusion protocols.

The presence of alpha thalassemia in newborns is indicated by elevated levels of Hb Barts. Alpha thalassemia genes in black patients are generally of no clinical significance. Patients with Hb H disease require care by a hematologist. Asian patients with alpha thalassemia trait need counseling for the potential reproductive risk of Hb H disease or hydrops fetalis.

Carrier Identification. Followup of the child identified as heterozygous for a hemoglobinopathy requires no specialized medical care. However, there are several social and genetic counseling implications that should be recognized when designing a program for notification. To maintain confidentiality, results should be released only to the parents, the hospital, and the patient's physician. Information provided should explain that the carrier state is not a disease, that there may be implications for other family members, and that depending on results of family studies, future children may be at risk for a clinically significant hemoglobinopathy. A referral source for family testing and counseling should be clearly identified and obtainable through the network.

What future research directions are indicated?

Improved screening techniques for sickle cell disease and other hemoglobinopathies would be highly desirable. Research in several new methodologies presently under development, including high pressure liquid chromatography, immunologic techniques using monoclonal antibodies, and DNA analysis from whole blood samples, should be encouraged. This latter technique could result in the definition of the alpha and beta genotype of the patient and completely circumvent the problem of high levels of fetal hemoglobin at birth. Automated processing of neonatal blood samples and computer generated reporting of screening results should also be explored for future diagnostic screening techniques. Each technique should be assessed for its technical adequacy with regard to reproducibility, sensitivity, specificity, and predictive values of screening tests for sickle cell diseases and other hemoglobinopathies.

Further analysis of the optimal components of networks of care for the newborn with sickle cell anemia is desirable. Standardization and evaluation of protocols used in these programs should be encouraged. The impact of the screening, followup, and treatment on the physical, social, cognitive, and emotional development of the child should be studied. The effect of neonatal diagnosis and counseling for sickle cell anemia on individual family members should also be assessed.

Further studies on the optimal management of the known potentially fatal complications of sickle cell anemia are required. First, a better definition of the dose, route of administration, type, and duration of penicillin therapy for prophylaxis of pneumococcal sepsis is necessary. In addition, the role of pneumococcal vaccine in sickle cell patients over age 2 should be assessed. Development of a pneumococcal vaccine effective at an earlier age should be encouraged. The mechanisms of susceptibility to infection in sickle cell patients should be investigated. More research is needed to determine the child at risk for splenic sequestration crises.

Studies of the potential effect of neonatal diagnosis on management of other hemoglobinopathies (including hemoglobin E-beta thalassemia and homozygous alpha and beta thalassemia) are required. These studies will necessitate the development of new and more effective methods for the diagnosis of alpha and beta thalassemia in the newborn than are currently available.

The impact of neonatal diagnosis on the reproductive choices in families at risk for all hemoglobinopathies should be evaluated.

Optimal methods for educating individuals and families at risk for sickle cell diseases and other hemoglobinopathies should be studied. The studies should include an analysis of the relevant aspects of these conditions, neonatal screening, and issues related to the process or counseling and followup. Research projects should evaluate the best method of educating and counseling both the families of trait newborns proximal to the birth of the child and the child itself, in the long run.

Conclusions

1. Effective intervention in children with sickle cell disease provides a major impetus for neonatal screening. Prophylactic penicillin therapy provided in a setting of comprehensive care has been found to significantly reduce the morbidity and mortality of patients with pneumococcal sepsis.

2. Reliable, simple, and cost-effective techniques for mass screening of neonates are available and have demonstrated validity.

3. The benefits of screening are so compelling that universal screening should be provided. State law should mandate the availability of these services while permitting parental refusal.

4. Centralization of laboratory services improves efficiency and decreases the probability of error.

5. To be effective, neonatal screening must be part of a comprehensive program for the care of sickle cell patients and their families. These services must include a network of providers who ensure optimal medical care, psychosocial support, and genetic counseling. Such followup capabilities should be in place before screening is instituted.

6. Further research should focus on the following: improving and evaluating the technology for screening; defining the impact of screening on the physical, social, cognitive, and emotional development on the child and on family members; assessing other methods of management of infection; and providing optimal education of individuals and families at risk.

In summary, the panel concludes that every child should be screened for hemoglobinopathies to prevent the potentially fatal complications of sickle cell disease during infancy.

Part Six

Pregnancy in Mothers with Special Concerns

Chapter 21

Information for Rh-Negative Women

Screening Recommendations

Rh blood typing and antibody screening is recommended for all pregnant women at their first prenatal visit. Repeat antibody screening at 24-28 weeks' gestation is recommended for unsensitized Rh-negative women.

Burden of Suffering

Rh incompatibility exists when a rh-negative woman is pregnant with a rh-positive fetus, which occurs in up to 9-10% of pregnancies, depending on race.

If no preventive measures are taken, 0.7-1.8% of these women will become isoimmunized antenatally, developing rh antibody through exposure to fetal blood; 8-17% will become isoimmunized at delivery, 3-6% after spontaneous or elective abortion, and 2-5% after amniocentesis. In subsequent rh-positive pregnancies of isoimmunized women, maternal rh antibody will cross the placenta into the fetal circulation and hemolyze red cells. Without treatment, 25-30% of these offspring will have some degree of hemolytic anemia and hyperbilirubinemia, and another 20-25% will be hydropic and often will die either in utero or in the neonatal period.

From the NIH Homepage, prepared for the U.S. Preventive Services Task Force by Carolyn DiGuiseppi, MD, MPH.

Since the introduction of routine postpartum prophylaxis in the 1960s, the crude incidence of rh isoimmunization in the U.S. and Canada has fallen from 9.1-10.3 cases to 1.3 cases/1,000 total births. Hemolytic disease of the fetus or newborn due to rh isoimmunization (also called erythroblastosis fetalis) now accounts for only 4-5 deaths/ 100,000 total births, although this may be an underestimate as early intrauterine deaths are not always reported.

Even before the introduction of prophylaxis, however, a decline in fetal and neonatal mortality from rh hemolytic disease was occurring due to declines in both incidence and case fatality rates. It has been estimated that 30-40% of the recent decline in disease incidence is attributable to smaller family size, since the incidence of rh hemolytic disease increases with increasing birth order.

Since the 1940s, the case fatality rate has fallen from about 50% to 2-6%. This decline can be attributed in part to the trend toward smaller families, since the first affected infant in a family generally has less severe disease. The decline has also been associated with the introduction of interventions such as amniotic fluid spectrophotometry, exchange transfusion, amniocentesis, intrauterine fetal transfusion, and improved care of both the mother and the premature erythroblastotic infant.

Accuracy of Screening Tests

Hemagglutination is the established reference standard for the determination of rh blood type. The indirect antiglobulin (Coombs) test (IAGT) is the reference standard for detecting anti-rh antibody in women who are sensitized to rh-positive blood. The IAGT will also detect other maternal antibodies that may cause hemolytic disease.

Effectiveness of Early Detection

The early detection of rh-negative blood type in the pregnant woman is of substantial benefit if the patient is not yet isoimmunized and the father is not known to be rh-negative. Administration of rh immunoglobulin [or Rho (D) immune globulin (human)] to an unsensitized rh-negative woman after delivery of a rh-positive fetus will prevent maternal isoimmunization and consequent hemolytic disease in subsequent rh-positive offspring.

Treatment by Rh Immunoglobulin

The efficacy of rh immunoglobulin prophylaxis was convincingly demonstrated in a series of controlled clinical trials in the early 1960s.

Information for Rh-Negative Women

Despite a variety of minor flaws in study design, these trials showed that isoimmunization did not occur in any of the women who received a full dose of rh immunoglobulin postpartum and who were unsensitized when it was administered. These findings led to the introduction of routine postpartum prophylaxis following licensure of rh immunoglobulin in 1968.

Time series studies have since shown a dramatic decline in the incidence of rh isoimmunization, from 13-14% in the mid-1960s to 1-2% in the mid-1970s, although as described above, at least some of this decline is probably attributable to smaller family size.

The most frequent cause of apparent failure of postpartum prophylaxis is antenatal isoimmunization, which happens in 0.7-1.8% of pregnant women at risk. Although sample selection and other design features were not optimal, nonrandomized controlled trials have shown that the administration of rh immunoglobulin at 28 weeks' gestation, when combined with postpartum administration, reduces the incidence of isoimmunization to 0.2% of women at risk.

Risk Factors for Isoimmunization

Since rh isoimmunization during pregnancy is caused by transplacental hemorrhage, the risk of isoimmunization increases whenever such hemorrhage is likely to occur, including after abortion, amniocentesis, chorionic villus sampling (CVS), cordocentesis, ectopic pregnancy, fetal manipulation (e.g., external version procedures) or surgery, antepartum hemorrhage, antepartum fetal death, and stillbirth. Studies documenting the effectiveness of rh immunoglobulin prophylaxis are available for only a few of these indications, however.

In a nonrandomized trial of rh immunoglobulin after amniocentesis, control rh-negative women delivering rh-positive infants were more likely to become isoimmunized than were those receiving rh immunoglobulin (5.2% vs. 0%), although because of small numbers this difference was not statistically significant. Case series describing rh immunoglobulin administration after amniocentesis have demonstrated isoimmunization rates as low as 0-0.5%.

In a case series of rh immunoglobulin after induced abortion, isoimmunization occurred in 0.4%, compared to 2.6% among a series of patients, described by the same authors, who did not receive rh immunoglobulin.

The preliminary results from a randomized controlled trial of rh immunoglobulin after CVS showed that among rh-negative women delivering rh-positive infants, similar rates of isoimmunization were seen in both intervention (2.3%) and control (1.1%) groups; insufficient details are provided to ensure baseline comparability between the two groups, however. Rh-negative women who received rh immunoglobulin experienced twice as many unintended fetal losses as did controls (6.9% vs. 3.8%), but this difference was not statistically significant. No studies evaluating the use of rh immunoglobulin after other obstetric procedures or after obstetric complications were found.

Dosage of Rh Immunoglobulin

The standard postpartum dose of Rh immunoglobulin (300 micro-g) contains sufficient rh antibodies to prevent sensitization to at least 15 mL of rh-positive fetal red blood cells (RBCs), or approximately 30 mL of fetal blood; a "minidose" (50 micro-g) prevents sensitization to 2.5 mL of rh-positive fetal RBCs. For women with transplacental hemorrhages, the risk of rh isoimmunization developing after the full postpartum rh immunoglobulin dose is 30-35%. The incidence of fetal-maternal hemorrhage is 0.1-0.7% for all rh-negative pregnancies, but it is 1.7-2.5% after complicated vaginal and cesarean deliveries, and 4.5% after stillbirth.

There are several available methods for detecting excess fetomaternal hemorrhage. Acid elution (Kleihauer-Betke) is both sensitive and specific when done correctly, but it is subject to substantial laboratory and technologist error. Flow cytometry is also highly sensitive and specific, but it is technically difficult to perform.

The erythrocyte rosette test is simple to perform and highly sensitive (99-100%) for the presence of Rh-positive fetal RBCs, but its specificity is low so positive results must be confirmed by more specific tests such as acid elution and flow cytometry.

In clinical practice, combined antenatal and postnatal prophylaxis will prevent isoimmunization in 96% of women at risk. The remaining cases are due to failure to give rh immunoglobulin when indicated, isoimmunization that occurred before the widespread availability of rh immunoglobulin, administration of an insufficient dose, or treatment failure (i.e., isoimmunization occurring before 28 weeks or transplacental hemorrhage too large or too late in pregnancy to be prevented by the standard antepartum dose). Human error causes 22-50% of these cases.

While clinicians almost always administer rh immunoglobulin postpartum or after induced abortion, administration rates have been documented to be lower for other obstetric procedures and complications: 81-88% after spontaneous abortion, 36-60% after ectopic pregnancy, 31% after antepartum hemorrhage, and 14% after amniocentesis.

Information for Rh-Negative Women

Adverse Effects of Rh Immunoglobulin

Rh immunoglobulin has few adverse effects. Some fetuses will become weakly direct antiglobulin-positive following antenatal administration, but resulting anemia and hyperbilirubinemia in the newborn are very rare. All plasma for rh immunoglobulin production is screened for infectious diseases as required by the Food and Drug Administration; no cases of human immunodeficiency virus (HIV) infection from rh immunoglobulin have been reported. The evidence is therefore compelling that early detection and prophylaxis of the unsensitized rh-negative woman is both safe and effective in preventing isoimmunization and thus in preventing Rh hemolytic disease.

Treatment of Isoimmunized Women

Early detection is also beneficial for rh-negative women who are already isoimmunized and are carrying rh-positive offspring, because early intervention may improve clinical outcome. Decisions to intervene depend on the validity of screening tests in predicting the degree of fetal anemia. Obstetric history, maternal antibody titers, and ultrasound are currently used to determine the need for more invasive tests during isoimmunized pregnancies, but in the absence of hydrops none of these reliably distinguishes mild from severe hemolytic disease. Immunologic tests on maternal serum show promise in predicting disease severity. In the third trimester, serial amniotic fluid spectrophotometry has been found to correctly predict disease severity (i.e., cord hemoglobin and need for neonatal therapy) in 94-99% of cases. In the second trimester, however, this test has insufficient sensitivity or specificity for predicting the need for intervention.

Determination of fetal hemoglobin and rh blood type by ultrasound-guided cordocentesis, which can be performed in the second trimester, quantifies the degree of anemia, can be followed by transfusion if indicated, and allows referral of those with rh-negative babies to routine care. Case series, however, have demonstrated complication rates of 2-7% and procedure-related fetal mortality rates of 0.5-1%. DNA amplification in amniotic cells and chorionic villus samples appears to be effective in determining fetal rh blood type early in pregnancy, without the risk associated with invading the fetomaternal circulation.

In the presence of severe fetal anemia, early intervention appears to offer substantial improvement in clinical outcome. Current perinatal survival after ultrasound-guided intravascular transfusion at experienced centers is 62-86% for hydropic fetuses and 90% for those without hydrops. Once pulmonary maturity is established, the fetus can be delivered early and exchange transfusion performed with only 1% mortality risk.

Recommendations of Other Groups

The American College of Obstetricians and Gynecologists (ACOG) and the U.S. Public Health Service Expert Panel on the Content of Prenatal Care recommend rh blood typing and antibody screening at the first prenatal visit and repeat rh antibody screening at 24-28 weeks of pregnancy for rh-negative women. Both groups recommend offering rh immunoglobulin to all unsensitized rh-negative women at 28 weeks of gestation, and to those at increased risk of sensitization because of delivery of a rh-positive infant, antepartum hemorrhage, spontaneous or induced abortion, amniocentesis, external version procedures, or ectopic pregnancy, within 72 hours of the event. ACOG also recommends Rh immunoglobulin administration to unsensitized rh-negative women who have CVS, cordocentesis, antepartum fetal death, fetal surgery, or transfusion of rh-positive blood products. ACOG recommends measuring fetal blood cell levels in the mother when antepartum placental hemorrhage occurs.

The Canadian Task Force on the Periodic Health Examination recommends rh blood typing and antibody screening at the first prenatal visit, before elective procedures such as amniocentesis and therapeutic abortion in which there is the possibility of fetal bleed, between 24 and 28 weeks if the mother is rh-negative, and within 72 hours of delivery. They recommend administration of rh immunoglobulin to unsensitized women at 28 weeks and postpartum, and after amniocentesis or induced abortion.

Discussion

Although the burden of suffering from this disease is now low, the incidence was at least 10/1,000 live births before the introduction of preventive measures in the 1960s. There is excellent evidence for the efficacy and effectiveness of blood typing, anti-rh antibody screening, and postpartum rh immunoglobulin prophylaxis. Although ante-partum prophylaxis offers some additional benefit, some critics argue that the total impact of antepartum prophylaxis on the incidence of rh disease is relatively small, making it approximately 16 times less cost-effective than a program consisting only of postpartum treatment. Other studies support the cost-effectiveness of antepartum prophylaxis. The cost-effectiveness of rh immunoglobulin after obstetric procedures and complications is unknown.

Clinical Intervention

Rh blood typing and antibody testing is recommended for all pregnant women at their first prenatal visit, including visits for elective abortion. Unless the father is known to be Rh-negative, a repeat Rh antibody test is recommended for all unsensitized Rh-negative women at 24-28 weeks' gestation, followed by the administration of a full (300 micro-g) dose of Rh immunoglobulin if they are antibody-negative. If a Rh-positive infant is delivered, the dose should be repeated postpartum, preferably within 72 hours after delivery. Unless the father is known to be Rh-negative, a full dose of Rh immunoglobulin is recommended for all unsensitized Rh-negative women after elective abortion (50 micro-g before 13 weeks) and amniocentesis. There is currently insufficient evidence to recommend for or against the routine administration of Rh immunoglobulin after other obstetric procedures or complications such as chorionic villus sampling, ectopic pregnancy termination, cordocentesis, fetal surgery or manipulation (including external version), antepartum placental hemorrhage, antepartum fetal death, and stillbirth.

References

Mollison PL, Engelfriet CP, Contreras M. Blood transfusion in clinical medicine. 8th ed. Oxford: Blackwell Scientific Publications, 1987.

Huchcroft S, Gunton P, Bowen T. Compliance with postpartum Rh isoimmunization prophylaxis in Alberta. Can Med Assoc J 1985; 133:871-875.

Bowman JM. Controversies in Rh prophylaxis. Am J Obstet Gynecol 1985; 151:289-294.

Tannirandorn Y, Rodeck CH. New approaches in the treatment of haemolytic disease of the fetus. Baillieres Clin Haematol 1990; 3:289-320.

Centers for Disease Control. Rh hemolytic disease—Connecticut, United States,1970-1979. MMWR 1981; 30:13-15.

Baskett TF, Parsons ML. Prevention of Rh(D) alloimmunization: a cost-benefit analysis. Can Med Assoc J 1990;142:337-339.

Bowman JM, Pollock J. Rh immunization in Manitoba: progress in prevention and management. Can Med Assoc J 1983; 129:343-345.

Wysowki DK, Flynt JW, Goldberg MF, et al. Rh hemolytic disease: epidemiologic surveillance in the United States,1968 to 1975. JAMA 1979; 242:1376-1379.

Bowman JM, Chown B, Lewis M. Rh isoimmunization, Manitoba,1963-75. Can Med Assoc J 1977; 116: 282-284.

Clarke CA. Preventing rhesus babies: the Liverpool research and follow up. Arch Dis Child 1989; 64:1734-1740.

Adams MM, Marks JS, Gustafson J, et al. Rh hemolytic disease of the newborn: using incidence observations to evaluate the use of Rh immune globulin. Am J Public Health 1981; 71:1031-1035.

Walker RH, ed. Technical manual. 10th ed. Arlington, VA: American Association of Blood Banks, 1990.

American College of Obstetricians and Gynecologists. Management of isoimmunization in pregnancy. Technical Bulletin no. 148. Washington, DC: American College of Obstetricians and Gynecologists, 1990.

Chown B, Duff AM, James J, et al. Prevention of primary Rh immunization: first report of the Western Canadian Trial,1966-1968. Can Med Assoc J 1969; 100:1021-1024.

Pollack W, Gorman JG, Freda VJ, et al. Results of clinical trials of RhoGAM in women. Transfusion 1968; 8:151-153.

Prevention of Rh-haemolytic disease: results of the clinical trial. A combined study from centres in England and Baltimore. BMJ 1966; 2:907-914.

Freda VJ, Gorman JG, Pollack W. Prevention of Rh hemolytic disease: ten years' clinical experience with Rh immune globulin. N Engl J Med 1975; 292:1014-1016.

Davey MG, Zipursky A. McMaster conference on prevention of Rh immunization. Vox Sang 1979; 36:50-64.

Bowman JM, Chown B, Lewis M. Rh isoimmunization during pregnancy: antenatal prophylaxis. Can Med Assoc J 1978; 118:623-627.

Tovey LA, Stevenson BJ, Townley A. The Yorkshire antenatal anti-D immunoglobulin trial in primigravidae. Lancet 1983; 2:244-246.

Trolle B. Prenatal Rh-immune prophylaxis with 300micro-g immune globulin anti-D in the 28th week of pregnancy. Acta Obstet Gynecol Scand 1989; 68:45-47.

American College of Obstetricians and Gynecologists. Prevention of D isoimmunization. Technical Bulletin no. 147. Washington, DC: American College of Obstetricians and Gynecologists, 1990.

Daffos F, Capella-Pavlovsky M, Forestier F. Fetal blood sampling during pregnancy with use of a needle guided by ultrasound: a study of 606 consecutive cases. Am J Obstet Gynecol 1985; 153:655-660.

Blakemore KJ, Baumgarten A, Schoenfeld-Dimaio M, et al. Rise in maternal serum alpha-fetoprotein concentration after chorionic villus sampling and the possibility of isoimmunization. Am J Obstet Gynecol 1986; 155:988-993.

Medical Research Council. An assessment of the hazards of amniocentesis. Br J Obstet Gynaecol 1978; 85(Suppl2):1-42.

Crane JP, Rohland B, Larson D. Rh immune globulin after genetic amniocentesis: impact on pregnancy outcome. Am J Med Genet 1984; 19:763-768.

Brandenburg H, Jahoda MGJ, Pijpers L, et al. Rhesus sensitization after midtrimester genetic amniocentesis. Am J Med Genet 1989; 32:225-226.

Tabsh KMA, Lebherz TB, Crandall BF. Risks of prophylactic anti-D immunoglobulin after second-trimester amniocentesis. Am J Obstet Gynecol 1984; 149:225-226.

Simonovits I. Efficiency of anti-D IgG prevention after induced abortion. Vox Sang 1974; 26:361-367.

Simonovits I, Timar I, Bajtai G. Rate of Rh immunization after induced abortion. Vox Sang 1980; 38:161-164.

Smidt-Jensen S, Philip J. Comparison of transabdominal and transcervical CVS and amniocentesis: sampling success and risk. Prenat Diagn 1991; 11:529-537.

Pollack W, Ascari WQ, Kochesky RJ, et al. Studies on Rh prophylaxis: 1. Relationship between doses of anti-Rh and size of antigenic stimulus. Transfusion 1971; 11:333-339.

Bowman JM. Historical overview: hemolytic disease of the fetus and newborn. In: Kennedy MS, Wilson SM, Kelton JG, eds. Perinatal transfusion medicine. Arlington, VA: American Association of Blood Banks, 1990.

Ness PM, Baldwin ML, Niebyl JR. Clinical high-risk designation does not predict excess fetal-maternal hemorrhage. Am J Obstet Gynecol 1987; 156:154-158.

Feldman N, Skoll A, Sibai B. The incidence of significant fetomaternal hemorrhage in patients undergoing cesarean section. Am J Obstet Gynecol 1990; 163:855-858.

Bayliss KM, Keuck BD, Johnson ST, et al. Detecting fetomaternal hemorrhage: a comparison of five methods. Transfusion 1991; 31:303-307.

Stedman CM, Baudin JC, White CA, et al. Use of the erythrocyte rosette test to screen for excessive fetomaternal hemorrhage in Rh-negative women. Am J Obstet Gynecol 1986; 154:1363-1369.

Bowman JM, Pollock JM. Failures of intravenous Rh immune globulin prophylaxis: an analysis of the reasons for such failures. Transfus Med Rev 1987; 1:101-112.

Tovey LAD. Haemolytic disease of the newborn—the changing scene. Br J Obstet Gynaecol 1986; 93:960-966.

Grimes DA, Ross WC, Hatcher RA. Rh immunoglobulin utilization after spontaneous and induced abortion. Obstet Gynecol 1977; 50:261-263.

Grimes DA, Geary FH Jr, Hatcher RA. Rh immunoglobulin utilization after ectopic pregnancy. Am J Obstet Gynecol 1981; 140:246-249.

Information for Rh-Negative Women

Thornton JG, Page C, Foote G, et al. Efficacy and long term effects of antenatal prophylaxis with anti-D immunoglobulin. BMJ 1989; 298:1671-1673.

Centers for Disease Control. Lack of transmission of human immunodeficiency virus through Rho(D) immune globulin (human). MMWR 1987; 36:728-729.

Nicolaides KH, Fontanarosa M, Gabbe SG, et al. Failure of ultrasonographic parameters to predict the severity of fetal anemia in rhesus isoimmunization. Am J Obstet Gynecol 1988; 158: 920-926.

Nance SJ, Nelson JM, Horenstein J, et al. Monocyte monolayer assay: an efficient noninvasive technique for predicting the severity of hemolytic disease of the newborn. Am J Clin Pathol 1989; 92:89-92.

Zupanska B, Brojer E, Richards Y, et al. Serological and immunological characteristics of maternal anti-Rh(D) antibodies in predicting the severity of haemolytic disease of the newborn. Vox Sang 1989; 56:247-253.

Bowman JM. Rh erythroblastosis fetalis 1975. Semin Hematol 1975; 12:189-207.

Liley AW. Errors in the assessment of hemolytic disease from amniotic fluid. Am J Obstet Gynecol 1963; 86:485-494.

Nicolaides KH, Rodeck CH, Mibashan RS, et al. Have Liley charts outlived their usefulness? Am J Obstet Gynecol 1986; 155:90-94.

Ananth U, Queenan JT. Does midtrimester delta OD450 of amniotic fluid reflect severity of Rh disease? Am J Obstet Gynecol 1989; 161:47-49.

Daffos F. Access to the other patient. Semin Perinatol 1989; 13:252-259.

Pielet BW, Socol ML, MacGregor SN, et al. Cordocentesis: an appraisal of risks. Am J Obstet Gynecol 1988; 159:1497-1500.

Bennett PR, Le Van Kim C, Colin Y, et al. Prenatal determination of fetal RhD type by DNA amplification. N Engl J Med 1993; 329:607-610.

Poissonnier MH, Brossard Y, Demedeiros N, et al. Two hundred intrauterine exchange transfusions in severe blood incompatibilities. Am J Obstet Gynecol 1989; 161:709-713.

Harman CR, Bowman JM, Manning FA, et al. Intrauterine transfusion—intraperitoneal versus intravascular approach: a case-control comparison. Am J Obstet Gynecol 1990; 162:1053-1059.

Watts DH, Luthy DA, Benedetti TJ, et al. Intraperitoneal fetal transfusion under direct ultrasound guidance. Obstet Gynecol 1988; 71:84-88.

U.S. Public Health Service Expert Panel on the Content of Prenatal Care. Caring for our future: the content of prenatal care. Washington, DC: Public Health Service, Department of Health and Human Services, 1989. (NIH Publication No. 90-3182.)

Canadian Task Force on the Periodic Health Examination. Canadian guide to clinical preventive health care. Ottawa: Canada Communication Group, 1994: 116-125.

Urbaniak SJ. Rh(D) haemolytic disease of the newborn: the changing scene. BMJ 1985; 291:4-6.

Nusbacher J, Bove JR. Rh immunoprophylaxis: is antepartum therapy desirable? N Engl J Med 1980; 303:935-937.

Torrance GW, Zipursky A. Cost-effectiveness of antepartum prevention of Rh immunization. Clin Perinatol 1984; 11:267-281.

Chapter 22

Pregnancy in Women with Asthma

Introduction

Asthma is one of the most common illnesses that complicate pregnancy. Asthma may occur for the first time during pregnancy, or it may change during pregnancy; about one-third of pregnant women with asthma experience worse asthma during pregnancy, one-third remain the same, and one-third improve. In any case, pregnant women with asthma need treatment to control their asthma and thus protect their health and the health of their fetus. Asthma is a chronic, persistent disease of the airways characterized by exacerbations of coughing, wheezing, chest tightness, and difficult breathing that are usually reversible, but that can be severe and sometimes fatal. Recent studies demonstrated that inflammation is a critical factor in the pathogenesis of asthma, and therefore asthma therapy is predicated on medications to reverse and prevent this abnormality.

Pregnant women with asthma require long-term management to maintain lung function and blood oxygenation to ensure the oxygen supply to the fetus. Uncontrolled asthma during pregnancy can produce serious maternal and fetal complications. Maternal complications include preeclampsia, gestational hypertension, hyperemesis gravidarum, vaginal hemorrhage, toxemia, and induced and complicated labors. Fetal complications include increased risk of perinatal mortality, intrauterine growth retardation, preterm birth, low birth

---

Excerpts from NIH Publication No. 93-3279, September 1993

weight, and neonatal hypoxia. When asthma is properly controlled, however, pregnant women with asthma can maintain a normal pregnancy with little or no increased risk to themselves or their fetuses.

The goals of therapy for pregnant women with asthma are to control symptoms, including nocturnal symptoms; maintain normal or near-normal pulmonary function; maintain normal activity levels, including exercise; prevent acute exacerbations of asthma; avoid any adverse effects from asthma medications; and deliver a healthy infant. To achieve these goals, the Working Group on Asthma and Pregnancy strongly recommends that asthma be as aggressively treated in pregnant women as it is in nonpregnant women. Underestimation of asthma severity and undertreatment of exacerbations are two common errors that may lead to adverse maternal and fetal outcomes.

Asthma care should be integrated with obstetric care. Effective management of asthma includes ongoing management to prevent asthma exacerbations and control chronic symptoms, and early intervention to relieve acute exacerbations. There are four integral components of effective asthma management:

Use Objective Measures for Assessment and Monitoring.

Maternal lung function. Objective measures of lung volumes or flow rates are essential for assessing and monitoring the severity of asthma in order to make appropriate therapeutic recommendations. Using an office spirometer in the initial assessment of all pregnant patients being evaluated for asthma, and periodically thereafter as appropriate, is recommended. The single best measure of pulmonary function for assessing severity is forced expiratory volume in 1 second (FEV1).

Peak expiratory flow rate (PEFR), which can be measured reliably with inexpensive portable peak flow meters, correlates well with FEV1. Home peak expiratory flow monitoring should be considered for patients who take medications daily. Regular monitoring can help detect early signs of deterioration, indicate when asthma therapy might be changed, and assess response to therapy. Women with asthma may have minimal symptoms but still have abnormal pulmonary function tests and potentially impaired fetal oxygenation. Peak flow measurement will also help differentiate asthma from other causes of dyspnea during pregnancy.

Fetal monitoring. Fetal evaluation is based on objective measurements made by different techniques used according to gestational age and risk factors. Early (12 to 20 weeks) sonography provides a benchmark for progressive fetal growth. Sequential sonographic evaluations of fetal growth are indicated in second and third trimesters if asthma is moderate or severe or if growth retardation is suspected. Electronic fetal heart rate monitoring and ultrasonic determinations of fetal behavior in the third trimester should be used as needed to ensure fetal well-being. For many third-trimester patients weekly fetal assessment is sufficient, but frequency should increase if fetal problems are suspected. Daily maternal recording of fetal activity, or "kick counts," should be encouraged.

Immediate antepartum fetal assessment is indicated in asthma exacerbations with an incomplete or poor response to therapy or with significant maternal hypoxemia. One reasonable approach to antepartum fetal assessment is continuous electronic fetal heart rate monitoring.

When women with asthma are admitted in labor, careful fetal monitoring is essential. Intensive fetal monitoring (either continuous electronic tent auscultation) is recommended for those patients who enter labor with uncontrolled or severe asthma and with a nonreassuring admission test of fetal assessment or other risk factors.

Avoid or Control Asthma Triggers.

The identification and control of triggers—factors that induce airway inflammation or precipitate asthma exacerbations—are important in controlling asthma during pregnancy. Avoiding exposure to identified allergens and irritants can reduce asthma symptoms, airway hyperresponsiveness, and the need for medication. In addition, eliminating all exposure to tobacco smoke is important for pregnant women with asthma. Although immunotherapy should not be started during pregnancy, ongoing immunotherapy may be continued to reduce the response to a specifically identified allergen.

Establish Medication Plans for Chronic Management of Asthma and for Managing Exacerbations Using Preferred Medications

Chronic Management of Asthma. Asthma is a disease that varies among patients, and the degree of severity may change for individual patients from 1 month or season to the next or during pregnancy. Therefore, specific therapeutic regimens must be tailored to individual needs and circumstances. A stepwise approach to pharmacological therapy, in which the number and frequency of medications are increased with increasing asthma severity, permits this flexibility. Once control of asthma is sustained for several weeks or months, a reduction in therapy—a step down—can be carefully considered because the aim of pharmacotherapy is to use the least medication to maintain control. The stepwise approach presented with detailed recommendations in this chapter emphasizes that anything more than mild occasional asthma requires daily therapy with inhaled anti-inflammatory agents, either cromolyn sodium or beclomethasone. Further, all patients must have inhaled beta2-agonists to relieve symptoms, but it is essential that patients should not rely on frequent use of bronchodilator agents to control their asthma. An increased need for inhaled beta2-agonist is an indication that the asthma is deteriorating and anti-inflammatory therapy should be instituted or increased.

An extensive review of the animal and human studies on the effects of asthma medications found few risks of adverse effects to the fetus. The known risks of uncontrolled asthma are far greater than the known risks to the mother or fetus from asthma medications.

Managing Exacerbations. Anticipatory or early intervention is important in treating acute exacerbations. This reduces the likelihood of an episode progressing to severe airway obstruction with impaired maternal/fetal oxygenation. Every patient needs to have a written action plan for recognizing and responding early to signs of worsening asthma. The action plan indicates how to increase medications in response to decreased PEFR or increased symptoms and how to obtain medical advice at any time.

Patients should not delay seeking medical help in the emergency department or hospital if any of the following occur: therapy does not provide rapid improvement, the improvement is not sustained, there is further deterioration, the asthma exacerbation is severe, or the fetal kick count decreases.

Treatment in the emergency department or hospital emphasizes intensified administration of inhaled beta2-agonists, oxygen supplementation, and the early introduction of systemic corticosteroids.

Monitoring is essential because, in the presence of a moderate to severe exacerbation, deterioration can be rapid and a decrease in maternal PaO_2 (especially below 60 mmHg) and fetal PaO_2 can result in profoundly decreased fetal oxygen saturation and fetal hypoxia. Furthermore, fetal distress can occur even in the absence of maternal hypotension or hypoxia. Aggressive monitoring of fetal well-being is essential during critical maternal illness.

Managing Asthma During Labor and Delivery. The patient's regularly scheduled asthma medications should be continued during labor and delivery. The patient's PEFR should be taken upon admission to labor and delivery and, subsequently, every 12 hours. Asthma is often quiescent during labor and delivery. However, if asthma symptoms develop, PEFR should be monitored after asthma treatments. The patients should be kept well hydrated and be provided adequate analgesia to limit the risk of bronchospasm. Patients who have required chronic systemic corticosteroids during pregnancy should be given hydrocortisone to treat for possible adrenal suppression.

Narcotic analgesics that cause histamine release should be avoided; fentanyl is a preferred agent. Lumbar epidural analgesia reduces oxygen consumption and minute ventilation during first and second stages of labor, which offers patients with asthma considerable benefit. If a general anesthetic is necessary, preanesthetic use of atropine and glycopyrrolate may provide bronchodilatory effect. For induction of anesthesia, ketamine is the agent of choice. Low concentrations of halogenated anesthetics can provide bronchodilation to the patient with asthma.

For labor induction, oxytocin is the drug of choice. Prior to term, the use of 15 methyl prostaglandin F2-alpha should be avoided because it may cause bronchospasm; use of prostaglandin E2 suppositories or gel has not been reported to cause bronchospasm.

For postpartum hemorrhage, oxytocin is the recommended agent. If additional agents are required, methylergonovine as well as ergonovine should be avoided if possible because they may cause bronchospasm. If their use is unavoidable, pretreatment with methylprednisolone is recommended. If prostaglandin treatment is necessary, the safest analog is E2, which is less likely to cause bronchospasm.

The treatment of preterm labor in a patient already receiving asthma medication creates the risk of dangerous drug interactions. During an asthma exacerbation, uterine contractions are common and usually do not progress to preterm labor. Successful treatment of the exacerbation will usually abate the contractions. If tocolytic therapy is necessary, care should be taken to avoid the use of more than one type of beta2-agonist. Magnesium sulfate is recommended to treat uterine contractions if the patient is already taking a systemic beta2-agonist for her asthma.

Educate Pregnant Patients to Develop a Partnership in Asthma Management.

It is of the greatest importance for pregnant women with asthma to understand that they are "breathing for two." These women need information on how to properly control and manage their asthma during pregnancy to reduce the risk to the fetus. Concerns of pregnant women need to be elicited and addressed. Open communication, joint development of a treatment plan by the clinician and patient, and encouragement of the family's efforts to improve prevention and treatment of the patient's symptoms will assist in promoting maternal and fetal safety and well-being. Providing support to pregnant women with asthma during this potentially anxious time is important.

Impact of Asthma on Fetal Oxygenation

Changes in maternal respiratory, cardiovascular, and circulatory systems during pregnancy influence fetal oxygenation and acid base status. This section looks at these physiological alterations and their clinical implications.

Respiratory System Changes

A relative hyperventilation during pregnancy is seen beginning in the first trimester, with minute ventilation increasing up to 48 percent by term. This change is due to an increase in tidal volume; respiratory rate is relatively unchanged during pregnancy, so tachypnea in pregnancy (respirations more than 20 per minute) is an abnormal finding that must be investigated. Increased tidal volume change is due principally to increased placental progesterone production, which also accounts for a sensation of shortness of breath ("dyspnea of pregnancy") that is common in pregnancy. The hyperventilation of pregnancy is associated with significant changes in arterial blood gas with a resting arterial carbon dioxide tension (PCO_2) below 35 mmHg. This chronic respiratory alkalosis is partially compensated for by increased renal bicarbonate excretion. Total oxygen consumption and basal metabolic rate also increase by 20 percent and 15 percent, respectively, accounting for increased maternal oxygen tension, which is also common in normal pregnancy. Normal values of PO_2 range from 106 to 108 mmHg during the first trimester and decrease slightly in the third trimester (Prowse & Gaensler, 1965; Templeton & Kelman, 1976).

Pregnancy in Women with Asthma

Oxygenization is significantly influenced by postural effects. Twenty-five percent of pregnant women experience arterial oxygen tensions of less than 90 mmHg in the supine position, and there is also an increased likelihood of developing increased alveolar-arterial oxygen gradients in the supine, compared to the upright, position.

In terms of pulmonary function, the following are seen by term: a decrease in residual volume, functional residual capacity, expiratory reserve volume, and total lung capacity; an increase in inspiratory capacity; and no change in vital capacity or forced expiratory volume in 1 second (FEV1). All the changes just discussed have the potential for profound impact upon the clinical interpretation of pulmonary function studies and blood gas measurements in the pregnant woman with asthma and must be clearly kept in mind in the clinical interpretation of such data. In general, however, those measurements of pulmonary function in common clinical use (such as respiratory rate or FEV1) do not change with pregnancy, so any changes in these measures should be considered abnormalities and treated as such.

Recent information suggests that during painful labor there is relative hypoventilation between contractions resulting in decreased maternal PO2. With normal pulmonary function, the fetal implications of this phenomenon are negligible. However, this information forms a rationale for the liberal use of oxygen in laboring patients with any degree of respiratory impairment. Maternal oxygen saturation must remain greater than 95 percent to assure adequate fetal oxygenation (Clark, 1990).

Cardiovascular System Changes

During normal pregnancy, resting cardiac output is significantly increased by 6 weeks gestation, peaking at 30 to 50 percent over nonpregnant values by the early part of the third trimester (Clark et al., 1989). This increase is a result of increases in both heart rate and stroke volume and is sustained throughout the pregnancy. In the third trimester, cardiac output is significantly decreased in either the supine or standing positions. Up to 10 percent of women may experience the "supine hypotensive syndrome," a marked drop in blood pressure resulting from venacaval occlusion in the supine position (Holmes, 1960). Supine hypotension can have important maternal hemodynamic consequences and, because of decreased uterine perfusion, may result in fetal hypoxia and bradycardia. Thus recumbent pregnant women should avoid the supine position and favor the lateral decubitus or lateral tilt position.

Further significant increases in cardiac output are seen in the peripartum period. Labor is associated with an additional 1 to 2 liters per minute by the second stage (Ueland & Hansen, 1969). This increase may be minimized by having the patient labor in the lateral recumbent position with epidural anesthesia (Clark et al., 1991). In the immediate postpartum period, cardiac output is increased further, by up to 40 to 50 percent (Ueland et al., 1969), as a result of the "autotransfusion" phenomenon—the release of venacaval obstruction and expulsion of blood from the utero/placental bed into the central circulation. Thus the period of maximum risk for patients with compromised cardiovascular function is during the peripartum period. Cesarean section does not appear to reduce this risk.

Circulatory System Changes

Blood Volume. Blood volume increases markedly in pregnancy, with an increase in plasma volume at term averaging 40 to 50 percent over nonpregnant values (Clark et al., 1989). This increase, due to estrogen stimulation of aldosterone, begins as early as 4 to 6 weeks gestation, plateaus at approximately 32 to 34 weeks gestation, and then remains unchanged until delivery. There is a concomitant increase in red cell mass, erythropoiesis being stimulated by chorionic somatomammotrophin, progesterone, and possibly prolactin. Because red cell mass is increased 20 to 25 percent as opposed to the greater increase in plasma volume, a "physiologic anemia" of pregnancy may be produced. In absolute terms, it is estimated that blood volume in single pregnancies is increased 1,600 cc, with an average 2,000 cc increase observed by 32 weeks in twin gestations.

Blood pressure. Systolic and diastolic arterial blood pressure decrease until midpregnancy and gradually return to nonpregnant values by term (Wilson et al., 1980). These changes appear to be secondary to hormonally mediated decreases in systemic vascular resistance. Thus blood pressures that might be considered frankly hypotensive in the adult male may be normal in the pregnant female, especially during the second trimester of pregnancy. In evaluating blood pressure in the seriously ill pregnant patient with asthma, a comparison of prenatal blood pressure records is important.

Other hemodynamic changes. Systemic vascular resistance falls by the second trimester, rising toward normal by late third trimester. However, even in the late third trimester, systemic vascular

Pregnancy in Women with Asthma

resistance is decreased by 20 percent compared to nonpregnant controls (Clark et al., 1989). Similarly, pulmonary vascular resistance falls 35 percent by late pregnancy compared to nonpregnant values. Left ventricular stroke work index, pulmonary capillary wedge pressure, and central venous pressure all remain unchanged. The pulmonary-capillary-wedge pressure/colloid-oncotic pressure gradient decreases significantly, however, by the third trimester of pregnancy. This predisposes the pregnant woman to pulmonary edema, either because of increased intravascular pressure (i.e., increased fluid overload) or increased pulmonary capillary permeability.

Intrauterine growth retardation and adverse perinatal outcome have been associated with asthma during pregnancy. For this reason, all patients with moderate or severe asthma or uncontrolled asthma during pregnancy should have serial ultrasound assessment of fetal growth as well as antepartum fetal heart rate assessment during the late third trimester of pregnancy.

The Effect of Asthma on Mother and Fetus

Epidemiologic Studies

Two large epidemiologic studies published in the early 1970's most clearly define the potential adverse effects of maternal asthma on pregnancy and the infant. One study (Bahna & Bjerkedal, 1972) described pregnancy outcomes in 381 women with asthma compared to a control population of 112,530 pregnant women with no medical illness. There was a statistically significant increase in preterm births and low birth weight infants, decreased mean birth weight, increased neonatal mortality, and increased neonatal hypoxia in the pregnancies of women with asthma compared to control pregnancies. The study also found a statistically significant increase in hyperemesis gravidarum, vaginal hemorrhage, and toxemia as well as a significant increase in induced and complicated labors in pregnant women with asthma versus control pregnant women. The study did not find an increased incidence of congenital malformations.

The second study (Gordon et al., 1970) compared the pregnancy outcome of 277 women with asthma to the pregnancy outcome of the entire cohort population of 30,861 women. This study found a statistically significant increase in perinatal mortality in pregnant women with asthma versus pregnant women without asthma. Neonatal mortality was not specifically reported in this series. Maternal "chronic hypertensive disease" was present in three of the eight cases of fetal death. The data also suggested that pregnant women with severe asthma were at particularly high risk.

Subsequent controlled studies have reported increases in low birth weight infants (Lao & Huengsburg, 1990), chronic hypertension (Dombrowski et al., 1986), and preeclampsia (Stenius-Aamiala et al., 1988) in pregnant women with asthma compared to pregnant women without asthma. In addition to fetal morbidity and mortality, severe asthma during pregnancy may be a cause of maternal mortality (Gordon et al., 1970; Schaefer & Silverman, 1961; Williams, 1967). These epidemiological studies have found that pregnant women with asthma have increased risk of perinatal mortality, prematurity, intrauterine growth retardation, gestational hypertension, and other adverse effects. These studies, however, do not define the mechanisms of the increased risk.

Mechanisms

Definition of the mechanisms of asthma's adverse effects on pregnancy would allow institution of optimal intervention strategy. Potential explanations for the adverse effects of maternal asthma on pregnancy and the neonate include: (1) poor asthma control, (2) asthma medications, (3) increased prevalence of cigarette smoking among pregnant women with asthma versus pregnant women without asthma (Dombrowski et al., 1986), (4) extrapulmonary autonomic nervous system abnormalities, such as uterine muscle hyperreactivity (Bertrand et al., 1985), and (5) an increased proportion of African Americans among asthma patients (Centers for Disease Control, 1990a) with associated excess perinatal morbidity (Centers for Disease Control, 1990b). The published data do not fully define the mechanism(s) of maternal asthma's potential adverse effects on pregnancy and the infant. However, available information does suggest that poor asthma control may be the most important factor (see Table 22.1). The information available also supports the important generalization that adequate asthma control during pregnancy is important in improving maternal/fetal outcome.

Effects of Pregnancy on Asthma

Epidemiology

A number of studies suggest that the course of asthma may change during pregnancy. In a combined series of 1,087 patients from the literature, the course of asthma was reported to improve in 36 percent,

Table 22.1. Relationship Between Poor Asthma Control and Perinatal Mortality/Morbidity

- Acute asthma may be associated with hypoxia, hypocapnia, and alkalosis.
- Maternal hypocapnia/alkalosis may impair fetal oxygenation.
- Relative maternal hypoxia is associated with lower infant birth weight in high altitude pregnancies.
- Chronic maternal hypoxia is associated with increased prevalences of prematurity and intrauterine growth retardation in women with uncorrected congenital heart disease.
- No increase in perinatal mortality occurred in recent studies in which asthma was managed by specialists (Stenius-Aamiala et al., 1988; Greenberger & Patterson, 1983; Schatz et al., 1975; Greenberger & Patterson, 1988).
- Lower mean birth weight was manifested by infants whose mothers were hospitalized for asthma during pregnancy (2,920 g) compared to infants whose mothers did not require emergency therapy for their gestational asthma (3,354 g) (Greenberger & Patterson, 1988).
- Impaired pulmonary function was associated with lower birth weight and asymmetric intrauterine growth retardation in infants of asthmatic mothers (Schatz et al., 1990).
- Acute asthma is associated with hypertension that improves with amelioration of the asthma.

* Modified from Schatz and Zeiger, 1991.

worsen in 23 percent, and remain unchanged in 41 percent (Gluck & Gluck, 1976). However, individual studies differed substantially in their results (Gluck & Gluck, 1976). This pattern is maintained in recent studies (Gluck & Gluck, 1976; Juniper et al., 1989; Schatz et al., 1988a; Stenius-Aamiala et al., 1988; White et al., 1989), in which 18 to 69 percent of patients improved while 6 to 42 percent worsened. There are at least two reasons for this variability: (1) the method by which the course of asthma was assessed and (2) the asthma severity of the population studied. Review of the data suggests that women with severe asthma prior to pregnancy are more likely to deteriorate during pregnancy (Gluck & Gluck, 1976; White et al., 1989). The variable effect of pregnancy on the course of asthma appears to be more than random fluctuations in the natural history of the disease because the changes generally revert toward the prepregnancy level of severity within 3 months postpartum (Schatz et al., 1988a). It is also of interest that asthma severity is often consistent among successive pregnancies in individual women (Schatz et al., 1988a; Williams, 1967).

Other Clinical Observations

A study that prospectively evaluated methacholine sensitivity in 16 pregnant women with asthma (Juniper et al., 1989) found a twofold improvement (decrease) in airway responsiveness during pregnancy compared to preconception and postpartum. An associated improvement in clinical asthma severity, as indicated by a reduction in minimum medication requirements, was also observed. Individually, 11 of 16 subjects demonstrated improved airway responsiveness. Change in responsiveness was not closely related to serum concentrations of progesterone or estriol.

Additional observations have identified factors contributing to worsening asthma during pregnancy. Upper respiratory tract infections appear to be the most common precipitants of asthma exacerbations during pregnancy (Williams, 1967). Patient noncompliance with medical regimens may also be associated with poor asthma control during pregnancy, especially among adolescents (Apter et al., 1989). The peak incidence of exacerbations appears to be between the 24th and 36th weeks of gestation (Gluck & Gluck, 1976), particularly in women whose asthma worsens with pregnancy (Schatz et al., 1988a). In contrast, women with asthma, in general, tend to experience fewer symptoms during weeks 37 to 40 of pregnancy than during any prior 4-week gestational period (Schatz et al., 1988a). Finally, asthma generally remains quiescent during labor and delivery. Ninety percent of 360 women with asthma in one study had no symptoms of asthma at all during labor and delivery (Schatz et al., 1988a). Of those who did, approximately half required no acute treatment, some used inhaled bronchodilators, and only two required intravenous aminophylline.

Mechanisms

The mechanisms responsible for the altered course of asthma during pregnancy are unknown and represent a fertile area for additional research. There are multiple biochemical, physiological, and psychological factors that could potentially ameliorate or exacerbate asthma during pregnancy (see Table 22.2). It seems probable that the importance of individual factors varies from individual to individual, and presumably a combination of these factors determines what effect, if any, pregnancy will have on the course of asthma.

Asthma Drugs in Pregnancy and Lactation

When considering the possible effects of drugs and disease on pregnancy, it is important to keep in mind the background incidence of adverse pregnancy outcome in the general population. For example, congenital anomalies are recognized in 3 to 8 percent of live-born infants, miscarriage occurs in 20 to 25 percent of clinically diagnosed pregnancies, and severe mental retardation occurs in 1 to 2 percent of births. In addition, although birth defects are the most dramatic evidence of embryogenesis gone amiss, other endpoints of abnormal development are equally significant. These include spontaneous abortion (miscarriage), fetal death (stillbirth), and functional abnormalities such as impairments in the nervous or immune systems. Growth retardation, preterm labor, and other obstetric complications are also developmental problems of clinical importance. The challenge is to determine whether a drug or disease exposure increases the incidence of adverse outcome over the background incidence.

It is also important to remember that drug-induced birth defects are unusual: Of the 3 to 8 percent of newborns with congenital anomalies, only 1 percent or fewer of these are attributable to drug exposures (Czeizel & Racz, 1990).

Physiologic Changes in Pregnancy Affecting Drug Distribution

With the profound physiologic changes that occur during pregnancy, it is reasonable to suppose that these changes affect the manner in which

Table 22.2. Physiologic Changes During Pregnancy That May Affect the Course of Asthma

Factors that may improve asthma:

- Progesterone-mediated bronchodilation
- Estrogen- or progesterone-mediated potentiation of beta-adrenergic bronchodilation
- Decreased plasma-histamine-mediated bronchoconstriction (due to increased circulating histaminase)
- Pulmonary effects of increased serum-free cortisol
- Glucocorticosteroid-mediated increased beta-adrenergic responsiveness
- Prostaglandin-E-mediated bronchodilation
- Prostaglandin-I_2-mediated bronchial stabilization
- Atrial-natriuretic-factor-induced bronchodilation
- Increased half-life or decreased protein binding of endogenous or exogenous bronchodilators.

Factors that may worsen asthma:

- Pulmonary refractoriness to cortisol effects because of competitive binding to glucocorticosteroid receptors by progesterone, aldosterone, or deoxycorticosterone
- Prostaglandin-F_2-alpha-mediated bronchoconstriction
- Decreased functional residual capacity with resultant airway closure during tidal breathing and altered ventilation-perfusion ratios
- Increased placental major basic protein reaching the lung
- Increased viral- or bacterial-respiratory-infection-triggered asthma exacerbations
- Increased gastroesophageal-reflux-induced asthma
- Increased stress
- Increased pulmonary capillary permeability.

* Modified from Schatz and Zeiger, 1991.

drugs are handled by the body. Pharmacokinetics is the study of drug absorption, distribution, metabolism, and elimination in the body. Although few therapeutic agents have been completely studied as to the effect of pregnancy on the drug's pharmacokinetics, the following changes have been shown to occur during pregnancy and are clinically relevant:

- **Reduction in plasma proteins.** This is largely caused by a decrease in serum albumin concentration (Dean et al., 1980). During pregnancy, drugs bound to serum albumin show a reduction in protein binding and a corresponding increase in the available free fraction of the drug (Connelly et al., 1990; Frederiksen et al., 1986; Gardner et al., 1987). This change in protein binding implies that for certain drugs plasma concentrations should be reduced or kept at the lower end of the therapeutic range during pregnancy (Connelly et al., 1990). For example, the protein binding of theophylline decreases by 10 to 15 percent during pregnancy; therefore, the therapeutic range for theophylline needs to be modified to account for the corresponding increase in the free fraction of theophylline. During pregnancy, theophylline plasma concentrations between 8 and 12 g/mL are therapeutically equivalent to concentrations of 10 to 15 g/mL in the nonpregnant patient.

- **Increased total body water and plasma volume.** Several studies, however, have shown that this change does not affect the volume of distribution for drugs if the weight of the patient is taken into consideration (Aldridge et al., 1981; Frederiksen et al., 1986; Gardner et al., 1987; Philipson, 1977; Philipson & Stiernstedt, 1982). Therefore, to achieve the therapeutic drug concentration usually recommended, the mg/kg dose should be calculated using the actual weight of the patient. For example, to calculate a loading dose of aminophylline or theophylline for a pregnant patient not previously receiving a methylxanthine, use the recommended 6-mg/kg regimen and the actual weight of the patient at the time therapy is instituted.

- **Decreased gastrointestinal motility.** This change does not affect the overall absorption of even poorly absorbed drugs, such as ampicillin (Philipson, 1977); however, the time to peak drug concentration is prolonged, and the peak concentration is lower

(Philipson, 1977). This may in part explain the observation that an oral dose of 500 mg of ampicillin during pregnancy gives a plasma peak concentration 40 percent lower than in a nonpregnant patient, and the peak concentration occurs approximately 1 hour later.

- **Altered drug elimination.** Pregnancy can alter the manner in which drugs are eliminated from the body, with the greatest effect occurring in the last trimester of pregnancy. Renal elimination of drugs may increase for such drugs as theophylline, ampicillin, and cefuroxime due to the increase in glomerular filtration rate that occurs during pregnancy (Frederiksen et al., 1986; Philipson, 1977; Philipson & Stiernstedt, 1982). Metabolic elimination of drugs is less predictable; some drugs, such as methadone, have an increase in metabolic clearance (Pond et al., 1985) and others, including theophylline, have a decrease in metabolic clearance (Frederiksen et al., 1986; Gardner et al., 1987). Therefore, the elimination route and characteristics of each drug must be considered, and frequent use of therapeutic drug monitoring is indicated. Thus, because the overall elimination rate of intravenous methylxanthine decreases by 30 percent in the last trimester of pregnancy, the recommended dose for intravenously administered methylxanthine is a continuous infusion rate of 0.4 mg/kg/hr theophylline (or 0.5 mg/kg/hr aminophylline) in order to maintain serum theophylline concentrations within the range of 8-12 g/mL.

As a general rule most medications administered to pregnant women will cross the placenta and can be detected in fetal blood. However, extremely large molecular weight drugs, or highly polar compounds, such as heparin, do not effectively cross the placenta in measurable amounts.

Breast Feeding

Nearly all medications enter breast milk by diffusion from plasma. Milk concentrations are typically very low, and it is unusual for infants to receive a dose sufficient to produce toxic effects. Recommendations concerning drugs and breast feeding have been made by the American Academy of Pediatrics Committee on Drugs (1989) and by the World Health Organization (Bennett, 1988).

Table 22.3. Potential Fetal/Neonatal Adverse Effects of Asthma Drugs

Drug or Class	Effect
Systemic corticosteroids	Impaired fetal growth (about 300 to 400 g decrease in birth weight)
Theophylline	Fetal tachycardia with maternal plasma drug levels greater than 20 µg/mL. Neonatal jitteriness, vomiting, tachycardia with neonatal drug levels greater than 10 µg/mL. Neonatal effects are most often seen when maternal plasma drug levels are greater than 12 µg/mL.
Systemic beta$_2$-agonists	Fetal tachycardia. Neonatal tachycardia, hypoglycemia, tremor.
Topical sympathomimetic decongestants	Fetal heart rate alterations attributed to uterine vasoconstriction. Effect seen at high doses, perhaps only with overdosage.

Table 22.4. Drugs for Asthma and Associated Conditions That Generally Should Be Avoided During Pregnancy

- Alpha-adrenergic compounds (other than pseudoephedrine)
- Epinephrine
- Iodides
- Sulfonamides (in late pregnancy)
- Tetracyclines
- Quinalones

Figure 22.5. Management of Chronic Mild Asthma During Pregnancy

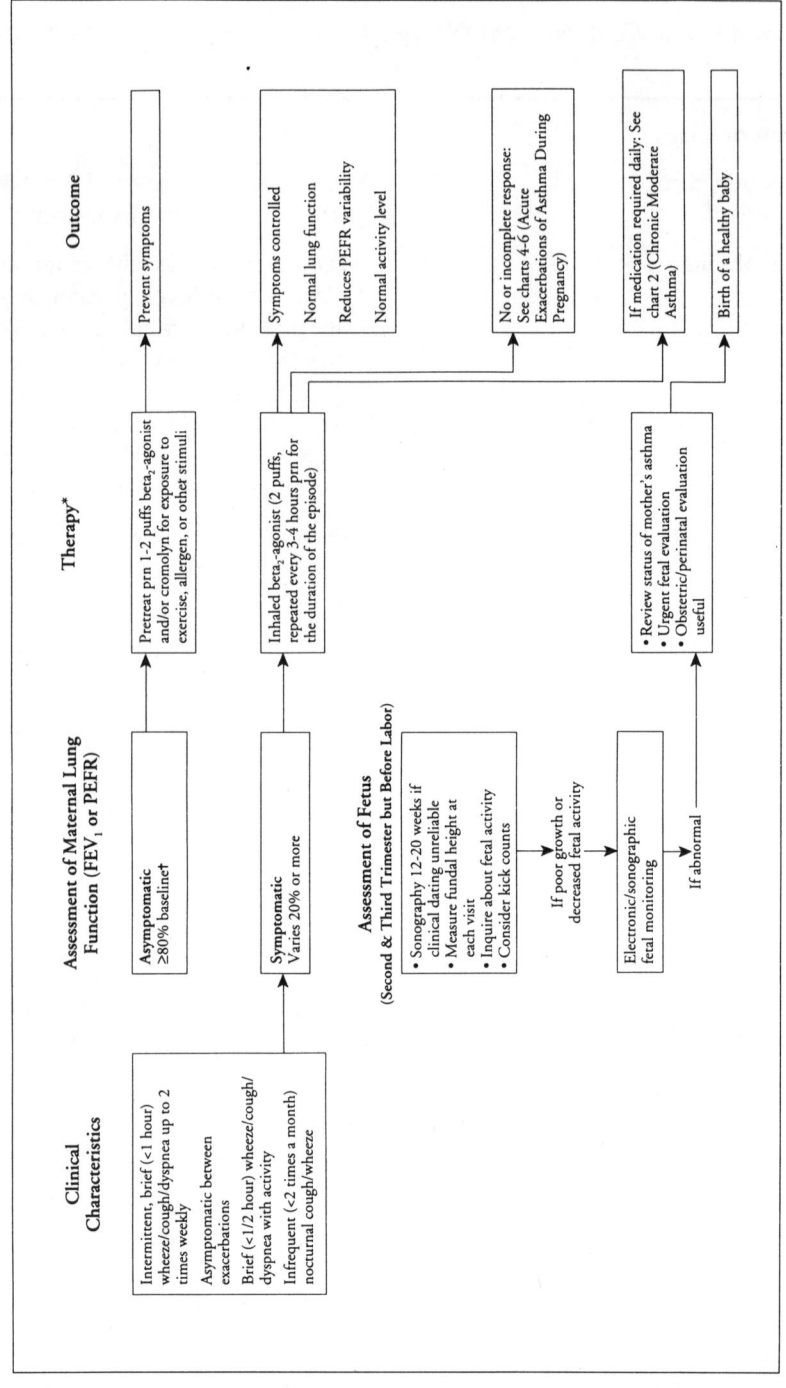

Pregnancy in Women with Asthma

Figure 22.6. Management of Chronic Moderate Asthma During Pregnancy

Clinical Characteristics	Assessment of Maternal Lung Function (FEV_1 or PEFR)	Therapy*	Outcome
Symptoms >1-2 times weekly Exacerbations affect sleep or activity level Exacerbations may last several days Occasional emergency care	60-80% baseline† (may be normal when asymptomatic) Varies 20-30% when symptomatic	**Anti-inflammatory agents** • Cromolyn (2 puffs qid) *or* • Inhaled corticosteroids (2-4 puffs bid, 168-336 µg/day) *and* **Inhaled beta$_2$-agonist** prn to tid/qid††	Symptoms controlled Pulmonary function values optimal for patient Reduced PEFR variability Normal activity level Rarely awakened at night Infrequent exacerbations Reduced frequency of prn inhaled beta$_2$-agonist
	Assessment of Fetus (Second & Third Trimester but Before Labor)	If symptoms persist **Additional therapy** • Increase inhaled corticosteroids *and/or* • Sustained release theophylline *and/or* • Oral beta$_2$-agonist	
	• Sonography for dating and growth evaluation • Measure fundal height at each visit • Daily kick counts • Consider serial antepartum fetal assessment beginning at 32 weeks		
	If poor growth or decreased fetal activity		
	Electronic/sonographic fetal monitoring	• Review status of mother's asthma • Urgent fetal evaluation • Obstetric/perinatal consultation useful	Birth of a healthy baby
	If abnormal		
Increasingly frequent symptoms	Varies more than 30% during worst exacerbations	**Oral corticosteroids** • Short course of oral prednisone followed by inhaled corticosteroids	Symptoms reduced Peak flow values stabilized Get specialist consultation
		See chart 3: Chronic Severe Asthma ▶ Get assessment by specialist	No or intermittent response

* All therapy must include patient education about prevention (including environmental control where appropriate) as well as control of symptoms.
† PEFR percent baseline refers to the norm for the individual, established by the clinician. This may be percent predicted based on standardized norms or percent of patient's personal best.
†† If exceed 3-4 doses a day, consider additional therapy other than inhaled beta$_2$-agonist.

Figure 22.7. Management of Chronic Severe Asthma During Pregnancy

Clinical Characteristics	Assessment of Maternal Lung Function (FEV₁ or PEFR)	Therapy*	Outcome
Continuous symptoms Limited activity level Frequent exacerbations Frequent nocturnal symptoms Occasional hospitalization and emergency treatment	<60% baseline† Highly variable: 20–30% changes with routine medicine Varies more than 50% during worst exacerbations	**Anti-inflammatory agents** • Inhaled corticosteroid 4–6 puffs bid or 2–5 puffs qid (336–840 µg/day) *with or without* —Cromolyn 2 puffs qid *with or without* • Oral sustained-released theophylline, *and/or* • Oral beta₂-agonist *and* • Inhaled beta₂-agonist prn qid†† *with* • Episodic extra beta₂-agonist (2–4 puffs MDI or nebulized treatment) for exacerbations *and* **Oral corticosteroids** • Burst for active symptoms (40 mg a day, single or divided dose, for 1 week, then tapered for 1 week) *Consider* • Daily or alternate day use (single dose a.m.)	Improved pulmonary function Reduced peak flow variability Almost normal activity Infrequent awakening at night Reduced frequency of exacerbations Reduced frequency of prn inhaled beta₂-agonist Reduced need for corticosteroid burst Reduced need for emergency department treatment

Assessment of Fetus (Second & Third Trimester but Before Labor)

- Sonograms for dating and growth evaluation
- Measure fundal height at each visit
- Daily kick counts
- Consider serial antepartum fetal assessment beginning at 32 weeks
- Perinatal consultation useful

If poor growth or decreased fetal activity → Electronic/sonographic fetal monitoring

If abnormal →
- Urgent fetal evaluation
- Perinatal consultation useful

• Review status of mother's asthma → Birth of a healthy baby

Note: Individuals with severe asthma should be evaluated by an asthma specialist.
* All therapy must include patient education about prevention (including environmental control where appropriate) as well as control of symptoms.
† PEFR percent baseline refers to the norm for the individual, established by the clinician. This may be percent predicted based on standardized norms or percent of patient's personal best.
†† If exceed 3–4 doses a day, consider additional therapy other than inhaled beta₂-agonist.

Pregnancy in Women with Asthma

Figure 22.8. Home Management of Acute Exacerbations of Asthma During Pregnancy

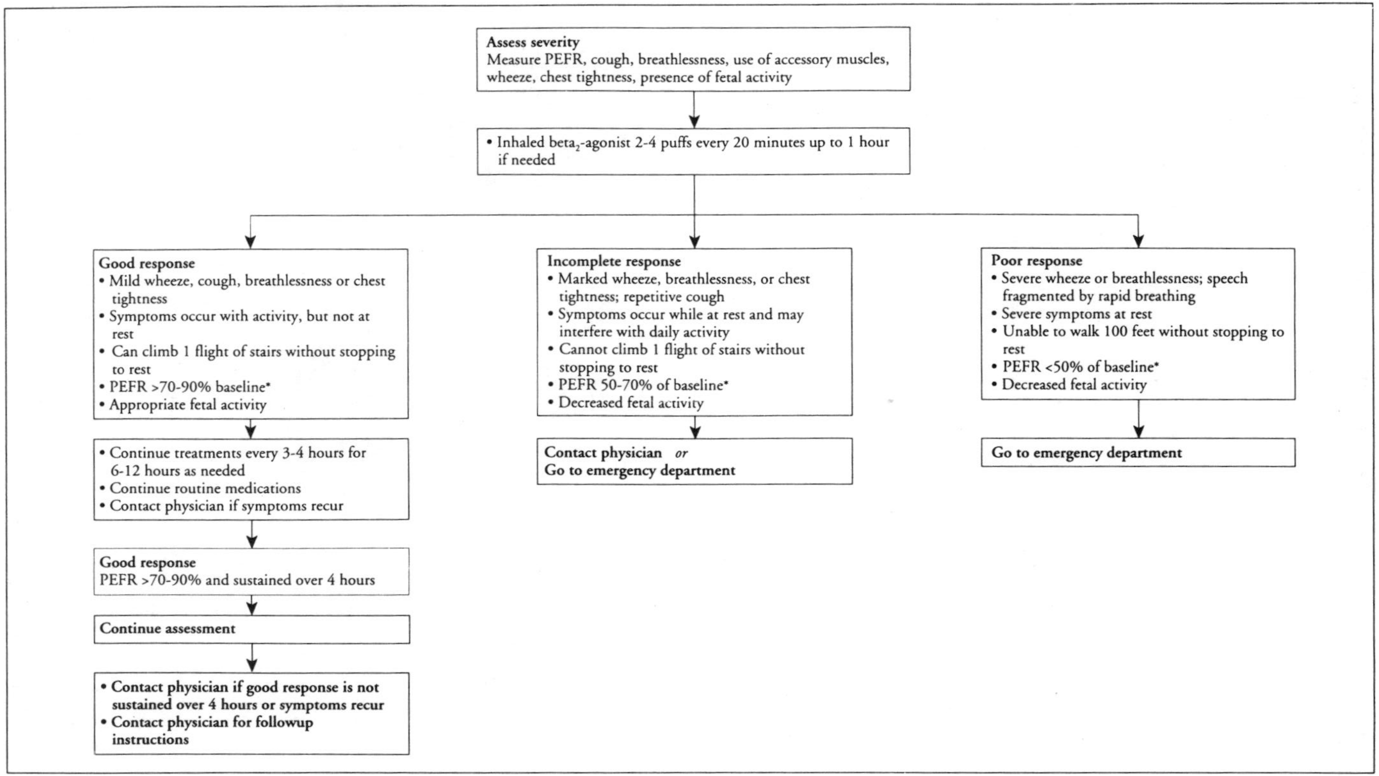

Assess severity
Measure PEFR, cough, breathlessness, use of accessory muscles, wheeze, chest tightness, presence of fetal activity

- Inhaled beta$_2$-agonist 2-4 puffs every 20 minutes up to 1 hour if needed

Good response
- Mild wheeze, cough, breathlessness or chest tightness
- Symptoms occur with activity, but not at rest
- Can climb 1 flight of stairs without stopping to rest
- PEFR >70-90% baseline*
- Appropriate fetal activity

Incomplete response
- Marked wheeze, breathlessness, or chest tightness; repetitive cough
- Symptoms occur while at rest and may interfere with daily activity
- Cannot climb 1 flight of stairs without stopping to rest
- PEFR 50-70% of baseline*
- Decreased fetal activity

Poor response
- Severe wheeze or breathlessness; speech fragmented by rapid breathing
- Severe symptoms at rest
- Unable to walk 100 feet without stopping to rest
- PEFR <50% of baseline*
- Decreased fetal activity

- Continue treatments every 3-4 hours for 6-12 hours as needed
- Continue routine medications
- Contact physician if symptoms recur

Contact physician *or*
Go to emergency department

Go to emergency department

Good response
PEFR >70-90% and sustained over 4 hours

Continue assessment

- Contact physician if good response is not sustained over 4 hours or symptoms recur
- Contact physician for followup instructions

* PEFR percent baseline refers to the norm for the individual, established by the clinician. This may be percent predicted based on standardized norms or percent of patient's personal best.

Figure 22.9. Emergency Department Management of Acute Exacerbations of Asthma During Pregnancy

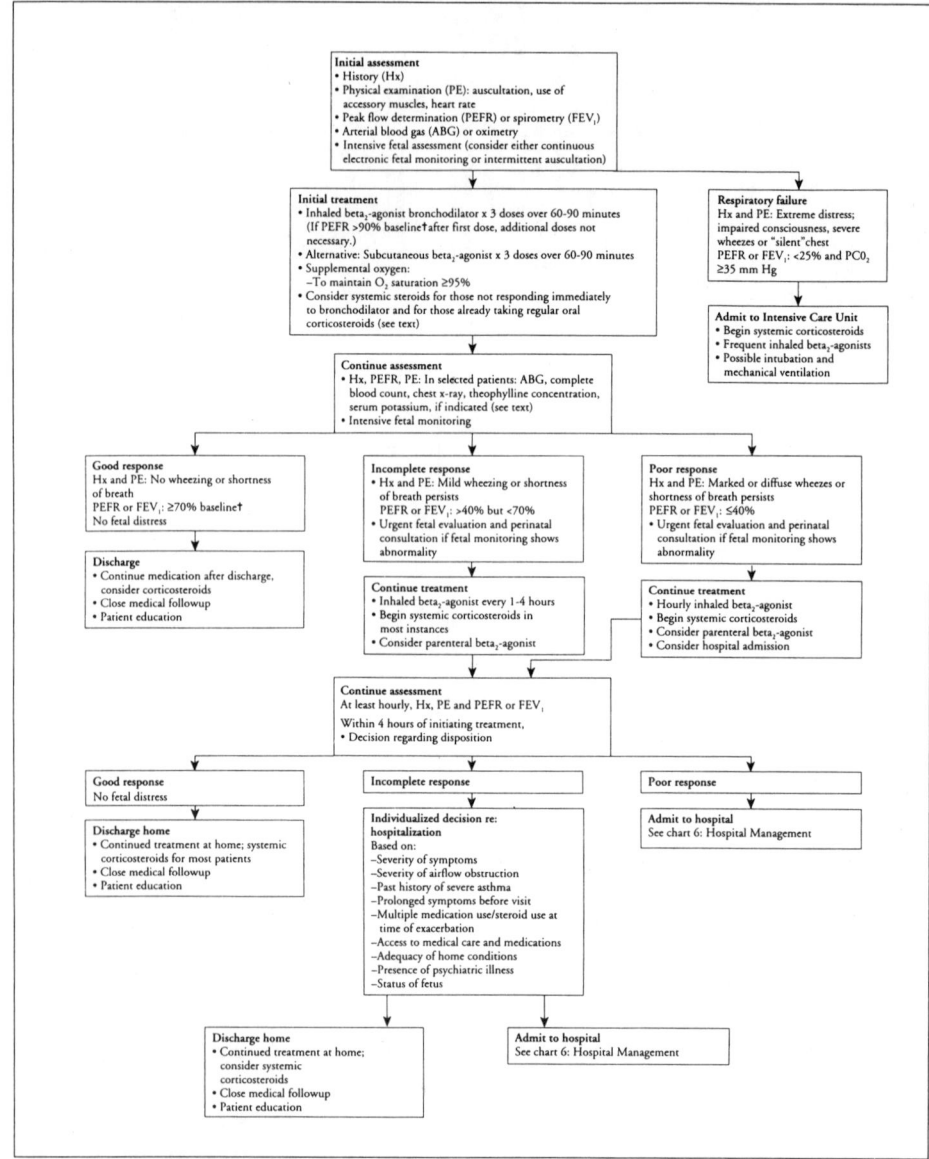

* Therapies are often available in a physician's office. However, most acute severe exacerbations of asthma require a complete course of therapy in an emergency department.

† PEFR percent baseline refers to the norm for the individual, established by the clinician. This may be percent predicted based on standardized norms or percent of patient's personal best.

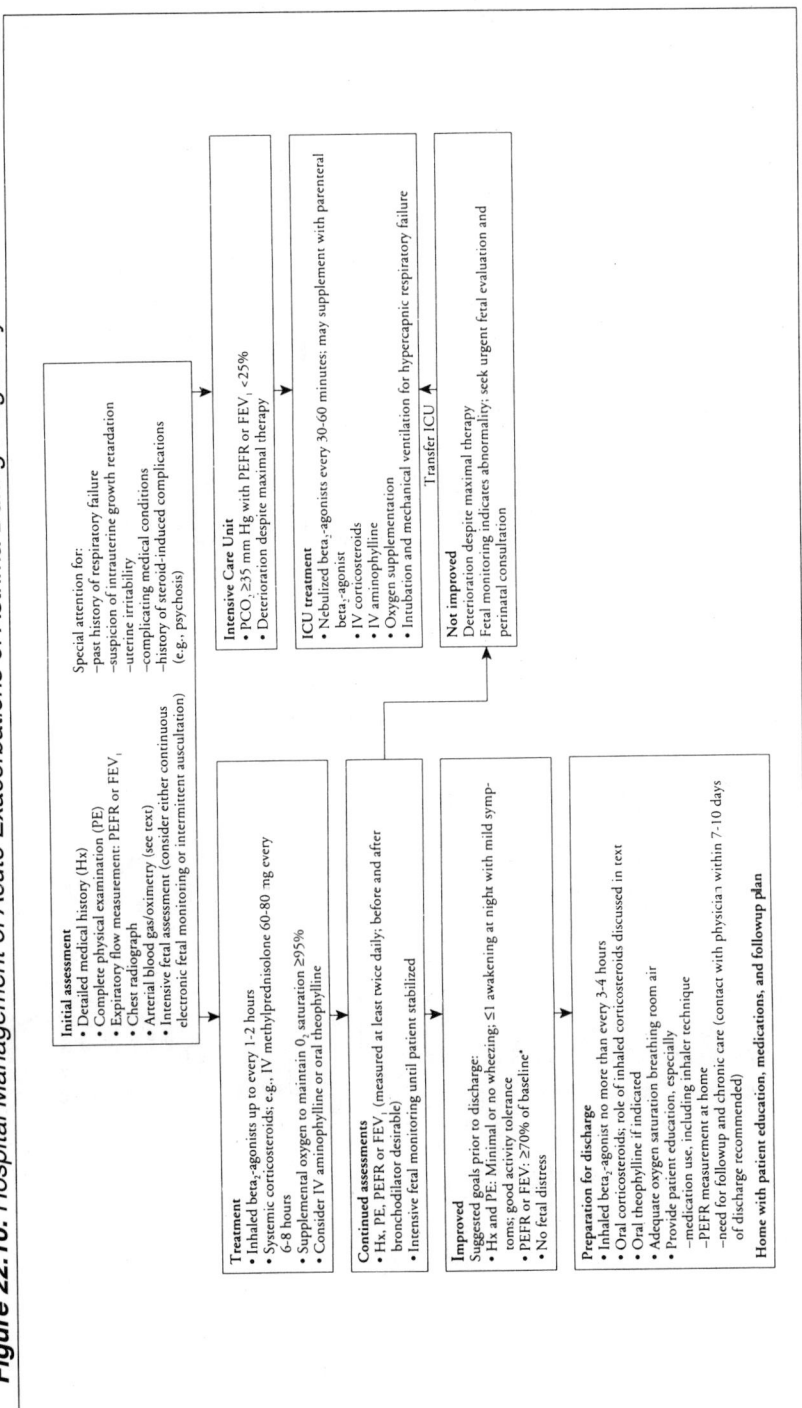

Figure 22.10. Hospital Management of Acute Exacerbations of Asthma During Pregnancy

* PEFR percent baseline refers to the norm for the individual, established by the clinician. This may be percent predicted based on standardized norms or percent of patient's personal best.

Figure 22.11. Management of Asthma During Labor

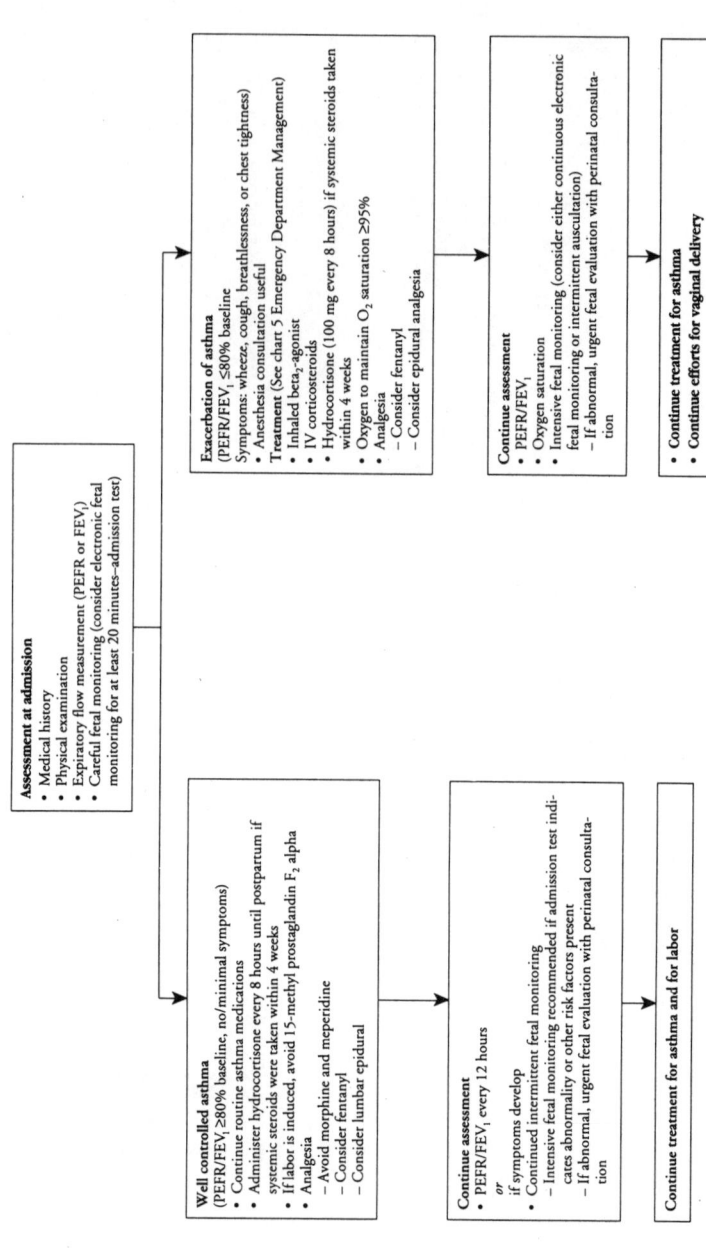

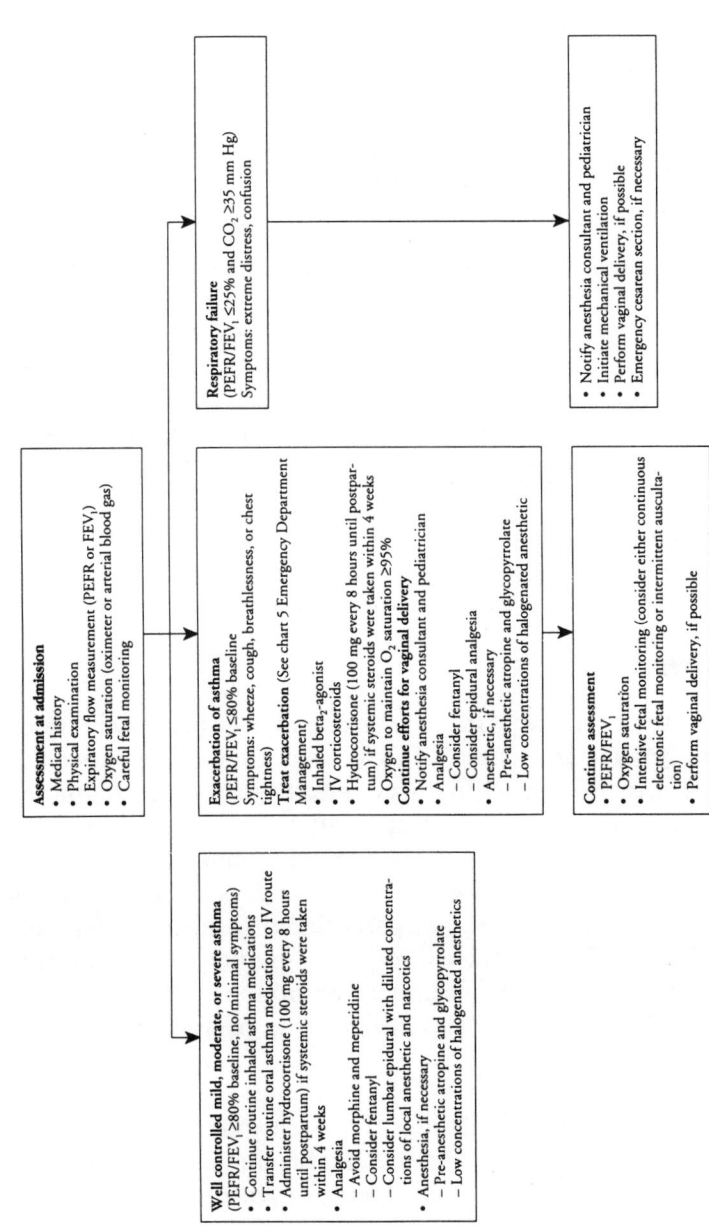

Figure 22.12. Management of Asthma During Delivery

Special Considerations

Hypertension

When a pregnant woman with asthma either has hypertension or develops hypertension, the pharmacologic management of the hypertension is best achieved by avoiding the use of beta-adrenergic antagonists (beta-blockers) because they may exacerbate the asthma.

Diabetes

If diabetes, either insulin-dependent or gestational, and asthma coexist during pregnancy, the overall management may be complicated because asthma medication may impair carbohydrate tolerance and worsen diabetes. Specifically, systemic beta2-agonists and systemic corticosteroids may cause hyperglycemia, which necessitates close monitoring of blood sugars and may increase the patient's insulin requirements. Although it would be best to avoid the use of these agents during the pregnancy of a woman with diabetes, asthma exacerbations may require systemic beta2-agonists and/or systemic steroids. Close communication among the physicians managing the asthma, the diabetes, and the pregnancy is necessary.

Rhinitis

Significant nasal symptoms occur in approximately 35 percent of randomly selected women (Mabry, 1980, 1986). Few data exist regarding the interrelationships between rhinitis and pregnancy. In one survey, preexisting rhinitis worsened during pregnancy in 34 percent of the women, improved in 15 percent, remained unchanged in 45 percent, and could not be evaluated in 6 percent (Schatz & Zeiger, 1991). It seems unlikely that gestational rhinitis would have any direct adverse effect on the course of pregnancy, but severe rhinitis can interfere with sleeping, eating, or emotional well-being. In addition, uncontrolled rhinitis or sinusitis during pregnancy may exacerbate coexisting asthma.

Diagnosis. Essentially, any of the recognized forms of rhinitis may occur during pregnancy, but the most common types appear to be allergic rhinitis, rhinitis medicamentosa, vasomotor rhinitis, and bacterial rhinosinusitis.

Allergic rhinitis is caused by an intranasal IgE-mediated reaction to inhaled allergens such as pollen, house-dust mites, mold spores, or animal dander. Prominent symptoms include sneezing, runny nose, nasal itching, and eye itching that may be exacerbated seasonably or by exposure to allergens (grass, house-dust mites, animal dander).

Rhinitis medicamentosa is the syndrome of rebound nasal congestion resulting from the overuse of topical vasoconstricting nose sprays. It may complicate another underlying cause of chronic rhinitis or a viral upper respiratory infection.

Vasomotor rhinitis of pregnancy is a syndrome of nasal congestion and vasomotor instability limited to the gestational period. Symptoms in these women with this condition tend to be most prominent in the second half of pregnancy (Bende et al., 1989; Mohun, 1943) and usually disappear within 5 days postpartum (Mohun, 1943).

Treatment. Many women will be able to tolerate their nasal symptoms during pregnancy with little or no pharmacologic therapy. Although this may be desirable, especially during the first trimester, substantially bothersome symptoms warrant treatment. For patients with allergic rhinitis, as with allergic asthma, environmental control measures are important to reduce antigen exposure. Pharmacotherapy is reasonable if environmental control measures do not provide sufficient control. Intranasal cromolyn may be considered first, based on its topical effects and reassuring gestational animal and human data. For patients with allergic rhinitis inadequately controlled by intranasal cromolyn, antihistamine therapy (tripelennamine or chlorpheniramine) should be considered. Many patients with eosinophilic rhinitis will respond better to a combination of an antihistamine and pseudoephedrine than to either drug alone.

An alternative to oral therapy for allergic rhinitis during pregnancy is intranasal corticosteroid therapy. Although there is no published experience on the use of these medications intranasally during pregnancy, some authors consider these medications to be preferable to oral medications for allergic rhinitis during pregnancy due to their topical application (Norman, 1983). Intranasal beclomethasone is recommended, beginning with two sprays in each nostril twice daily and then tapering to the lowest effective dose.

Although discontinuation of the topical vasoconstrictor is the most important treatment of rhinitis medicamentosa, intolerable congestion frequently results. Addition of intranasal beclomethasone (two sprays in each nostril twice daily) usually allows comfortable discontinuation of the offending vasoconstricting spray.

Two nonpharmacologic approaches may be useful for patients with vasomotor rhinitis during pregnancy. A buffered saline nose spray may be helpful for the nasal dryness, nasal bleeding, and vascular congestion associated with pregnancy. Exercise (commensurate with the pregnancy) may also be useful because exercise leads to physiologic nasal vasoconstriction. When pharmacologic therapy is required, pseudoephedrine is recommended.

Sinusitis

Bacterial rhinosinusitis may complicate another underlying cause of rhinitis or may follow a viral upper respiratory infection. The incidence of sinusitis in pregnancy has been reported to be 1.5 percent, an apparent sixfold increased incidence over the nonpregnant population (Sorri et al., 1980).

Diagnosis. The diagnosis of sinusitis during pregnancy is often made empirically based on clinical findings of posterior nasal drainage, sinus distribution pain, and purulent discharge lasting more than 5 to 7 days. A high index of suspicion must be maintained for bacterial sinusitis during pregnancy because as many as half of pregnant women with documented sinusitis may lack the classic clinical findings (Sorri et al., 1980). Sinus radiographs should be used during pregnancy when indicated, such as when a clinically diagnosed sinus infection is not responding to antibiotic therapy or when a probable clinical diagnosis cannot be made without radiologic confirmation.

Treatment. Cultures of sinus aspirates obtained during pregnancy have shown the most common sinus pathogens to be Hemophilus influenza and Streptococcus pneumonae (Sorri et al., 1980). Data on the use of antibiotics during pregnancy have been reviewed (Hamod & Khouzomi, 1988). Amoxicillin is the initial antibiotic of choice in the management of sinusitis during pregnancy in women who are not allergic to penicillin. Erythromycin is recommended for the penicillin-allergic patient with gestational sinusitis, and the addition of sulfisoxazole may be considered in early or midpregnancy if the patient is not responding in 5 to 7 days. Experience suggests that 3 weeks of therapy is superior to a 10- to 14-day course with regard to preventing the development of recurrent sinusitis during pregnancy. Oxymetazoline nose spray or drops (for up to 5 days) and pseudoephedrine may also be helpful as adjunctive and symptomatic therapy of gestational bacterial rhinosinusitis.

An appropriate cephalosporin, amoxicillin/beta-lactamase inhibitor, erythromycin, or erythromycin plus sulfisoxazole (in early or midpregnancy) may be considered for women with unequivocal clinical sinusitis who do not respond to amoxicillin. If improvement does not occur, sinus films should be obtained, and sinus irrigation may be necessary as both a diagnostic and therapeutic modality.

Anaphylaxis

Any agent that can cause anaphylaxis in the nonpregnant state could potentially lead to anaphylaxis in the susceptible or sensitized pregnant patient. Maternal hypoxemia and hypotension caused by anaphylaxis may be catastrophic to the mother and the fetus (Entman & Moise, 1984; Erasmus et al., 1982). Thus management of anaphylaxis during pregnancy must be aggressive and expeditious, and all anaphylactic reactions should be considered potentially severe or life threatening until resolved.

Treatment. Because of the altered circulatory and respiratory physiology during pregnancy, adequate intravascular volume repletion and oxygenation are particularly important in the management of anaphylaxis during pregnancy to prevent both maternal and fetal complications. Epinephrine (0.3 cc of 1:1000 intramuscularly [IM]) is the initial pharmacologic treatment of choice and may be repeated every 10 to 15 minutes. If the reaction is due to a cutaneous injection or sting, a tourniquet should be placed above the site, 0.1 cc epinephrine should be injected at the site of the injection or sting, and 0.3 cc epinephrine should be injected into the opposite arm. Unless the reaction resolves promptly after the first epinephrine injection, diphenhydramine 50 mg IM (i.v. with hypotension) should be administered. For persistent symptoms, cimetidine 300 mg i.v. should be given. For persistent wheezing, nebulized beta2-agonists may be administered, and for recalcitrant hypotension, plasma expanders are indicated. In cases of extreme hypotension where tissue perfusion may be inadequate, intravenous epinephrine (1:10,000) may be considered.

References

Abboud T, Raya J, Sadri S, Grobler N, Stine L, Miller F. Fetal and maternal cardiovascular effects of atropine and glycopyrrolate. Anesth Analg 1983 Apr;62(4):426-30.

Abboud TK, Read J, Miller F, Chen T, Valle R, Hendriksen EH. Use of glycopyrrolate in the parturient: effect on the maternal and fetal heart and uterine activity. Obstet Gynecol 1981 Feb;57(2):224-7.

Adamsons K, Mueller-Heubach E, Myers RE. Production of fetal asphyxia in the rhesus monkey by administration of catecholamines to the mother. Am J Obstet Gynecol 1971 Jan 15;109(2):248-62.

Akerlund M, Bengtsson LP, Carter AM. A technique for monitoring endometrial or decidual blood flow with an intra-uterine thermistor probe. Acta Obstet Gynecol Scand 1975;54(5):469-77.

Aldridge A, Bailey J, Neims AH. The disposition of caffeine during and after pregnancy. Semin Perinatol 1981 Oct;5(4):310-4.

American Academy of Pediatrics Committee on Drugs. Transfer of drugs and other chemicals into human milk. Pediatrics 1989 Nov;84(5):924-36.

American Thoracic Society. Standards for the diagnosis and care of patients with chronic obstructive pulmonary disease (COPD) and asthma. Am Rev Respir Dis 1987;136:225-43.

Apter AJ, Greenberger PA, Patterson R. Outcomes of pregnancy in adolescents with severe asthma. Arch Intern Med 1989 Nov;149(11):2571-5.

Arcuri PA, Gautieri RF. Morphine-induced fetal malformations: 3. Possible mechanisms of action. J Pharm Sci 1973 Oct;62(10):1626-34.

Arwood LL, Dasta JF, Friedman C. Placental transfer of theophylline: two case reports. Pediatrics 1979 Jun;63(6):844-6.

Aselton P, Jick H, Milunsky A, Hunter JR, Stergachis A. First-trimester drug use and congenital disorders. Obstet Gynecol 1985 Apr;65(4): 451-5.

Back KC, Newberne JW, Weaver LC. A toxicopathologic study of endobenzyline bromide, a new cholinergic blocking agent. Toxicol Appl Pharmacol 1961 Jul;3(4):422-30.

Bahna SL, Bjerkedal T. The course and outcome of pregnancy in women with bronchial asthma. Acta Allergol 1972 Dec;27(5):397-406.

Baillie P, Meehan FP, Tyzack AJ. Treatment of premature labour with orciprenaline. Br Med J 1970 Oct 17;4(5728):154-5.

Banerjee BN, Woodard G. Teratologic evaluation of metaproterenol in the rhesus monkey (Macaca mulatta). Toxicol Appl Pharmacol 1971 Dec;20(4):562-4.

Baxi LV, Gindoff PR, Pregenzer GJ, Parras MK. Fetal heart rate changes following maternal administration of a nasal decongestant. Am J Obstet Gynecol 1985 Dec 1;153(7):799-800.

Bende M, Hallgårde U, Sjögren C. Occurrence of nasal congestion during pregnancy. Am J Rhinol 1989 Fall;3(4):217-9.

Bennett PN. Drugs and human lactation. New York: Elsevier, 1988.

Berlin CM Jr. Excretion of methylxanthines in human milk. Semin Perinatol 1981 Oct;5(4):389-94.

Bertrand JM, Riley SP, Popkin J, Coates AL. The long-term pulmonary sequelae of prematurity: the role of familial airway hyperreactivity and the respiratory distress syndrome. N Engl J Med 1985 Mar;312(12):742-5.

Bongiovanni AM, McPadden AJ. Steroids during pregnancy and possible fetal consequences. Fertil Steril 1960 Mar-Apr;11(2):181-6.

Bonica J. Principles and practice of obstetric analgesia and anesthesia. Philadelphia: FA Davis Company, 1972:24.

Brenner BE. Bronchial asthma in adults: presentation to the emergency department. Pt 1: Pathogenesis, clinical manifestations, diagnostic evaluation, and differential diagnosis. Am J Emerg Med 1983a Jul;1(1):50-70.

Brenner BE. Bronchial asthma in adults: presentation to the emergency department. Pt 2: Sympathomimetics, respiratory failure, recommendations for initial treatment, indications for admission, and summary. Am J Emerg Med 1983b Nov;1(3):306-33.

Briggs GG, Freeman RK, Yaffe SJ. Drugs in pregnancy and lactation. 3rd ed. Baltimore: Williams & Wilkins, 1990:237-8, 520-1.

Bruyere HJ Jr, Fallon JF, Gilbert EF. External malformations in chick embryos following concomitant administration of methylxanthines and beta-adrenomimetic agents: 1. Gross pathologic features. Teratology 1983 Oct;28(2):257-69.

Bueker ED, Platner WS. Effect of cholinergic drugs on development of chick embryo. Proc Soc Exp Biol Med 1956 Apr;91(4):539-43.

Cederqvist LL, Merkatz IR, Litwin SD. Fetal immunoglobulin synthesis following maternal immunosuppression. Am J Obstet Gynecol 1977 Nov 15;129(6):687-90.

Centers for Disease Control. Asthma—United States, 1980-1987. MMWR 1990a Jul 27;39(29):493-7.

Centers for Disease Control. Low birthweight—United States, 1975-1987. MMWR 1990b Mar 9;39(9):148-51.

Chester SW. Pregnancy and the treatment of hay fever, allergic rhinitis, and pollen asthma. Ann Allergy 1950 Nov-Dec;8(6):772-3, 798.

Chestnut DH, Pollack KL, Laszewski LJ, Bates JN, Choi WW. Continuous epidural infusion of bupivacaine-fentanyl during the second stage of labor. Anesthesiology 1989 Sep;71(3A):A841.

Cheung MO, Gilbert EF, Bruyere HJ Jr, Ishikawa S, Hodach RJ. Chronotropism and blood flow patterns following teratogenic doses of catecholamines in 5-day-old chick embryos. Teratology 1977 Dec;16(3):327-43.

Clark B, Clarke AJ, Bamford DG, Greenwood B. Nedocromil sodium preclinical safety evaluation studies: a preliminary report. Eur J Respir Dis 1986;69(147 Suppl):248-51.

Clark EB, Hu N, Dooley JB. The effect of isoproterenol on cardiovascular function in the stage 24 chick embryo. Teratology 1985 Feb; 31(1):41-7.

Clark NC. Asthma self-management education: research and implications for clinical practice. Chest 1989 May;95(5):1110-3.

Clark SL. Shock in the pregnant patient. Seminar Perinatol 1990;14:52-8.

Clark SL, Cotton DB, Lee W, et al. Central hemodynamic assessment of normal term pregnancy. Am J Obstet Gynecol 1989;161:1439-42.

Clark SL, Cotton DB, Pivarnik JM, et al. Position change and central hemodynamic profile during normal third-trimester pregnancy and postpartum. Am J Obstet Gynecol 1991;164:883-7.

Connelly TJ, Ruo TI, Frederiksen MC, Atkinson AJ Jr. Characterization of theophylline binding to serum proteins in pregnant and nonpregnant women. Clin Pharmacol Ther 1990 Jan;47(1):68-72.

Corssen G, Gutierrez J, Reves JG, Huber FC Jr. Ketamine in the anesthetic management of asthmatic patients. Anesth Analg 1972 Jul-Aug;51(4):588-96.

Cote CJ, Meuwissen HJ, Pickering RJ. Effects on the neonate of prednisone and azathioprine administered to the mother during pregnancy. J Pediatr 1974 Sep;85(3):324-8.

Cottle MK, Van Petten GR, van Muyden P. Effects of phenylephrine and sodium salicylate on maternal and fetal cardiovascular indices and blood oxygenation in sheep. Am J Obstet Gynecol 1982 May 15;143(2):170-6.

Cox JS, Beach JE, Blair AM, et al. Disodium cromoglycate (Intal). Adv Drug Res 1970;5:115-96.

Crawford JS. Bronchospasm following ergometrine [letter]. Anesthesiology 1980 Apr;35(4):397-8.

Czeizel A, Racz J. Evaluation of drug intake during pregnancy in the Hungarian Case-Control Surveillance of Congenital Anomalies. Teratology 1990;42(5):505-12.

Dean M, Stock B, Patterson RJ, Levy G. Serum protein binding of drugs during and after pregnancy in humans. Clin Pharmacol Ther 1980 Aug;28(2):253-61.

Derbes VJ, Sodeman WA. Reciprocal influences of bronchial asthma and pregnancy. Am J Med 1946 Oct;1(4):367-75.

Diaz DM, Diaz SF, Marx GF. Cardiovascular effects of glycopyrrolate and belladonna derivatives in obstetric patients. Bull NY Acad Med 1980 Mar;56(2):245-8.

Dombrowski MP, Bottoms SF, Boike GM, Wald J. Incidence of preeclampsia among asthmatic patients lower with theophylline. Am J Obstet Gynecol 1986 Aug;155(2):265-7.

Doyle LW, Kitchen WH, Ford GW, Rickards AL, Kelly EA. Antenatal steroid therapy and 5-year outcome of extremely low birth weight infants. Obstet Gynecol 1989 May;73(5 Pt 1):743-6.

Einarson TR, Leeder JS, Koren G. A method for meta-analysis of epidemiological studies. Drug Intell Clin Pharm 1988 Oct;22(10): 813-24.

Entman SS, Moise KJ. Anaphylaxis in pregnancy. South Med J 1984 Mar;77(3):402.

Erasmus C, Blackwood W, Wilson J. Infantile multicystic encephalomalacia after maternal bee sting anaphylaxis during pregnancy. Arch Dis Child 1982 Oct;57(10):785-7.

Fanta CH, Rossing TH, McFadden ER Jr. Emergency room treatment of asthma: relationships among therapeutic combinations, severity of obstruction, and time course of response. Am J Med 1982 Mar;72(3):416-22.

Fanta CH, Rossing TH, McFadden ER Jr. Glucocorticoids in acute asthma: a critical controlled trial. Am J Med 1983 May;74(5):845-51.

Fanta CH, Rossing TH, McFadden ER Jr. Treatment of acute asthma. Is combination therapy with sympathomimetics and methylxanthines indicated? Am J Med 1986 Jan;80(1):5-10.

Feldman CH, Clark NM, Evans D. The role of health education in medical management of asthma. Clin Rev Allergy 1987;5:195-205.

Findlay JW, Butz RF, Sailstad JM, Warren JT, Welch RM. Pseudoephedrine and triprolidine in plasma and breast milk of nursing mothers. Br J Clin Pharmacol 1984 Dec;18(6):901-6.

Fitzsimons R, Greenberger PA, Patterson R. Outcome of pregnancy in women requiring corticosteroids for severe asthma. J Allergy Clin Immunol 1986 Aug;78(2):349-53.

Frederiksen MC, Ruo TI, Chow MJ, Atkinson AJ Jr. Theophylline pharmacokinetics in pregnancy. Clin Pharmacol Ther 1986 Sep;40(3):321-8.

Fung DL. Emergency anesthesia for asthma patients. Clin Rev Allergy 1985 Feb;3(1):127-41.

Gal TJ, Suratt PM. Atropine and glycopyrrolate effects on lung mechanics in normal man. Anesth Analg 1981 Feb;60(2):81-90.

Gardner MJ, Schatz M, Cousins L, Zeiger R, Middleton E, Jusko WJ. Longitudinal effects of pregnancy on the pharmacokinetics of theophylline. Eur J Clin Pharmacol 1987;32(3):289-95.

Gluck JC, Gluck P. The effects of pregnancy on asthma: a prospective study. Ann Allergy 1976 Sep;37(3):164-8.

Gordon M, Niswander KR, Berendes H, Kantor AG. Fetal morbidity following potentially anoxigenic obstetric conditions: 7. Bronchial asthma. Am J Obstet Gynecol 1970 Feb;106(3):421-9.

Greenberger P, Patterson R. Safety of therapy for allergic symptoms during pregnancy. Ann Intern Med 1978 Aug;89(2):234-7.

Greenberger PA, Patterson R. Beclomethasone diproprionate for severe asthma during pregnancy. Ann Intern Med 1983 Apr;98(4):478-80.

Greenberger PA, Patterson R. The outcome of pregnancy complicated by severe asthma. Allergy Proc 1988 Sep-Oct;9(5):539-43.

Hagerdal M, Morgan CW, Sumner AE, Gutsche BB. Minute ventilation and oxygen consumption during labor with epidural analgesia. Anesthesiology 1983 Nov;59(5):425-7.

Hamod KA, Khouzami VA. Antibiotics in pregnancy. In: Niebyl JR, ed. Drug use in pregnancy. 2nd ed. Philadelphia: Lea and Febiger, 1988: 29-36.

Harris JB, Weinberger MM, Nassif E, Smith G, Milavetz G, Stillerman A. Early intervention with short courses of prednisone to prevent progression of asthma in ambulatory patients incompletely responsive to bronchodilators. J Pediatr 1987 Apr;110(4):627-33.

Harrison BD, Stokes TC, Hart GJ, Vaughn DA, Ali NJ, Robinson AA. Need for intravenous hydrocortisone in addition to oral prednisolone in patients admitted to hospital with severe asthma without ventilatory failure. Lancet 1986 Jan 25;1(8474):181-4.

Heinonen OP, Slone D, Shapiro S. Birth defects and drugs in pregnancy. Littleton, MA: Publishing Sciences Group, 1977.

Hollmen AI, Jouppila R, Albright GA, Jouppila P, Vierola H, Koivula A. Intervillous blood flow during caesarean section with prophylactic ephedrine and epidural anaesthesia. Acta Anaesth Scand 1984 Aug;28(4):396-400.

Holmes F. Incidence of the supine hypotensive syndrome in late pregnancy. J Obstet Gynaecol Brit Emp 1960;67:254-8.

Horowitz DA, Jablonski WJ, Mehta KA. Apnea associated with theophylline withdrawal in a term neonate. Am J Dis Child 1982 Jan;136(1):73-4.

Janz D, Fuchs U. Are anti-epileptic drugs harmful when given during pregnancy? Ger Med Mon 1964;9(1):20-2.

Jensen K. Pregnancy and allergic diseases. Acta Allergol 1953;6:44-53.

Josephson GW, MacKenzie EJ, Lietman PS, Gibson G. Emergency treatment of asthma: a comparison of two treatment regimens. JAMA 1979 Aug 17;242(7):639-43.

Juniper EF, Daniel EE, Roberts RS, Kline PA, Hargreave FE, Newhouse MT. Improvement in airway responsiveness and asthma severity during pregnancy: a prospective study. Am Rev Respir Dis 1989 Oct;140(4):924-31.

Kanto J, Virtanen R, Iisalo E, Maenpaa K, Liukko P. Placental transfer and pharmacokinetics of atropine after a single maternal intravenous and intramuscular administration. Acta Anaesth Scand 1981 Apr;25(2):85-8.

Katz FH, Duncan BR. Entry of prednisone into human milk [letter]. N Engl J Med 1975 Nov 27;293(22):1154.

Katz VL, Thorp JM Jr, Bowes WA Jr. Severe symmetric intrauterine growth retardation associated with the topical use of triamcinolone. Am J Obstet Gynecol 1990 Feb;162(2):396-7.

Kivalo I, Saarikoski S. Placental transmission of atropine at full-term pregnancy. Br J Anaesth 1977 Oct;49(10):1017-21.

Korsch BM, Gozzi EK, Francis V. Gaps in doctor-patient communication: 1. Doctor-patient interaction and patient satisfaction. Pediatrics 1968 Nov;42(5):855-71.

Kraus AM. Congenital cataract and maternal steroid injection. J Pediatr Ophthalmol 1975 May;12(2):107-8.

Lao TT, Huengsburg M. Labour and delivery in mothers with asthma. Eur J Obstet Gynecol Reprod Biol 1990 May-Jun;35(2-3):183-90.

Littenberg B, Gluck EH. A controlled trial of methylprednisolone in the emergency treatment of asthma. N Engl J Med 1986 Jan 16;314(3):150-2.

Mabry RL. Intranasal steroid injection during pregnancy. South Med J 1980 Sep;73(9):1176-9.

Mabry RL. Rhinitis of pregnancy. South Med J 1986 Aug;79(8):965-71.

Maietta AL. The management of the allergic patient during pregnancy. Ann Allergy 1955 Sep-Oct;13(5):516-22.

Maren TH, Ellison AC. The teratological effect of certain thiadiazoles related to acetazolamide, with a note on sulfanilamide and thiazide diuretics. Johns Hopkins Med J 1972 Feb;130(2):95-104.

McFadden ER Jr. Therapy of acute asthma. J Allergy Clin Immunol 1989 Aug;84(2):151-8.

McKenzie SA, Selley JA, Agnew JE. Secretion of prednisolone into breast milk. Arch Dis Child 1975 Nov;50(11):894-6.

Mellin GW. Drugs in the first trimester of pregnancy and the fetal life of homo sapiens. Am J Obstet Gynecol 1964 Dec 1;90(7 Pt 2):1169-80.

Mellins RB. Patient education is key to successful management of asthma. J Rev Respir Dis 1989;(Suppl):S47-S52.

Metzger WJ, Turner E, Patterson R. The safety of immunotherapy during pregnancy. J Allergy Clin Immunol 1978 Apr;61(4):268-72.

Mohun M. Incidence of vasomotor rhinitis during pregnancy. Arch Otolaryngol 1943;37:699-709.

National Asthma Education Program Expert Panel on the Management of Asthma. Guidelines for the diagnosis and management of asthma. Bethesda, MD: U.S. Department of Health and Human Services, National Heart, Lung, and Blood Institute. 1991.

National Asthma Education Program Expert Panel on the Management of Asthma. Executive summary: guidelines for the diagnosis and management of asthma. Bethesda, MD: U.S. Department of Health and Human Services, National Heart, Lung, and Blood Institute. 1991.

Needs CJ, Brooks PM. Antirheumatic medication in pregnancy. Br J Rheumatol 1985 Aug;24(3):282-90.

Norman PS. The John Sheldon memorial lecture: review of nasal therapy: update. J Allergy Clin Immunol 1983 Nov;72(5 Pt 1):421-32.

Ohguro Y, Kiyohara A, Mijagawa A, Imamura S, Koyama K, Hara T. Pharmacological and toxicological studies on beclometasone dipropionate. Yamaguchi Igaku 1970 Mar;19(1):65-86.

Onnen I, Barrier G, dAthis P, Sureau C, Olive G. Placental transfer of atropine at the end of pregnancy. Eur J Clin Pharmacol 1979 Jul;15(6):443-6.

Ost L, Wettrell G, Bjorkhem I, Rane A. Prednisolone excretion in human milk. J Pediatr 1985 Jun;106(6):1008-11.

Philipson A. Pharmacokinetics of ampicillin during pregnancy. J Infect Dis 1977 Sep;136(3):370-6.

Philipson A, Stiernstedt G. Pharmacokinetics of cefuroxime in pregnancy. Am J Obstet Gynecol 1982 Apr 1;142(7):823-8.

Pirson Y, Van Lierde M, Ghysen J, Squifflet JP, Alexandre GP, van Ypersele de Strihou C. Retardation of fetal growth in patients receiving immunosuppressive therapy [letter]. N Engl J Med 1985 Aug 1;313(5):328.

Pond SM, Kreek MJ, Tong TG, Raghunath J, Benowitz NL. Altered methadone pharmacokinetics in methadone-maintained pregnant women. J Pharmacol Exp Ther 1985 Apr;233(1):1-6.

Prowse CM, Gaensler EA. Respiratory and acid-base changes during pregnancy. Anesthesiology 1965;20:381-92.

Rayburn WF. Prostaglandin E2 gel for cervical ripening and induction of labor: a critical analysis. Am J Obstet Gynecol 1989 Mar;160(3):529-34.

Rayburn WF, Anderson JC, Smith CV, Appel LL, Davis SA. Uterine and fetal Doppler flow changes from a single dose of a long-acting intranasal decongestant. Obstet Gynecol 1990 Aug;76(2):180-2.

Robson JM, Sullivan FM, Smith RL, eds. Embryopathic activity of drugs. Boston: Little Brown, 1965. 110 p.

Ron M, Hochner-Celnikier D, Menczel J, Palti Z, Kidroni G. Maternal-fetal transfer of aminophylline. Acta Obstet Gynecol Scand 1984;63(3):217-8.

Roodenburg PJ, Wladimiroff JW, Van Weering HK. Effect of maternal intravenous administration of atropine (0.5 mg) on fetal breathing and heart pattern. Contr Gynecol Obstet 1979;6:92-7.

Rossing TH, Fanta CH, Goldstein DH, Snapper JR, McFadden ER Jr. Emergency therapy of asthma: comparison of the acute effects of parenteral and inhaled sympathomimetics and infused aminophylline. Am Rev Respir Dis 1980 Sep;122(3):365-71.

Rubin JD, Loffredo C, Correa-Villasenor A, Ferencz C. Prenatal drug use and congenital cardiovascular malformations. Teratology 1991 May;43(5):423.

Sakai T, Owaki Y, Noguchi Y. Reproduction studies of pirbuterol hydrochloride [abstract]. In: Shepard TH, ed. Catalog of Teratogenic Agents. 6th ed. Baltimore: Johns Hopkins University Press, 1989: 512.

Saxen I. Cleft palate and maternal diphenhydramine intake [letter]. Lancet 1974 Mar 9;1(854):407-8.

Schaefer G, Silverman F. Pregnancy complicated by asthma. Am J Obstet Gynecol 1961 Jul; 82(1):182-91.

Schatz M, Harden K, Forsythe A, et al. The course of asthma during pregnancy, post partum, and with successive pregnancies: a prospective analysis. J Allergy Clin Immunol 1988a Mar;81(3):509-17.

Schatz M, Patterson R, Zeitz S, O'Rourke J, Melam H. Corticosteroid therapy for the pregnant asthmatic patient. JAMA 1975 Aug;233(7):804-7.

Schatz M, Zeiger RS. Management of asthma, rhinitis, and anaphylaxis during pregnancy. Curr Obstet Gynecol 1991;1:65.

Schatz M, Zeiger RS, Harden KM, et al. The safety of inhaled beta-agonist bronchodilators during pregnancy. J Allergy Clin Immunol 1988b Oct;82(4):686-95.

Schatz M, Zeiger RS, Hoffman CP. Intrauterine growth is related to gestational pulmonary function in pregnant asthmatic women: Kaiser-Permanente Asthma and Pregnancy Study Group. Chest 1990 Aug;98(2):389-92.

Schulman BA. Active patient orientation and outcomes in hypertensive treatment. Med Care 1979 Mar;17(3):267-80.

Scott JR. Fetal growth retardation associated with maternal administration of immunosuppressive drugs. Am J Obstet Gynecol 1977 Jul 15;128(6):668-76.

Sears MR, Taylor PR, Print CG, et al. Regular inhaled beta-agonist treatment in bronchial asthma. Lancet 1990;336:1391-6.

Shim CS, Williams MH Jr. Evaluation of the severity of asthma: patients versus physicians. Am J Med 1980 Jan;68(1):11-3.

Siegel D, Sheppard D, Gelb A, Weinberg PF. Aminophylline increases the toxicity but not the efficacy of an inhaled beta-adrenergic agonist in the treatment of acute exacerbations of asthma. Am Rev Respir Dis 1985 Aug;132(2):283-6.

Smith CV, Rayburn WF, Anderson JC, Duckworth AF, Appel LL. Effect of a single dose of oral pseudoephedrine on uterine and fetal Doppler blood flow. Obstet Gynecol 1990 Nov;76(5 Pt 1):803-6

Smith NT, Corbascio AN. The use and misuse of pressor agents. Anesthesiology 1970 Jul;33(1):58-101.

Soares de Moura RS. Effect of terbutaline on the human fetal placental circulation. Br J Obstet Gynaecol 1981 Jul;88(7):730-3.

Sobrevilla LA, Cassinelli MT, Carcelen A, Malaga JM. Human fetal and maternal oxygen tension and acid-base status during delivery at high altitude. Am J Obstet Gynecol 1971;111:1111-8.

Sorri M, Hartikainen-Sorri AL, Karja J. Rhinitis during pregnancy. Rhinology 1980 Jun;18(2):83-6.

Stec GP, Greenberger P, Ruo TI, et al. Kinetics of theophylline transfer to breast milk. Clin Pharmacol Ther 1980 Sep;28(3):404-8.

Stenius-Aarniala B, Piirila P, Teramo K. Asthma and pregnancy: a prospective study of 198 pregnancies. Thorax 1988 Jan;43(1):12-8.

Stewart JJ. Gastrointestinal drugs. In: Wilson JT, ed. Drugs in breast milk. England: MTP Press Limited, 1981: 65-71.

Templeton A, Kelman GR. Maternal blood gases (PAO2-PaO2), physiological shunt, and VD/VT in normal pregnancy. Br J Anaesth 1976;48:1001-4.

Towers CV, Rojas JA, Lewis DF, Asrat T, Nageotte MP, Briggs GG. Usage of prostaglandin E2 (PGE2) in patients with asthma. Am J Obstet Gynecol 1991 Jan;164(1 Pt 2):295.

Ueland K, Hansen JM. Maternal cardiovascular dynamics: III. Labor and delivery under local and caudal analgesia. Am J Obstet Gynecol 1969;103:8-18.

Ueland K, Novy MJ, Peterson EN, Metcalfe J. Maternal cardiovascular dynamics: IV. The influence of gestational age on the maternal cardiovascular response to posture and exercise. Am J Obstet Gynecol 1969;104:856-64.

White RJ, Coutts II, Gibbs CJ, MacIntyre C. A prospective study of asthma during pregnancy and the puerperium. Respir Med 1989 Mar;83(2):103-6.

Widdicombe JG, ed. Supplement: airway hyperreactivity from the International Symposium on Airway Hyperreactivity, October 26 to 28, 1988, Sendai, Japan. Am Rev Respir Dis 1991 Mar;143(3 Pt 2):S1-S82.

Williams DA. Asthma and pregnancy. Acta Allergol 1967;22:311-23.

Wilson J. Use of sodium cromoglycate during pregnancy. J Pharm Med 1982;8:45-51.

Wilson M, Morganti AA, Zervoudakis I, et al. Blood pressure, the renin-aldosterone system and sex steroids throughout normal pregnancy. Am J Med 1980;68:97-104.

Woolcock AJ. Use of corticosteroids in treatment of patients with asthma. J Allergy Clin Immunol 1985;19:33-7

Yeh TF, Pildes RS. Transplacental aminophylline toxicity in a neonate [letter]. Lancet 1977 Apr 23;1(8017):910.

Younker D, Clark R, Tessem J, Joyce TH 3d, Kubicek M. Bupivacaine-fentanyl epidural analgesia for a parturient in status asthmaticus. Can J Anaesth 1987 Nov;34(6):609-12.

Yurchak AM, Jusko WJ. Theophylline secretion into breast milk. Pediatrics 1976 Apr;57(4):518-20.

Zilianti M, Aller J. Action of orciprenaline on uterine contractility during labor, maternal cardiovascular system, fetal heart rate, and acid-base balance. Am J Obstet Gynecol 1971 Apr 1;109(7):1073-9.4

Good News and Great Tips for Pregnant Women with Asthma

Congratulations! Your pregnancy is an exciting event, and your visit to the doctor shows you care about staying healthy. You are breathing for two now, and you need to keep your asthma under control. By taking the steps listed in this handout, you can control your asthma and protect your baby.

If you do not take these steps, you could lose control of your asthma. Asthma symptoms such as coughing, chest tightness, wheezing, and shortness of breath can keep your baby from getting enough oxygen to grow well. Your baby could be less healthy and smaller when born, or could even be born too early. But these things do not need to happen! Asthma can be controlled so you can have a normal pregnancy, labor, and delivery and a healthy baby!

Here are the steps you can take to control your asthma and protect your baby:

Work with your doctor and other health care providers.

- Keep your appointments.
- Ask all the questions you have. Writing them down before each visit is a good idea. It helps you remember them all.
- Tell your doctor about any wheezing, coughing, or shortness of breath that you have.
- Tell your doctor if you notice any changes in your asthma.
- Tell your doctor any concerns you have about your medicines or the other parts of your treatment plan.
- Make sure you know what your doctor wants you to do before you leave the office.

Take your medicines.

- Follow directions exactly about when to take your asthma medicines and how much medicine to take.

- Don't stop taking your asthma medicines unless your doctor directs you.

- Get your doctor's okay before you take ANY new medicines or over-the-counter drugs (drugs you choose yourself at the store, such as headache, cough, or cold medicine).

Remember: Using asthma medicine during pregnancy is much safer than letting your asthma get out of control. Such asthma medicines as inhaled beta-agonists, cromolyn, and inhaled steroids are safe for pregnant women when you take them as directed by your doctor. So, take your medicines and control your asthma!

Watch your asthma and treat symptoms fast.

Pregnancy is a time of change. Your asthma can change too and can get worse, better, or stay the same. If this is your first pregnancy, there is no way to predict what will happen with your asthma. If you have been pregnant before, your asthma is most likely to change—or not change—the same way it did with your last pregnancy. It is very important for you to watch your asthma closely.

- Use a peak flow meter each day so you can find any changes in your asthma and act early.

- Know how to tell if your asthma is getting worse. Make a list with your doctor of the ways you can tell if your asthma is getting worse.

- Make a plan with your doctor for dealing with any sign that your asthma is getting worse. Use it.

Stay away from your asthma triggers.

Your asthma triggers are those things that you know make your asthma worse. House dust mites or damp places, animals, tobacco smoke, and very cold air are some examples of asthma triggers. You can stay away from some triggers. For other triggers, you can take action to keep them from bothering your asthma.

Do not smoke or stay around people who smoke.

- Cigarette smoke makes it more likely that you will have asthma episodes.

Pregnancy in Women with Asthma

- Smoking during your pregnancy makes it more likely that your baby will be born too early and too small. Your baby is more likely to be sick more often, too.

- If babies breathe in other people's smoke, the babies' lungs will not grow and work as well as they should. The baby is likely to have more colds and earaches.

- When babies live with people who smoke, they have a greater chance of developing asthma.

- If you smoke, now is the time to stop! Your doctor or nurse will help you. Ask them.

Answers to Some Common Questions

Are asthma medicines safe for pregnant women? Yes, asthma medicines are safe when you take them as directed by your doctor. It is very important for your baby's health that you keep your asthma under good control!

Can I exercise? Yes! You can exercise. Exercise is important and you should be able to be physically active without having asthma symptoms. Talk to your doctor about this.

Can I take allergy shots? Yes. Allergy shots can be continued if you were getting them before you were pregnant. But allergy shots should not be started for the first time while you are pregnant.

Should I get flu shots? You can get flu shots. These are made from dead viruses that will not harm you or your baby. Flu shots are often recommended for people who have asthma. Ask your doctor.

What happens if I get an asthma episode (or "attack") during labor or delivery? Asthma episodes usually do not occur during labor and delivery. If asthma symptoms do occur, you will receive prompt treatment and you and your baby will be watched carefully. Your asthma will be controlled so you can have a normal labor and delivery.

Will my breast milk be safe for my baby? Yes. Very little asthma medicine will get to your baby through your breast milk. The small amount in breast milk will not harm your baby.

Will my baby have asthma? Perhaps. A child is more likely to have asthma when one or both parents have asthma or allergies.

Chapter 23

Pre-Gestational Diabetes

Introduction

When a woman who is known to have diabetes becomes pregnant, she is said to have pre-gestational diabetes. When a woman develops diabetes during pregnancy or is first recognized as having this condition during pregnancy, she is said to have gestational diabetes. Each year, approximately 10,000 infants are born to women with pre-gestational diabetes, and 60,000 to 90,000 infants are born to women with gestational diabetes.

The factor most important to the outcome of pregnancy is how well the mother's glucose level is controlled before and during pregnancy. When women with diabetes receive optimal care, the perinatal mortality rate for their offspring approaches the corresponding rate for the general population. However, when pregnant women with diabetes do not receive expert treatment, the perinatal mortality rate for their offspring more than doubles.

Offspring of women with diabetes are at increased risk of macrosomia, hypoglycemia, respiratory distress syndrome, and congenital malformations. Current statistics, although limited, suggest that the mortality rates of infants of mothers with diabetes is approximately 7 percent. In diabetes centers that have experience in intensive treatment, however, mortality rates are closer to 2 percent. It is becoming clear that pregnancy counseling and management are critical and that

---

Excerpts from NIH Publication No's. 93-3464 and 88-1587 and Research Resources Reporter, November 1990 by M. Elisabeth Tracey

normal glycemia at the time of conception will decrease the rate of fetal anomalies, which currently account for 40 percent of neonatal deaths. There is a need both for educational efforts and disease surveillance in the health care community to clearly establish the problems and the effects of interventions.

Background

Metabolic changes. Normal pregnancy is characterized by increasing insulin resistance, which is probably due to human placental lactogen, a growth-hormone-like protein secreted by the placenta. Although pregnant women develop compensatory hyperinsulinemia, postprandial glucose levels increase significantly throughout pregnancy. During late pregnancy, fasting glucose levels fall because of increased glucose consumption by the placenta and the fetus.

Human placental lactogen reaches its peak late in pregnancy; during the third trimester, insulin requirements rise. Gestational diabetes most often appears during this period of maximum insulin resistance, and ketoacidosis may be seen—particularly in patients with insulin-dependent diabetes mellitus who do not increase their insulin dose appropriately.

Effect on the fetus. Because glucose crosses the placenta by facilitated diffusion, maternal hyperglycemia produces fetal hyperglycemia. Fetal hyperinsulinemia occurs in response to this abnormal metabolic environment. Hyperinsulinemia, combined with hyperglycemia, leads to excessive fetal growth. It may also contribute to intrauterine fetal death, delayed fetal pulmonary maturation, and neonatal hypoglycemia.

The incidence of major congenital malformations is increased approximately fourfold among infants of women with pre-gestational diabetes. Approximately 9% of pregnancies complicated by pre-gestational diabetes result in the birth of infants with central nervous system, cardiac, renal, skeletal, and other malformations. Major malformations may occur in 20% to 25% of infants born to women with very poor glycemia control during organogenesis, as evidenced by markedly elevated glycosylated hemoglobin levels during the first trimester.

Other factors that may increase the risk for fetal anomalies include early age at onset of maternal diabetes and microvascular disease in the mother. The earlier the age at onset of pre-gestational diabetes, the worse the prognosis is for successful pregnancy.

Pre-Gestational Diabetes

Effect on the mother. Pregnancy may be associated with exacerbation of diabetic eye disease, especially in women with unrecognized or untreated proliferative diabetic retinopathy. Diabetic women with nephropathy and hypertension are at greater risk for preeclampsia and fetal growth retardation than are women without nephropathy. Death has been reported among pregnant women with diabetes and coronary artery disease.

Caring for the Patient with Pre-Gestational Diabetes

Prevention

The outcome of pregnancy complicated by pre-gestational diabetes is improved when care begins before conception. Each visit with a woman of childbearing age who has diabetes should be considered a pre-conceptional visit. Discuss family planning and ask the patient her thoughts about a future pregnancy.

Results of a glycosylated hemoglobin test provide overall assessment of glycemic control. Pregnancy should be deferred until excellent glycemic control is achieved, as indicated by a normal or near normal glycosylated hemoglobin level. Counsel patients about nutrition and teach them how to monitor their blood glucose levels and how to adjust their insulin treatment.

For patients who are planning to become pregnant, establish baseline data that can be used to assess maternal and perinatal risk, including the following:

- History of diabetic ketoacidosis and severe hypoglycemia.
- Blood pressure measurement.
- Eye examination.
- Quantitative assessment of renal function and urinary protein or albumin excretion.
- Electrocardiogram (if indicated).

Patients whose pregnancy is complicated by diabetes often experience significant emotional and financial stresses. Assess the patient's emotional or psychosocial support and financial resources through discussion with the patient, her partner, and her family.

Emphasize the dangers of smoking and of consuming alcohol when pregnant.

Treatment

Health care team. An experienced health care team is required to care for a patient with pregestational diabetes. The team should include the following persons:

- An obstetrician or a specialist in maternal-fetal medicine.
- An internist or diabetologist.
- A pediatrician or neonatologist.
- A diabetes educator.
- A dietitian.
- A social worker.

Every effort should be made to refer patients to medical centers that can provide comprehensive support. If such referral is not possible, members of the health care team should frequently consult with each other by telephone.

Glucose level. Excellent control of maternal diabetes is a critical objective both before and during pregnancy. During normal pregnancy, mean maternal plasma glucose levels rarely exceed 120 mg/dL and range from fasting levels of 60 mg/dL to 2-hour postprandial levels of 120 mg/dL. Use these values as the therapeutic objective for patients whose pregnancies are complicated by pregestational diabetes.

Diet. During the latter half of pregnancy, the patient with pregestational diabetes needs to eat approximately 35 kilocalories per kilogram of her ideal pre-pregnancy body weight each day, or approximately 2200 to 2400 calories per day. A weight gain of 24 to 28 pounds is recommended for most patients; however, for obese patients with noninsulin-dependent diabetes mellitus, the preferred daily dietary intake is 25 kilocalories per kilogram of ideal pre-pregnancy body weight, or approximately 1600 to 1800 calories per day.

The calories should be derived as follows: approximately 50% from complex carbohydrates, 30% from fats, and 20% from proteins. Patients will require three meals and up to three snacks each day. A bedtime snack is particularly important to decrease the risk of nocturnal hypoglycemia.

Pre-Gestational Diabetes

Monitoring. Patients with insulin-treated diabetes should monitor their blood glucose levels at least four times a day either before or 2 hours after each meal and at bedtime. Before breakfast, patients should test for ketones in their urine. Ask patients to record results in a log book and to note any changes in diet and exercise and any problems with hypoglycemia.

Measure the glycosylated hemoglobin level at least once each trimester to assess overall glycemic control.

Insulin therapy. Patients treated with oral hypoglycemic agents should be switched to insulin before they become pregnant. Human insulin should generally be used. Patients with insulin-treated diabetes require an individualized insulin regimen based on their exercise plan and blood glucose levels.

Most patients will require at least two injections a day of a mixture of intermediate-acting (NPH or lente) and short-acting (regular) insulin. Selected patients may be treated with multiple daily injections (that is, regular insulin before each meal and an injection of intermediate- or long-acting (ultralente) insulin at bedtime). For some patients, continuous subcutaneous insulin infusion is an option, but it appears to offer no significant advantage over multiple daily injections. Patients who prefer the flexibility offered by the pump may be started on such therapy, and those who have used a pump before pregnancy may continue to do so.

Fetal assessment. Maintain a program of fetal assessment throughout pregnancy. Measure the maternal serum alpha-fetoprotein level at 16 weeks of gestation to screen for neural tube defects and other fetal anomalies. Perform a detailed ultrasonographic examination at 16 to 18 weeks of gestation. If indicated, assess the fetal cardiac structure by echocardiography at 20 weeks of gestation. When performed by experienced professionals, such tests allow detection of most major fetal malformations. If an anomaly is found skilled counseling must be provided for the patient.

During the third trimester, assessment of fetal growth and well-being becomes most important. Fetal growth may be evaluated by serial ultrasonographic examination every 4 to 6 weeks. Fetal well-being may be determined by a variety of techniques, including the following:

- Maternal monitoring of fetal activity.

- Antepartum heart rate testing by using the nonstress or contraction stress test.

- Biophysical profile that includes an ultrasonographic evaluation of fetal activity, fetal breathing movements, fetal tone, and amniotic fluid volume.

Although these tests may be initiated at 28 weeks of gestation, they are most often begun at 32 weeks and performed once or twice a week until delivery.

Delivery. If the patient maintains excellent glucose control, if her blood pressure is normal, and if antepartum fetal testing shows no evidence of fetal compromise, delivery may occur at term. If delivery is planned before term, assess fetal pulmonary maturation by measuring the ratio of amniotic fluid lecithin to sphingomyelin (L/S) and the level of acidic phospholipid phosphatidyglycerol. If ultrasound suggests excessive fetal size, delivery by cesarean section may be elected.

Delivery must take place where expert maternal and neonatal care are available. Breast-feeding should be encouraged.

Postpartum care. In the immediate postpartum period, reassess the patient's meal plan and adjust her treatment program. Maternal insulin requirements fall significantly, usually to—or even below—prepregnancy levels.

During the patient's postpartum follow-up visit, encourage her to diet, if necessary, to achieve her ideal body weight. Contraception should be discussed. Low-dose oral contraceptives or a progestin-only pill may be offered to patients who have no evidence of hypertension or vascular disease. For patients with hypertension or vascular disease, a barrier method of contraception, such as a diaphragm, is preferred. If the patient has completed her family or if she has serious vascular disease, sterilization should be discussed.

Patient Education Principles

- Emphasize the importance of pre-pregnancy care.

- Work with the patient, her partner, her family, and other health care providers to improve the patient's nutrition, exercise program, and glucose control.

- Recommend that conception be delayed until the patient's blood glucose control is excellent and the glycosylated hemoglobin level is normal or near normal.

Pre-Gestational Diabetes

- Explain the risks of birth defects and adverse perinatal outcomes and the need for fetal surveillance.

- Recommend that the patient's vascular condition be thoroughly evaluated before she becomes pregnant. Explain that pregnancy may exacerbate advanced diabetic retinopathy but generally does not permanently worsen diabetic nephropathy.

- Explain that, overall, pregnancy does not shorten the life expectancy of a woman with diabetes but does increase her risk for hypoglycemia and ketoacidosis and for associated mortality.

- Inform patients with coronary atherosclerosis that their risks for morbidity or mortality may be greater during pregnancy.

- Discuss the emotional and financial demands of pregnancy with the patient, her partner, and her family.

- Inform patients about lifestyle elements—such as drinking alcoholic beverages and smoking—that increase the risk for a poor outcome of pregnancy. Emphasize that patients will need to modify such behaviors before becoming pregnant.

Prevention of Spontaneous Abortion in Diabetic Pregnancies

Good glycemic control decreases the rate of spontaneous abortion in diabetic pregnancies, according to researchers at the University of Cincinnati College of Medicine in Ohio. "Our studies have shown that the rate of spontaneous abortion in women with insulin-dependent diabetes mellitus (IDDM) is about 30 percent, or roughly twice that of the normal population," says principal investigator Dr. Menachem Miodovnik, associate professor in obstetrics and gynecology.

"Through a series of studies we have shown that very good glycemic control in early pregnancy can reduce the rate of spontaneous abortions and will probably reduce the number of birth defects as well," Dr. Miodovnik says.

The investigators monitored the glycemic status of the women by determining whether certain proteins found in the blood were glycosylated—had sugar molecules attached. "We looked at the concentration of glycohemoglobin A_1 (Hb A_1), a normal variant of hemoglobin that reflects the concentration of blood glucose during the preceding 4 to 8 weeks; at glycosylated serum albumin, which reflects glucose status during the previous 2 to 4 weeks; and at glycosylated serum total proteins, which reflect control in the previous 1 to 2 weeks," explains Dr. Miodovnik. "Looking at all of these proteins allows us to assess glucose status at conception, in early pregnancy, and close to the abortive event itself."

In a study of 68 IDDM women during 84 pregnancies the researchers found that the concentration of glycohemoglobin A_1 was significantly higher in women who had spontaneous abortions than in women who had successful pregnancies. In contrast, the concentrations of total glycosylated serum proteins and glycosylated serum albumin did not differ between the two groups of women. "What this tells us is that it is the glycemic control in very early pregnancy or even preconception that is important in determining whether a spontaneous abortion will occur, since glycohemoglobin A_1 reflects glucose status in the previous 4 to 8 weeks," explains Dr. Miodovnik.

To evaluate whether careful glycemia control was capable of reducing the incidence of spontaneous abortion, Dr. Miodovnik and Dr. Francis Mimouni, associate professor of pediatrics, and their colleagues recruited 45 insulin-dependent diabetic women with two consecutive pregnancies. The women were recruited before the ninth week of pregnancy. Blood glucose measurements were made both before eating and 90 minutes after eating at each weekly visit to the clinic, and glycohemoglobin A_1 concentrations were measured at 9 weeks of pregnancy. Diabetes management included a split dosage regimen of insulin, including both a short and intermediate acting insulin, along with dietary regulation.

"Our results have given us four classes of patients," explains Dr. Miodovnik. "One class contains 20 women who had a successful pregnancy followed by another successful pregnancy, a second class contains 15 women who had an abortion followed by a successful pregnancy. The last two classes contain five women who had a successful pregnancy followed by an abortion and three women who had two abortions, respectively. We included only the first two classes in the statistical analysis, and we found that the abortion/successful pregnancy patients had a significant decrease in Hb A_1 and average postprandial blood glucose from the first to the second pregnancy, which resulted in a 50-percent reduction in the abortion rate."

Dr. Miodovnik believes this reduction in the spontaneous abortion rate owes much of its success to patient education and close management. "Today we use glucometers with memory chips to measure blood sugar as often as eight times a day, and for our patients who live some

Pre-Gestational Diabetes

distance from the clinic we use modems to transmit the information. We also start educating them as early as possible, preferably before they become pregnant, on good diabetes management. In fact, now we have a program for teenagers and parents and try to get them in as early as we can," he explains.

The investigators believe that there might be an association between poor glycemic control and malformations in infants of diabetic women. "We have observed for quite a long time that babies of mothers with IDDM have a much higher rate of malformations than do offspring of normal mothers," says Dr. Mimouni. In 165 first pregnancies there were 13 infants with malformation (7.9 percent), including live-born infants and stillbirths. "Because all spontaneous abortions in that study occurred between 9 and 15 weeks of gestation—a time period believed to be associated with major malformations in the fetus—we suggest that such malformations are the cause of the higher spontaneous abortion rate in IDDM mothers, and that good glycemic control will reduce the rates of both malformations and abortions," he says. Neither maternal age nor duration of diabetes had a significant impact on the rate of spontaneous abortion.

According to Dr. Mimouni, "Cardiac problems occur most frequently. In addition, some very rare malformations occur much more frequently in these infants than in normal infants. One example is the caudal regression syndrome in which the sacrum (a bone situated between the two hip bones) can actually be completely missing. This defect may be accompanied by severe deformation of the lower limbs."

The malformations in the recent study were associated with elevated $Hb\ A_1$ concentrations at approximately 9 weeks of pregnancy and the presence of blood vessel disorders, or vasculopathies, in the retina or kidney of the mother. "We're not sure of the exact role played by maternal vascular disease in producing congenital malformations," says Dr. Mimouni. "The significance of elevated $Hb\ A_1$ may be the same as in animal studies that have shown a teratogenic (malformation-producing) effect of hyperglycemia, although other studies have shown hypoglycemia to be even more teratogenic."

Insulin that has crossed the placenta and magnesium deficiency in the diabetic women may be two additional causes of birth defects and spontaneous abortions. Dr. Mimouni notes that "it is well known that diabetic women are at risk of magnesium deficiency predominantly due to increased urinary magnesium losses. Because of the very important role magnesium plays in the function of enzymes and critical metabolic processes, magnesium deficiency could contribute to lethal fetal malformations and spontaneous abortions," he says.

Dr. Miodovnik is currently working on a study looking at "strict" versus "customary" glycemic control in pregnant IDDM women. Factors to be assessed include pregnancy outcome, complications of pregnancy, and the influence of hypoglycemic episodes on spontaneous abortion and malformation rates. Dr. Mimouni adds that the glucometers will allow separate analysis of the influence of hypoglycemic and hyperglycemic periods. Both physicians agree that identifying the exact mechanisms of malformation and spontaneous abortion in insulin-dependent diabetic women will help more of them achieve successful pregnancies and bear healthy children.

This work was supported by the General Clinical Research Centers Program of the National Center for Research Resources and by the National Institute of Child Health and Human Development.

Accomplishments and Future Directions in Research

Women with diabetes risk serious complications of pregnancy and a threefold increased incidence of congenital anomalies in their babies. Clinical studies have shown that meticulous regulation of blood glucose during the second and third trimester of pregnancy reduces the frequency and severity of most complications of pregnancy to those associated with nondiabetic pregnancies. Preliminary studies suggest that careful control of diabetes before and during the initial 12 weeks of pregnancy, when the baby's organs are being formed, will reduce the occurrence of birth defects. The opportunity exists for more fundamental research into the causes of the increase in birth defects in infants of mothers with diabetes, now the most common cause of death in these babies.

Accomplishments

The progress made over the past 10 years in the field of diabetes and pregnancy stands as a model for the possibilities for improvement in all areas of diabetes and its complications. Perinatal mortality in the best centers devoted to care of the pregnant woman with diabetes has fallen from 6.5 percent in the mid-1970's to 2.1 percent in the mid-1980's. Because 50 percent of this perinatal mortality rate is attributable to major congenital malformations, the corrected perinatal mortality is approximately 1 percent, approaching that seen in the general population without diabetes. Pregnancy is the one area of human diabetes in which meticulous metabolic control has been conclusively shown to be effective.

Pre-Gestational Diabetes

The achievement of near-normal glucose profiles in pregnant women with IDDM has been made possible by new and improved technologies such as self blood glucose monitoring in the home setting and the development of optimal insulin delivery systems. The improvement in perinatal mortality is partially due to the development of better approaches to judge fetal maturation and, in particular, the ability of the neonate's lungs to permit survival. Overall, fetal maturation now is judged by a combination of electrocardiographic and ultrasonographic procedures, and improved techniques permit accurate assessment of pulmonary maturation. This combined approach has allowed the woman with diabetes to deliver the infant vaginally and close to term, thus decreasing the mortality and morbidity associated with respiratory distress syndrome, hypoglycemia, hypocalcemia, erythremia, and hyperbilirubinemia. The highly sophisticated technology now available in neonatal intensive care units also has aided survival in those infants born prematurely. Advances in respiratory equipment, for example, have allowed treatment for the respirator-dependent newborn infant without necessarily subjecting the baby to the risk of retrolental fibroplasia. The importance of gestational diabetes as a cause of stillbirths has led to the initiation of universal screening with glucose tolerance tests of all pregnant women in the third trimester. With improved case finding and strategies specific for the woman with gestational diabetes, improvement already has been noted in obstetrical outcome.

Ongoing Research

Considerable progress has been achieved in the field of diabetes and pregnancy in the last decade. Maternal mortality is now similar both for women with diabetes and for women in the general population, and fetal mortality has fallen significantly in the best centers devoted to care of women whose pregnancies are complicated by diabetes. However, higher incidences of congenital anomalies, macrosomia, late intrauterine death, and respiratory distress syndrome remain a significant problem in pregnant women with diabetes.

The NICHD supports a broad range of research related to the effects of diabetes on maternal and child health, including three multidisciplinary centers that focus on pregnancy in women with diabetes. These centers are providing important information on the prevention of perinatal morbidity and mortality related to diabetes.

Metabolic studies are providing insight into carbohydrate and protein metabolism of the newborn. Centers have examined the effects of the abnormal intrauterine environment in maternal diabetes, the effects of intrauterine exposure to insulin, and glucose production by newborn infants. Animal studies have shown that exposure to insulin accelerates fetal growth.

An important ongoing research project in one of the pregnancy centers is the development of an implantable open-loop insulin infusion system for treatment of IDDM. The system delivers insulin into the peritoneum in a preprogrammed fashion, which the patient can adjust according to periodic blood glucose measurement and anticipated caloric intake. The system is expected to facilitate strict metabolic control, which is especially important during pregnancy to reduce birth defects and excess infant mortality.

Future Research Directions

The remarkable improvements cited above should provide added incentive to the research needs for the next 10 years. Although not strictly a "research" issue, one clear priority is to bring to all women with diabetes that level of care that has been shown to afford the best possible prognosis. The Federal Government's role may be to designate specialized regional centers that are designed to encourage care of pregnant women with diabetes and to support public and professional education initiatives, with possible use of reimbursement formulas.

The preliminary findings that the incidence of congenital malformations can be reduced in infants born to women with diabetes if meticulous metabolic control is initiated *before* conception must be translated into common clinical practice. Reliable techniques to detect the presence of serious malformations in the fetus must be developed; this would permit rational counseling on the possibility of therapeutic abortion. Starting with suitable animal models, studies must be conducted to determine whether inadvertent but repeated hypoglycemia will have serious adverse effects on the fetus such as damage at the time of organogenesis or damage to the rapidly developing brain later in gestation. The mechanism by which the diabetic milieu causes abnormalities of overall fetal growth and development (including failure of fetal pulmonary maturation) needs to be defined in precise biochemical and physiologic terms. Evidence now is emerging that the pathway involves a functional deficiency of arachidonic acid during organogenesis, which may, in turn, be associated with a depletion of tissue myoinositol. These observations need to be confirmed and extended, because the myoinositol data would indicate that the mechanism for diabetic embryopathy is analogous to the putative pathway that is hypothesized to be responsible for diabetic neuropathy and retinopathy. Exploration should continue of alternate hypotheses such as the role of various metabolites and growth factors or inhibitors. Animal models would appear to be highly suitable for these studies, especially the use of the whole embryo culture technique. Progress in this area should be followed by clinical trials that use an intervention strategy based on more precise knowledge of the teratogenic mechanism.

Further improvements must be made in the treatment programs for women with diabetes. Complicated regimens for optimal insulin delivery need to be simplified and made more flexible. Explorations should be made of technologies such as glucose monitors with built-in memories and algorithms to guide insulin dose adjustment. Markers other than glycosylated hemoglobin to guide optimal pregnancy therapy need to be developed. The possible use of other glycosylated serum proteins with a shorter half-life may prove to be of use; standards and norms for pregnancy will need to be defined. For women with gestational diabetes, an improved, simplified approach to screening must be developed and validated to replace the time-consuming and costly method now used. Once the diagnosis of gestational diabetes is made, safe and simplified treatment programs must be devised and evaluated. Methods to validate these programs would include newer approaches to nutrition prescriptions, the evaluation of exercise as adjunct therapy, and the development and testing of safe oral hypoglycemic agents.

Closely related to the issue of pregnancy is the assessment of the safety and efficacy of contraception programs for women with diabetes. Giving the woman with diabetes a choice of contraceptive methods could help to plan pregnancy so as to achieve optimal metabolic control from preconception to delivery.

The long-term issues of diabetes in pregnancy should be explored. These issues include the effects of pregnancy on the diabetic woman's risk of development or progression of diabetic nephropathy and diabetic retinopathy. The possibilities have been raised that infants of mothers with diabetes are at increased risk for the development of obesity and neurologic dysfunction and for the future onset of diabetes.

Additional Reading

Freinkel N, Dooley SL, Metzger BE. Care of the pregnant woman with insulin-dependent diabetes mellitus. *New England Journal of Medicine.* 1985;313:96-101.

Fuhrmann K, Reiher H. Semmler K, Fischer F. Fischer M, Glockner E. Prevention of congenital malformations in infants of insulin-dependent diabetic mothers. *Diabetes Care.* 1983;6:219-223.

Gabbe SG. Management of diabetes mellitus in pregnancy. *American Journal of Obstetrics and Gynecology.* 1985;153:824-828.

Greene MF, Hare JW, Cloherty JP, et al. First-trimester hemoglobin A_1 and risk for major malformation and spontaneous abortion in diabetic pregnancy. *Teratology.* 1989;39:225-231.

Landon MB, Gabbe SG. Glucose monitoring and insulin administration in the pregnant diabetic patient. *Clinical Obstetrics and Gynecology.* 1985;28:496-506.

Menon, R. K., Cohen, R. M., Sperling, M. A., et al., Transplacental passage of insulin in pregnant women with insulin-dependent diabetes mellitus: Its role in fetal macrosomia. *New England Journal of Medicine* 323:309-315, 1990.

Mills JL, Knopp RH, Simpson JL, et al. Lack of relation of increased malformation rates in infants of diabetic mothers to glycemic control during organogenesis. *New England Journal of Medicine.* 1988;318:671-676.

Mills JL, Simpson JL, Driscoll SG, et al. Incidence of spontaneous abortion among normal women and insulin-dependent diabetic women whose pregnancies were identified within 21 days of conception. *New England Journal of Medicine.* 1988;319:1617-1623.

Miodovnik, M., Mimouni, F., Siddiqi, T. A., et al., Spontaneous abortions in repeat diabetic pregnancies: A relationship with glycemic control. *Obstetrics and Gynecology* 75:75-78, 1990.

Miodovnik, M., Mimouni, F., Dignan, P. S. J., et al., Major malformations in infants of IDDM women. Vasculopathy and early first-trimester poor glycemic control. *Diabetes Care* 11:713-718, 1988.

Miodovnik, M., Mimouni, F., Tsang, R. C., et al., Glycemic control and spontaneous abortion in insulin dependent diabetic women. *Obstetrics and Gynecology* 68:366-369, 1986.

Miodovnik, M., Lavin, J. P., Knowles, H. C., et al., Spontaneous abortion among insulin-dependent diabetic women. *American Journal of Obstetrics and Gynecology* 150:372-376, 1984.

Mimouni, F., Miodovnik, M., Tsang, R. C., et al., Decreased maternal serum magnesium concentration and adverse fetal outcome in insulin-dependent diabetic women. *Obstetrics and Gynecology* 70:85-88, 1987.

Schwartz R. The infant of the diabetic mother. In: Davidson JK, ed. *Clinical Diabetes Mellitus.* New York: Thieme, 1986.

Steel JM. Prepregnancy counseling and contraception in the insulin-dependent diabetic patient. *Clinical Obstetrics and Gynecology.* 1985;28:553-566.

Chapter 24

Pre-Gestational Hypertension

The prevalence of chronic hypertension in pregnancy (that is, in those hypertensive women who become pregnant) is not known. It differs widely in different geographic areas, but is probably present in 1 to 5 percent of all pregnancies.

Women with essential hypertension often experience reductions in blood pressure during the first two trimesters; failure for this to occur is an unfavorable prognostic sign.

Definition of Chronic Hypertension

Chronic hypertension is defined as hypertension that is present and observable prior to pregnancy, or that is diagnosed before the 20th week of gestation. Hypertension is defined as a blood pressure equal to or greater than 140/90 mm Hg. Hypertension that is diagnosed for the first time during pregnancy and that persists beyond the 42nd day postpartum is also classified as chronic hypertension.

Management of Preexisting Chronic Hypertension in Pregnancy

Counseling

Hypertensive women considering pregnancy should be counseled prior to conception. They should be informed of the high likelihood of

---

Excerpts from NIH Publication No. 91-3029, 1991

a favorable outcome in most cases of mild to moderate essential hypertension. They should be aware of the increased risk of superimposed preeclampsia and of the possible complications if preexisting renal disease or systemic illness is present.

It is helpful to inform women prior to pregnancy of possible adjustments in lifestyle that may be necessary during pregnancy if the blood pressure is elevated—specifically, the possibility that restricted activity, bed rest, or even hospitalization may be advisable.

Patients with intrinsic renal disease who are normotensive and have minimal renal dysfunction usually do well in pregnancy. However, those with azotemia (creatinine >2 mg/dL or some say 1.5 mg/dL) and hypertension should be advised of a number of risks. These include a high incidence of superimposed preeclampsia, increased perinatal morbidity and mortality, and the possibility that maternal renal function may deteriorate further as a result of the pregnancy. These concerns are especially applicable to women with renal transplants, in whom pregnancy should be undertaken only after consultation with a nephrologist with expertise in this area.

Nonpharmacologic Treatment of Chronic Hypertension

Close medical supervision is the mainstay of management of pregnant women with chronic hypertension. It is preferable to control the blood pressure without medication when possible. In patients with diastolic blood pressure from 90 to 99 mm Hg, this goal is not difficult to attain, since blood pressure falls in most pregnant women during the first and second trimesters.

The strategies for nonpharmacologic therapy of hypertension during pregnancy differ from those in nonpregnant individuals. Whereas weight reduction and exercise might benefit a nonpregnant individual, these measures are not encouraged during pregnancy. Although there are no studies that address the issue of exercise in hypertensive pregnancy, given the theoretical concerns regarding the role of the uteroplacental blood flow in the pathogenesis of preeclampsia, women with chronic hypertension should not be encouraged to participate in vigorous exercise.

Restriction of Activity. Bed rest is a good means of maximizing uteroplacental blood flow during pregnancy and is considered established therapy in preeclampsia. In chronic hypertension, its effectiveness has not been well studied, but it is an integral feature of management. Rest has been shown to reduce premature labor, lower

Pre-Gestational Hypertension

blood pressure, and promote diuresis. Strict bed rest is rarely necessary. However, all pregnant women with elevated blood pressure, whatever the cause, should be advised to limit their activities when possible, and set aside time during the day when they can be "off their feet."

Although many women may find it difficult to restrict their activity, it is helpful to explain the benefits to the patient prior to pregnancy so she can make adjustments in child care, her job, and other responsibilities. In patients with mild to moderate hypertension, restriction of activity may be effective in lowering blood pressure, and antihypertensive medications may be avoided. In patients with severe hypertension, it is usually advisable to hospitalize them for bed rest and medication when necessary.

Diet. Weight reduction may be helpful in reducing blood pressure in nonpregnant individuals, but it cannot be recommended during pregnancy. If a hypertensive woman is overweight and planning a pregnancy, then weight reduction prior to pregnancy is advisable.

Hypertensive pregnant women have lower plasma volume than normotensives, and some studies suggest that the severity of hypertension correlates with the degree of plasma volume contraction. For this reason, sodium restriction is generally not recommended during pregnancy. If, however, a pregnant women with chronic hypertension is known to have salt-sensitive hypertension and she has been successfully treated with a low-salt diet prior to pregnancy, then it is reasonable to continue some sodium restriction during pregnancy. Patients with renal disease and reduced creatinine clearances are more likely to require sodium restriction for blood pressure control, and this should be continued during pregnancy. The amounts of weight gained during the pregnancy may be an indication of whether salt intake is appropriate.

Preliminary studies have shown that dietary calcium supplementation lowers blood pressure in pregnant and nonpregnant individuals. However, there are insufficient data to recommend its use for hypertension treatment.

Home Blood Pressure Monitoring. The rationale for close observation of the pregnant hypertensive woman is that changes in clinical status (such as development of superimposed preeclampsia) can be recognized before they become severe. This is easier to accomplish if patients are instructed to take their blood pressures at home and keep a record of the readings. They can then contact medical personnel if the blood pressure rises significantly before a scheduled visit.

Home monitoring of blood pressure is often helpful since it will enable the patient to determine how much limitation of activity is necessary to keep her blood pressure controlled. This technique also helps discriminate truly elevated blood pressure from labile blood pressure increases common in young patients. Patients who are candidates for home blood pressure monitoring should have formal instruction on the correct technique for blood pressure determination. In addition, their equipment should be periodically checked for accuracy. Preliminary data on home blood pressure monitoring during pregnancy suggest that it is a useful adjunct to the care of the pregnant woman.

Alcohol and Tobacco. The use of alcohol and tobacco during pregnancy should be discouraged strongly. Both have a deleterious effect on the fetus and mother. Excessive consumption of alcohol can aggravate hypertension or raise blood pressure in the mother de novo.

Rationale for Pharmacologic Treatment

The majority of women with chronic hypertension in pregnancy have mild to moderate elevations in blood pressure, and therefore the risk of acute cardiovascular complications is extremely low. In the small percentage of women who have severe hypertension, the increased risk of cerebral hemorrhage, cardiac failure, and myocardial infarction necessitates close monitoring and aggressive treatment during pregnancy.

Although there is increased perinatal morbidity and mortality when the mother has chronic hypertension, most pregnancies in these women result in healthy, full-term infants. Women with chronic hypertension are at increased risk of developing superimposed preeclampsia, and there is evidence that most, if not all, of the increased perinatal morbidity and mortality associated with chronic hypertension is attributable to this complication. The literature is conflicting, however. Some studies have shown that babies born to women with chronic hypertension in pregnancy who do not develop superimposed preeclampsia do as well as those born to normotensive women. Other studies report a higher perinatal loss in uncomplicated hypertensive pregnancy (compared with normotensive), especially with higher levels of blood pressure.

The objective in treating a pregnant woman with chronic hypertension is to minimize the short-term risks to the mother of elevated blood pressure while avoiding therapeutic maneuvers that compromise fetal well-being. The specific goals for the mother are to prevent

Pre-Gestational Hypertension

cardiovascular complications of severe hypertension and, if possible, to prevent preeclampsia. When maternal blood pressure reaches diastolic levels of equal to or greater than 100 mm Hg, treatment should be instituted to avoid hypertensive vascular damage. Some experts feel at least nonpharmacologic treatment is warranted at diastolic blood pressures of equal to or greater than 90 mm Hg.

The indications for treatment of hypertension (at diastolic blood pressures of 90-99 mm Hg) during pregnancy are less clear. In the nonpregnant individual, treatment of mild to moderate hypertension is recommended for prevention of long-term cardiovascular consequences of elevated blood pressure.

To date, clinical trials and clinical experience have not given us a conclusive answer to the question, "Does treatment of chronic hypertension prevent preeclampsia?" Many of the clinical trials of antihypertensive therapy in chronic hypertension have evaluated treatment begun in the third trimester. This is largely a consequence of the fact that blood pressure falls in most women during the first trimester, reaching its nadir by midpregnancy. This phenomenon occurs in chronic hypertensives as well, and since most patients have only mild hypertension to begin with, by midpregnancy the majority will be normotensive. Therefore, it is frequently not until the third trimester, when the blood pressure rises, that treatment is begun. If superimposed preeclampsia in the chronic hypertensive is associated with the same placental pathology as in pure preeclampsia, then the definitive morphological changes are already present by 20 weeks. Thus, one would not expect antihypertensives begun in the third trimester to alter these changes. To complicate matters, patients enrolled in clinical trials that have started treatment in the third trimester are frequently a heterogeneous population—and include patients with transient hypertension, preeclampsia, and chronic hypertension.

There are almost no data available that would either support or dispute the notion that early treatment of chronic hypertension (in the first half of pregnancy) prevents superimposed preeclampsia. Carefully conducted clinical trials are needed to resolve this issue.

It is not uncommon for a pregnant woman with chronic hypertension to be hospitalized because of elevated blood pressure. Early treatment of hypertension in pregnancy may reduce the need for such hospitalization, but it may obscure the diagnosis of superimposed preeclampsia, since a rise in blood pressure may be the first sign of this condition. It is particularly important to monitor women being treated for hypertension during pregnancy for signs of preeclampsia since this condition is associated with adverse fetal outcome.

Fetal Well-Being. With regard to fetal well-being, several studies suggest, but do not conclusively demonstrate, benefits of treating mild to moderate hypertension during pregnancy. In the largest published clinical trial demonstrating a reduction in perinatal mortality in mothers treated with methyldopa, the major intake of patients was during the second trimester, with a significant proportion entering earlier in the first half of pregnancy. Since the beneficial outcome was due to a decrease in midtrimester pregnancy losses, it is not clear whether lowering blood pressure was responsible for the improved outcome. Given the potential hazards of antihypertensive treatment during pregnancy (the possibility that medication may reduce placental blood flow, or adversely affect the fetus) treatment of hypertension (at diastolic levels of 90-99 mm Hg) must be undertaken cautiously, weighing the risks and benefits of treatment for both mother and child at all times. Excessive blood pressure reduction is to be avoided, and a conservative approach is recommended.

Drug Treatment of Chronic Preexisting Hypertension

The goal of treating chronic hypertension during pregnancy is the reduction of maternal risk and perhaps that of the fetus. With this goal in mind it is mandatory to establish not only the efficacy of drugs to reduce blood pressure but also the acute and long-range effects of these drugs on fetal well-being, especially (based on the mechanism of action of many antihypertensive drugs) long-range neurological effects. So far only one drug—methyldopa—meets these criteria. Thus, if feasible, methyldopa therapy should be chosen in pregnancy. If this drug is ineffective or cannot be tolerated (which happens not infrequently), alternative therapy is determined by guidelines based on limited clinical experience and rational choices based on the mechanisms by which the drugs act. It is important to point out that, in spite of theoretical concerns, none of the drugs currently used to treat hypertension other than the angiotensin converting enzyme (ACE) inhibitors have been demonstrated to increase perinatal morbidity or mortality within the limits of acute followup. The following categories of antihypertensive agents are addressed alphabetically.

Angiotensin Converting Enzyme Inhibitors. This new class of antihypertensive agents, which act in part by inhibiting conversion of angiotensin I to angiotensin II, has become popular in the treatment of essential hypertension and hypertension associated with renal disease in nonpregnant patients because of its minimal side effects. Although no teratogenic effects have been observed in animals with these drugs, they do lower uterine blood flow and reduce fetal survival in pregnant rabbits and sheep, perhaps by decreasing uterine PGE2 and PGI2 synthesis. Acute renal failure with lethal consequences has also been described in the neonates of women treated with ACE inhibitors in the last trimester. Because other antihypertensive agents are available, it is recommended that ACE inhibitors should be avoided during pregnancy.

Beta-Adrenergic Blocking Agents. Evidence is accumulating that beta-adrenergic blocking drugs are useful and sufficiently safe in treating preexisting hypertension during pregnancy. There is also evidence that the combined alpha- and beta-blocking agent labetalol (alpha and beta antagonism ratio 1:4) is relatively safe and effective in pregnancy. Most studies to date demonstrate equal effectiveness when beta adrenoreceptor antagonists and the combined alpha- and beta-blocker labetalol are compared to methyldopa.

Finally, despite a growing and reassuring literature of controlled trials with beta and combined beta and alpha adrenoreceptor agents, we must interject a note of caution. Most studies were relatively small and gestational age at entry was usually 29 to 33 weeks, leaving unanswered the possibility that treatment of larger numbers of patients and/or a longer duration of drug administration may reveal adverse effects. For instance, Butters et al. suggest that the long-term use of beta-blockers predisposes to major growth retardation. Finally, while some prefer beta-adrenergic blockers because they cause less somnolence than methyldopa, others continue to favor the alpha2 agonists because of concern that beta-blocking agents, which cross the placenta, may interfere with interpretation of fetal heart rate, as well as the theoretical possibility that beta-blockers compromise the ability of the fetus to withstand hypoxic stress.

Calcium Channel Blockers. Calcium channel blockers have been used to treat essential hypertension for many years in Europe and recently have been introduced into the United States. Nifedipine, which has a greater effect on vascular smooth muscle than on the myocardium, has proven promising in treating hypertension. However, it is teratogenic in rats when given in doses 30 times the maximum recommended human dose. There are very few studies of its use throughout human pregnancy, although these drugs are used in later pregnancy as treatment for preterm labor without adverse consequences.

Centrally Acting Alpha-Adrenergic Inhibitors. Methyldopa and clonidine are the two most commonly used central adrenergic antagonists and both are used during pregnancy. Clonidine is a centrally acting adrenergic inhibitor that inhibits sympathetic output from the central nervous system. The effect of methyldopa is more complex, but it also inhibits central sympathetic discharge. Methyldopa was the first antihypertensive agent used in the treatment of hypertension during pregnancy, so the experience with it is the longest. Followup studies of children born to mothers taking methyldopa throughout pregnancy have revealed normal mental and physical development in these children at 10 years of age. Methyldopa given to women with essential hypertension has been demonstrated to reduce the number of midtrimester abortions without affecting neonatal survival or fetal growth.

Methyldopa causes somnolence in many individuals. However, its demonstrated safety for the fetus in long-term followup makes this the initial drug of choice in the management of chronic hypertension in pregnant women and the benchmark against which other antihypertensive agents must be tested.

Diuretics. The use of diuretic agents in pregnancy is controversial. The primary concern is theoretical. It is known that preeclampsia is associated with a reduction of plasma volume and that fetal outcome is worse in chronically hypertensive women who fail to expand plasma volume. Whether this is a cause-and-effect relationship is not clearly established. Nonetheless, women using diuretics from early pregnancy do not increase their blood volume to the degree usually occurring in normal pregnancy. This theoretical concern must be tempered by extensive experience in several well-controlled studies with the prophylactic use of diuretics in normotensive gravidas in which no excess of perinatal mortality or morbidity was evident. A meta-analysis of nine randomized trials comprising over 7,000 subjects revealed a decrease in the tendency of these women to develop edema and/or hypertension and confirmed no increased incidence of adverse fetal effects. Based on the theoretical concerns, diuretics are usually not used as first-line drugs. However, if their use is indicated, they are safe and efficacious agents, can markedly potentiate the response to other antihypertensive agents, and are not contraindicated in pregnancy except in settings where uteroplacental perfusion is already reduced (preeclampsia and intrauterine growth retardation).

Although data concerning the use of diuretics in pregnant women with essential hypertension are sparse, this committee concluded that gestation does not preclude use of saluretic drugs to reduce or control blood pressure in women whose hypertension predated conception or manifested prior to midpregnancy.

Vasodilators. Hydralazine is a vasodilator that is relatively ineffective when used alone because of the reflex tachycardia with increased cardiac output that occurs with its use. However, when hydralazine is combined with a beta-adrenergic blocking agent, the reflex tachycardia is prevented, and the combination is quite effective in reducing blood pressure. Hydralazine is used extensively, usually with methyldopa, in treating preexisting hypertension in pregnancy and is considered to be safe for mother and fetus by most obstetricians. Still, one survey in Scandinavia has reported fetal thrombocytopenia. Therefore, its use as a first-line drug in treating pregnant women with chronic preexisting hypertension should be limited.

Summary

Although this working group endorses judicious antihypertensive therapy for pregnant women with preexisting essential (chronic) hypertension (diastolic blood pressures of equal to or greater than 90 mm Hg), there is no good existing evidence that the use of antihypertensive therapy improves fetal survival. Methyldopa may prevent mid-gestational losses.

Certain Hypertension Drugs Dangerous for Pregnant Women

Pregnant women who take angiotensin-converting enzyme (ACE) inhibitors, drugs used to treat high blood pressure, should consult their doctors about switching treatment. Using the drugs past the first three months of pregnancy could result in significant harm and even death to the fetus.

At FDA's request, the six U.S. companies that manufacture the drugs sent a letter in March to doctors emphasizing the risks when women in the second and third trimesters of pregnancy take ACE inhibitors. In addition, FDA announced that all ACE inhibitors would be required to carry a boxed warning on the label.

The companies that manufacture ACE inhibitors are Bristol-Myers Squibb (Capoten, Capozide, Monopril), Ciba-Geigy (Lotensin), Hoechst-Roussel Pharmaceuticals (Altace), ICI Pharmaceuticals Group (Zestril, Zestoretic), Merck-Sharp & Dohme (Vasotec, Vasotec I.V., Vaseretic, Prinivil, Prinzide), and Parke-Davis (Accupril).

FDA's actions were prompted by continuing reports of fetal damage, including kidney failure and face or skull deformities, caused by these hypertension drugs. Although labeling for the products has for several years warned of the risks, more than 50 cases of fetal harm have been reported over the past several years.

In addition, very limited epidemiological evidence from Tennessee and Michigan Medicaid data bases indicates that fetal injury from exposure to ACE inhibitors in the second and third trimesters may be as high as 10 to 20 percent. FDA Commissioner David A. Kessler, M.D., noted, "The additional warnings will allow the safe use of ACE inhibitors by women who need them while helping to assure that women who become pregnant while taking these drugs promptly seek alternative treatment."

Pharmacists are being asked to counsel women of childbearing age who are taking ACE inhibitors about the risks and are being provided with warning stickers to place directly on the prescription bottles. Women taking ACE inhibitors who become pregnant should continue to take the medication because uncontrolled hypertension is dangerous to both mother and fetus, but they should consult their doctors immediately. There appears to be no risk to fetuses when the drugs are taken during the first trimester.

Recommended Laboratory Tests

Most women presenting with hypertension prior to gestation week 20 have (or will develop) essential hypertension. Some of these patients will be under the care of primary physicians and will have been screened for signs of secondary hypertension. Pregnant women with preexisting or early gestational hypertension are among the population where secondary hypertension is more apt to be found, e.g., renal disease, renovascular hypertension, primary aldosteronism, Cushing's syndrome, and pheochromocytoma. Thus, further evaluation is warranted even for minimal suspicion. For example, pheochromocytoma, although rare, has a propensity to manifest or be activated by pregnancy, and it is associated with high maternal mortality when undiagnosed. Thus, suspicion warrants performance of a screening test to detect pheochromocytoma—for example, 24-hour excretion rate of vanillylmandelic acid (VMA) or metanephrines, or plasma norepinephrine and epinephrine levels.

Baseline determinations of renal function (serum creatinine, uric acid) and platelet count can be compared with values in later pregnancy to help determine if blood pressure increases at this time are the usual physiological increase in blood pressure or the onset of preeclampsia. Since these fetuses are at high risk for the development of intrauterine growth retardation, baseline sonography for dating and fetal size are indicated prior to 20 weeks gestation.

References

Chesley LC: Hypertensive Disorders In Pregnancy. New York: Appleton-Century-Crofts, 1978.

The 1988 Joint National Committee: The 1988 Report of the Joint Committee on Detection, Evaluation, and Treatment of High Blood Pressure. Arch Intern Med 1988;148: 1023-1038.

Ellison GT, Mansberger JA, Mansberger AR Jr.: Malignant recurrent pheochromocytoma during pregnancy: case report and review of the literature. Surgery 1988;103: 484-489.

Schenker JG, Chowers I: Pheochromocytoma and pregnancy. Review of 89 cases. Obstet Gynecol Surv 1971;26: 739-747.

Packham DK, Fairley KF, Ihle BU, Whitworth JA, Kincaid-Smith P: Comparison of pregnancy outcome between normotensive and hypertensive women with primary glomerulonephritis. Clin Exp Hypertens 1987-1988;B6: 387-399.

Hou SH, Grossman SD, Madias NE: Pregnancy in women with renal disease and moderate renal insufficiency. Am J Med 1985;78: 185-194.

Lindheimer MD, Katz AI: Gestation in women with kidney disease: prognosis and management. Clin Obstet Gynaecol (Bailliére) 1987;1: 921-937.

Papiernik E, Kaminski M: Multifactorial study of the risk of prematurity at 32 weeks of gestation. 1. A study of the frequency of 30 predictive characteristics. J Perinat Med 1974;2: 30-36.

Gallery ED, Hunyor SN, Gyory AZ: Plasma volume contraction: A significant factor in both pregnancy-associated hypertension (pre-eclampsia) and chronic hypertension in pregnancy. Q J Med 1979;48: 593-602.

Palomaki JF, Lindheimer MD: Sodium depletion simulating deterioration in a toxemic pregnancy. N Engl J Med 1970;282: 88-89.

Kawasaki N, Matsui K, Ito M, et al: Effect of calcium supplementation on the vascular sensitivity to angiotensin II in pregnant women. Am J Obstet Gynecol 1985;153: 576-582.

Villar J, Repke J, Belizan JM, Pareja G: Calcium supplementation reduces blood pressure during pregnancy: results of a randomized controlled clinical trial. Obstet Gynecol 1987;70: 317-322.

Rayburn WF, Zuspan FP, Piehl EJ: Self-monitoring of blood pressure during pregnancy. Am J Obstet Gynecol 1984;148: 159-162.

Page EW, Christianson R: The impact of mean arterial blood pressure in the middle trimester upon the outcome of pregnancy. Am J Obstet Gynecol 1976;125: 740-745.

Friedman EA, Neff RK: Pregnancy Hypertension: A Systematic Evaluation of Clinical Diagnostic Criteria. Littleton, MA: PSG Publishing Co., 1977.

Dunlop JCH: Chronic hypertension and perinatal mortality. Proc R Soc Med 1966;59: 838-841.

Leather HM, Humphreys DM, Baker P, Chadd MA: A controlled trial of hypotensive agents in hypertension in pregnancy. Lancet 1968;2: 488-490.

Rubin PC, Butters L, Clark DM, et al: Placebo controlled trial of atenolol in treatment of pregnancy-associated hypertension. Lancet 1983;1: 431-434.

Landesman R, McLarn WD, Ollstein RN, Mendelsohn B: Reserpine in toxemia of pregnancy. Obstet Gynecol 1957;9: 377-383.

Fletcher AE, Bulpitt CJ: A review of clinical trials in pregnancy. In: Rubin PC (ed), Hypertension in Pregnancy. New York: Elsevier, 1988, pp 186-201.

Redman CW, Beilin LJ, Bonnar J, Ounsted MK: Fetal outcome in trial of antihypertensive treatment in pregnancy. Lancet 1976;2: 753-756.

Ferris TF, Weir EK: Effect of captopril on uterine blood flow and prostaglandin E synthesis in the pregnant rabbit. J Clin Invest 1983;71: 809-815.

Schubiger G, Flury G, Nussberger J: Enalapril for pregnancy-induced hypertension: acute renal failure in a neonate. Ann Intern Med 1988;108: 215-216. Published erratum appears in Ann Int Med 1988;108: 777.

Rosa FW, Bosco LA, Graham CF, Milstien JB, Dreis M, Creamer J: Neonatal anuria with maternal angiotensin-converting enzyme inhibition. Obstet Gynecol 1989;74: 371-374.

Scott AA, Purohit DM: Neonatal renal failure: a complication of maternal antihypertensive therapy. Am J Obstet Gynecol 1989;160: 1223-1224.

Knott PD, Thorpe SS, Lamont CAR: Congenital renal dysgenesis possibly due to captopril. Lancet 1989;1: 451.

Barron WM, Murphy MD, Lindheimer MD: Management of hypertension during pregnancy. In: Laragh JH and Brenner BM (eds), Hypertension, Diagnosis and Management. New York: Raven Press, 1990, pp 1809-1827.

Redman CW: A controlled trial of the treatment of hypertension in pregnancy: labetalol compared with methyldopa, In Riley A, Symonds EM (eds), Investigation of Labetalol in the Management of Hypertension in Pregnancy, International Congress Series 591. Amsterdam, Excerpta Medica, 1982, pp 101-110.

Sibai BM, Gonzalez AR, Mabie WC, Moretti M: A comparison of labetalol plus hospitalization versus hospitalization alone in the management of preeclampsia remote from term. Obstet Gynecol 1987;70: 323-327.

Sibai BM, Mabie WC, Villar M, Shamsa F, Anderson GD: A comparison of no medication vs. methyldopa or labetalol in chronic hypertension during pregnancy. Am J Obstet Gynecol 1990;162: 960-966.

Butters L, Kennedy S, Rubin P: Atenolol and fetal weight in chronic hypertension. Abstract. Clin Exp Hypertens 1989;B8: 468.

Constantine G, Beevers DG, Reynolds AL, Luesley DM: Nifedipine as a second line antihypertensive drug in pregnancy. Br J Obstet Gynaecol 1987;94: 1136-1142.

Ulmsten U: Treatment of normotensive and hypertensive patients with preterm labor using oral nifedipine, a calcium antagonist. Arch Gynecol 1984;236: 69-72.

Fidler J, Smith V, Fayers P, DeSwiet M: Randomized controlled comparative study of methyldopa and oxprenolol in treatment of hypertension in pregnancy. Br Med J 1983;286: 1927-1930.

Kincaid-Smith P, Bullen M, Mills J: Prolonged use of methyldopa in severe hypertension in pregnancy. Br Med J 1966;1: 274-276.

Redman CW: Treatment of hypertension in pregnancy. Kidney Int 1980;18: 267-278.

Ounsted M, Cockburn J, Moar VA, Redman CW: Maternal hypertension with superimposed pre-eclampsia: effects on child development at 7-1/2 years. Br J Obstet Gynaecol 1983;90: 644-649.

Hays PM, Cruikshank DP, Dunn LJ: Plasma volume determination in normal and pre-eclamptic pregnancies. Am J Obstet Gynecol 1985;151: 958-966.

Arias F, Zamora J: Antihypertensive treatment and pregnancy outcome in patients with mild chronic hypertension. Obstet Gynecol 1979;53: 489.

Sibai BM, Grossman RA, Grossman HG: Effects of diuretics on plasma volume in pregnancies with long-term hypertension. Am J Obstet Gynecol 1984;150: 831-835.

Kraus GW, Marchese JR, Yen SSC: Prophylactic use of hydrochlorothiazide in pregnancy. JAMA 1966;198: 1150-1154.

Collins R, Yusuf S, Peto R: Overview of randomised trials of diuretics in pregnancy. Br Med J 1985;290: 17-23.

Widerlov E, Karlman I, and Storsater J. Hydralazine-induced neonatal thrombocytopenia. Letter. New Engl J Med 1980;301: 1235.

Chapter 25

Multiple Pregnancy

Chapter Contents

Section 25.1—Twins or More 466
Section 25.2—Rates of Twin Births 481

Section 25.1

Twins or More

Reprinted by Permission of Matria Healthcare, copyright 1991.

Twin pregnancies occur more often than you might expect. In fact, 2% of pregnancies produce twins. You might be surprised to learn that approximately one in every 1,500 births are triplets, quadruplets or more.

Sometimes a "twins or more.." pregnancy is referred to as a "multiple gestation", "multiple pregnancy" or "multiple birth". This simply means more than one baby is born to a mother. These babies may be identical or fraternal.

What is the difference between identical and fraternal twins?

Identical twins are just that. Identical copies of each other. Identical twins occur when one fertilized egg divides into two embryos, and then grows and develops into a separate baby. Identical twins are always of the same sex and genetic makeup. They will share the same placenta, and they may share the same amniotic sac, but they will grow individually. Identical twins account for approximately one-third of multiple births.

Fraternal twins develop when two different eggs are released from the ovary or ovaries and become fertilized separately by different sperm. Fraternal twins can be either the same sex or opposite sex. they have different genetic make-ups, and are no more alike than other brothers and sisters.

If a women is carrying triplets or more, the babies can be any combination of identical and fraternal.

Why do multiple gestations occur?

Identical twins are just a twist of fate... a chance cell division. Fraternal twins, on the other hand, are more likely to occur to women who:

Multiple Pregnancy

- Have twins in their families
- Have taken fertility drugs or had in vitro fertilization
- Belong to certain ethnic groups. (For example, Blacks have a 20% higher rate of twins and a 75% higher incidence of triplets than Caucasians).
- Are over age 35; or
- Become pregnant soon after discontinuing use of birth control pills.

What kind of care and treatments should I receive during my pregnancy?

As with any pregnancy, getting the proper prenatal care is the key to promoting the health of both you and your babies. Be sure to keep all of your scheduled office appointments as recommended by your obstetrician. Your doctor will want to check frequently on the growth and development of your babies. Also, remember to check with your doctor before taking any medicine, even a "home remedy".

At each office visit your blood pressure, weight and a urine specimen will be checked. The doctor or nurse will also listen to the babies' heartbeats. Later, starting at about 4 months gestation, the height of your uterus will be measured to help indicate the babies growth. There are other special tests that your physician may order periodically, such as:

1. Ultrasound: an ultrasound uses sound waves to show a "picture" of the baby. this test can show the babies' positions and help estimate their sizes, weights and gestational age.

2. Glucose Challenge Test and Glucose Tolerance Test: Glucose challenge and glucose tolerance tests let the obstetrician know if diabetes or high blood sugar is a problem during this pregnancy. These tests are frequently performed during the 6th month of pregnancy or at about 24-28 weeks of gestation. Usually a Glucose Challenge Test (GCT) is done first. A Glucose Tolerance Test (GTT) is then performed only if necessary.

3. Non-Stress Test: This test, also known as an NST, may be done during the third trimester of your pregnancy to monitor

the babies' heart rates. This test helps your doctor to determine if the babies are responding normally to their special environment. It is considered a measure of fetal well-being.

What can I do to reduce physical stress and strain?

- Good posture helps reduce back strain.

- Try to avoid making sudden or "jerky" movements which will add stress to your abdomen and back.

- Lower yourself by squatting instead of bending over from the waist.

- Use a pillow to support you lower back while sitting.

- Elevate your feet to increase circulation and help reduce minor swelling of your ankles.

- Avoid lifting or pushing heavy objects. Do not lift more than 35 pounds at a time. Young children should be encouraged to climb up on your lap. Try not to carry them around unnecessarily.

- Use your arms and legs to help push you back up on feet from a sitting position.

- Blood circulation to your babies is best if you rest or sleep lying on your side. When lying down, you may find it more comfortable to bend your knees slightly and place a pillow between them. To raise up, use your arms to push yourself upward before standing up. Sit on the side of the bed with your feet dangling to be sure you have your balance.

- Use additional pillows to help support your abdomen, buttocks and shoulders.

- It is very important for you to take care of yourself. Whenever you feel the need to rest, do so. Enlist the help of your husband, children or friends whenever possible.

What can I do to nourish my babies?

Good nutrition combined with adequate weight gain during your pregnancy can help keep you healthy. and give your babies the best start in life. You will need increased amounts of many nutrients, especially iron,

Multiple Pregnancy

calcium, zinc, protein, folic acid and vitamin B6. By making careful food choices and taking a multivitamin mineral pill you can meet your needs and your babies' needs. A daily food guide will help you choose the right foods. Request an appointment with a registered dietitian (RD) to work out the details to fit our personal needs.

What kinds of food and how much do I need to eat?

The daily food guide will help you to select foods wisely. Select at least the minimum number of servings from each group on a daily basis. If you are unable to drink milk then try to choose cheese instead. If you have difficulty digesting meats, try to ear more dry beans, nuts or sunflower seeds. Very often it may be easier to digest meats if eaten in stews or soups.

In addition to your food intake, you will need to increase the amount of fluids you consume. Try fluids which provide some nutrition, such as milk, fruit juices and hearty soups. You may drink fruit juices diluted with water. If you are gaining weight too slowly add more milk products to your snacks, and eat more than the minimum number of servings.

Daily Food Guide

Food Group—Protein Rich Foods
Provide protein, iron, zinc, and B-vitamins for growth of muscles, bone, blood, and nerves. Vegetable protein provides fiber to prevent constipation.

Example Foods—One Serving Equals
1 egg, cooked
1 oz. chicken, turkey, lamb, ham, lean beef
1 oz. fish
2 oz. shellfish
2 oz. tuna fish
7 medium oysters
3 medium clams
3 medium sardines
1/4 cup cottage cheese
1/2 cup cooked, dry beans, lentils or split peas
3 oz. tofu
1/2 cup baked beans
2 tablespoons peanut butter

1 oz. or 1/3 cup peanuts
1 1/2 oz. or 1/3 cup other nuts
1/2 cup hummus
1 oz. seeds, sunflower

Minimum Number of Servings Needed Daily
Twins—9
Triplets—11
Quads—12

Food Group—Milk Products
Provide protein and calcium to build strong bones, teeth, healthy nerves and muscles and to promote normal blood clotting.

Example Foods—One Serving Equals
8 oz. fluid milk, 1% or 2%
8 oz. yogurt, plain
8 oz. milkshake
1 1/2 oz. hard cheese: cheddar, Swiss, Jack, Mozarella
4 tablespoons parmesan cheese
1 1/2 cups frozen yogurt
1 cup pudding or custard 1 1/2 cups ice cream

Minimum Number of Servings Needed Daily
Twins—4
Triplets—5
Quads—6

Food Group—Grains and Cereals
Provide carbohydrates and B-vitamins for energy and healthy nerves. Also provide iron for healthy blood. Whole grains provide fiber to prevent constipation.

Example Foods—One Serving Equals
1 slice whole grain, enriched bread
1/2 bagel, bun, roll or pita
1/2 English muffin
1 small tortilla, corn or flour
3/4 cup cold cereal
1/2 cup granola or hot cereal
1/2 cup oatmeal, cooked
6-8 medium crackers
4 graham cracker squares

Multiple Pregnancy

4 tablespoons wheat germ
3 cups popcorn, 1/2 cup cooked noodles, rice or pasta
1 small muffin, 1 4-inch pancake or waffle

Minimum Number of Servings Needed Daily
Twins—8
Triplets—9
Quads—10
*Select whole grain sources whenever possible.

Food Group—Vitamin C Rich Foods
Provide vitamin C to prevent infection and to promote wound healing and iron absorption. Also provide fiber to prevent constipation.

Example Foods—One Serving Equals
6 oz. juice: orange, grapefruit, tomato, vegetable cocktail
1/2 cup strawberries
1/2 grapefruit
1/2 cantaloupe
1/2 cup papaya
1 medium mango
1 kiwi or guava
2 medium tangerines
1 medium orange
1/2 cup brocolli
1/2 cup tomato puree
1/2 cup sweet peppers
1/2 cup cauliflower
1/2 cup cooked cabbage
2 tomatoes

Minimum Number of Servings Needed Daily
Twins—2
Triplets—2
Quads—3

Food Group-Vitamin A Rich Foods
Provide beta-carotene and vitamin A to prevent infection and to promote wound healing and night vision. Also provide fiber to prevent constipation.

Example Foods—One Serving Equals
6 oz. juice: apricot nectar, vegetable juice cocktail

1/4 cup dried apricots
1/4 small mango
3 raw apricots
1/4 medium cantaloups
1/2 cup carrots
2 whole tomatoes
1/2 cup spinach, cooked
1/2 cup cooked Swiss chard, collards, kale
1/2 cup cooked yams
1/2 cup pumpkin, sweet potato, or winter squash

Minimum Number of Servings Needed Daily
Twins—1
Triplets—2
Quads—2

Food Group—Other Fruits and Vegetables
Provide carbohydrates for energy and fiber to prevent constipation.

Example Foods—One Serving Equals
6 oz. fruit juice: apple, pear, grape, cranberry
1 medium banana, peach
1/4 cup raisins
1/2 cup pineapple
1/2 cup berries, cherries
1/2 cup watermelon
1 cup lettuce
1/2 cup fresh mixed fruit
1/2 artichoke
1 medium plum, pear
1/2 cup chopped corn, potato, squash, peas, green beans, asparagus

Minimum Number of Servings Needed Daily
Twins—4
Triplets—5
Quads—6

Food Group—Unsaturated Fats
Provide vitamin E to protect tissue.

Example Foods—One Serving Equals
1/4 medium avocado
1 teaspoon margarine

Multiple Pregnancy

1 teaspoon mayonnaise
1 teaspoon vegetable oil
2 teaspoons salad dressing (mayo)
1 tablespoon salad dressing (oil)
5 large olives

Minimum Number of Servings Needed Daily
Twins—4
Triplets—5
Quads—6

How might my eating habits change?

The hormones of pregnancy can decrease your appetite and cause stomach upset. You may experience discomforts such as stomach fullness, nausea, heartburn and constipation. Some suggestions for prevention and remedies are discussed below.

It may be helpful to eat smaller amounts more often. For example, instead of eating 2 meals and 1 snack, you may find it easier to eat 3 medium-sized meals and 3 or 4 snacks during the day, evening or even in the middle of the night. Eating protein rich foods (cheese, cottage cheese, meats, yogurt) in the morning and at bedtime may help prevent dizziness, headache or nausea.

Suggestions to Relieve Discomforts

Nausea and Vomiting

Prevention.

- Eat several small meals
- Eat protein rich foods several times daily
- Drink fluids and liquids between meals
- Avoid greasy, acidic or strongly flavored foods
- Snack on dry, starchy foods such as crackers, cereals, rice, pasta, or potatoes.

Remedies.

- Replace fluids with chicken broth, tea or Gatorade
- Try popsicles, jello or carbonated drinks
- Check with your doctor about trying Vitamin B6.

Heartburn

Prevention.

- Eat several smaller meals
- Avoid stomach irritants such as coffee and cigarettes
- Avoid gas-producing foods (garlic, peppers, onions, cabbage)
- Avoid greasy or spicy food
- Sit up or walk after meals if possible

Remedies.

- Sip carbonated water
- Eat a spoonful of yogurt, heavy cream or milk
- Check with your doctor about which specific antacids would be safe

Constipation

Prevention

- Drink lots of fluids (50 oz./day)
- Eat high fiber foods: fruits, vegetables and grains (prunes, corn, oatmeal, berries, beans, bran, cereal, apples, peas and applesauce)

Remedies

- Drink hot liquids in the morning and before meals
- Check with your doctor about trying laxatives

What kinds of food should I avoid?

Avoid:

- Larger amounts of coffee or caffeinated beverages (limit to 1 or 2 cups per day).

- Alcoholic beverages

- Large amounts of cola beverages due to phosphates which decrease calcium absorption

- Raw fish, meats or poultry, and unpasteurized milk products

Multiple Pregnancy

How much weight will I need to gain?

The amount of weight you will need to gain depends on your weight and height before pregnancy. In general, women who begin pregnancy underweight should gain more, and women who begin pregnancy overweight may safely gain somewhat less. The amount of weight you gain depends on several factors, such as the type of food chosen, the amount of food, and the activity level. *The most important goal is to eat a very good quality diet by following the daily food guide.*

Here are some guidelines for weight gain during pregnancy:

Twins

- Overall range recommended is 35 to 45 lbs.
- Underweight mother may gain closer to 45 lbs.
- Overweight mother may gain closer to 35 lbs. or more

Triplets

- No recommended weight gain officially
- Expect to gain 50 to 55 lbs.

Quadruplets

- No recommended weight gain officially
- Expect 60 lbs or more

When should I gain the weight?

How you gain the weight is as important as how much you gain. Weight gain should be continuous throughout your pregnancy. It is important to avoid weight loss or poor weight gain in the last 6 months of pregnancy. Some studies found a link between slowed weight gain and preterm birth.

Twins

- Gain about 1 1/2 pounds each week during the last 6 months of pregnancy
- Avoid weight loss or low weight gain

Triplets

- Gain about 2 pounds each week during the last 6 months of pregnancy
- Avoid weight loss or low weight gain

Will I be able to carry my babies to full term?

Multiple pregnancies have a higher rate of preterm (premature) labor and delivery. You can help reduce your risk by receiving prenatal care, following the instructions of your health care professionals, eating a balanced diet, getting plenty of rest and promptly reporting any problems.

The following are common signs and symptoms of preterm labor. Some of these symptoms, such as backache, can occur as a normal part or pregnancy. However, if you notice a change in what feels normal for you, please notify your doctor or nurse.

1. Uterine contractions
2. Menstrual-like cramps
3. Low, dull backache
4. Pelvic or thigh pressure
5. Vaginal discharge
6. A general feeling that something is not right

Recognizing signs and symptoms of preterm labor can help you receive timely treatment for controlling contractions so the pregnancy can continue until the babies are fully developed and "mature".

Generally, the longer babies stay in their natural incubator, their mother, the better their chances are for a healthy start. Additional weeks, even days, help the development of the babies' lungs and hearts and assures their long term health. This is particularly important in multiple gestation pregnancies since there is greater potential for an early delivery. Remember, please call your doctor promptly if you are experiencing any of these symptoms.

What will happen if I should go into preterm labor?

Research has shown that women with multiple gestation pregnancies may experience increased contractions. These contractions could be signs of early labor and (if undetected) could lead to premature delivery.

Multiple Pregnancy

Having some uterine activity before 37 weeks of pregnancy is normal. However, if your contractions are occurring more than once every 15 minutes (4 or more per hour) you should call your doctor right away.

If you experience preterm labor, your obstetrician will prescribe the treatment that is best for you.

Just in case, you may want to pack your hospital bag during your sixth month. Include toiletries, night gown or pajamas, a robe, slippers and a magazine or book.

What can I do if I need help coping?

If you feel the need for emotional support, ask your doctor about the availability of a medical social worker or local support group. There is also a list of helpful organizations at the end of this text.

Support groups can be an invaluable resource for you. Most of the women in the support groups are mothers of multiples and have had experiences similar to those you are currently facing. They will be happy to help you talk through your specific concerns.

Points to Remember

Feeling comfortable and informed about yourself can reduce some of the stresses that you may experience during this pregnancy. Don't be afraid to call on family and friends for help, and take advantage of all offers of assistance. Your job is to help those babies receive a healthy start.

Be an active participant in your own care. Keep the lines of communication open between you and your obstetrician. Be aware of what is normal for your pregnancy and discuss any questions with your health care provider.

Eat well, take it easy, and enjoy!

Support Groups/Organizations and Other Resources Serving Multiples and Their Families

- **Sidelines National Support Network** is a non-profit foundation offering support and encouragement for women and their families experiencing a high-risk pregnancy. Phone support, national and local newsletters, educational literature, and practical suggestions for making bedrest more comfortable are available. Contact Candace Hurley, Executive Director, at (714) 497-2265.

- **The Triplet Connection** is a support service for expectant and new parents of higher multiples. They provide a vitally important packet of information to expectant parents on diet, ways to prevent preterm birth, and other educational materials. Quarterly newsletters address the needs of multiples of all ages. Call the Triplet Connection at (209) 474-0885.

- **Twin Services** is a health education and service agency providing publications, services and telephone advice in English or Spanish for families of multiple births as well as for health care professionals. Monday through Friday, 10:00 a.m. to 4:00 p.m. Pacific Time. Call (415) 474-3073 or (415) 644-0863 or write to Twin Services, Post Office Box 10066, Berkeley, CA 94709.

- **Parent Care, Inc.** is an international organization of parents of premature and high-risk infants. For more information, write 9041 Colgate Street, Indianapolis, IN 46268-1210 or call (317) 872-9913.

- **International Twins Association, Inc.** is a non-profit organization promoting spiritual, intellectual, and social growth of twins. For more information about ITA and their annual convention, contact Jerry VanDenBerg at 259 Calvin Avenue, Holland, MI 49423 or call (616) 396-6269.

- **La Leche League** holds monthly meetings for pregnant and breastfeeding women. Babies are welcome. For more information call (800) LA-LECHE (525-3243).

- **Mothers of Supertwins (M.O.S.T.)** is a non-profit organization serving parents of higher multiples; triplets, quads, or quints. They publish a newsletter and offer networking across the country. For more information, write to Post Office Box 951, Brentwood, NY 11717 or call (516) 434-MOST (6678).

- **Mothers of Twins Clubs (MOTC)** are local non-profit groups offering support and information for twin and supertwin moms through meetings and social events. Contact your local hospital for more information.

Multiple Pregnancy

- **The National Organization of Mothers of Twins Clubs, Inc. (NOMOTC)** is a non-profit nationwide network of clubs which shares information, concerns and advice, and focuses on education and research. For more information, write to NOMOTC, Post Office Box 23188, Albuquerque, NM 87192-1188 or call (505) 275-0955.

- **"Our Newsletter" and Network** offers support and information for parents who have lost one or all of their multiples. Contact "our Newsletter" c/o Jean Kollantai, Post Office Box 1064, Palmer, AK 996645 or call (907) 745-2706.

- **Bittersweet,** located in Minneapolis is a group for grieving parents of a multiple or multiples. Contact Barbara Schaak, R.N. for more information (612) 854-1997.

Books

Alexander, T.P. *Make Room for Twins: A Complete Guide to Pregnancy, Delivery and the Childhood Years.* New York: Bantam Books, 1987. BLB.

Clegg, A. and Woollett, A. *Twins: From Conception to Five Years.* New York: Van Nostrand Reinhold, 1983. BLB.

Friedrich, E. and Rowland, C. *The Parents Guide to Raising Twins.* New York: St. Martin's Press, 1984. BLB.

Gromada,K. *Mothering Multiples: Breastfeeding and Caring for Twins.* La Leche League Publication #267. 1985. BLB.

Novotny, P.P. *The Joy of Twins.* New York: Crown Publishers, 1988. BLB

Magazines

Double Talk: (A quarterly newsletter) $8/year. P.O. box 412, Amelia, OH 45102; (513) 753-7117.

Twins (A bi-monthly magazine with a regular column of prematurity.) $18/year, P.O. Box 12045, Overland Park, KS 66212; (800) 821-5533, ext. 30.

Mail Order

Parents of multiples are quick to learn that catalog shopping is the fastest and easiest way to get things done in a hurry. Here is a list of manufacturers that will send out a catalogue at your request. When ordering, always enquire about a twin discount.

A Baby Carriage (800) 228-TWIN
McGills (Twins) (402) 592-0000
Olesen's Mill Direct (800) 537-4979
One Step Ahead (800) 274-8440
Preemie Store (800) O SO-TINY
Preemie Wear (800) 992-TINY
T.L.C. (Preemie) (800)7555-4852
Play Fair Toys (800) 824-7255
Just For Kids (800) 654-6963
Child Craft (800) 631-5657
After the Stork (800) 333-KIDS
Nurse Mate for Twins (800) 526-2594
The Right Start (800) LITTLE 1
Mainly Multiples (800) 388-TWIN
Twincerely Yours (904) 394-5493
Perfectly Safe (800) 837-KIDS
Biobottoms (800) 766-1254

References

California Department of Health Services. Nutrition During Pregnancy and the Postpartum Period. A manual for Health Care Professionals. Maternal and Child Health Branch, WIC Supplemental Food Branch, June 1990.

Sahakian V, Rouse D, Sipes S, Rose N, and Niebyl J. Vitamin B6 Is Effective Therapy for Nausea and Vomiting of Pregnancy: A Randomized Double-Blind Placebo Controlled study. Obstet Gynecol. 78: 33, 1991.

Institute of Medicine, National Academy of Sciences, Nutrition During Pregnancy. National Academy Press, Wash., D.C., 1990.

Luke B. 1987. Twin Births: Influence of Maternal Weight on Intrauterine Growth and Prematurity. Fed. Proc., Fed. Am..Sec.Exp.Biol. 46: 1015.

Konwinski T, Gerard C, Hult AM, Papiernik-Berkhauer E, 1974. Maternal pregestational weight and multiple pregnancy duration. Acta Genet Med Gemollol Suppl. 22: 44-47

Nutrition information provided by: Erica P. Gunderson, MS, MPH, RD, Perinatal Nutrition Specialist, California Medical Center, San Francisco, California.

Section 25.2

Rates of Twin Births

Morbidity and Mortality Weekly Report, February 1997

During 1980-1994, the number of twin births in the United States increased by 42%, from 68,339 to 97,064, and the twin birth rate (i.e., the number of twin births to total live births) increased 30%, from 18.9% to 24.6 per 1,000 live births. These increases are important because the risks for preterm birth, low birthweight (LBW), long-term disability, and early death are greater for twins than for singletons.

State-Specific Twin Birth Rates

To estimate state-specific rates of twin births, CDC analyzed data from the U.S. certificates of birth for 1992-1994. This report presents the findings of this analysis of these data, which indicate that state-specific rates of twin births varied substantially, and the variations reflect factors other than state-specific differences in maternal age distributions.

In this analysis, twin births were defined as individual live births in twin deliveries, rather than sets of twins (e.g., a delivery resulting in one live birth and one stillbirth is reported as one birth from a twin delivery). Because the type of twin (i.e., monozygotic—resulting from the fertilization of one ovum, or dizygotic—resulting from the fertilization of two ova) is not listed on birth certificates, this analysis could not distinguish between twin types. To improve the reliability of the state-specific estimates of rates of twin births, data from 1992-1994 were combined. Because rates of twin births increased with maternal age, state-specific rates were standardized to the U.S. maternal age distribution for 1992-1994 to account for differing age distributions.

During 1992-1994, the rate of twin births in the United States was 24.0 per 1000 live births. Among the 50 states and the District of Columbia, rates ranged from 19.8 (Idaho and New Mexico) to 27.7 (Connecticut and Massachusetts). Rates were highest for the New England, Middle Atlantic, and East North Central Region.

The 10 highest rates were reported for Connecticut, Massachusetts, New Jersey, Rhode Island, Illinois, Michigan, New York, Delaware, Ohio, and Maryland. In general, rates for states in the South and West were substantially lower than the overall rate for the United States; in particular, six of the 10 states in the Mountain region (New Mexico, Idaho, Utah, Montana, Arizona, and Wyoming) accounted for the lowest rates.

In general, in states with rates of twin births higher than the overall rate for the United States, the maternal age distribution was older than that for the United States overall. Consequently, rates in these states were generally decreased after standardization. However, rates for nine of the 10 states with the highest observed rates remained significantly higher than the U.S. rate even after standardization. For five of these states (Connecticut, Massachusetts, Illinois, Michigan, and Ohio), rates ranked among the 10 highest after standardization. The persistent differences between rates for these states and the overall rate for the United States primarily reflected higher rates among mothers aged over 25. Age-specific rates for states with the highest rates generally were similar to U.S. rates for mothers younger than 25 years but higher for mothers over 25 years.

The state-specific variation in rates of twin births also reflected state-specific differences in racial/ethnic composition, although in some states the small numbers of twin births for which detailed age and racial/ethnic information was listed precluded reliable standardization. For 1994, the twin birth rate among non-Hispanic white mothers was 24.3; among non-Hispanic black mothers, 28.3; and among Hispanic mothers, 18.6. However, accounting for these differences does not completely account for variation in twin births. For example, even after simultaneously adjusting for maternal age, race, and Hispanic origin, rates of twin births for Connecticut and Massachusetts remained significantly higher than the rate for the United States overall.

Multiple Pregnancy

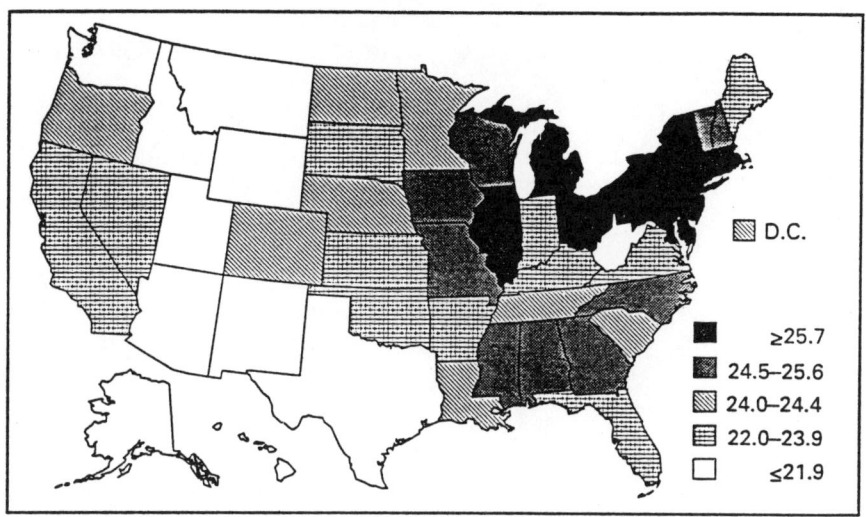

*Per 1000 live births.

Figure 25.1. Rate of Twin Births (per 1000 live births), by State—United States, 1992-1994

Chapter 26

Pregnancy in Women with Sickle Cell Anemia

Purpose of This Text

This text can help you understand sickle cell disease and how it can affect your child.

The best way to help your baby is to learn as much as you can about the disease, the problems it can cause, and what you can do to care for your baby. Talk about [these issues] and your baby's health care choices with your doctor and others who know about sickle cell disease. Working together, you can give your child the best possible care.

You will find a description of the kinds of problems a baby with sickle cell disease may have [in the section titled "How Are Babies Affected?"]. Remember when you read it that not all babies will have all of these problems. At the [end of this chapter], you will find a list of terms often used by doctors and nurses when they talk about sickle cell disease.

What Is Sickle Cell Disease?

Sickle cell disease is an inherited disorder of the red blood cells. Red blood cells carry oxygen to all parts of the body by using a protein called hemoglobin. Normal red blood cells contain only normal hemoglobin and are shaped like doughnuts. These cells are very flexible and move easily through small blood vessels.

Agency for Health Care Policy and Research (AHCPR) Pub. No. 93-0564, 1993

But in sickle cell disease, the red blood cells contain sickle hemoglobin, which causes them to change to a curved shape (sickle shape) after oxygen is released. Sickled cells become stuck and form plugs in the small blood vessels. This blockage of blood flow can damage the tissue. Because there are blood vessels in all parts of the body, damage can occur anywhere in the body.

Types of Sickle Cell Disease

There are several forms of sickle cell disease. The most common is sickle cell anemia. Your doctor or nurse will tell you what kind of sickle cell disease your baby has. Be sure to write down the name so that you can refer to it if your baby has to go to a new doctor or clinic.

The most common types of sickle cell disease are:

- Sickle cell anemia
- Hemoglobin SC disease
- Sickle beta-thalassemia

How Are Babies Affected?

Babies with sickle cell disease may have:

- *Anemia* (a low number of red blood cells). People with anemia may tire easily.

- *Aplastic crisis*. Babies with sickle cell disease may stop making red blood cells for a short time. Signs include paleness, less activity than normal, fast breathing, and fast heartbeat. A baby with these signs must be seen quickly by the doctor.

- *Hand-and-foot syndrome*. Babies with sickle cell disease may have pain and swelling in their hands or feet.

- *Painful episodes* (mostly in the arms, hands, legs, feet, or abdomen). This happens when sickle cells plug blood vessels and block the flow of blood. Doctors call this a painful episode, event, or crisis.

- *Severe infections*. The child with sickle cell anemia is at great risk for serious infections—such as sepsis (a blood stream infection), meningitis, and pneumonia. The risk of infection is increased because the spleen does not function normally.

Pregnancy in Women with Sickle Cell Anemia

- *Splenic sequestration crisis.* The spleen is the organ that filters blood. In children with sickle cell disease, the spleen can enlarge rapidly from trapped red blood cells. This condition is called splenic sequestration crisis and can be life-threatening.

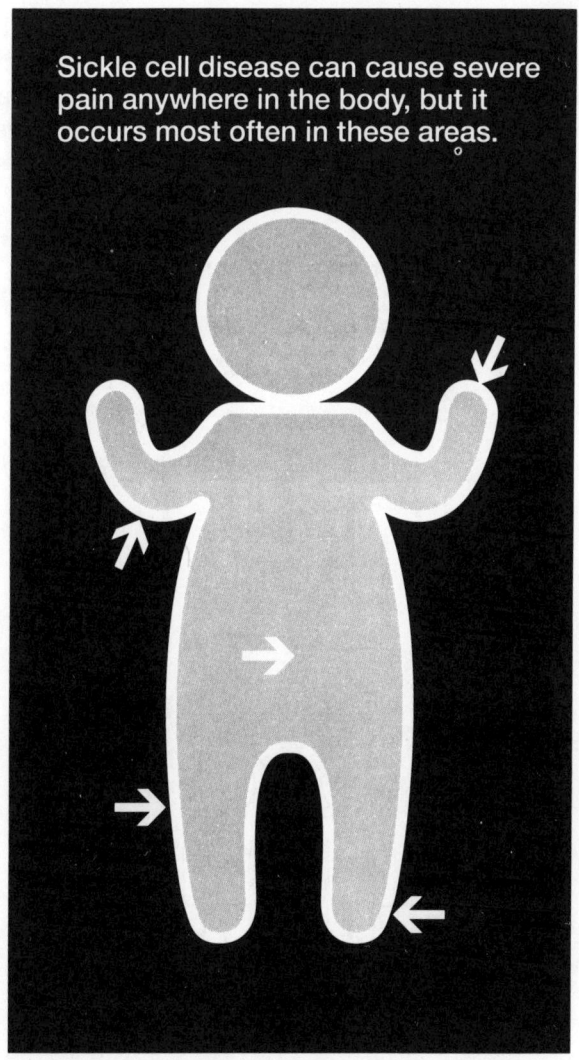

Figure 26.1. Areas of the body commonly affected by sickle cell disease.

- *Stroke.* This happens when blood vessels in the brain are blocked by sickled red blood cells. Signs include seizure, weakness of the arms and legs, speech problems, and loss of consciousness. A baby with any of these signs must be seen quickly by a doctor.

Who Is Affected?

In the United States, most people who have sickle cell disease are African Americans. About 1 in 375 African-American children has sickle cell disease. Hispanic Americans from the Caribbean, Central America, and parts of South America may also have the disease. Sickle cell disease is also found in individuals from Turkey, Greece, Italy, the Middle East, or East India.

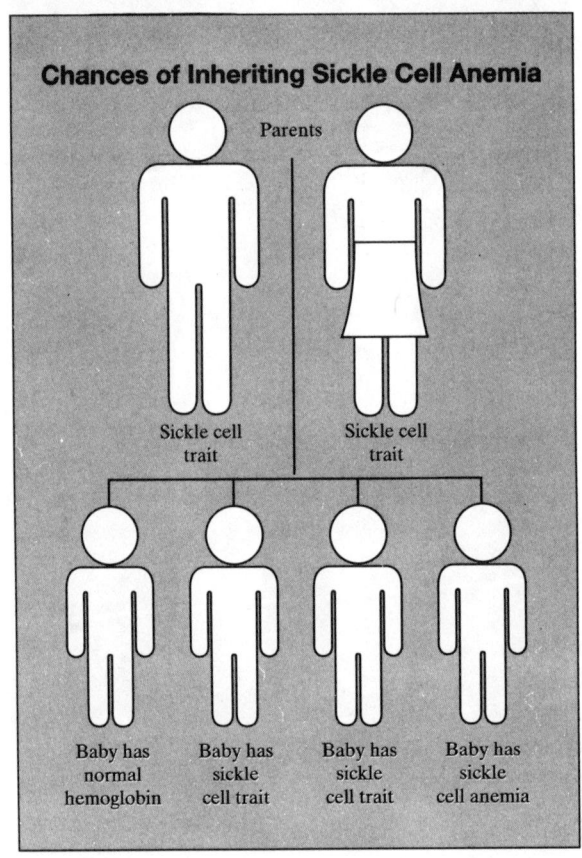

Figure 26.2. Pattern of inheritance for sickle cell anemia

Pregnancy in Women with Sickle Cell Anemia

What Causes Sickle Cell Disease?

All forms of sickle cell disease are inherited. Children inherit genes for the disease from their parents.

Genes are substances within the father's sperm and the mother's egg that determine all of the physical characteristics of a baby. Children inherit the genes for hemoglobin from their parents. Persons who inherit both normal and sickle hemoglobin have sickle cell trait. Sickle cell trait is not a disease and does not change to disease. The individual sperm or egg from a person with sickle cell trait may contain either a gene for normal hemoglobin or a gene for sickle hemoglobin.

When both parents have sickle cell trait, for each pregnancy, the chances are:

- 1 in 4 that the baby will have only normal hemoglobin.
- 2 in 4 that the baby will have both normal and sickle hemoglobin (sickle cell trait).
- 1 in 4 that the baby will have only sickle hemoglobin (sickle cell anemia).

The inheritance of other forms of sickle cell disease can be explained by your doctor.

How Do I Know If My Baby Has Sickle Cell Disease?

All newborn babies should be tested for sickle cell disease. Many States have screening programs that test babies born in the hospital within a few days of birth. A blood sample is taken from the baby's heel for the sickle cell test, as well as screening tests for several other medical conditions.

If the test shows your baby might have sickle cell disease, the doctor will do the test again to make sure. The doctor may ask one or both parents for blood samples to test. If your baby has sickle cell disease, the doctor will tell you as soon as possible.

What If My Baby Has Sickle Cell Disease?

If your baby has sickle cell disease, the doctor will help you find the best medical care for your child. This care could be provided by your family doctor, a pediatrician (children's doctor), or a pediatric hematologist (children's blood specialist), or a special sickle cell clinic. You also may want to see a counselor who can talk with you about your chances of having another baby with sickle cell disease.

Sickle cell disease is not just a medical problem. You may have many concerns about your baby and your family—for example, how to cope with your feelings and how to pay the medical bills. Your doctor or nurse can talk with you about your concerns. They also can help you find a local social service agency to assist you. In many areas there are sickle cell support groups, as well as community organizations that offer testing, education, and support to families affected by sickle cell disease.

How Can I Help My Baby?

The best way to help your baby is to learn as much as you can about the disease and to make sure your baby gets the best health care possible. The child with sickle cell disease has special needs and must have regular medical care to stay as healthy as possible. The doctor or nurse will explain how often to bring your baby for medical care and what you can do if your baby becomes ill.

By 2 months of age, your baby should start taking penicillin by mouth twice each day. **It is very important to give the medicine exactly as the doctor tells you.** This will help prevent life-threatening infections. Penicillin should be continued until at least 5 years of age.

Also by 2 months of age, your baby will get a shot to protect against *H. influenzae*, a type of bacteria that causes an infection which can be dangerous to people with sickle cell disease. The baby also will need a shot to protect against hepatitis B, a liver disease. At age 2, your child should receive pneumococcal vaccine. Your child should have all the other shots that children normally receive.

Here are some of the most important things you need to know about caring for a baby with sickle cell disease:

- **If your baby has a fever (over 101 degrees), you must get medical help right away.** A fever in a child with sickle cell disease can be a sign of serious medical problems. Always take your baby's temperature when your baby appears sick. Your doctor will tell you what to do if your baby has a fever.

- If any new doctor or health care provider sees your baby for any reason, explain that your baby has sickle cell disease.

- A good diet is very important for all babies. Ask your doctor or other health care provider about the right foods and liquids for your baby. Make sure your baby drinks plenty of liquids. Find out if your baby also should have vitamins or iron.

Pregnancy in Women with Sickle Cell Anemia

- Make sure your baby does not become overheated or chilly. Keep your baby warm. Cold baths or cold air can slow the baby's blood flow and cause problems.

If your baby is sick, you must get medical help right away. Any sign of illness in a child with sickle cell disease can be serious. Your baby needs to see the doctor quickly if the baby:

- Is breathing fast or having a problem with breathing
- Coughs frequently
- Is cranky and cries more than usual
- Screams when touched
- Is very tired or has little energy
- Is very weak
- Vomits
- Does not want to eat
- Has diarrhea
- Has fewer wet diapers
- Has pain or swelling in the abdomen
- Has swollen hands or feet
- Has pale blue or grey lips or skin

Questions to Ask

You should always feel free to ask any question about sickle cell disease and how it affects you and your family. Here are some questions you may want to ask the doctor, nurse, counselor, or social worker.

- What does my baby have? How did he or she get it?
- What do I have? How did I get it? How will it affect me and my family?
- How often does my baby need to see you?
- What medicine does my baby need? What do I need to know about giving it?
- What should my baby eat and drink?
- Is there anything my baby should not do?
- How can I tell if my baby gets sick?
- What should I do, and who should I call, if my baby gets sick?
- What other help is available to my family?

Additional Resources

To learn more about sickle cell disease and how to cope with it, contact:

National Association for Sickle Cell Disease
3345 Wilshire Boulevard, Suite 1106
Los Angeles, CA 90010-1880
Telephone: (800) 421-8453

Additional organizations that can provide help include:

California State Department of Health
Children's Medical Services Branch
Sacramento, CA 95814
Telephone: (916) 654-0499

Cincinnati Comprehensive Sickle Cell Center
Children's Hospital Medical Center
Cincinnati, OH 45229
Telephone: (513) 559-4200

Clinical Center Communications
9000 Rockville Pike
Building 10, Room 1C255
Bethesda, MD 20892
Telephone: (301) 496-2563

Education Programs Associates
1 West Campbell Ave, Building D
Campbell, CA 95008
Telephone: (408) 374-1210

Howard University
Comprehensive Sickle Cell Center
2121 Georgia Ave.
Washington DC 20059
Telephone: (202) 806-7930

March of Dimes Birth Defects Foundation
1275 Mamaroneck Avenue
White Plains, NY 10605
(For faster service, look in the telephone book for a local March of Dimes chapter in your area)

Pregnancy in Women with Sickle Cell Anemia

Mid-South Sickle Cell Center
Le Bonheur Children's Medical Center
Memphis, TN 38103
Telephone: (901) 522-6792

Mississippi State Department of Health
Genetics Division
P.O. Box 1700
Jackson, MS
Telephone: (601) 960-7619

National Maternal and Child Health Clearinghouse
8201 Greensboro Drive, Suite 600
McLean, VA 22102
Telephone: (703) 821-8955

New York State Department of Health
Newborn Screening Program
Wadsworth Center for Laboratories and Research
P.O. Box 509
Albany, NY 12201-0509
Telephone: (518) 473-7552

Northern California Comprehensive Sickle Cell Center
San Francisco, CA 94110
Telephone: (510) 428-3651

Texas Department of Health
Newborn Screening Program
1100 West 49th St.
Austin, TX 78756-3199
Telephone: (512) 458-7111

This is not a complete list. Check with your state or local health department or sickle cell agency for more information.

Common Sickle Cell Terms

Your doctor, nurse, or other caregiver may use these terms in talking with you about sickle cell disease and your child.

Acute chest syndrome. A serious condition caused by infection or trapped red blood cells in the lungs. Fast or difficult breathing, chest pain, and coughing are signs of acute chest syndrome in the child with sickle cell disease. A child with acute chest syndrome usually will have to go to the hospital for treatment.

Anemia. A reduced number of red blood cells. Anemia occurs in persons with sickle cell disease because sickled red blood cells do not live as long as normal red blood cells. A child with sickle cell disease cannot make red blood cells fast enough to keep up with the rapid breakdown, so the person with sickle cell disease has fewer red blood cells than normal and is anemic.

Aplastic crisis. Occurs when a child's bone marrow temporarily stops producing red blood cells. A child with aplastic crisis may appear pale and be tired and less active than usual.

Capillaries. Tiny blood vessels where sickle-shaped blood cells may get trapped and cause problems.

Gene. The biological units that are passed from both parents to a child. Genes determine all of the child's characteristics—for example, hair, eye, and skin color, foot size, height—and whether the child will have sickle cell disease or another inherited disease.

Haemophilus influenzae. A type of bacteria that causes infection and can lead to serious problems in the child with sickle cell disease. Babies must receive a special vaccine beginning at 2 months of age to protect them from this condition.

Hand-and-foot syndrome. Pain and swelling of the hands and feet caused by sickle-shaped red blood cells that plug blood vessels in the hands and feet. Often this will be the baby's first problem caused by sickle cell disease.

Hemoglobin. A molecule found in red blood cells that carries oxygen from the lungs to other parts of the body.

Pain event or painful episode. Pain caused by plugging of blood vessels by sickled blood cells. Pain is most often felt in the arms, legs, back, and abdomen. The pain may last only a few hours or as long as a week or two. The pain may be mild or so severe that pain medicine is needed. The number of pain events a person has may vary greatly.

Pregnancy in Women with Sickle Cell Anemia

Sepsis. The presence of infection in the blood stream.

Sickle cell anemia. The most common form of sickle cell disease. Other types of sickle cell disease include hemoglobin SC disease and sickle beta-thalassemia; there are also other, less common types of sickle cell disease.

Sickle cell disease. A group of inherited disorders in which anemia is present and sickle hemoglobin is produced.

Sickle cell trait. The condition in which a person has both normal and sickle hemoglobin in the red cells as a result of inheriting a normal hemoglobin gene and a gene for sickle hemoglobin. Sickle cell trait is not a disease and does not change to sickle cell disease. Persons with sickle cell trait may pass the sickle gene to their children.

Sickled cells. In children with sickle cell disease, hemoglobin molecules in red blood cells stick to one another and cause the red cells to become crescent or sickle shaped. Sickled cells cannot pass easily through tiny blood vessels.

Splenic sequestration crisis. Occurs when a large portion of the child's blood becomes trapped in the spleen. Early signs include paleness, an enlarged spleen, and pain in the abdomen.

Streptococcus pneumoniae. A bacteria that causes a very serious type of pneumonia in children with sickle cell disease. Twice daily doses of penicillin by mouth, starting at about 2 months of age, can help to prevent this life-threatening infection in children with sickle cell anemia and sickle beta-thalassemia.

For More Information

The information in this booklet was taken from the *Clinical Practice Guideline on Sickle Cell Disease: Screening, Diagnosis, Management, and Counseling in Newborns and Infants*. The guideline was written by a panel of experts sponsored by the Agency for Health Care Policy and Research. Other guidelines on common health problems also are being developed.

For more information about guidelines, or to order extra copies of this [text], contact:

Agency for Health Care Policy and Research
Publications Clearinghouse
P.O. Box 8547
Silver Spring, MD 20907

Or call 1-800-358-9295 (for callers outside the US, only: 301-495-3453) weekdays, 9 a.m. to 5 p.m., Eastern time.

Chapter 27

Pregnancy in Women with Lupus

Definition

Lupus is a chronic, autoimmune disease which causes inflammation of various parts of the body, especially the skin, joints, blood and kidneys. The body's immune system normally makes proteins called antibodies to protect the body against viruses, bacteria and other foreign materials. These foreign materials are called antigens. In an autoimmune disorder such as lupus, the immune system loses its ability to tell the difference between foreign substances (antigens) and its own cells and tissues. The immune system then makes antibodies directed against "self." These antibodies, called "auto-antibodies, react with the "self" antigens to form immune complexes. The immune complexes build up in the tissues and can cause inflammation, injury to tissues, and pain.

More people have lupus than AIDS, cerebral palsy, multiple sclerosis, sickle-cell anemia and cystic fibrosis combined. LFA market research data show that between 1,400,000 and 2,000,000 people reported to have been diagnosed with lupus. (Study conducted by Bruskin/Goldring Research, 1994.) For most people, lupus is a mild disease affecting only a few organs. For others, it may cause serious and even life-threatening problems. Thousands of Americans die each year from lupus-related complications.

What is Lupus; Pregnancy and Lupus. ©Lupus Foundation of America, Inc. Reprinted with permission.

Types of Lupus

There are three types of lupus: discoid, systemic, and drug-induced. Discoid lupus is always limited to the skin. It is identified by a rash that may appear on the face, neck and scalp. Discoid lupus is diagnosed by examining a biopsy of the rash. In discoid lupus the biopsy will show abnormalities that are not found in skin without the rash. Discoid lupus does not generally involve the body's internal organs. Therefore, the ANA test, a blood test used to detect systemic lupus, may be negative in patients with discoid lupus. However, in a large number of patients with discoid lupus, the ANA test is positive, but at a low level or "titer."

In approximately 10 percent of the people with lupus, discoid lupus can evolve into the systemic form of the disease, which can affect almost any organ or system of the body. This cannot be predicted or prevented. Treatment of discoid lupus will not prevent its progression to the systemic form. Individuals who progress to the systemic form probably had systemic lupus at the outset, with the discoid rash as their main symptom.

Systemic lupus is usually more severe than discoid lupus, and can affect almost any organ or system of the body. For some people, only the skin and joints will be involved. In others, the joints, lungs, kidneys, blood or other organs and/or tissues may be affected. Generally, no two people with systemic lupus will have identical symptoms. Systemic lupus may include periods in which few, if any, symptoms are evident (remission) and other times when the disease becomes more active (flare). Most often when people mention "lupus," they are referring to the systemic form of the disease.

Drug-induced lupus occurs after the use of certain prescribed drugs. The symptoms of drug-induced lupus are similar to those of systemic lupus. The drugs most commonly connected with drug-induced lupus are hydralazine (used to treat high blood pressure or hypertension) and procainamide (used to treat irregular heart rhythms). However, not everyone who takes these drugs will develop drug-induced lupus. Only about 4 percent of the people who take these drugs will develop the antibodies suggestive of lupus. Of those 4 percent, only an extremely small number will develop overt drug-induced lupus. The symptoms usually fade when the medications are discontinued.

Although drug-induced lupus and discoid lupus share features of systemic lupus, the rest of this chapter primarily discusses systemic lupus.

Pregnancy in Women with Lupus

Cause

The cause(s) of lupus is unknown, but environmental and genetic factors are involved. While scientists believe there is a genetic predisposition to the disease, it is known that environmental factors also play a critical role in triggering lupus. Some of the environmental factors that may trigger the disease are: infections, antibiotics (especially those in the sulfa and penicillin groups), ultraviolet light, extreme stress, and certain drugs.

Although lupus is known to occur within families, there is no known gene or genes which are thought to cause the illness. Only 10 percent of lupus patients will have a close relative (parent or sibling) who already has or may develop lupus. Statistics show that only about 5 percent of the children born to individuals with lupus will develop the illness.

Lupus is often called a "woman's disease" despite the fact that many men are affected. Lupus can occur at any age, and in either sex, although it occurs 10-15 times more frequently among adult females than among adult males. The symptoms of the disease are the same in men and women. People of African, American Indian, and Asian origin are thought to develop the disease more frequently than Caucasian women, but the studies that led to this result are small and need corroboration.

Hormonal factors may explain why lupus occurs more frequently in females than in males. The increase of disease symptoms before menstrual periods and/or during pregnancy support the belief that hormones, particularly estrogen, may be involved. However, the exact hormonal reason for the greater prevalence of lupus in women, and the cyclic increase in symptoms, is unknown.

Pregnancy and Lupus

Since lupus primarily affects young women, pregnancy often becomes a crucial question. Years ago, all medical texts said that lupus patients could not have children, and if they become pregnant, they should have therapeutic abortions. Clearly, these early conclusions are wrong. Currently, 50 percent of all lupus pregnancies are completely normal, and 25 percent deliver normal babies prematurely. Fetal loss, due to spontaneous abortion (miscarriage) or death of the baby accounts for the remaining 25 percent. While not all of the problems of pregnancy with Lupus have been solved, pregnancies are possible, and normal children are the rule.

While it is certainly possible for lupus patients to have children, pregnancy may not be easy. It is important to note that although many lupus pregnancies will be completely normal, all lupus pregnancies should be considered "high risk." "High risk" is a term commonly used by obstetricians to indicate that solvable problems may occur and must be anticipated. Pregnant lupus patients should be managed by obstetricians who are thoroughly familiar with high risk pregnancies and work in close concert with the woman's primary physician. Delivery should be planned at a hospital that has access to a unit specializing in the care of premature newborns. SLE mothers should not attempt home delivery, or be overly committed to "natural" childbirth, since treatable complications during delivery are frequent. However, under close observation, the risk to the mother's health is lessened, and healthy babies can be born.

Will Pregnancy Flare My Lupus?

Although older medical texts suggest that SLE flares are common in pregnancy, recent studies indicate that flares are uncommon and are usually easily treated. In fact, 6-15 percent of lupus patients will actually experience an improvement in lupus symptoms during pregnancy. Flares most often occur during the first or second trimester, or during the two months immediately after delivery. Most of the flares tend to be mild. The most common symptoms of these flares are arthritis, rashes and fatigue. Approximately 33 percent of lupus patients will have a decrease in platelet count during pregnancy, and about 20 percent will have an increase in or new occurrence of protein in the urine.

Women who conceive after 5-6 months of remission are less likely to experience a lupus flare than those who get pregnant while their lupus is active. Lupus nephritis before conception also increases the chance of experiencing a lupus flare during pregnancy.

It is important to distinguish the symptoms of a lupus flare from the normal body changes that occur during pregnancy. For example, because the ligaments that hold the joints together normally soften in pregnancy, fluid may accumulate in the joints, especially in the knees, and cause swelling. Although this may suggest an increase in inflammation due to lupus, it may simply be the swelling that occurs during a normal pregnancy. Similarly, lupus rashes may appear to worsen during pregnancy, but this is usually due to an increased blood flow to the skin that is common in pregnancy (the "blush" of a pregnant woman). Many women also experience new hair growth during pregnancy, followed by a dramatic loss of hair after delivery. Although hair loss is certainly a symptom of active SLE, this again is most likely a result of the changes that occur during a normal pregnancy.

When Is the Best Time to Get Pregnant?

The answer is simple: when you are at your healthiest. Women in remission have much less trouble than do women with active disease. Their babies do much better, and everyone worries less.

Good health rules are essential: rest well, take medications as prescribed, visit your doctor(s) regularly, don't smoke, don't drink, and certainly don't use "recreational" drugs.

Why Are Frequent Doctor Visits So Important in a Lupus Pregnancy?

Frequent doctor visits are important in any high risk pregnancy because many conditions which may occur can be prevented or treated more easily, if found early.

About 20 percent of lupus patients will have a sudden increase in blood pressure, protein in the urine, or both during pregnancy. This is called toxemia of pregnancy (or preeclampsia, or pregnancy-induced hypertension). It is a serious condition, and will require immediate treatment and usually immediate delivery. Toxemia is more common in older women, in black women, in women with twins, in women with kidney disease, in women with high blood pressure, and in women who smoke. Serum complement and blood platelet count may be abnormal in these cases. Since complement levels and blood platelet counts are also abnormal during SLE flares, it may be difficult for the doctor to be certain that a flare is not causing these symptoms. If toxemia is promptly treated the woman should be in no danger, but there is a high risk that the baby will die if it is not rapidly delivered. If toxemia is ignored, both the woman and her baby are in danger.

As pregnancy progresses it is often wise for the doctor to check the baby's growth with sonograms (which are harmless). The doctor should also regularly check the baby's heart beat. Abnormalities in either the baby's growth or heart beat may be the first signs of trouble that can be treated.

Can I Take Medications During Pregnancy?

It is always unwise to take unnecessary medications during pregnancy. However, necessary medications should not be discontinued. Most medications commonly taken by SLE patients are safe to use during pregnancy. Prednisone, Prednisolone, and probably methylprednisolone (Medrol) do not get through the placenta and are safe for the baby. Specifically, dexamethasone (Decodrol, Hexadrol) and betamethasone (Celestone) do reach the baby and are used **ONLY** when it is necessary to treat the baby as well. For example, these medications might be used to help the baby's lungs mature more rapidly if the baby will be premature. Aspirin is safe (but see the FDA warning below); it is often used to protect against a complication known as toxemia of pregnancy. Preliminary reports suggest that azathioprine (Imuran) and hydroxychloroquine (Plaquenil) do not harm babies but the final word is not yet in on these. Cyclophosphamide (Cytoxan) is definitely harmful if taken during the first three months of pregnancy.

Editor's note: The September, 1990 issue of the *FDA Consumer* draws attention to the FDA's warning to pregnant women not to take aspirin during the last three months of pregnancy without a physician's consent. As of September 1991, all oral and rectal nonprescription aspirin and drugs containing aspirin must carry this warning. The article notes that aspirin can impede fetal circulation and uterine contractions, causing damage to the fetus and complicating delivery. This warning is similar to one issued earlier for nonprescription medication containing ibuprofen. The FDA decided to issue the warning based on recommendations from its Advisory Review Panel on OTC (over-the-counter) Internal Analgesic and Antirheumatic Drug Products which is composed of non-government experts.

What about "Prophylactic" (Preventative) Treatment with Prednisone?

A few doctors feel that all pregnant women with lupus should take small doses of Prednisone to prevent early abortion. However, there are no confirmed data that this is necessary. Similarly, some physicians feel steroids should be given or increased after the baby is born to prevent "post partum flare." Again, there is no evidence that this is necessary in most cases either. For patients recently on steroids, however, "stress" steroid is usually given during labor to supplement what the mother can't make herself.

What Are Anti-phospholipid Antibodies and Why Are They Important?

About 33 percent of lupus patients have antibodies that interfere with the function of the placenta. These antibodies are called anti-phospholipid antibodies, the lupus anticoagulant or anti-cardiolipin antibodies. These antibodies may cause blood clots, including blood clots in the placenta, that prevent the placenta from growing and functioning normally. This usually occurs during the second trimester. Since the placenta is the passageway for nourishment from the mother to the baby, the baby's growth slows. The baby can be delivered at this time and will be normal if it is big enough.

Treatment for lupus patients who have these antibodies is still being tested. Aspirin, Prednisone, Heparin and plasmapheresis have all been suggested as possible therapies. However even with the use of such medications, these antibodies may still lead to miscarriage.

Will My Baby Be Normal?

Prematurity is the greatest danger to the baby. About 50 percent of lupus pregnancies end before 9 months, usually because of the complications previously discussed. Babies born after 30 weeks or over 3 pounds usually do well. Premature babies may have difficulty breathing, may develop jaundice, and may become anemic. In modern neonatal units, these problems can be easily treated. Babies weighing more than three pounds at birth grow normally. Even babies as small as 1 pound, 4 ounces have survived and have been healthy in every way, but the outcome is uncertain for babies of this size. There are no congenital abnormalities that occur only to babies of lupus patients (except as described below), and no unusual frequency of mental retardation.

Will My Baby Have Lupus?

About 33 percent of lupus patients have an antibody known as anti-Ro or anti-SSA antibody. About 10 percent of women with Anti-Ro antibodies, or about 3 percent of all lupus women, will have a baby with a syndrome known as neonatal lupus. Neonatal lupus is not SLE. Neonatal lupus consists of a transient rash, transient blood count abnormalities, and a special type of heart beat abnormality. If the heart best abnormality occurs, which is very rare, it is treatable, but it is permanent. Neonatal lupus is the only type of congenital abnormality found in children of mothers with lupus. For babies with neonatal lupus who do not have the heart problem, there is no trace of the disease by 3-6 months of age, and it does not recur. Even babies with the heart beat abnormality problem grow normally. If a mother has had one child with neonatal lupus, there is about a 25 percent chance of having another child with the same problem.

Will I Have to Have a Caesarian Section?

Very premature babies, babies showing signs of stress, babies of mothers with low platelets, and babies of mothers who are very ill are almost always delivered by Caesarian section. This is often both the safest and fastest method of delivery in these cases. Usually the decision about type of delivery is not made in advance because the specific circumstances at the time of delivery are the determining factors.

Can I Breast-feed?

Although breast feeding is possible for lupus patients, breast milk may not come if the baby is born very prematurely because very premature babies are not strong enough to suckle, and thus, cannot draw the milk. However, milk can be pumped from the breast to feed a premature baby if the baby is not strong enough to suckle and the mother wishes to do this. Plaquenil and the cytotoxic drugs (Cytoxan, Imuran) are passed through the milk to the baby. Some medications, such as Prednisone, may prevent milk from being produced. If you are taking any medication it is best not to breast feed; but if your doctor approves, you may.

Who Will Care for the Baby?

Prospective parents often do not ask what will happen after the baby is born if the mother is ill and unable to care for the child. Since it is likely that a lupus patient will have future periods of illness, it is wise to think of this possibility in advance and to have plans for alternate child-care (spouse, grandparent, etc.) if needed.

Chapter 28

Breast Cancer and Pregnancy

Disease Description

Breast cancer is the most common cancer in pregnant and postpartum women occurring in about one in 3,000 pregnancies. The average patient is between 32-38 years of age and, with many women choosing to delay childbearing, it is likely that the incidence of breast cancer during pregnancy will increase.

Diagnosis

The natural tenderness and engorgement of the breasts of pregnant and lactating women may hinder detection of discrete masses, and therefore, early diagnosis of breast cancer. Delays in diagnosis are common, with an average reported delay of 5 to 15 months from the onset of symptoms. Because of this delay, cancers are typically detected at a later stage than in a nonpregnant, age-matched population. To detect breast cancer, pregnant and lactating women should practice self-examination and undergo a breast examination as part of the routine prenatal examination by a doctor.

If an abnormality is found, diagnostic approaches such as ultrasound and mammography may be used. With proper shielding, mammography poses little risk of radiation exposure to the fetus. However, mammograms should only be used to evaluate dominant masses and to locate occult carcinomas in the presence of other suspicious physical findings. Since 25% of mammograms in pregnancy

From NIH Homepage, National Cancer Institute, April 1997

may be negative in the presence of cancer, a biopsy is essential for the diagnosis of suspicious lesions. Diagnosis may be safely accomplished with a fine needle aspiration or excisional biopsy under local anesthesia.

Staging

Procedures used for staging of breast cancer should be modified to avoid radiation exposure to the fetus in pregnant women. Nuclear scans cause fetal radiation exposure. If such scans are essential for evaluation, hydration and Foley catheter drainage of the bladder can be used to prevent retention of radioactivity. Timing of the exposure to radiation relative to the gestational age of the fetus may be more critical than the actual dose of radiation delivered. Radiation exposure during the first trimester can lead to congenital malformations, especially microcephaly. Doses greater than 100 rad may produce congenital abnormalities in 100% of cases. Doses of 10 rad may result in fewer defects. A chest x-ray delivers 0.008 rad, and a bone scan delivers 0.1 rad.

Chest x-rays with abdominal shielding are considered safe, but as with all radiologic procedures, they should be used only when essential for making treatment decisions. For the diagnosis of bone metastases, a bone scan is preferable to a skeletal series because the bone scan delivers a smaller amount of radiation and is more sensitive. Evaluation of the liver can be performed with ultrasound, and brain metastases can be diagnosed with an MRI, both of which avoid fetal radiation exposure. However, no data evaluating the safety of MRI during pregnancy are available. Carcinogenesis in the fetus exposed to radiation is another consideration.

Breast cancer pathology is similar in age-matched pregnant and nonpregnant women. Hormone receptor assays are usually negative in pregnant breast cancer patients, but this may be the result of receptor binding by high serum estrogen levels associated with the pregnancy. However, enzyme immunocytochemical receptor assays are more sensitive than competitive binding assays. A study by Elledge et al. using binding methods indicated similar receptor positivity between pregnant and nonpregnant women with breast cancer. The study concluded that increased estrogen levels during pregnancy could result in a higher incidence of receptor positivity detected with immunohistochemistry than is detected by radio-labeled ligand binding, due to competitive inhibition by high levels of endogenous estrogen.

Overall survival of pregnant women with breast cancer may be worse than in nonpregnant women at all stages. However, the decreased overall survival in this patient population may be due primarily to delayed diagnosis.

Termination of pregnancy has not been shown to have any beneficial effect on breast cancer outcome and is not usually considered as a therapeutic option. However, termination of pregnancy may be considered, based on the age of the fetus, if maternal treatment options, such as chemotherapy and radiotherapy, are significantly limited by the continuation of the pregnancy.

Treatment Recommendations

Early Stage Cancer (Stages I and II)

Surgery is recommended as the primary treatment for breast cancer in pregnant women. Since radiation in therapeutic doses may expose the fetus to potentially harmful scatter radiation, modified radical mastectomy is the treatment of choice. Conservative surgery with postpartum radiotherapy has been used for breast preservation. If adjuvant chemotherapy is necessary, it should not be given during the first trimester to avoid the risk of teratogenicity.

Chemotherapy given after the first trimester is generally not associated with a high risk of fetal malformation, but may be associated with premature labor and fetal wastage. If considered necessary, chemotherapy may be given after the first trimester, but should generally be postponed until after delivery. Data on the immediate and long-term effects of chemotherapy on the fetus are limited.

Studies using adjuvant hormonal therapy alone or in combination with chemotherapy for breast cancer in pregnant women are also limited. Therefore, no conclusion has been reached regarding these options. Radiotherapy, if indicated, should be withheld until after delivery since it may be harmful to the fetus at any stage of development.

Late Stage Disease (Stages III and IV)

First-trimester radiotherapy should be avoided. Chemotherapy may be given after the first trimester as discussed above. Because the mother may have a limited life span (most studies show a 5-year survival rate of 10% in pregnant patients with stages III and IV disease), and there is a risk of fetal damage with treatment during the first trimester, issues regarding continuation of the pregnancy should be discussed with the patient and her family. Therapeutic abortion does not improve prognosis.

Lactation

Suppression of lactation does not improve prognosis. However, if surgery is planned, lactation should be suppressed to decrease the size and vascularity of the breasts. It should also be suppressed if chemotherapy is to be given because many antineoplastics (specifically cyclophosphamide and methotrexate) given systemically may occur in high levels in breast milk and this would affect the nursing baby. In general, women receiving chemotherapy should not breast-feed.

Fetal Consequences of Maternal Breast Cancer

No damaging effects on the fetus from maternal breast cancer have been demonstrated and there are no reported cases of maternal-fetal transfer of breast cancer cells.

Consequences of Pregnancy in Patients with a History of Breast Cancer

Pregnancy does not appear to compromise the survival of women with a prior history of breast cancer, based on limited retrospective data, and no deleterious effects have been demonstrated in the fetus. Some physicians recommend that patients wait two years after diagnosis before attempting to conceive. This allows early recurrence to become manifest, which may influence the decision to become a parent. Little is known about pregnancy after bone marrow transplantation and high-dose chemotherapy with or without total-body irradiation. In one report of pregnancies after bone marrow transplant for hematologic disorders, a 25% incidence of preterm labor and low birth weight for gestational age infants was noted.

References

Hoover HC: Breast cancer during pregnancy and lactation. Surgical Clinics of North America 70(5): 1151-1163, 1990.

Clark RM, Chua T: Breast cancer and pregnancy: the ultimate challenge. Clinical Oncology (Royal College of Radiologists) 1(1): 11-18, 1989.

Barnavon Y, Wallack MK: Management of the pregnant patient with carcinoma of the breast. Surgery, Gynecology and Obstetrics 171(4): 347-352, 1990.

Gallenberg MM, Loprinzi CL: Breast cancer and pregnancy. Seminars in Oncology 16(5): 369-376, 1989.

Elledge RM, Ciocca DR, Langone G, et al.: Estrogen receptor, progesterone receptor, and HER-2/neu protein in breast cancers from pregnant patients. Cancer 71(8): 2499-2506, 1993.

Guinee VF, Olsson H, Moller T, et al.: Effect of pregnancy on prognosis for young women with breast cancer. Lancet 343(8913): 1587-1589, 1994.

Petrek JA, Dukoff R, Rogatko A: Prognosis of pregnancy-associated breast cancer. Cancer 67(4): 869-872, 1991.

Harvey JC, Rosen PP, Ashikari R, et al.: The effect of pregnancy on the prognosis of carcinoma of the breast following radical mastectomy. Surgery, Gynecology and Obstetrics 153: 723-725, 1981.

Petrek JA: Pregnancy safety after breast cancer. Cancer 74(1): 528-531, 1994.

von Schoultz E, Johansson H, Wilking N, et al.: Influence of prior and subsequent pregnancy on breast cancer prognosis. Journal of Clinical Oncology 13(2): 430-434, 1995.

Sanders JE, Hawley J, Levy W, et al.: Pregnancies following high-dose cyclophosphamide with or without high-dose busulfan or total-body irradiation and bone marrow transplantation. Blood 87(7): 3045-3052, 1996.

Chapter 29

Pregnancy in Women with Hodgkin's Disease

Since Hodgkin's disease affects primarily young adults, most oncologists will eventually face the dilemma of how to provide therapy to a pregnant woman while minimizing the risk to the fetus. Treatment choice must be individualized, taking into consideration the mother's wishes, the severity and pace of the Hodgkin's disease, and the length of the remaining pregnancy. Since general guidelines can never substitute for clinical judgment, oncologists should be prepared to alter the initial plans when necessary.

Treatment in the First Trimester

Oncologists usually counsel therapeutic abortion for women with Hodgkin's disease who are in the first trimester. If the Hodgkin's disease presents in early stage above the diaphragm and appears to be growing slowly, patients can be followed carefully with plans to induce delivery early and proceed with definitive therapy. Alternatively, these patients can receive radiotherapy with proper shielding. Investigators at M.D. Anderson reported no congenital abnormalities in 16 babies delivered after the mothers had received supradiaphragmatic radiation while shielding the uterus with five half-value layers of lead. Chemotherapy administered in the first trimester is associated with congenital abnormalities in up to one-third of infants. However, in one series, there were no adverse effects in 14 children of mothers who

---

From NIH Homepage, National Cancer Institute publication, March 1997

received MOPP or ABVD during gestation, 5 of whom began treatment during the first trimester.

Consequently, some women may opt to continue the pregnancy and agree to radiotherapy or chemotherapy if immediate treatment is required.

Treatment in the Second and Third Trimesters

In the second half of pregnancy, most patients can be followed carefully, postponing therapy until induction of delivery at 32 to 36 weeks. If chemotherapy is mandatory prior to delivery, such as for patients with symptomatic advanced stage disease, vinblastine alone (given at 6 milligrams per square meter intravenously every two weeks until induction of delivery) may be considered as it has never been associated with fetal abnormalities in the second half of pregnancy. Steroids are also employed both for their antitumor effect as well as for hastening fetal pulmonary maturity. As an alternative, a short course of radiation can also be used prior to delivery in cases of respiratory compromise due to a rapidly enlarging mediastinal mass. Combination chemotherapy may be safe in the second half of pregnancy but should be avoided except in unusual circumstances. In any case, a full course of chemotherapy should follow delivery.

In one study, the 20-year survival of pregnant women with Hodgkin's disease was not different from nonpregnant women matched for similar stage of disease, age at diagnosis, and calendric year of treatment. The long-term effects on progeny after chemotherapy in utero are unknown, although present evidence tends to be reassuring.

References

Woo SY, Fuller LM, Cundiff JH, et al.: Radiotherapy during pregnancy for clinical stages IA-IIA Hodgkin's disease. International Journal of Radiation Oncology, Biology, Physics 23(2): 407-412, 1992.

Thomas PR, Peckham MJ: The investigation and management of Hodgkin's disease in the pregnant patient. Cancer 38(3): 1443-1451, 1976.

Aviles A, Diaz-Maqueo JC, Talavera A, et al.: Growth and development of children of mothers treated with chemotherapy during pregnancy: current status of 43 children. American Journal of Hematology 36: 243-248, 1991.

Jacobs C, Donaldson SS, Rosenberg SA, et al.: Management of the pregnant patient with Hodgkin's disease. Annals of Internal Medicine 95(6): 669-675, 1981.

Nisce LZ, Tome MA, He S, et al.: Management of coexisting Hodgkin's disease and pregnancy. American Journal of Clinical Oncology 9(2): 146-151, 1986.

Lishner M, Zemlickis D, Degendorfer P, et al.: Maternal and foetal outcome following Hodgkin's disease in pregnancy. British Journal of Cancer 65: 114-117, 1992.

Chapter 30

AIDS and Pregnancy

Chapter Contents

Section 30.1—HIV Testing and Counseling for
  Pregnant Women 516
Section 30.2—Pregnancy and HIV: Is AZT the
  Right Choice for You and Your Baby? 530

Section 30.1

HIV Testing and Counseling for Pregnant Women

Excerpts from Morbidity and Mortality Weekly Report, July 7, 1995

Introduction

During the past decade, human immunodeficiency virus (HIV) infection has become a leading cause of morbidity and mortality among women, the population accounting for the most rapid increase in cases of acquired immunodeficiency syndrome (AIDS) in recent years. As the incidence of HIV infection has increased among women of childbearing age, increasing numbers of children have become infected through perinatal (i.e., mother to infant) transmission; thus, HIV infection has also become a leading cause of death for young children. To reverse these trends, HIV education and services for prevention and health care must be made available to all women. Women who have HIV infection or who are at risk for infection need access to current information regarding:

1. early interventions to improve survival rates and quality of life for HIV-infected persons.
2. strategies to reduce the risk for perinatal HIV transmission, and
3. management of HIV-infection in pregnant women and perinatally exposed or infected children.

Results from a randomized, placebo-controlled clinical trial have indicated that the risk for perinatal HIV transmission can be substantially reduced by administration of zidovudine (ZDV [also referred to as AZT]) to HIV-infected pregnant women and their newborns. To optimally benefit from this therapy, HIV-infection must be diagnosed in these women before or during early pregnancy.

AIDS and Pregnancy

The U.S. Public Health Service (PHS) encourages all women to adopt behaviors that can prevent HIV infection and to learn their HIV status through counseling and voluntary testing. Ideally, women should know their HIV infection status before becoming pregnant. Thus, sites serving women of childbearing age (e.g., physicians' offices, family planning clinics, sexually transmitted disease clinics, and adolescent clinics) should counsel and offer voluntary HIV testing to women, including adolescents regardless of whether they are pregnant. Because specific services must be offered to HIV-infected pregnant women to prevent perinatal transmission, PHS is recommending routine HIV counseling and voluntary testing of all pregnant women so that interventions to improve the woman's health and the health of her infant can be offered in a timely and effective manner.

The recommendations in this report were developed by PHS as guidance to:

1. encourage HIV-infected pregnant women to learn their infection status.
2. advise infected pregnant women of methods for preventing perinatal, sexual, and other modes of HIV transmission.
3. facilitate appropriate follow-up for HIV-infected women, their infants, and their families, and
4. help uninfected pregnant women reduce their risk for acquiring HIV infection.

Increased availability of HIV counseling, voluntary testing, and follow-up medical and support services is essential to ensure successful implementation of these recommendations. These services can be optimally delivered through a readily available medical system with support services designed to facilitate ongoing care for patients.

Background Information

HIV Infection and AIDS in Women and Children

HIV infection is a major cause of illness and death among women and children. Nationally, HIV infection was the fourth leading cause of death in 1993 among women 25-44 years of age and the seventh leading cause of death in 1992 among children 1-4 years of age. Blacks and Hispanics have been disproportionately affected by the HIV epidemic. In 1993, HIV infection was the leading cause of death among black women 25-44 years of age and the third leading cause of death among Hispanic women in this age group. In 1991, HIV infection was the second leading cause of death among black children 1-4 years of age in New Jersey, Massachusetts, New York, and Florida and among Hispanic children in this age group in New York (CDC, unpublished data).

By 1995, CDC had received reports of more than 58,000 AIDS cases among adult and adolescent women and more than 5,500 cases among children who acquired HIV infection perinatally. Approximately one half of all AIDS cases among women have been attributed to injecting-drug use and one third to heterosexual contact. Nearly 90% of cumulative AIDS cases reported among children and virtually all new HIV infections among children in the United States can be attributed to perinatal transmission of HIV. An increasing proportion of perinatally acquired AIDS cases has been reported among children whose mothers acquired HIV infection through heterosexual contact with an infected partner whose infection status and risk factors were not known by the mother.

Data from the National Survey of Childbearing Women indicate that in 1992, the estimated national prevalence of HIV infection among childbearing women was 1.7 HIV-infected women per 1,000 childbearing women. Approximately 7,000 HIV-infected women gave birth annually for the years 1989-1992. Given a perinatal transmission rate of 15%-30%, an estimated 1,000-2,000 HIV-infected infants were born annually during these years in the United States. Although urban areas, especially in the northeast, generally have the highest seroprevalence rates, data from this survey have indicated a high prevalence of HIV infection among childbearing women who live in some rural and small urban areas particularly in the southern states.

Perinatal Transmission of HIV

HIV can be transmitted from an infected woman to her fetus or newborn during pregnancy, during labor and delivery, and during the postpartum period (through breastfeeding), although the percentage of infections transmitted during each of these intervals is not precisely known. Although transmission of HIV to a fetus can occur as early as the 8th week of gestation, data suggest that at least one half of perinatally transmitted infections from non-breastfeeding women occur shortly before or during the birth process. Breastfeeding may increase the rate of transmission by 10%-20%.

Several prospective studies have reported perinatal transmission rates ranging from 13% to 40%. Transmission rates may differ among

AIDS and Pregnancy

studies depending on the prevalence of various factors that can influence the likelihood of transmission. Several maternal factors have been associated with an increased risk for transmission, including low CD4+ T-lymphocyte counts, high viral titer, advanced HIV disease, the presence of p24 antigen in serum, placental membrane inflammation, intrapartum events resulting in increased exposure of the fetus to maternal blood, breastfeeding, low vitamin A levels, premature rupture of membranes, and premature delivery. Factors associated with a decreased rate of HIV transmission have included cesarean section delivery, the presence of maternal neutralizing antibodies, and maternal zidovudine therapy.

HIV Prevention and Treatment Opportunities for Women and Infants

HIV counseling and testing for women of childbearing age offer important prevention opportunities for both uninfected and infected women and their infants. Such counseling is intended to:

1. assist women in assessing their current or future risk for HIV infection.
2. initiate or reinforce HIV risk reduction behavior, and
3. allow for referral to other HIV prevention services (e.g., treatment for substance abuse and sexually transmitted diseases) when appropriate.

For infected women knowledge of their HIV infection status provides opportunities to

1. obtain early diagnosis and treatment for themselves and their infants.
2. make informed reproductive decisions.
3. use methods to reduce the risk for perinatal transmission.
4. receive information to prevent HIV transmission to others, and
5. obtain referral for psychological and social services, if needed.

Interventions designed to reduce morbidity in HIV-infected persons require early diagnosis of HIV infection so that treatment can be initiated before the onset of opportunistic infections and disease progression. However, studies indicate that many HIV-infected persons do not know they are infected until late in the course of illness. A survey of persons diagnosed with AIDS between January 1990 and December

1992 indicated that 57% of the 2,081 men and 62% of the 360 women who participated in the survey gave illness as the primary reason for being tested for HIV infection; 36% of survey participants first tested positive within 2 months of their AIDS diagnosis.

Providing HIV counseling and testing services in gynecologic and prenatal and other obstetric settings presents an opportunity for early diagnosis of HIV infection because many young women frequently access the health-care system for obstetric or gynecologic-related care. Clinics that provide prenatal and postnatal care, family planning clinics, sexually transmitted disease clinics, adolescent-health clinics, and other health-care facilities already provide a range of preventive services into which HIV education, counseling, and voluntary testing can be integrated. When provided appropriate access to ongoing care, HIV-infected women can be monitored for clinical and immunologic status and can be given preventive treatment and other recommended medical care and services.

Diagnosis of HIV infection before or during pregnancy allows women to make informed decisions regarding prevention of perinatal transmission. Early in the HIV epidemic, strategies to prevent perinatal HIV transmission were limited to either avoiding pregnancy or avoiding breastfeeding (for women in the United States and other countries that have safe alternatives to breast milk). More recent strategies to prevent perinatal HIV transmission have focused on interrupting in utero and intrapartum transmission. Foremost among these strategies has been administration of ZDV to HIV-infected pregnant women and their newborns (see next section). The ZDV regimen caused minimal adverse effects among both mothers and infants; the only adverse effect after 18 months of follow-up was mild anemia in the infants that resolved without therapy. As a result of these findings, PHS issued recommendations regarding ZDV therapy to reduce the risk for perinatal HIV transmission. In addition, the Food and Drug Administration (FDA) has approved the use of ZDV for this therapy.

Despite the substantial benefits and short-term safety of the ZDV regimen, however, the results of the trial present several unresolved issues, including:

1. the long-term safety of the regimen for both mothers and infants.
2. ZDV's effectiveness in women who have different clinical characteristics (e.g., CD4+ T-lymphocyte count and previous ZDV use) than those who participated in the trial, and

AIDS and Pregnancy

3. the likelihood of the mother's adherence to the lengthy treatment regimen.

The PHS recommendations for ZDV therapy emphasize that HIV-infected pregnant women should be informed of both benefits and potential risks when making decisions to receive such therapy. Discussions of treatment options should be noncoercive—the final decision to accept or reject ZDV treatment is the responsibility of the woman. Decisions concerning treatment can be complex and adherence to therapy, if accepted, can be difficult; therefore, good rapport and a trusting relationship should be established between the healthcare provider and the HIV-infected woman.

Several other possible strategies to reduce the risk for perinatal HIV transmission are under study or are being planned, however, their efficacies have not yet been determined. These strategies include:

1. administration of HIV hyperimmune globulin to infected pregnant women and their infants
2. efforts to boost maternal and infant immune responses through vaccination.
3. virucidal cleansing of the birth canal before and during labor and delivery.
4. modified and shortened anti-retroviral regimens
5. cesarean section delivery, and
6. vitamin A supplementation.

Knowledge of HIV infection status during pregnancy also allows for early identification of HIV-exposed infants, all of whom should be appropriately tested, monitored and treated. Prompt identification and close monitoring of such children (particularly infants) is essential for optimal medical management. Approximately 10%-20% of perinatally infected children develop rapidly progressive disease and die by 24 months of age. Pneumocystis carinii pneumonia (PCP) is the most common opportunistic infection in children who have AIDS and is often fatal. Because PCP occurs most commonly among perinatally infected children 3-6 months of age effective prevention requires that children born to HIV-infected mothers be identified promptly, preferably through prenatal testing of their mothers, so that prophylactic therapy can be initiated as soon as possible. CDC and the National Pediatric & Family HIV Resource Center have published revised guidelines for prophylaxis against PCP in children that recommend that all children born to HIV-infected mothers be placed on prophylactic therapy at 4-6 weeks of age. Careful follow-up of these children to promptly diagnose other potentially treatable HIV-related conditions (e.g., severe bacterial infections or tuberculosis) can prevent morbidity and reduce the need for hospitalization. Infants born to HIV-infected women also require changes in their routine immunization regimens as early as 2 months of age.

Despite the potential benefits of HIV counseling and testing to both women and their infants, some persons have expressed concerns about the potential for negative effects resulting from widespread counseling and testing programs in prenatal and other settings. These concerns include the fear that a) such programs could deter pregnant women from using prenatal-care services if testing is not perceived as voluntary and b) women who have been tested but who choose not to learn their test results may be reluctant to return for further prenatal care. Other potential negative consequences following a diagnosis of HIV infection can include loss of confidentiality, job- or health-care-related discrimination and stigmatization, loss of relationships, domestic violence, and adverse psychological reactions. Although cases of discrimination against HIV-infected persons and loss of confidentiality have been documented, data concerning the frequency of these events for women are limited. Reported rates of abandonment, loss of relationships, severe psychological reactions, and domestic violence have ranged from 4% to 13%. Providing infected women with or referring them to psychological, social, or legal services may help minimize such potential risks and enable women to benefit from the many health advantages of early HIV diagnosis.

Counseling and Testing Strategies

Guidelines published in 1985 regarding HIV counseling and testing of pregnant women recommended a targeted approach directed to women known to be at increased risk for HIV infection (e.g., injecting-drug users and women whose sex partners were HIV-infected or at risk for infection). However, several studies have indicated that counseling and testing strategies that offer testing only to those women who report risk factors fail to identify and offer services to many HIV-infected women (i.e., 50%-70% of infected women in some studies). Women may be unaware of their risk for infection if they have unknowingly had sexual contact with an HIV-infected person. Other women may refuse testing to avoid the stigma often associated with high-risk sexual and injecting-drug-use behaviors.

AIDS and Pregnancy

Because of the advances in prevention and treatment of opportunistic infections for HIV-infected adults and children during the past 10 years, several professional organizations have recommended a more widespread approach of offering HIV counseling and testing for pregnant women. This approach can be applied nationally to all pregnant women or to women in limited geographic areas based on the prevalence of HIV infection among childbearing women in those areas. However, a counseling and testing recommendation based on a prevalence threshold (e.g., one HIV-infected woman per 1,000 childbearing women) could delay or discourage implementation of counseling and testing services in areas (e.g., states) where prevalence data are inadequate, outdated, or unavailable, and would miss substantial numbers of HIV-infected pregnant women in areas with lower seroprevalence rates but high numbers of births (e.g., California). A prevalence-based approach also could lead to potentially discriminating testing practices, such as singling out a geographic area or racial/ethnic group. A universal approach of offering HIV counseling and testing to all pregnant women regardless of the prevalence of HIV infection in their community or their risk for infection provides a uniform policy that will reach HIV-infected pregnant women in all populations and geographic areas of the United States. Although this universal approach will necessitate increased resources (e.g., funding), effective implementation of HIV counseling and testing services for pregnant women and the ensuing medical interventions will reduce HIV-related morbidity in women and their infants and could ultimately reduce medical costs.

Counseling and testing policies also must address issues associated with provision of consent for testing. Data from universal routine HIV counseling and voluntary testing programs in several areas indicate that high test-acceptance levels can be achieved without mandating testing. Mandatory testing may increase the potential for negative consequences of HIV testing and result in some women avoiding prenatal care altogether. In addition, mandatory testing may adversely affect the patient-provider relationship by placing the provider in an enforcing rather than facilitating role. Providers must act as facilitators to adequately assist women in making decisions regarding HIV testing and ZDV preventive therapy. Although few studies have addressed the issue of acceptance of HIV testing, higher levels of acceptance have been found in clinics where testing is voluntary but recommended by the health-care provider than in clinics that use a non-directive approach to HIV testing (i.e, patients are told the test is available, but testing is neither encouraged nor discouraged).

Recommendations

The following recommendations have been developed to provide guidance to health-care workers when educating women about HIV infection and the importance of early diagnosis of HIV. The recommendations are based on the advances made in treatment and prevention of HIV infection and stress the need for a universal counseling and voluntary testing program for pregnant women. These recommendations address a) HIV-related information needed by infected and uninfected pregnant women for their own health and that of their infants, b) laboratory considerations involved in HIV testing of this population, and c) the importance of follow-up services for HIV-infected women, their infants, and other family members.

HIV Counseling and Voluntary Testing of Pregnant Women and Their Infants

- Health-care providers should ensure that all pregnant women are counseled and encouraged to be tested for HIV infection to allow women to know their infection status both for their own health and to reduce the risk for perinatal HIV transmission. Counseling should include information regarding the risk for HIV infection associated with sexual activity and injecting-drug use, the risk for transmission to the woman's infant if she is infected, and the availability of therapy to reduce this risk. HIV counseling, including any written materials, should be linguistically, culturally, educationally, and age appropriate for individual patients.

- HIV testing of pregnant women and their infants should be voluntary. Consent for testing should be obtained in accordance with prevailing legal requirements. Women who test positive for HIV or who refuse testing should not be a) denied prenatal or other health-care services, b) reported to child protective service agencies because of refusal to be tested or because of their HIV status, or c) discriminated against in any other way.

- Health-care providers should counsel and offer HIV testing to women as early in pregnancy as possible so that informed and timely therapeutic and reproductive decisions can be made. Specific strategies and resources will be needed to communicate with women who may not obtain prenatal care because of

AIDS and Pregnancy

homelessness, incarceration, undocumented citizenship status, drug or alcohol abuse, or other reasons.

- Uninfected pregnant women who continue to practice high-risk behaviors (e.g., injecting-drug use and unprotected sexual contact with an HIV-infected or high-risk partner) should be encouraged to avoid further exposure to HIV and to be retested for HIV in the third trimester of pregnancy.

- The prevalence of HIV infection may be higher in women who have not received prenatal care. These women should be assessed promptly for HIV infection. Such an assessment should include information regarding prior HIV testing, test results, and risk history. For women who are first identified as being HIV infected during labor and delivery, health-care providers should consider offering intrapartum and neonatal ZDV according to published recommendations. For women whose HIV infection status has not been determined, HIV counseling should be provided and HIV testing offered as soon as the mother's medical condition permits. However, involuntary HIV testing should never be substituted for counseling and voluntary testing.

- Some HIV-infected women do not receive prenatal care, choose not to be tested for HIV, or do not retain custody of their children. If a woman has not been tested for HIV, she should be informed of the benefits to her child's health of knowing her child's infection status and should be encouraged to allow the child to be tested. Counselors should ensure that the mother provides consent with the understanding that a positive HIV test for her child is indicative of infection in herself. For infants whose HIV infection status is unknown and who are in foster care, the person legally authorized to provide consent should be encouraged to allow the infant to be tested (with the consent of the biologic mother, when possible) in accordance with the policies of the organization legally responsible for the child and with prevailing legal requirements for HIV testing.

- Pregnant women should be provided access to other HIV prevention and treatment services (e.g., drug-treatment and partner-notification services) as needed.

Interpretation of HIV Test Results

- HIV antibody testing should be performed according to the recommended algorithm, which includes the use of an EIA to test for antibody to HIV and confirmatory testing with an additional, more specific assay (e.g., Western blot or IFA). All assays should be performed and conducted according to manufacturers' instructions and applicable state and federal laboratory guidelines.

- HIV infection (as indicated by the presence of antibody to HIV) is defined as a repeatedly reactive EIA and a positive confirmatory supplemental test. Confirmation or exclusion of HIV infection in a person with indeterminate test results should be made not only on the basis of HIV antibody test results, but with consideration of a) the person's medical and behavioral history, b) results from additional virologic and immunologic tests when performed, and c) clinical follow-up. Uncertainties regarding HIV infection status, including laboratory test results, should be resolved before final decisions are made concerning pregnancy termination, ZDV therapy, or other interventions.

- Pregnant women who have repeatedly reactive EIA and indeterminate supplemental tests should be retested immediately for HIV antibody to distinguish between recent seroconversion and a negative test result. Additional tests (e.g., viral culture, PCR, or p24 antigen test) to diagnose or exclude HIV infection may be required for women whose test results remain indeterminate—especially women who have behavioral risk factors for HIV, have had recent exposure to HIV, or have clinical symptoms compatible with acute retroviral illness. In such situations, confirmation by an FDA-licensed IFA kit may be helpful because IFA is less likely to yield indeterminate results than Western blot.

- Women who have negative EIAs and those who have repeatedly reactive EIAs but negative supplemental tests should be considered uninfected.

Recommendations for HIV-Infected Pregnant Women

- HIV-infected pregnant women should receive counseling as previously recommended. Post-test HIV counseling should include an explanation of the clinical implications of a positive

AIDS and Pregnancy

HIV antibody test result and the need for, benefit of, and means of access to HIV-related medical and other early intervention services. Such counseling should also include a discussion of the interaction between pregnancy and HIV infection, the risk for perinatal HIV transmission and ways to reduce this risk, and the prognosis for infants who become infected.

- HIV-infected pregnant women should be evaluated according to published recommendations to assess their need for antiretroviral therapy, antimicrobial prophylaxis, and treatment of other conditions. Although medical management of HIV infection is essentially the same for pregnant and nonpregnant women, recommendations for treating a patient who has tuberculosis have been modified for pregnant women because of potential teratogenic effects of specific medications (e.g., streptomycin and pyrazinamide). HIV-infected pregnant women should be evaluated to determine their need for psychological and social services.

- HIV-infected pregnant women should be provided information concerning ZDV therapy to reduce the risk for perinatal HIV transmission. This information should address the potential benefit and short-term safety of ZDV and the uncertainties regarding a) long-term risks of such therapy and b) effectiveness in women who have different clinical characteristics (e.g., CD4+ T-lymphocyte count and previous ZDV use) than women who participated in the trial. HIV-infected pregnant women should not be coerced into making decisions about ZDV therapy. These decisions should be made after consideration of both the benefits and potential risks of the regimen to the woman and her child. A woman's decision not to accept treatment should not result in punitive action or denial of care.

- HIV-infected pregnant women should receive information about all reproductive options. Reproductive counseling should be nondirective. Health-care providers should be aware of the complex issues that HIV-infected women must consider when making decisions about their reproductive options and should be supportive of any decision.

- To reduce the risk for HIV transmission to their infants, HIV-infected women should be advised against breastfeeding.

Support services should be provided when necessary for use of appropriate breast-milk substitutes.

- To optimize medical management, positive and negative HIV test results should be available to a woman's health-care provider and included on both her and her infant's confidential medical records. After obtaining consent, maternal health-care providers should notify the pediatric-care providers of the impending birth of an HIV-exposed child, any anticipated complications, and whether ZDV should be administered after birth. If HIV is first diagnosed in the child, the child's health-care providers should discuss the implication of the child's diagnosis for the woman's health and assist the mother in obtaining care for herself. Providers are encouraged to build supportive healthcare relationships that can facilitate the discussion of pertinent health information. Confidential HIV-related information should be disclosed or shared only in accordance with prevailing legal requirements.

- Counseling for HIV-infected pregnant women should include an assessment of the potential for negative effects resulting from HIV infection (e.g., discrimination, domestic violence, and psychological difficulties). For women who anticipate or experience such effects, counseling also should include a) information on how to minimize these potential consequences, b) assistance in identifying supportive persons within their own social network, and c) referral to appropriate psychological, social, and legal services. In addition, HIV-infected women should be informed that discrimination based on HIV status or AIDS regarding matters—such as housing, employment, state programs, and public accommodations (including physicians' offices and hospitals) is illegal.

- HIV-infected women should be encouraged to obtain HIV testing for any of their children born after they became infected or, if they do not know when they became infected, for children born after 1977. Older children (i.e., children older then 12 years of age) should be tested with informed consent of the parent and assent of the child. Women should be informed that the lack of signs and symptoms suggestive of HIV infection in older children may not indicate lack of HIV infection; some perinatally infected children can remain asymptomatic for several years.

AIDS and Pregnancy

Recommendations for Follow-Up of Infected Women and Perinatally Exposed Children

- Following pregnancy, HIV-infected women should be provided ongoing HIV-related medical care, including immune-function monitoring, anti-retroviral therapy, and prophylaxis for and treatment of opportunistic infections and other HIV-related conditions. HIV-infected women should receive gynecologic care, including regular Pap smears, reproductive counseling, information on how to prevent sexual transmission of HIV, and treatment of gynecologic conditions.

- HIV-infected women (or the guardians of their children) should be informed of the importance of follow-up for their children. These children should receive follow-up care to determine their infection status, to initiate prophylactic therapy to prevent PCP, and, if infected, to determine the need for anti-retroviral and other prophylactic therapy and to monitor disorders in growth and development, which often occur before 24 months of age. HIV-infected children and other children living in households with HIV-infected persons should be vaccinated according to published recommendations for altered schedules.

- Because the identification of an HIV-infected mother also identifies a family that needs or will need medical and social services as her disease progresses, health-care providers should ensure that referrals to these services focus on the needs of the entire family.

For More Information

See Volume 4 of the Health Reference Series. Other sources of information included:

The National Institute of Child Health and Human Development. Telephone (301) 496-5133

The Pediatric AIDS Foundation. Telephone (310) 3995-9051

The National Pediatric HIV Resource Center. Telephone 1-800-362-0071

National AIDS Hotline. Staffed 24 hours a day, 7 days a week. Telephone 1-800-342-AIDS

American Academy of Pediatrics/Pediatric AIDS Coalition. Telephone (202) 662-7460

Section 30.2

Pregnancy and HIV: Is AZT the Right Choice for You and Your Baby?

DHSS Publication No. 96-0007, December 1995

If you know that you have HIV infection, you should:

- Tell your health care provider that you HIV.
- Talk with your doctor or nurse about the risks and benefits for you and your baby if you take AZT.

If you are pregnant and have HIV or AIDS, you may pass the virus to your baby. Taking AZT can lessen the chance that HIV will pass to your baby.

AZT is a medicine used to treat HIV infection. AZT is also called zidovudine or ZDV.

This text talks about the choice you have to take or not take AZT while you are pregnant. It also gives questions to ask your doctor, nurse, or other health care provider. Then you can make up your own mind about what is best for you and your baby.

Babies and HIV Infection

HIV stands for human immunodeficiency virus. HIV causes AIDS. As yet, there is no cure for either HIV or AIDS. Some babies who have HIV become very sick and die in their first year. Others live longer

AIDS and Pregnancy

but may still get sick. A baby can get HIV from an HIV-infected mother in three ways:

1. During pregnancy.
2. During delivery.
3. After delivery through breast feeding.

The chances are about one in four that HIV will pass from a mother to her baby before or during birth. This is only an average. No one can tell you for sure what your baby's chances are.

After delivery, your health care provider will ask for your consent to test your baby for HIV. Many babies can be diagnosed as either HIV-infected or not infected by 6 months of age. In some cases, it takes up to 18 months to know for sure if a baby has HIV.

If you have HIV and are pregnant, the most important thing you can do is to see your health care provider early and often during your pregnancy.

What You Should Know About AZT

AZT is one of the medicines that work against HIV. AZT may slow down the virus and the effects it has on your body.

Many people who have HIV feel better while taking AZT. Sometimes AZT causes problems such as upset stomach, anemia (low blood), headache, or muscle soreness. These problems usually go away when AZT is stopped or the dose is lowered. Talk to your health care provider.

What We Have Learned About Babies and AZT

You may have heard about a research study by the National Institutes of Health called the 076 study. 076 is the number NIH gave to the study. The 076 study found that women with HIV who took AZT were much less likely to pass the virus to their babies.

Here are the facts:

- More than 500 pregnant women with HIV took part in the study.
- Half of the mothers and babies did not take AZT.
- The other half of the women took AZT, and their babies were given AZT for 6 weeks after they were born.
- Three of every 12 babies born to women who did not take AZT got HIV.
- One of every 12 babies born to mothers who took AZT got HIV.

About the women in the AZT Study

The women in the AZT study:

- Began prenatal care early.
- Had HIV and began the study between 14 weeks (3 1/2 months) and 34 weeks (8 1/2 months) of pregnancy.
- Were 15 to 43 years old (average age 25).
- Were African-American (about 50 percent of the women), Hispanic (about 33 percent), and white (about 17 percent).
- Had not taken AZT for their own health before the study.
- Had T-cell counts over 200 at the start of the study. More than half had T-cell counts over 500.

What Are T Cells?

T cells are white blood cells that protect the body from "germs" such as viruses and bacteria. T cells are also called T-helper cells and CD4 cells.

When HIV enters the body, it infects the T cells. The virus kills these cells slowly. As more and more T cells die, the body loses its ability to fight infection.

Counting the number of T cells in a person's blood is one way to find out how well the person's body can fight infection. A normal T-cell count is about 1,000.

Questions and Answers About the AZT Study

1. *How was AZT given to the women and babies in the study?*

The women and babies in the 076 study took AZT in three stages:

- During pregnancy: The women took one AZT pill five times each day.
- During labor and delivery: The women were given AZT through an IV.
- Right after birth: The babies were given AZT syrup four times a day for 6 weeks.

2. *Did AZT cause problems for the women?*

Taking AZT did not seem to make the women in this study any sicker than the women who did not take AZT. Studies are being done to see if the women have any long-term problems.

AIDS and Pregnancy

3. Did AZT cause problems for the babies?

AZT did not cause any serious problems for the babies in the 076 study.

- AZT did not cause birth defects or cause babies to be born early.
- Babies born to women who did and did not take AZT were about the same size.
- Some of the AZT babies became anemic. The anemia went away soon after AZT was stopped.
- Babies born to women in both groups have been followed to at least 1 year of age. Growth and development are about the same for all babies.
- Studies are being done to see if AZT causes any long-term problems for the babies.

4. What do these results mean for me?

The results of the AZT study are very hopeful. But, we do not know if AZT will work the same for women and babies who are not like the women and babies in the study.

5. Is there anything else I can do?

- Do not breast feed your baby. HIV can pass to your baby through breast milk.
- Your baby should be given a medicine when he or she is 4 to 6 weeks old to help prevent pneumonia.

Other Studies Are in Progress

- Studies are underway to see if other methods will lower the chances that HIV will pass from mothers to babies.
- It is too soon to know if these methods will work.
- To find out more about this research, call 1-800-TRIALS-A (1-800-874-2572).

Talking With Your Health Care Provider

Here are some questions to ask your health care provider about using AZT:

1. Could AZT help me and my baby?
2. Will AZT make me or my baby sick?

3. What if I am taking other medicines?
4. What if I use drugs or alcohol?
5. Will I need to keep taking AZT after I have my baby?
6. When will I know if my baby has HIV?
7. What if I need to take AZT later on for myself?
8. How will I pay for my care?

Thinking About AZT

Here are some important points to keep in mind as you make a decision about using AZT:

- HIV can be passed from mother to baby.
- Babies who are infected with HIV may become very sick. Some may die during their first year of life.
- With AZT you can lower the chance that you baby will get HIV.
- With AZT the chance that your baby will get HIV is lowered from about 3 out of 12 (25 percent) to 1 out of 12 (8 percent).
- Even if you take AZT, there is a small chance that your baby might get the virus.
- Taking AZT may cause anemia in your baby. The anemia will go away after the AZT is stopped.
- In the 076 study, AZT did not cause birth defects or problems in the growth or development of babies during the first year of life.
- Although AZT does not appear to cause any short-term problems for mothers or babies, no one knows if there will be any long-term problems.

You Can Find Out More

Call the HIV/AIDS Treatment Information Service:

1-800-448-0440 (English and Spanish)
1-800-243-7012 (TTY/TDD)

You may qualify for Medicaid. Ask how you can find out more about Medicaid. Or, you can write to:

Pregnancy and HIV
CDC National AIDS Clearinghouse
P.O. Box 6003
Rockville, MD 20849-6003

Part Seven

Disorders of Pregnancy

Chapter 31

Ectopic Pregnancy

Chapter Contents

Section 31.1—Ectopic Pregnancy Explained 538
Section 31.2—Ectopic Pregnancy in the United
 States, 1990-1992 542

Section 31.1

Ectopic Pregnancy Explained

Reprinted by permission of William Morrow & Company, Inc. from *Mayo Clinic Complete Book of Pregnancy and Baby's First Year.* Copyright 1994 by Mayo Foundation for Medical Education and Research

An ectopic pregnancy is one in which the fertilized egg attaches itself in a place other than inside the uterus. Almost all (more than 95 percent) ectopic pregnancies occur in a fallopian tube; hence the term "tubal" pregnancy. Rarely, the egg may implant elsewhere, such as in the abdomen, ovary or cervix.

Because the narrow fallopian tubes are not designed to hold a growing embryo, the fertilized egg in a tubal pregnancy cannot develop normally. Eventually, the thin walls of the tube stretch to the point of bursting. If this happens, a woman is in danger of life-threatening blood loss (hemorrhage).

During the 1980s, the rate of ectopic pregnancy increased. Ectopic pregnancy now occurs in about seven of every 1,000 reported pregnancies in the United States. Even so, death from ectopic pregnancy is rare, occurring in fewer than one of every 2,500 cases. This low rate is largely a result of new techniques to detect ectopic pregnancy at an early stage, when the risk to the pregnant woman is much lower.

What causes it and who's at risk?

Most cases of ectopic pregnancy are caused by an inability of the fertilized egg to make its way through a fallopian tube into the uterus. This is often caused by an infection or inflammation of the tube which has caused it to become partly or entirely blocked. Scar tissue left behind from a previous infection or an operation on the tube may also impede the egg's movement. Previous surgery in the pelvic area or on the tubes can also cause adhesions (bands of tissue that bind together surfaces inside the abdomen or the tubes). A condition called endometriosis, in which tissue like that normally lining the uterus is

Ectopic Pregnancy

found outside the uterus, can also cause blockage of a fallopian tube. Another possible cause is an abnormality in the shape of the tube, which may be caused by abnormal growths or a birth defect.

Most ectopic pregnancies occur in women 35 to 44 years of age. The major risk factor for ectopic pregnancy is pelvic inflammatory disease (PID). This is an infection of the uterus, fallopian tubes or ovaries. The risk of ectopic pregnancy is also higher in women who have had any of the following:

- Previous ectopic pregnancy
- Surgery on a fallopian tube
- Several induced abortions
- Infertility problems or medication to stimulate ovulation

What are the symptoms?

In many cases, a pregnant woman and her doctor may not at first have any reason to suspect an ectopic pregnancy. The early signs of pregnancy, such as a missed period and other symptoms and signs, also occur in ectopic pregnancies.

Pain is usually the first sign of an ectopic pregnancy. The pain may be in the pelvis, abdomen or even the shoulder and neck (due to blood from a ruptured ectopic pregnancy building up under the diaphragm). Pain from an ectopic pregnancy is usually described as sharp and stabbing. It may come and go or vary in intensity.

Other warning signs of ectopic pregnancy include:

- Vaginal bleeding
- Gastrointestinal symptoms
- Dizziness or light-headedness

Although there may be other reasons for any of these symptoms, they should be reported to your doctor.

How is it diagnosed?

If your doctor suspects an ectopic pregnancy, she or he will probably first perform a pelvic exam to locate pain, tenderness or a mass in the abdomen. Lab tests may then be ordered. The most useful of these is the measurement of hCG. In a normal pregnancy, the level of this hormone approximately doubles about every two days during the first 10 weeks. In an ectopic pregnancy, however, the rate of this increase is much slower. An hCG level that is lower than what would be expected for the stage of the pregnancy is one reason to suspect an ectopic pregnancy.

The hCG level may be tested several times over a certain period to determine whether it is increasing at a normal rate. Progesterone is another hormone that can be measured to help in the diagnosis of ectopic pregnancy. Low levels of this hormone may indicate that a pregnancy is abnormal. Further tests will be needed to confirm whether the pregnancy is ectopic and, if it is, where it is located.

Ultrasound exams may also be used to help determine whether a pregnancy is ectopic. With this technique, a device called a transducer, which emits high-frequency sound waves, is moved over the abdomen or inserted into the vagina. The sound waves bounce off internal organs and create an image that can be viewed on a TV-like screen. With this procedure, your doctor may be able to see whether the uterus contains a developing fetus.

A procedure called culdocentesis is occasionally used to aid in diagnosing ectopic pregnancy. This technique involves inserting a needle into the space at the very top of the vagina, behind the uterus and in front of the rectum. The presence of blood in this area may indicate bleeding from a ruptured fallopian tube.

What's the treatment?

Treatment of ectopic pregnancy usually consists of surgery to remove the abnormal pregnancy. Surgery is generally scheduled soon after an ectopic pregnancy is diagnosed. At one time, a major operation was needed for ectopic pregnancy. General anesthesia was used, and the pelvic area was opened with a large incision. Now, however, it is often possible to remove an ectopic pregnancy with a less extensive technique called laparoscopy.

In this procedure, a small incision is made in the lower abdomen, near or in the navel. The surgeon then inserts a long, thin instrument, called a laparoscope, into the pelvic area. This instrument is a hollow tube with a light on one end. Through it, the internal organs can be viewed and other instruments can be inserted. Sometimes a second small incision is made in the lower abdomen, through which surgical instruments can be placed. The laparoscope allows the surgeon to remove the ectopic pregnancy and repair or remove the affected fallopian tube. Laparoscopy may be performed possibly with local anesthesia but more likely with regional or general anesthesia.

Ectopic Pregnancy

A fallopian tube that has ruptured from an ectopic pregnancy usually must be removed. Less extensive surgery can be done if the ectopic pregnancy has been found early, before the tube has been stretched too much or has burst. In these instances, it may be possible to remove the ectopic pregnancy and repair the tube, allowing it to continue to function.

Occasionally, a medication called methotrexate can be used to dissolve an ectopic pregnancy. This medication may be used either with or without laparoscopy, depending on how far the pregnancy has developed.

What about the future?

After treatment for an ectopic pregnancy, your doctor will want to see you on a regular basis to recheck your hCG level until it reaches zero. An hCG level that remains high could indicate that the ectopic tissue was not entirely removed. If this is the case, you may need additional surgery or medical management with methotrexate.

The outlook for future pregnancies after an ectopic pregnancy depends mainly on the extent of the surgery that was done. Although the chances of having a successful pregnancy are lower if you've had an ectopic pregnancy, they are still good—perhaps as high as 60 percent—if the fallopian tube has been spared. Even if one fallopian tube has been removed, an egg can be fertilized in the other tube. The chances of having a successful pregnancy with one tube removed may be more than 40 percent.

If you've had one ectopic pregnancy, though, you're more likely to have another one. And the risk increases with the number of ectopic pregnancies. If you've had an ectopic pregnancy, talk to your doctor before becoming pregnant again so that together you can plan your care.

Section 31.2

Ectopic Pregnancy in the United States, 1990-1992

Morbidity and Mortality Weekly Report, January 27, 1995

Ectopic pregnancy is the leading cause of pregnancy-related death during the first trimester. Women who have one ectopic pregnancy are at increased risk for another such pregnancy and for future infertility. In the United States, the reported number of hospitalizations for ectopic pregnancy increased from 17,800 in 1970 to 88,400 in 1989. This report summarizes trends in hospitalizations for ectopic pregnancy in the United States during 1990-1992 and presents the incidence of ectopic pregnancy in 1992, based on aggregated inpatient and outpatient data.

Data about hospitalizations for ectopic pregnancy were obtained from CDC's National Hospital Discharge Survey (NHDS), a national probability sample of inpatient admissions to non-institutional general and short-stay hospitals (excluding federal, military, and Veterans Administration hospitals). Data for outpatient diagnosis and treatment of ectopic pregnancy were obtained from CDC's National Hospital Ambulatory Medical Care Survey (NHAMCS), a national probability sample of visits to the emergency and outpatient departments of hospitals with the same characteristics as those sampled in NHDS. Because the actual numbers of ectopic pregnancy in NHAMCS were insufficient to provide a reliable point estimate, data from NHAMCS and NHDS were combined to create an aggregate estimate of ectopic pregnancies treated in both inpatient and outpatient settings in 1992. Data for women treated as outpatients who were subsequently admitted to the hospital were excluded from the combined estimate to avoid double counting. Data were weighted to represent the U.S. civilian, non-institutionalized population, and 95% confidence intervals (CIs) were calculated using standard errors generated by SUDAAN.

Based on NHDS, the estimated number of hospitalizations for ectopic pregnancy in 1990 was 64,400 (95% CI=54,100-74,800) (rate:

Ectopic Pregnancy

11.4 per 1000 reported pregnancies i.e., ectopic, legal abortions, and live births); in 1991, 55,600 (95% CI=45,800-65,500) (rate: 10.0); and in 1992, 58,200 (95% CI=48,600-67,700) (rate: 10.6).

Based on aggregated data from NHDS and NHAMCS, the estimated total number of ectopic pregnancies in 1992 was 108,800 (95% CI=83,600-134,000) (rate: 19.7 per 1000 reported pregnancies) (Figure 31.1).

In 1992, ectopic pregnancies accounted for approximately 2% of reported pregnancies, and ectopic pregnancy-related deaths accounted for 9% of all pregnancy-related deaths. The findings in this report indicate that, for 1992, the estimated total number of ectopic pregnancies, based on aggregated NHDS and NHAMCS data, was 47% higher than that based on hospitalizations only. Analysis of the estimated number of ectopic pregnancies, based only on hospitalizations, indicates a decline since the late 1980s. This decline may reflect the shift toward treating ectopic pregnancy in an outpatient setting. This

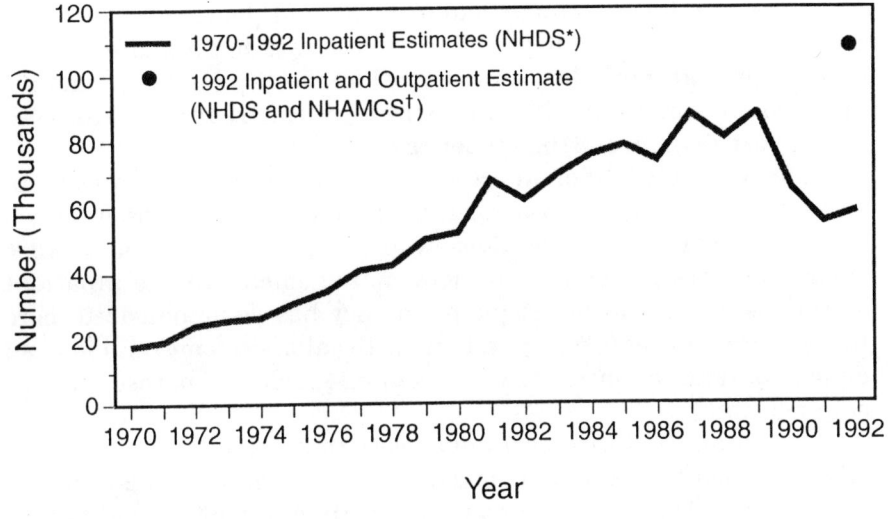

*National Hospital Discharge Survey.
†National Hospital Ambulatory Medical Care Survey.

Figure 31.1. Number of Ectopic Pregnancies—United States, 1990-1992

hypothesis is supported by the estimated total number of ectopic pregnancies, which suggests that incidence—instead of declining in the late 1980s—may have increased steadily since 1970. The increased occurrence of ectopic pregnancy in the United States is consistent with the trend in increased prevalence of important risk factors for ectopic pregnancy, including chlamydia and other sexually transmitted infections, induction of ovulation, and tubal sterilization.

This report is the first to document the incidence of ectopic pregnancy by including information about patients managed and treated on an outpatient basis. Although the addition of the outpatient reports has substantially improved the accuracy of this estimate for 1992, the NHAMCS database does not include patients examined and treated exclusively in physician offices. Therefore, the estimates in this report may underestimate the true incidence of ectopic pregnancy in the United States in 1992.

Outpatient management of ectopic pregnancy—which was first reported in 1987—is believed to have increased in association with the early detection of unruptured ectopic pregnancies as the result of sensitive radioimmunoassays for human chorionic gonadotropin and high-resolution transvaginal ultrasound. Outpatient treatment may include laparoscopic salpingectomy or salpingostomy, or methotrexate therapy. In particular, outpatient pharmacologic treatment of ectopic pregnancy with methotrexate has resulted in decreased patient morbidity, a preservation of reproductive capability, and—when compared with inpatient surgical treatment—an estimated cost savings of $10,000 per case.

Approximately half of all ectopic pregnancies reported in 1992 involved hospitalization. However, it is unknown whether these women required hospitalization because of more severe disease or because their providers preferred inpatient management. In the inpatient setting, management of ectopic pregnancy has de-emphasized more invasive procedures (e.g., laparotomy with salpingectomy) and instead emphasized more conservative procedures, such as laparoscopy with salpingostomy.

The findings in this report underscore that surveillance and other efforts to monitor national trends in ectopic pregnancy must include women who are treated or managed in both inpatient and outpatient settings. Despite substantial improvements in diagnosis and treatment of ectopic pregnancy, strategies to prevent this condition are needed. Other priorities include increased characterization of risk factors and etiology, and development and implementation of effective interventions.

References

Goldner TE, Lawson HW, Xia Z, Atrash HK. Surveillance for ectopic pregnancy—United States, 1970-1989. In: CDC surveillance summaries (December). MMWR 1993;42(no. SS-6): 73-85.

Cunningham FG, MacDonald PC, Gant NF, Leveno KJ, Gilstrap LC. Williams obstetrics. 19th ed. Norwalk, Connecticut: Appleton-Century Crofts, 1993: 706.

NCHS. Advanced report of final mortality statistics, 1992. Hyattsville, Maryland: US Department of Health and Human Services, Public Health Service, CDC,1994. (Monthly vital statistics report; vol 43, no. 6, suppl).

CDC. Sexually transmitted disease surveillance, 1992. Atlanta: US Department of Health and Human Services, Public Health Service, CDC, July 1993.

Churgay CA, Apgar BS. Ectopic pregnancy: an update on technologic advances in diagnosis and treatment. Prim Care 1993; 20: 629-38.

Loffer FD. Outpatient management of ectopic pregnancies. Am J Obstet Gynecol 1987;156: 1467-72.

Ory SJ. New options for diagnosis and treatment of ectopic pregnancy. JAMA 1992; 267:534-7.

Carson SA, Buster JE. Ectopic pregnancy. N Engl J Med 1993;329: 1174-81.

Stovall TG, Ling FW, Buster JE. Outpatient chemotherapy of unruptured ectopic pregnancy. Fertil Steril 1989;51: 435-8.

Crenin MD, Washington AE. Cost of ectopic pregnancy management: surgery versus methotrexate. Fertil Steril 1993; 60: 963-9.

Chapter 32

Molar Pregnancy

What Is Molar Pregnancy?

Gestational trophoblastic tumor (molar pregnancy), a rare cancer in women, is a disease in which cancer (malignant) cells grow in the tissues that are formed following conception (the joining of sperm and egg). Gestational trophoblastic tumors start inside the uterus, the hollow, muscular, pear-shaped organ where a baby grows. This type of cancer occurs in women during the years when they are able to have children. There are two types of gestational trophoblastic tumors: hydatidiform mole and choriocarcinoma.

If you have hydatidiform mole (also called molar pregnancy), the sperm and egg cells have joined, but there is no baby developing in the uterus. Instead, the tissue that is formed resembles grape-like cysts. Hydatidiform mole does not spread outside of the uterus to other parts of the body.

If you have choriocarcinoma, the tumor may have started from a hydatidiform mole or from tissue that remains in the uterus following an abortion or delivery of a baby. Choriocarcinoma can spread from the uterus to other parts of the body. A very rare type of gestational trophoblastic tumor starts in the uterus where the placenta was attached. This type of cancer is called placental-site trophoblastic disease.

Gestational trophoblastic tumor is not always easy to find. In its early stages, it may look like a normal pregnancy. You should see your

---

NCI Cancerfax 208/01163.

doctor if you have bleeding from the vagina, if your uterus gets bigger after you have given birth or had an abortion, or if you are pregnant and you do not feel the baby move at the expected time.

If you have symptoms, your doctor may use several tests to see if you have gestational trophoblastic tumor, usually beginning by giving you an internal (pelvic) exam. Your doctor will feel for any lumps or strange feeling in the shape or size of the uterus. Your doctor may then do an ultrasound, a test that uses sound waves to find tumors. A blood test will also be done to look for high levels of a hormone called beta HCG (beta human chorionic gonadotropin). This hormone is present during normal pregnancy, but if you are not pregnant and the hormone is still found in your blood, it can be a sign of gestational trophoblastic tumor.

Your chance of recovery (prognosis) and choice of treatment depend on the type of gestational trophoblastic tumor you have, whether it has spread to other places, and your general state of health.

Stages of Gestational Trophoblastic Tumor

Once gestational trophoblastic tumor has been found, more tests will be done to find out if the cancer has spread from inside the uterus to other parts of the body (staging). Your doctor needs to know the stage of your disease to plan treatment. The following stages are used for gestational trophoblastic tumor:

- **Hydatidiform mole.** Cancer is found only in the space inside the uterus. If the cancer is found in the muscle of the uterus, it is called an invasive mole (choriocarcinoma destruens).

- **Placental-site gestational trophoblastic tumor.** Cancer is found in the place where the placenta was attached and in the muscle of the uterus.

- **Non-metastatic.** Cancer cells have grown inside the uterus from tissue remaining following treatment of a hydatidiform mole or following an abortion or delivery of a baby. Cancer has not spread outside the uterus.

- **Metastatic, good prognosis.** Cancer cells have grown inside the uterus from tissue remaining following treatment of a hydatidiform mole or following an abortion or delivery of a baby. The cancer has spread from the uterus to other parts of the

Molar Pregnancy

body. Metastatic gestational trophoblastic tumors are considered good prognosis or poor prognosis.

Metastatic gestational trophoblastic tumor is considered good prognosis if all of the following are true:

1. Your last pregnancy was less than 4 months ago.
2. The level of beta HCG in your blood is low.
3. Cancer has not spread to your liver or brain.
4. You have not received chemotherapy earlier.

- **Metastatic, poor prognosis.** Cancer cells have grown inside the uterus from tissue remaining following treatment of a hydatidiform mole or following an abortion or delivery of a baby. The cancer has spread from the uterus to other parts of the body.

Metastatic gestational trophoblastic tumor is considered poor prognosis if any the following are true:

1. Your last pregnancy was more than 4 months ago.
2. The level of beta HCG in your blood is high.
3. Cancer has spread to your liver or brain.
4. You have received chemotherapy earlier and the cancer did not go away.
5. The tumor began after you completed a normal pregnancy.

- **Recurrent.** Recurrent disease means that the cancer has come back (recurred) after it has been treated. It may come back in the uterus or in another part of the body.

Treatment Options Overview

How Gestational Trophoblastic Tumor Is Treated

There are treatments for all patients with gestational trophoblastic tumor. Two kinds of treatment are used: surgery (taking out the cancer) and chemotherapy (using drugs to kill cancer cells). Radiation therapy (using high-energy x-rays to kill cancer cells) may be used in certain cases to treat cancer that has spread to other parts of the body.

Your doctor may take out the cancer using one of the following operations:

- Dilation and curettage (D & C) with suction evacuation is stretching the opening of the uterus (the cervix) and removing the material inside the uterus with a small vacuum-like device. The walls of the uterus are then scraped gently to remove any material that may remain in the uterus. This is used only for molar pregnancies.

- Hysterectomy is an operation to take out the uterus. In the treatment of this disease, the ovaries usually are not removed.

- Chemotherapy uses drugs to kill cancer cells. It may be taken by pill or put into the body by a needle in a vein or muscle. It is called a systemic treatment because the drugs enter the bloodstream, travel through the body, and can kill cancer cells outside the uterus. Chemotherapy may be given before or after surgery or alone.

- Radiation therapy uses high-energy x-rays to kill cancer cells and shrink tumors. Radiation may come from a machine outside the body (external beam radiation therapy) or from putting materials that produce radiation (radioisotopes) through thin plastic tubes into the area where the cancer cells are found (internal radiation).

Treatment by Stage

Treatment of gestational trophoblastic tumor depends on the stage of your disease, your age, and your overall condition.

You may receive treatment that is considered standard based on its effectiveness in a number of patients in past studies, or you may choose to go into a clinical trial. Not all patients are cured with standard therapy and some standard treatments may have more side effects than are desired. For these reasons, clinical trials are designed to find better ways to treat cancer patients and are based on the most up-to-date information.

Hydatidiform Mole. Your treatment my be one of the following:

- Removal of the mole using dilation and curettage (D & C) and suction evacuation.

- Surgery to remove the uterus (hysterectomy).

Molar Pregnancy

- Following surgery, your doctor will follow you closely with regular blood tests to make sure the level of beta HCG in your blood falls to normal levels. If the blood level of beta HCG increases or does not go down to normal, you will have more tests to see whether the tumor has spread. Your treatment will then depend on whether you have non-metastatic disease or metastatic disease (see the treatment sections on metastatic or non-metastatic disease).

Placental-Site Gestational Trophoblastic Tumor. Your treatment will probably be surgery to remove the uterus (hysterectomy).

Non-Metastatic Gestational Trophoblastic Tumor. Your treatment may be one of the following:

- Chemotherapy.
- Surgery to remove the uterus (hysterectomy) if you no longer wish to have children.

Good Prognosis Metastatic Gestational Trophoblastic Tumor. Your treatment may be one of the following:

- Chemotherapy
- Surgery to remove the uterus (hysterectomy) followed by chemotherapy.
- Chemotherapy followed by hysterectomy if cancer remains following chemotherapy.

Poor Prognosis Metastatic Gestational Trophoblastic Tumor. Your treatment will probably be chemotherapy. Radiation therapy may also be given to places where the cancer has spread, such as the brain.

Recurrent Gestational Trophoblastic Tumor. Your treatment will probably be chemotherapy.

Chapter 33

Understanding Gestational Diabetes

(For the purpose of this text the words sugar and glucose are used synonymously.)

Approximately 3 to 5 percent of all pregnant women in the United States are diagnosed as having gestational diabetes. These women and their families have many questions about this disorder. Some of the most frequently asked questions are: What is gestational diabetes and how did I get it? How does it differ from other kinds of diabetes? Will it hurt my baby? Will my baby have diabetes? What can I do to control gestational diabetes? Will I need a special diet? Will gestational diabetes change the way or the time my baby is delivered? Will I have diabetes in the future?

This text will address these and many other questions about diet, exercise, measurement of blood sugar levels, and general medical and obstetric care of women with gestational diabetes. It must be emphasized that these are general guidelines and only your health care professional(s) can tailor a program specific to your needs. You should feel free to discuss any concerns you have with your doctor or other health care provider, as no one knows more about you and the condition of your pregnancy.

What is gestational diabetes and what causes it?

Diabetes (actual name is diabetes mellitus) of any kind is a disorder that prevents the body from using food properly. Normally, the

---

NIH Publication No. 93-2788, February 1993

body gets its major source of energy from glucose, a simple sugar that comes from foods high in simple carbohydrates (e.g., table sugar or other sweeteners such as honey, molasses, jams, and jellies, soft drinks, and cookies), or from the breakdown of complex carbohydrates such as starches (e.g., bread, potatoes, and pasta). After sugars and starches are digested in the stomach, they enter the blood stream in the form of glucose (see Figure 33.1).

The glucose in the blood stream becomes a potential source of energy for the entire body, similar to the way in which gasoline in a service station pump is a potential source of energy for your car. But, just as someone must pump the gas into the car, the body requires some assistance to get glucose from the blood stream to the muscles and other tissues of the body. In the body, that assistance comes from a hormone called insulin. Insulin is manufactured by the pancreas, a gland that lies behind the stomach. Without insulin, glucose cannot get into the cells of the body where it is used as fuel. Instead, glucose accumulates in the blood to high levels and is excreted or "spilled" into the urine through the kidneys.

When the pancreas of a child or young adult produces little or no insulin we call this condition juvenile-onset diabetes or Type I diabetes

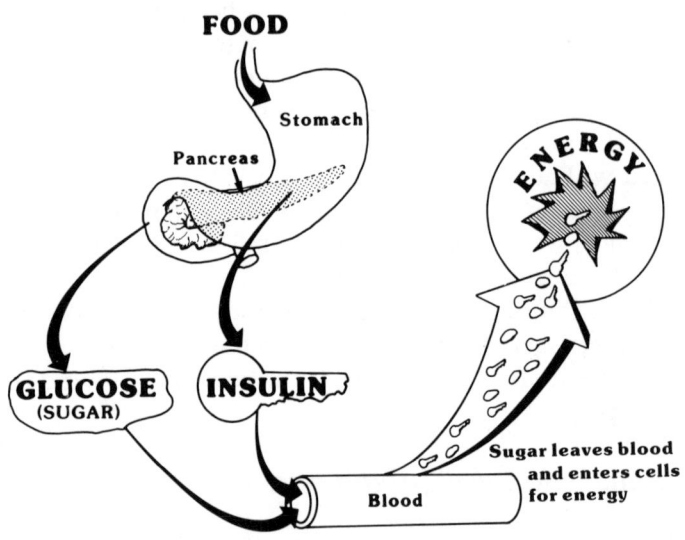

Figure 33.1. Insulin: The Key to Turning Food into Energy

Understanding Gestational Diabetes

(insulin-dependent). This is not the type of diabetes you have. Unlike women with Type I diabetes, women with gestational diabetes have plenty of insulin. In fact, they usually have more insulin in their blood than women who are not pregnant. However, the effect of their insulin is partially blocked by a variety of other hormones made in the placenta, a condition often called insulin resistance.

The placenta performs the task of supplying the growing fetus with nutrients and water from the mother's circulation. It also produces a variety of hormones vital to the preservation of the pregnancy. Ironically, several of these hormones such as estrogen, cortisol, and human placental lactogen (HPL) have a blocking effect on insulin, a "contra-insulin" effect. This contra-insulin effect usually begins about midway (20 to 24 weeks) through pregnancy. The larger the placenta grows, the more these hormones are produced, and the greater the insulin resistance becomes. In most women the pancreas is able to make additional insulin to overcome the insulin resistance. When the pancreas makes all the insulin it can and there still isn't enough to overcome the effect of the placenta's hormones, gestational diabetes results. If we could somehow remove all the placenta's hormones from the mother's blood, the condition would be remedied. This, in fact, usually happens following delivery.

How does gestational diabetes differ from other types of diabetes?

There are several different types of diabetes. Gestational diabetes begins during pregnancy and disappears following delivery. Another type is referred to as juvenile-onset diabetes (in children) or Type I (in young adults). These individuals usually develop their disease before age 20. People with Type I diabetes must take insulin by injection every day. Approximately 10 percent of all people with diabetes have Type I (also called insulin-dependent diabetes).

Type II diabetes or noninsulin-dependent diabetes (formerly called adult-onset diabetes) is also characterized by high blood sugar levels, but these patients are often obese and usually lack the classic symptoms (fatigue, thirst, frequent urination, and sudden weight loss) associated with Type I diabetes. Many of these individuals can control their blood sugar levels by following a careful diet and exercise program, by losing excess weight, or by taking oral medication. Some, but not all, need insulin. People with Type II diabetes account for roughly 90 percent of all diabetics.

Who is at risk for developing gestational diabetes and how is it detected?

Any woman might develop gestational diabetes during pregnancy. Some of the factors associated with women who have an increased risk are:

- obesity
- a family history of diabetes
- having given birth previously to a very large infant, a stillbirth, or a child with a birth defect
- having too much amniotic fluid (polyhydramnios).

Also, women who are older than 25 are at greater risk than younger individuals. Although a history of sugar in the urine is often included in the list of risk factors, this is not a reliable indicator of who will develop diabetes during pregnancy. Some pregnant women with perfectly normal blood sugar levels will occasionally have sugar detected in their urine.

The Council on Diabetes in Pregnancy of the American Diabetes Association strongly recommends that all pregnant women be screened for gestational diabetes. Several methods of screening exist. The most common is the 50-gram glucose screening test. No special preparation is necessary for this test, and there is no need to fast before the test. The test is performed by giving 50 grams of a glucose drink and then measuring the blood sugar level 1-hour later. A woman with a blood sugar level of less than 140 milligrams per deciliter (mg/dl) at l-hour is presumed not to have gestational diabetes and requires no further testing. If the blood sugar level is greater than 140 mg/dl the test is considered abnormal or "positive." Not all women with a positive screening test have diabetes. Consequently, a 3-hour glucose tolerance test must be performed to establish the diagnosis of gestational diabetes.

If your physician determines that you should take the complete 3-hour glucose tolerance test, you will be asked to follow some special instructions in preparation for the test. For 3 days before the test, eat a diet that contains at least 150 grams of carbohydrates each day. This can be accomplished by including one cup of pasta, two servings of fruit, four slices of bread, and three glasses of milk every day. For 10 to 14 hours before the test you should not eat and not drink anything but water. The test is usually done in the morning in your physician's office or in a laboratory. First, a blood sample will be drawn to measure

Understanding Gestational Diabetes

your fasting blood sugar level. Then you will be asked to drink a full bottle of a glucose drink (100 grams). This glucose drink is extremely sweet and occasionally makes some people feel nauseated. Finally, blood samples will be drawn every hour for 3 hours after the glucose drink has been consumed. The normal values for this test are shown in Figure 33.2.

If two or more of your blood sugar levels are higher than the diagnostic criteria, you have gestational diabetes. This testing is usually performed at the end of the second trimester or the beginning of the third trimester (between the 24th and 28th weeks of pregnancy) when insulin resistance usually begins. If you had gestational diabetes in a previous pregnancy or there is some reason why your physician is unusually concerned about your risk of developing gestational diabetes you may be asked to take the 50-gram glucose screening test as early as the first trimester (before the 13th week). Remember, merely having sugar in your urine or even having an abnormal blood sugar on the 50-gram glucose screening test does not necessarily mean you have gestational diabetes. The 3-hour glucose tolerance test must be abnormal before the diagnosis is made.

	Diagnostic Criteria Blood Glucose Level	Normal Mean Values* Blood Glucose Level
Fasting	105 mg/dl	80 mg/dl
1 hour	190 mg/dl	120 mg/dl
2 hour	165 mg/dl	105 mg/dl
3 hour	145 mg/dl	90 mg/dl

From 752 Unselected Pregnancies

Table 33.2. *3-Hour Glucose Tolerance Test for Gestational Diabetes. *Normal Mean Values from O'Sullivan J.B. Establishing Criteria for Gestational Diabetes.* Diabetes Care *3: 437-439, 1980.*

How does gestational diabetes affect pregnancy and will it hurt my baby?

The complications of gestational diabetes are manageable and preventable. The key to prevention is careful control of blood sugar levels just as soon as the diagnosis of gestational diabetes is made.

You should be reassured that there are certain things gestational diabetes does not usually cause. Unlike Type I diabetes, gestational diabetes generally does not cause birth defects. For the most part, birth defects originate sometime during the first trimester (before the 13th week) of pregnancy. The insulin resistance from the contra-insulin hormones produced by the placenta does not usually occur until approximately the 24th week. Therefore, women with gestational diabetes generally have normal blood sugar levels during the critical first trimester.

One of the major problems a woman with gestational diabetes faces is a condition the baby may develop called "macrosomia" Macrosomia means "large body" and refers to a baby that is considerably larger than normal. All of the nutrients the fetus receives come directly from the mother's blood. If the maternal blood has too much glucose, the pancreas of the fetus senses the high glucose levels and produces more insulin in an attempt to use the glucose. The fetus converts the extra glucose to fat. Even when the mother has gestational diabetes, the fetus is able to produce all the insulin it needs. The combination of high blood glucose levels from the mother and high insulin levels in the fetus results in large deposits of fat which causes the fetus to grow excessively large, a condition known as macrosomia. Occasionally, the baby grows too large to be delivered through the vagina and a cesarean delivery becomes necessary. The obstetrician can often determine if the fetus is macrosomic by doing a physical examination. However,

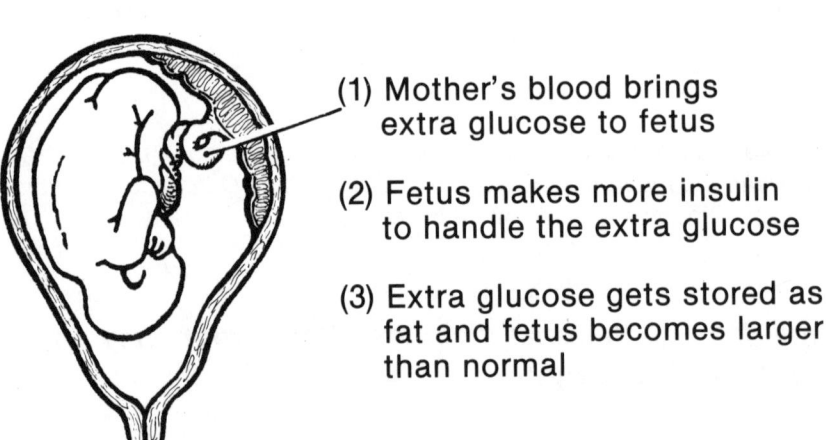

Figure 33.3. The Role of Maternal Glucose in Fetal Macrosomia.

Understanding Gestational Diabetes

in many cases a special test called an ultrasound is used to measure the size of the fetus. This and other special tests will be discussed later.

In addition to macrosomia, gestational diabetes increases the risk of hypoglycemia (low blood sugar) in the baby immediately after delivery. This problem occurs if the mother's blood sugar levels have been consistently high causing the fetus to have a high level of insulin in its circulation. After delivery the baby continues to have a high insulin level, but it no longer has the high level of sugar from its mother, resulting in the newborn's blood sugar level becoming very low. Your baby's blood sugar level will be checked in the newborn nursery and if the level is too low, it may be necessary to give the baby glucose intravenously. Infants of mothers with gestational diabetes are also vulnerable to several other chemical imbalances such as low serum calcium and low serum magnesium levels.

All of these are manageable and preventable problems. The key to prevention is careful control of blood sugar levels in the mother just as soon as the diagnosis of gestational diabetes is made. By maintaining normal blood sugar levels, it is less likely that a fetus will develop macrosomia, hypoglycemia, or other chemical abnormalities.

What can be done to reduce problems associated with gestational diabetes?

In addition to your obstetrician, there are other health professionals who specialize in the management of diabetes during pregnancy including internists or diabetologists, registered dietitians, qualified nutritionists, and diabetes educators. Your doctor may recommend that you see one or more of these specialists during your pregnancy. In addition, a neonatologist (a doctor who specializes in the care of newborn infants) should also be called in to manage any complications the baby might develop after delivery.

One of the essential components in the care of a woman with gestational diabetes is a diet specifically tailored to provide adequate nutrition to meet the needs of the mother and the growing fetus. At the same time the diet has to be planned in such a way as to keep blood glucose levels in the normal range (60 to 120 mg/dl). Specific details about diet during pregnancy are discussed later.

An obstetrician, diabetes educator, or other health care practitioner can teach you how to measure your own blood glucose levels at home to see if levels remain in an acceptable range on the prescribed diet. The ability of patients to determine their own blood sugar levels with easy-to-use equipment represents a major milestone in the management of diabetes, especially during pregnancy. The technique called "self blood glucose monitoring" (discussed in detail later) allows you to check your blood sugar levels at home or at work without costly and time-consuming visits to your doctor. The values of your blood sugar levels also determine if you need to begin insulin therapy sometime during pregnancy. Short of frequent trips to a laboratory, this is the only way to see if blood glucose levels remain under good control.

What is self blood glucose monitoring?

Once you are diagnosed as having gestational diabetes, you and your health care providers will want to know more about your day-to-day blood sugar levels. It is important to know how your exercise habits and eating patterns affect your blood sugars. Also, as your pregnancy progresses, the placenta will release more of the hormones that work against insulin. Testing your blood sugar level at important times during the day will help determine if proper diet and weight gain have kept blood sugar levels normal or if extra insulin is needed to help keep the fetus protected.

Self blood glucose monitoring is done by using a special device to obtain a drop of your blood and test it for your blood sugar level. Your doctor or other health care provider will explain the procedure to you. Make sure that you are shown how to do the testing before attempting it on your own. Some items you may use to monitor your blood sugar levels are:

Lancet—a disposable, sharp needle-like sticker for pricking the finger to obtain a drop of blood.

Lancet device—a spring-loaded finger sticking device.

Test strip—a chemically treated strip to which a drop of blood is applied.

Color chart—a chart used to compare against the color on the test strip for blood sugar level.

Glucose meter—a device which "reads" the test strip and gives you a digital number value.

Your health care provider can advise you where to obtain the self-monitoring equipment in your area. You may want to inquire if any

Understanding Gestational Diabetes

places rent or loan glucose meters, since it is likely you won't be needing it after your baby is born.

How often and when should I test?

You may need to test your blood several times a day. Generally, these times are fasting (first thing in the morning before you eat) and 2 hours after each meal. Occasionally, you may be asked to test more frequently during the day or at night. As each person is an individual, your health care provider can advise the schedule best for you.

How should I record my test results?

Most manufacturers of glucose testing products provide a record diary, although some health care providers may have their own version. A Self Blood Glucose Monitoring Diary is included at the end of this text.

You should record any test result immediately because it's easy to forget what the reading was during the course of a busy day. You should always have this diary with you when you visit your doctor or other health care provider or when you contact them by phone. These results are very important in making decisions about your health care.

Are there any other tests I should know about?

In addition to blood testing, you may be asked to check your urine for ketones. Ketones are by-products of the breakdown of fat and may be found in the blood and urine as a result of inadequate insulin or from inadequate calories in your diet. Although it is not known whether or not small amounts of ketones can harm the fetus, when large amounts of ketones are present they are accompanied by a blood condition, acidosis, which is known to harm the fetus. To be on the safe side, you should watch for them in your urine and report any positive results to your doctor.

How do I test for ketones?

To test the urine for ketones, you can use a test strip similar to the one used for testing your blood. This test strip has a special chemically treated pad to detect ketones in the urine. Testing is done by passing the test strip through the stream of urine or dipping the strip in and out of urine in a container. As your pregnancy progresses, you might find it easier to use the container method. All test strips are disposable and can be used only once. This applies to blood sugar test strips also. You cannot use your blood sugar test strips for urine testing, and you cannot use your urine ketone test strips for blood sugar testing.

When do I test for ketones?

Overnight is the longest fasting period, so you should test your urine first thing in the morning every day and any time your blood sugar level goes over 240 mg/dl on the blood glucose test. It is also important to test if you become ill and are eating less food than normal. Your health care provider can advise what's best for you.

Is it ever necessary to take insulin?

Yes, despite careful attention to diet some women's blood sugars do not stay within an acceptable range. A pregnant woman free of gestational diabetes rarely has a blood glucose level that exceeds 100 mg/dl in the morning before breakfast (fasting) or 2 hours after a meal. The optimum goal for a gestational diabetic is blood sugar levels that are the same as those of a woman without diabetes.

There is no absolute blood sugar level that necessitates beginning insulin injections. However, many physicians begin insulin if the fasting sugar exceeds 105 mg/dl or if the level 2 hours after a meal exceeds 120 mg/dl on two separate occasions. Blood sugar levels measured by you at home will help your doctor know when it is necessary to begin insulin. The ability to perform self blood glucose monitoring has made it possible to begin insulin therapy at the earliest sign of high sugar levels, thereby preventing the fetus from being exposed to high levels of glucose from the mother's blood.

Will my baby be healthy?

The ultimate concern of any expectant mother is, "Will my baby be all right?" There is an array of simple, safe tests used to assess the condition of the fetus before birth and these can be particularly valuable during a pregnancy complicated by gestational diabetes. Tests that may be given during your pregnancy include:

Ultrasound. Ultrasound uses short pulses of high-frequency, low-intensity sound waves to create images. Unlike x-rays, there is no

Understanding Gestational Diabetes

radiation exposure to the fetus. First used during World War II to detect enemy submarines below the surface of the water, ultrasound has since been used safely in obstetrics. Occasionally, the date of your last menstrual period is not sufficient to determine a due date. Ultrasound can provide an accurate gestational age and due date that may be very important if it is necessary to induce labor early or perform a cesarean delivery. Ultrasound can also be used to determine the position of the placenta if it is necessary to perform an amniocentesis (another test discussed later).

Fetal movement records. Recording fetal movement is a test you can do by yourself to help determine the condition of the baby. Fetal activity is generally a reassuring sign of well-being. Women are often asked to count fetal movements regularly during the last trimester of pregnancy. You may be asked to set aside specific times to lie down on your back or side and count the number of times the baby moves or kicks. Three or more movements in a 2-hour period is considered normal. Contact your obstetrician if you feel fewer than three movements to determine if other tests are needed.

Fetal monitoring. Modern instruments make it possible to monitor the baby's heart rate before delivery. Currently, there are two types of fetal monitors—internal and external. The internal monitor consists of a small wire electrode attached directly to the scalp of the fetus after the membranes have ruptured. The external monitor uses transducers secured to the mother's abdomen by an elastic belt. One transducer records the baby's heart rate by a sensitive microphone called a doppler. The other transducer measures the firmness of the abdomen during a contraction of the uterus. It is a crude measure of the strength and frequency of contractions. Fetal monitoring is the basis for the non-stress test and the oxytocin challenge test described below.

Non-stress test. The "non-stress" test refers to the fact that no medication is given to the mother to cause movement of the fetus or contraction of the uterus. It is often used to confirm the well-being of the fetus based on the principle that a healthy fetus will demonstrate an acceleration in its heart rate following movement. Fetal activity may be spontaneous or induced by external manipulation such as rubbing the mother's abdomen or making a loud noise above the abdomen with a special device. When movement of the fetus is noted, a recording of the fetal heart rate is made. If the heart rate goes up, the test is normal. If the heart rate does not accelerate, the fetus may merely be "sleeping"; if, after stimulation, the fetus still does not react, it may be necessary to perform a "stress test" (oxytocin challenge test).

Stress test (oxytocin challenge test). Labor represents a stress to the fetus. Every time the uterus contracts, the fetus is momentarily deprived of its usual blood supply and oxygen. This is not a problem for most babies. However, some babies are not healthy enough to handle the stress and demonstrate an abnormal heart rate pattern. This test is often done if the non-stress test is abnormal. It involves giving the hormone oxytocin (secreted by every mother when normal labor begins) to the mother to stimulate uterine contractions. The contractions are a challenge to the baby, similar to the challenge of normal labor. If the baby's heart rate slows down rather than speeds up after a contraction, the baby may be in jeopardy. The stress test is considered more accurate than the non-stress test. Nevertheless, it is not 100 percent fool-proof and your obstetrician may want to repeat it on another occasion to ensure its accuracy. Most women describe this test as mildly uncomfortable but not painful.

Amniocentesis. Amniocentesis is a method of removing a small amount of fluid from the amniotic sac for analysis. Either the fluid itself or the cells shed by the fetus into the fluid can be studied. In mid-pregnancy the cells in amniotic fluid can be analyzed for genetic abnormalities such as Down syndrome. Many women over the age of 35 have amniocentesis for just this reason. Another important use for amniocentesis late in pregnancy is to study the fluid itself to determine if the lungs of the fetus are mature and able to withstand early delivery. This information can be very important in deciding the best time for a woman with Type I diabetes to deliver. It is not done as frequently to women with gestational diabetes.

Amniocentesis can be performed in an obstetrician's office or on an outpatient basis in a hospital. For genetic testing, amniocentesis is usually performed around the 16th week when the placenta and fetus can be located easily with ultrasound and a needle can be inserted safely into the amniotic sac. The overall complication rate for amniocentesis is less than 1 percent. The risk is even lower during the third trimester when the amniotic sac is larger and easily identifiable.

Does gestational diabetes affect labor and delivery?

Most women with gestational diabetes can complete pregnancy and begin labor naturally. Any pregnant woman has a slight chance (about

Understanding Gestational Diabetes

5 percent) of developing preeclampsia (toxemia), a sudden onset of high blood pressure associated with protein in the urine, occurring late in pregnancy. If preeclampsia develops, your obstetrician may recommend an early delivery. When an early delivery is anticipated, an amniocentesis is usually performed to assess the maturity of the baby's lungs.

Gestational diabetes, by itself, is not an indication to perform a cesarean delivery, but sometimes there are other reasons your doctor may elect to do a cesarean. For example, the baby may be too large (macrosomia) to deliver vaginally, or the baby may be in distress and unable to withstand vaginal delivery. You should discuss the various possibilities for delivery with your obstetrician so there are no surprises.

Careful control of blood sugar levels remains important even during labor. If a mother's blood sugar level becomes elevated during labor, the baby's blood sugar level will also become elevated. High blood sugars in the mother produce high insulin levels in the baby. Immediately after delivery high insulin levels in the baby can drive its blood sugar level very low since it will no longer have the high sugar concentration from its mother's blood.

Women whose gestational diabetes does not require that they take insulin during their pregnancy, will not need to take insulin during their labor or delivery. On the other hand, a woman who does require insulin during pregnancy may be given insulin by injection on the morning labor begins, or in some instances, it may be given intravenously throughout labor. For most women with gestational diabetes there is no need for insulin after the baby is born and blood sugar level returns to normal immediately. The reason for this sudden return to normal lies in the fact that when the placenta is removed the hormones it was producing (which caused the insulin resistance) are also removed. Thus, the mother's insulin is permitted to work normally without resistance. Your doctor may want to check your blood sugar level the next morning, but it will most likely be normal.

Should I expect my baby to have any problems?

One of the most frequently asked questions is, "Will my baby have diabetes?" Almost universally the answer is no. However, the baby is at risk for developing Type II diabetes later in life, and of having other problems related to gestational diabetes, such as hypoglycemia (low blood sugar) mentioned earlier. If your blood sugars were not elevated during the 24 hours before delivery, there is a good chance that hypoglycemia will not be a problem for your baby. Nevertheless, a neonatologist (a doctor who specializes in the care of newborn infants) or other doctor should check your baby's blood sugar level and give extra glucose if necessary.

Another problem that may develop in the infant of a mother with gestational diabetes is jaundice. Jaundice occurs when extra red blood cells in the baby's circulation are destroyed, releasing a substance called bilirubin. Bilirubin is a pigment that causes a yellow discoloration of the skin (jaundice). A minor degree of jaundice is common in many newborns. However, the presence of large amounts of bilirubin in the baby's system can be harmful and requires placing the baby under special lights which help get rid of the pigment. In extreme cases, blood transfusions may be necessary.

Will I develop diabetes in the future?

For most women gestational diabetes disappears immediately after delivery. However, you should have your blood sugars checked after your baby is born to make sure your levels have returned to normal. Women who had gestational diabetes during one pregnancy are at greater risk of developing it in a subsequent pregnancy. It is important that you have appropriate screening tests for gestational diabetes during future pregnancies as early as the first trimester.

Pregnancy is a kind of "stress test" that often predicts future diabetic problems. In one large study more than one-half of all women who had gestational diabetes developed overt Type II diabetes within 15 years of pregnancy. Because of the risk of developing Type II diabetes in the future, you should have your blood sugar level checked when you see your doctor for your routine check-ups. There is a good chance you will be able to reduce the risk of developing diabetes later in life by maintaining an ideal body weight and exercising regularly.

Why is a special diet recommended?

A nutritionally balanced diet is always essential to maintaining a healthy mother and successful pregnancy. The foods you choose become the nutrient building blocks for the growth of the fetus. For a woman with gestational diabetes, proper diet alone often keeps blood sugar levels in the normal range and is generally the first step to follow before resorting to insulin injections. Careful attention should be paid to the total calories eaten daily, to avoid foods which increase blood sugar levels, and to emphasize the use of foods which help the

Understanding Gestational Diabetes

body maintain a normal blood sugar. A registered dietitian is the best person to help you with meal planning to meet your individual needs. Your physician can help you find a dietitian if this service is not a part of his or her office or clinic. Your local chapter of the American Dietetic Association or the American Diabetes Association can also help you locate a registered dietitian.

How much weight should I gain?

Of all questions asked by pregnant women, this is the most common. The answer is particularly important for women with gestational diabetes. The weight that you gain is a rough indication of how much

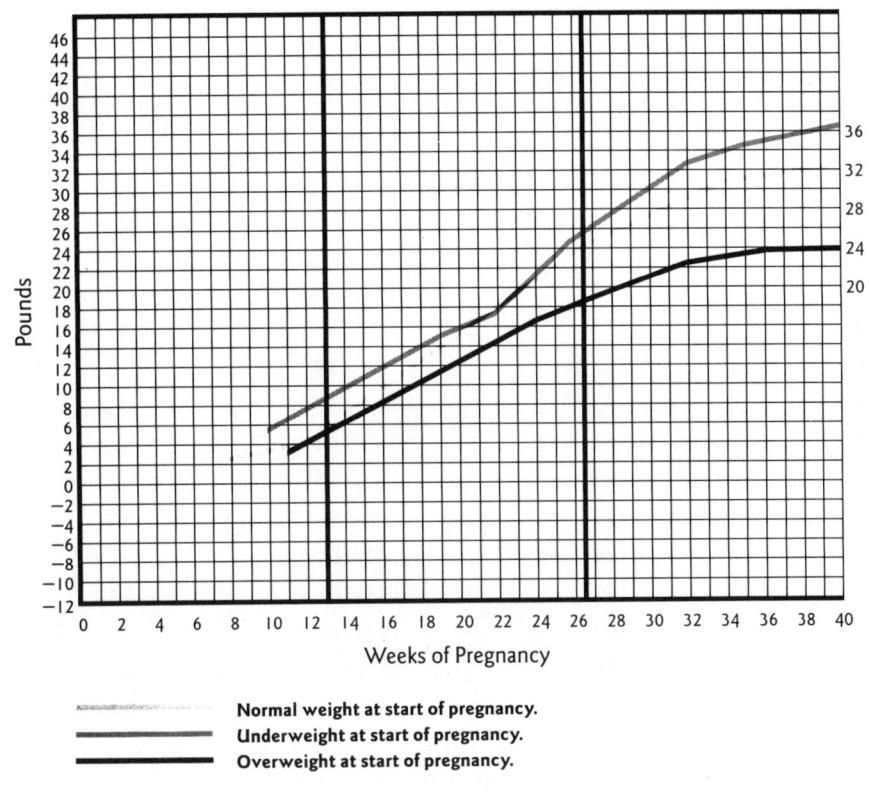

- - - - - Normal weight at start of pregnancy.
───── Underweight at start of pregnancy.
───── Overweight at start of pregnancy.

Adapted from Judith E. Brown. *Nutrition for Your Pregnancy.* University of Minnesota Press, 1983.

Figure 33.4. Prenatal Weight Gain Grid.

nutrition is available to the fetus for growth. An inadequate weight gain may result in a small baby who lacks protective calorie reserves at birth. This baby may have more illness during the first year of life. An excessive weight gain during pregnancy, however, has an insulin-resistant effect, just like the hormones produced by the placenta, and will make your blood sugar level higher.

The "optimal" weight to gain depends on the weight that you are before becoming pregnant (Figure 33.4.). Your pre-pregnancy weight is also a rough indication of how well-nourished you are before becoming pregnant. If you are at a desirable weight for your body size

Pre-pregnancy weight for height. Use this chart to determine if your pre-pregnancy weight is normal, underweight, or overweight.

Height without Shoes	Underweight If You Weighed This or Less	Normal Weight Range*	Overweight If You Weighed This or More
4'10"	88	89-108	109
4'11"	91	92-112	113
5'	94	95-115	116
5'1"	99	100-121	122
5'2"	104	105-127	128
5'3"	108	109-132	133
5'4"	113	114-138	139
5'5"	118	119-144	145
5'6"	123	124-150	151
5'7"	127	128-155	156
5'8"	132	133-161	162
5'9"	137	138-167	168
5'10"	142	143-173	174
5'11"	146	147-178	179
6'	151	152-184	185

*Normal weight for "thin-boned" women will be closer to the lower end of this range. For "big-boned" women, it will be closer to the higher end.

Reprinted with permission from: Judith E. Brown. *Nutrition for Your Pregnancy.* University of Minnesota Press, 1983.

Table 33.5. Pre-Pregnancy Weight

Understanding Gestational Diabetes

before you become pregnant, a weight gain of 24 to 27 pounds is recommended. If you are approximately 20 pounds or more above your desirable weight before pregnancy, a weight gain of 24 pounds is recommended. Many overweight women, however, have healthy babies and gain only 20 pounds. If you become pregnant when you are underweight, you need to gain more weight during the pregnancy to give your baby the extra nutrition he or she needs for the first year. You should gain 28 to 36 pounds, depending on how underweight you are before becoming pregnant. Figure 33.5. shows whether your pre-pregnancy weight is considered underweight, normal weight, or overweight.

Your nutrition advisor or health care provider can recommend an appropriate weight gain. How your weight gain is distributed is illustrated in Figure 33.6.

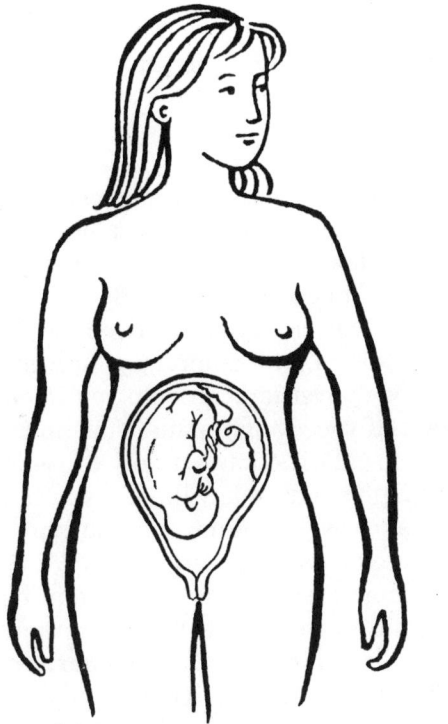

WEIGHT IN POUNDS	
7.5-8.5	FETUS
7.5	STORES OF FAT & PROTEIN
4.0	BLOOD
2.7	TISSUE FLUIDS
2.0	UTERUS
1.8	AMNIOTIC FLUID
1.5	PLACENTA & UMBILICAL CORD
1.0	BREASTS
28-29.0 POUNDS	

Figure 33.6. Distribution of Weight Gain During Pregnancy

Total recommended weight gain is often not as helpful as a weekly rate of gain. Most women gain 3 to 5 pounds during the first trimester (first 3 months) of pregnancy. During the second and third trimesters a good rate of weight gain is about three-quarters of a pound to one pound per week. Gaining too much weight (2 or more pounds per week) results in putting on too much body fat. This extra body fat produces an insulin-resistant effect which requires the body to produce more insulin to keep blood sugar levels normal. An inability to produce more insulin, as in gestational diabetes, causes your blood sugar levels to rise above acceptable levels. If weight gain has been excessive, often limiting weight gain to approximately three-quarters of a pound per week (3 pounds per month) can return blood sugar levels to normal. Fetal growth and development depend on proper nourishment and will be placed at risk by drastically reducing calories. However, you can limit weight gain by cutting back on excessive calories and by eating a nutritionally-sound diet that meets your needs and the needs of your baby. Remember that dieting and severely cutting back on weight gain may increase the risk of delivering prematurely. If blood sugar levels continue to go up and you are not gaining excessive weight or eating improperly, the safest therapy for the well-being of the fetus is insulin.

Occasionally, your weight may go up rapidly in the last trimester (after 28 weeks) and you may notice an increase in water retention, such as swelling in the feet, fingers, and face. If there is any question as to whether the rapid weight gain is due to eating too many calories or too much water retention, keeping records of how much food you eat and your exercise patterns at this time will be very helpful. By examining these patterns your nutrition advisor can help you determine which is causing the rapid weight gain. In addition, by examining your legs and body for signs of fluid retention, your physician can help you to determine the cause of your weight gain. If your weight gain is due to water retention, cutting back drastically on calories may actually cause more fluid retention. Bed rest and resting on your side will help you to lose the build-up of fluid. Limit your intake of salt (sodium chloride) and very salty foods, as they tend to contribute to water retention.

Marked fluid retention when combined with an increase in blood pressure and possibly protein in the urine are the symptoms of preeclampsia. This is a disorder of pregnancy that can be harmful to both the mother and baby. Inform your obstetrician of any rapid weight gain, especially if you are eating moderately and gaining more than 2 pounds per week. Should you develop preeclampsia, be especially careful to eat a well-balanced diet with adequate calories.

Understanding Gestational Diabetes

After being diagnosed as having gestational diabetes, many women notice a slower weight gain as they start cutting the various sources of sugar out of their diet. This seems to be harmless and lasts only 1 or 2 weeks. It may be that sweets were contributing a substantial amount of calories to the diet.

How should I eat during my pregnancy?

As with any pregnancy, it is important to eat the proper foods to meet the nutritional needs of the mother and fetus. An additional goal for women with gestational diabetes is to maintain a proper diet to keep blood sugars as normal as possible.

The daily need for calories increases by 300 calories during the second and third trimesters of pregnancy. If non-pregnant calorie intake was 1800 calories per day and weight gain was maintained, a calorie intake of 2100 calories per day is usual from 14 weeks until delivery. This is the equivalent of an additional 8 ounce glass of 2% milk and one-half of a sandwich (1 slice of bread, approximately 1 ounce of meat, and 1 teaspoon of margarine, mayonnaise, etc.) per day. The need for protein also increases during pregnancy. Make sure your diet includes foods high in protein, but not high in fat.

Most vitamins and minerals are also needed in larger amounts during pregnancy. This can be attained by increasing dairy products, especially those low in fat, and making sure you include whole grain cereals and breads, as well as fruits and vegetables in your diet each day. To make sure you get enough folate (a B vitamin critical during

TABLE 4. Protein Equivalents

Food	Grams of Protein
1 cup 2% milk	8
1 cup plain nonfat yogurt	8
1 ounce American processed cheese	7
1 ounce low-fat cheese	7
1 tbsp. peanut butter	7
1/4 cup cottage cheese	7
1/2 cup cooked dried beans	7
1 slice whole wheat bread	3
1/2 cup flaked cereal, bran or corn	3

Table 33.7. Protein Equivalents

pregnancy) and iron, your obstetrician will probably recommend a prenatal vitamin. Prenatal vitamins do not replace a good diet; they merely help you to get the nutrients you need. To absorb the most iron from your prenatal vitamin, take it at night before going to bed, or in the morning on an empty stomach.

The Daily Food Guide (Figure 33.8.) serves as a guideline for food sources that provide important vitamins and minerals, as well as carbohydrates, protein, and fiber during pregnancy. The recommended minimal servings per day appear in parentheses after each food group listed. This guide emphasizes foods that are low in fat and in sugar (discussed later).

The food guide is divided into six groups: milk and milk products; meat, poultry, fish, and meat substitutes; breads, cereals, and other starches; fruits; vegetables; and fats. Each group provides its own combination of vitamins, minerals, and other nutrients which play an important part in nutrition during pregnancy. Omitting the foods from one group will leave your diet inadequate in other nutrients. Plan your meals using a variety of foods within each food group, in the amounts recommended, and you'll be most likely to get all the vitamins, minerals, and other nutrients the fetus needs for growth and development.

Other Nutritional and Non-Nutritional Considerations

Alcohol. There is no known safe level of alcohol to allow during pregnancy. Daily heavy alcohol intake causes severe defects in development of the body and brain of the fetus, called Fetal Alcohol Syndrome. Even moderate drinking is associated with delayed fetal growth, spontaneous abortions, and lowered birth weight in babies. The Surgeon General's office warns: "Women who are pregnant or even considering pregnancy should avoid alcohol completely and should be aware of the alcohol content of food and drugs."

Salt. Salt restriction is no longer routinely advised during pregnancy. Recent research shows that during pregnancy the body needs salt to help provide the proper fluid balance. Your health care provider may recommend that you use salt in moderation.

Caffeine. Studies conflict on the potential danger of caffeine to the fetus. Caffeine is found primarily in coffee, tea, and some sodas (Figure 33.9.). Moderation is recommended. Talk to your doctor or other health professional about the maximum amount of caffeine recommended.

Understanding Gestational Diabetes

Table 33.8a. Daily Food Guide (Each item equals one serving)

Milk and Milk Products *(4 Servings Per Day)*	1 cup milk, skim or low-fat 1/3 cup powdered non-fat milk 1 cup reconstituted powdered non-fat milk 1½ oz. low-fat cheese* (no more than 6 grams of fat per ounce) 1 cup low-fat yogurt**	(high protein, calcium, vitamin D)
Meat, Poultry, Fish, and Meat Substitutes *(5-6 Servings Per Day)*	1 oz. cooked poultry, fish, or lean meat (beef, lamb, pork) 1 tbsp. peanut butter 1 egg 1/4 cup low-fat cottage cheese 1/2 cup cooked dried beans or lentils	(high protein, B vitamins, iron)
Breads, Cereals, and Other Starches *(5-6 Servings Per Day)*	1 slice whole grain bread 5 crackers 1 muffin, biscuit, pancake, or waffle 3/4 cup dry cereal, unsweetened 1/2 cup pasta (macaroni, spaghetti), rice, mashed potatoes, or cooked cereal 1/3 cup sweet potatoes or yams 1/2 cup cooked dried beans or lentils 1/2 bagel, 1/2 english muffin, or 1/2 flour tortilla 1 small baked potato 2 taco shells	(high complex carbohydrates) (emphasize whole grains, or use fortified or enriched) (a good source of protein, B-vitamins, fiber and minerals)

Table 33.8b. Daily Food Guide (Each item equals one serving)

Fruit *(2 servings per day)*	1/2 cup fresh fruit, 1/2 banana, or 1 medium-sized fruit (apple, orange)	(fresh fruit provides fiber)
	1/2 cup, orange, grapefruit, or other juice fortified with vitamin C	(include one vitamin C source daily)
	1/2 medium-sized grapefruit	
	1 cup strawberries	
	1/2 cup fresh apricots, nectarines, purple plums, cantaloup, or 4 halves dried apricots (vitamin A source)	
Vegetables*** *(2 servings per day)*	1/2 cup cooked or 1 cup raw: broccoli, spinach, carrots, (vitamin A source)	(include good vitamin A sources at least every other day)
	1/3 cup mixed vegetables	
Fats	1 tsp. butter or margarine	
	1 tsp. oil or mayonnaise	
	1 tbsp. regular salad dressing	
	2 tbsp. low-calorie salad dressing	
	1/4 cup nuts or seeds	

*1 oz. low-fat cheese can also be used as 1 serving from the Meat, Poultry, Fish, and Meat Substitutes group if sufficient calcium is already being provided from 4 servings.

**This refers to plain yogurt. Commercially fruited yogurt contains a lot of added sugar.

***Starchy vegetables such as corn, peas, and potatoes are included in Breads, Cereals, and Other Starches list.

Understanding Gestational Diabetes

Megavitamin. Megavitamins are defined as 10 times the Recommended Dietary Allowance (Dietary allowances established by the National Academy of Sciences—National Research Council) of vitamins and minerals and are not recommended for pregnant women. Although it is possible to get all of the necessary nutrients from food alone, your doctor may prescribe some prenatal vitamins and minerals. If taken regularly, along with a balanced diet, you will be getting all the vitamins and minerals needed during your pregnancy.

Smoking. Research has shown without question that smoking during pregnancy increases the risk of fetal death and preterm delivery, impairs fetal growth, and can lead to low birth weight. It is best to stop smoking entirely and permanently, or at the very least, to cut back drastically on the number of cigarettes you smoke.

What food patterns help keep blood sugar levels normal?

The following outlines food patterns which help to keep blood sugar levels within an acceptable range.

Avoid sugar and foods high in sugar. Most women with gestational diabetes, just like those without diabetes, have a desire for something sweet in their diet. In pregnant women, sugar is rapidly absorbed into the blood and requires a larger release of insulin to

Table 33.9. Caffeine Comparisons

TABLE 6. Caffeine Comparisons

Food	Serving	Amount of Caffeine
Regular coffee	8 oz.	80-200 mg.
Instant coffee	8 oz.	60-100 mg.
Decaffeinated coffee	8 oz.	3-5 mg.
Tea	8 oz.	60-65 mg.
Carbonated drinks, e.g., colas	12 oz.	30-65 mg.
Hot chocolate	8 oz.	13 mg.

maintain normal blood sugar levels. Without the larger release of insulin, blood sugar levels will increase excessively when you eat sugar-containing foods.

There are many forms of sugar such as table sugar, honey, brown sugar, corn syrup, maple syrup, turbinado sugar, high fructose corn syrup, and molasses. Generally, food that ends in "ose" is a sugar (e.g., sucrose, dextrose, and glucose).

Foods that usually contain high amounts of sugar include pies, cakes, cookies, ice cream, candy, soft drinks, fruit drinks, fruit packed in syrup, commercially fruited yogurt, jams, jelly, doughnuts, and sweet rolls. Many of these foods are high in fat as well.

Be sure to check the list of ingredients on food products. Ingredients are listed in order of amount. If an ingredient is first on the list, it is present in the highest amount. If some type of sugar is listed first, second, or third on the list of ingredients, the product should be avoided. If sugar is further down, fourth, fifth, or sixth, it probably will not cause your blood sugar levels to go up excessively.

Fruit juices should only be taken with a meal and limited to 6 ounces. Tomato juice is a good choice because it is low in sugar. Six ounces of most other juice (apple, grapefruit, orange) with no sugar added still contain approximately 4 to 5 teaspoons of sugar. However, these do not contain much of the fiber of a piece of fruit which normally would act to slow the absorption of sugar into the blood. If you drink juice frequently to quench your thirst during the day, a high blood sugar level may result. Use only whole fruit for snacks.

To help with the occasional sweet tooth that we all have, artificial sweeteners may be used in foods. Aspartame has been extensively tested for safety. Use during pregnancy has been approved by the Food and Drug Administration and by the American Medical Association's Review Board. However, aspartame has not been tested for long-term safety and has not been on the market very long. It may be best to avoid its use until more tests have been done.

Saccharin is not advised during pregnancy. Likewise, use of mannitol, xylitol, sorbitol, or other artificial sweeteners is not recommended until further research is done.

Fructose is a special type of sugar that is slowly absorbed into the system. A small amount of fructose can be used if your blood sugar levels are within normal range. However, fructose still has 4 calories per gram, as much as table sugar. High fructose corn syrup is part fructose and part corn syrup, making it very similar to table sugar in composition. It will raise blood sugar levels and should definitely be avoided.

Understanding Gestational Diabetes

Emphasize the use of complex carbohydrates. These include vegetables, cereal, grains, beans, peas, and other starchy foods. A well-balanced diet with plenty of fiber provided by vegetables, dried beans, cereals, and other starchy foods decreases the amount of insulin your body needs to keep blood sugars within a normal range. Anything that decreases the need for insulin is beneficial. The American Diabetes Association recommends that at least one-half of your calories come from complex carbohydrates. Starchy foods include pasta, rice, grains, cereals, crackers, bread, potatoes, dried beans, peas, and legumes. Also, contrary to popular belief, carbohydrates are not highly fattening when eaten in moderate amounts and without the rich sauces and toppings often added.

Emphasize foods high in dietary fiber. Fiber is the edible portion of foods of plant origin that is not digested (e.g., skins, membranes, seeds, bran). Foods with a high fiber content include whole grain cereals and breads, fruits, vegetables, and legumes (dried peas and beans). Fiber aids digestion and helps prevent constipation. The fiber found in fruits, vegetables, and legumes also helps keep your blood sugar level from becoming too high without requiring extra insulin.

Keep your diet low in fat. Some fat is needed to help with the absorption of certain vitamins and to provide the essential fatty acids necessary for fetal growth. A diet which is high in fat causes the insulin to react in a less efficient manner, necessitating more insulin to keep blood sugar levels within normal range. Foods high in saturated fats such as fatty meats, butter, bacon, cream (light, coffee, sour cream, etc.), and whole milk cheeses are likely to be high in total fat. Most foods with saturated fat are also high in cholesterol because they are fats from animal origin. However, foods such as crackers made with coconut, palm, or palm kernel oil can be high in saturated fats as well. Read labels carefully. Unsaturated fats are found in foods such as fish, margarine and vegetable oils. Keep your use of salad dressings to a minimum and whenever possible use those prepared with olive oil. To help keep the diet lower in fat, avoid adding extra fats such as rich sauces and creamy desserts, and bake or broil foods instead of frying them. Replacing fatty foods with those high in complex carbohydrates is also helpful.

Include a bedtime snack that is a good source of protein and complex carbohydrates. Women with gestational diabetes have a tendency toward lower than normal blood sugar levels during the night. This causes the body to increase its utilization of fats as a fuel source. As fat is used, ketones (discussed later) are produced as a by-product of the breakdown of fats, and in large amounts, may be harmful to the fetus. This can be prevented by having a bedtime snack that provides protein and complex carbohydrates such as starchy foods. Starch will stabilize your blood sugar level in the early night, while protein acts as a long-acting stabilizer. Examples of a bedtime snack are:

> 1 oz. American-processed cheese + 5 crackers
> 1/2 chicken sandwich on whole wheat bread
> 3 cups unbuttered popcorn + 1/4 cup nuts

Table 33.10. Sample Menu—2000 Calories

This diet is planned for women whose normal non-pregnant weight should be 130-135 lbs. For women who weigh less than 130 before pregnancy, the diet should contain fewer calories. Women who are overweight are at higher risk for gestational diabetes. Your health care provider can discuss this and help you make necessary changes.

BREAKFAST
1/2 grapefruit
3/4 cup oatmeal, cooked
1 tsp. raisins
1 cup 2% milk
1 whole wheat English muffin
1 tsp. margarine

LUNCH
Salad with:
   1 cup romaine lettuce
   1/2 cup kidney beans, cooked
   1/2 fresh tomato
1 oz. part skim mozzarella cheese
2 tbsp. low-calorie Italian dressing
1 bran muffin
1/2 cup cantaloupe chunks

AFTERNOON SNACK
2 rice cakes
6 oz. low-fat yogurt, plain
1/2 cup blueberries

DINNER
3/4 cup vegetable soup with
   1/4 cup cooked barley
3 oz. chicken, without skin
1 baked potato
1/2 cup cooked broccoli
1 piece whole wheat bread
1 tbsp. margarine
1 fresh peach

BEDTIME SNACK
1 apple
2 cups popcorn, plain
1/4 cup peanuts

Understanding Gestational Diabetes

If you need to take insulin, a bedtime snack is critical and you should not omit it. When taken by injection, insulin acts to lower blood sugar level, even during the night when meals are not eaten. A bedtime snack is protective against low blood sugars while sleeping or upon arising. If a bedtime snack causes heartburn, sleep with your head raised on pillows, and be careful that you are not eating too large a bedtime snack.

How do I plan meals?

A registered dietitian or qualified nutritionist can help you plan a meal pattern that is right for you. Most women with gestational diabetes need three meals and a bedtime snack each day. It is unwise for anyone who is pregnant to go long periods of time (greater than 5 hours) without eating, as this will produce ketones. Extra snacks are necessary if your schedule results in a long time between meals. Blood sugars will be easier to keep in the normal range if meal times and amounts (total calories) are evenly spaced. It's more likely that a higher blood sugar will result if the majority of calories are eaten at dinner, than if they are distributed more evenly throughout the day. If insulin injections prove necessary, the time at which meals are eaten and the amounts eaten should be approximately the same from day to day. Do not skip meals and snacks, as this often results in hypoglycemia (low blood sugar), which may be harmful to the fetus and makes you feel irritable, shaky, or may result in a headache.

What can be done to slow weight gain during pregnancy?

Gaining too much weight during pregnancy will make blood sugar levels higher than normal for women with gestational diabetes. Yet, for many pregnant women it is very difficult to gain weight slowly and still get all of the recommended nutrients. Luckily, fat, which is high in calories (9 calories per gram), is needed in only small amounts during pregnancy. Carbohydrates and protein, in contrast to fat, provide only 4 calories per gram. To cut calories without depriving the fetus of any necessary nutritional factors, it is best to avoid fats and fatty foods.

- Avoid high-fat meats. Choose lean cuts of beef, pork, and lamb. Emphasize more fish and poultry (without the skin).

- Avoid frying meat, fish, or poultry in added oil, shortening, or lard. Bake, broil, or roast instead.

- Avoid foods fried in oil such as chips, french fries, and doughnuts. Substitute pretzels, unbuttered popcorn, or breadsticks instead.

- Avoid using cream sauces and butter sauces, as well as salt pork for seasoning on vegetables. Season with herbs instead.

- Avoid using the fat drippings from meat or poultry for gravy. Use broth or bouillon instead and thicken with cornstarch.

- Avoid using mayonnaise or oil for salads. Use vinegar, lemon juice, or low-calorie salad dressings instead.

To help reduce calories choose low-fat dairy products. During pregnancy you need 1200 mg calcium daily to build the fetal skeleton without drawing from maternal calcium stores. Figure 33.11. points out foods in which the calcium content is almost the same, yet the calories are not due to the difference in fat content.

Table 33.11. Calorie Comparisons

Food	Calories
4-8 oz. glasses whole milk	600
4-8 oz. glasses 2% milk	480
4-8 oz. glasses skim milk	340
2-8 oz. glasses whole milk plus 3 oz. American processed cheese	600
2-8 oz. glasses 2% milk plus 3 oz. American processed cheese	540
2-8 oz. glasses skim milk plus 3 oz. American processed cheese	470

Understanding Gestational Diabetes

The difference between 600 calories and 340 calories is only 260 calories and may seem insignificant. Yet, if your diet is cut by 260 calories daily for 1 week, your weight gain slows down by approximately 1/2 pound per week. In other words, instead of gaining 2 pounds per week you will only gain 1 pound per week.

If cheese is a part of your daily diet, use low-fat cheeses such as low-fat cottage cheese, Neufchatel, mozzarella, farmers, and pot cheese. Avoid using cream cheese, as it has little protein and most of its calories come from fat.

Even though pregnancy can be a very hectic time, with little time for meal preparation, eat less and less often at "fast food" restaurants. Studies have shown that some foods from fast food restaurants average 40 to 60 percent of their calories from fat, and are quite high in calories (*Fast Food Facts: Nutritive and Exchange Values for Fast Food Restaurants.* Marion J. Franz. International Diabetes Center, Minneapolis, Minnesota. 1987, 54 pp). For example, chicken and fish that are coated with batter and deep-fried in fat may contain more fat and calories than a hamburger or roast beef sandwich.

Go lightly when using butter and margarine. Adding only an extra three pats of butter or margarine (same calories) daily could add an extra pound of weight gain next month. It may be better to emphasize the use of foods rich in complex carbohydrates that don't use butter, margarine, or cream sauce to make them palatable. Many people find rice, noodles, and spaghetti tasty without a lot of butter. Use a variety of spices and herbs (such as curry, garlic, and parsley) to flavor rice and tomato sauce to flavor pasta without additional fats.

It is also a good idea to eat small amounts frequently, thereby keeping the edge off your appetite. This will assist your "self-control" in avoiding large portions of food that you should not have. Avoid skipping meals or trying to cut back drastically on breakfast or lunch. It will leave you too hungry for the next meal to exercise any control. Your doctor or dietitian can help you determine how you can cut extra calories.

You may find it helpful to keep food records of what you eat, as most of us tend to forget or not realize the extent of our snacking. Recording everything you eat or drink tends to be a sobering and instructive experience. A Food and Exercise Record Sheet is included at the end of this text.

Be careful to maintain a weight gain of at least 1/2 pound per week, over several weeks, if you are in the second trimester (14 weeks or more of gestation). Cutting back more than this may increase the risk of having a low-birth-weight infant.

Is breast-feeding recommended?

Breast-feeding is strongly encouraged. For most women this represents the easiest way back to pre-pregnancy weight after delivery. The body draws on the calories stored during the first part of pregnancy to use in milk production. Approximately 800 calories per day are used during the first 3 months of milk production, and even more during the next 3 months. By 6 weeks after delivery, women who breast-feed usually have lost 4 pounds more than women who bottle-feed. This can be a very important factor, as it is strongly recommended that women with gestational diabetes return to their desirable body weight 4 to 5 months postpartum. As previously mentioned, maintaining a weight appropriate for your height and frame may reduce the risk of developing diabetes later in life.

In addition, breast-feeding has many advantages for your baby. Protection from infection and allergies are transferred to the baby through breast milk. This milk is also easier to digest than formula, and its minerals are better absorbed than those in formula.

Should I exercise?

A daily exercise program is an important part of a healthy pregnancy. Daily exercise helps you feel better and reduces stress. In addition, being physically fit protects against back pain, and maintains muscle tone, strength, and endurance. For women with gestational diabetes, exercise is especially important.

- Regular exercise increases the efficiency or potency of your body's own insulin. This may allow you to keep your blood sugar levels in the normal range while using less insulin.

- Moderate exercise also helps blunt your appetite, helping you to keep your weight gain down to normal levels. Maintaining the correct weight gain is very important in preventing high blood sugar levels.

Talk with your doctor about what exercise program is right for you. Your doctor can advise you about limitations, warning signs, and any special considerations. Generally, you can continue any exercise program or sport you participated in prior to pregnancy. Use caution, however, and avoid sports or exercises where you might fall, or that involve jolting. Pre-pregnancy bicycling, jogging, and cross-country

Understanding Gestational Diabetes

skiing are good exercises to continue during pregnancy. If you plan to start an exercise program during pregnancy, talk to your doctor before beginning and start slowly. Vigorous walking is good for women who need to start exercising and have not been active before pregnancy.

Exercising frequently, 4 to 5 days per week, is necessary to get the "blood sugar lowering" advantages of an exercise program. Don't omit a warm-up period of 5 to 10 minutes and a cool-down period of 5 to 10 minutes. Always stop exercising if you feel pain, dizziness, shortness of breath, faintness, palpitations, back or pelvic pain, or experience vaginal bleeding. Also, avoid vigorous exercise in hot, humid weather or if you have a fever. It is important to prevent dehydration during exercise, especially during pregnancy. The American College of Obstetricians and Gynecologists (ACOG) recommends drinking fluids prior to and after exercise, and if necessary, during the activity to prevent dehydration.

An ACOG report (*Home Exercise Program: Exercise During Pregnancy and the Postnatal Period*. American College of Obstetricians and Gynecologists May 1985, 6 pp.)issued in 1985, warned that target heart rates for pregnant and postpartum women should be set approximately 25 to 30 percent lower than rates for non-pregnant women. It may be that exercising too vigorously will direct blood flow away from the uterus and fetus. ACOG recommends that pregnant women measure their heart rate during activity and that maternal heart rate not exceed 140 beats per minute.

If you need to be on insulin during your pregnancy, take a few precautions. Because both insulin and exercise lower blood sugar levels, the combination can result in hypoglycemia or low blood sugar. You need to be aware that this is a potential problem, and you should be familiar with the symptoms of hypoglycemia (confusion, extreme hunger, blurry vision, shakiness, sweating). When exercising, take along sugar in the form of hard, sugar-sweetened candies just in case your blood sugar becomes too low. When on insulin, you should always carry some form of sugar for potential episodes of hypoglycemia.

It may be necessary for you to eat small snacks between meals if the exercise results in low blood sugar levels.

- One serving of fruit will keep blood sugars normal for most short-term activities (approximately 30 minutes).

- One serving of fruit plus a serving of starch will be enough for activities that last longer (60 minutes or more).

If you exercise right after a meal, eat the snack after the exercise. If the exercise is 2 hours or more after a meal, eat the snack before the exercise.

What happens if diet and exercise fail to control my blood sugars?

If your blood sugars tend to go over the acceptable levels (105 mg/dl or below for fasting, 120 mg/dl or below 2 hours after a meal) you may need to take insulin injections. Insulin is a protein and would be digested like any other protein in food if it were given orally. The needles used to inject insulin are extremely fine, so there is little discomfort. If insulin injections are necessary, you will be taught how to fill the syringe and how to do the injections yourself.

Your physician will calculate the amount of insulin needed to keep blood sugar levels within the normal range. It is very likely that the amount or dosage of insulin needed to keep your levels of blood sugar normal will increase as your pregnancy advances. This does not mean your gestational diabetes is getting worse. As any healthy pregnancy progresses, the placenta will grow and produce progressively higher levels of contra-insulin hormones. As a result you will likely need to inject more insulin to overcome their effect. Some women may even require two injections each day. This does not imply anything about the severity of the problem or the outcome of the pregnancy. The goal is to maintain normal blood sugar levels with whatever dosage of insulin is needed.

Can my blood sugar level go too low, and if so, what do I do?

Occasionally, your blood sugar level may get too low if you are taking insulin. This can happen if you delay a meal or exercise more than usual, especially at the time your insulin is working at its peak. This low blood sugar is called "hypoglycemia" or an "insulin reaction." This is a medical emergency and should be promptly treated, never ignored.

The symptoms of insulin reaction vary from sweating, shakiness, or dizziness to feeling faint, disoriented, or a tingling sensation. Remember, if you take insulin injections, you need to keep some form of sugar-sweetened candy in your purse, at home, at work, and in your car. In case of an episode of hypoglycemia, you will be prepared to treat it immediately. Be sure to eat something more substantial afterward. Also, report any insulin reactions or high blood sugar levels to your doctor right away in case an adjustment in your treatment needs to be made.

As you can see from reading this text, extra care, work, and commitment on the part of you and your spouse or partner are required to provide the special medical care necessary. Don't worry if you occasionally go off your diet or miss a planned exercise program. Your doctor and other health care professionals will work along with you to make sure you receive the specialized care that has resulted in dramatically improved pregnancy outcome.

An ounce of prevention is worth a pound of cure! Eat as directed. Exercise as directed. Monitor as directed. Do these things and you are doing your part toward a happy, healthy pregnancy.

Gestational Diabetes—A Personal Story

Sharon, 27 and expecting her first baby, was in her 18th week of pregnancy and feeling fine when her obstetrician told her that the routine blood screening test for glucose levels she had taken the week before identified her as a gestational diabetic.

If an expectant mother cannot metabolize (process) glucose (a form of sugar) properly, her fetus can receive too much glucose and grow too large. Glucose metabolism is altered during all pregnancies, but in women with gestational diabetes, erratic glucose metabolism is harmful to the fetus, causing problems during the pregnancy as well as during labor and delivery.

Because Sharon had always been healthy, she was shocked when her obstetrician told her that she was now considered a high-risk patient and would have to be closely monitored until her baby was born.

A team—including Sharon's obstetrician, the hospital's perinatal specialist, and a certified diabetic educator—began to work with her. They taught her how to monitor her glucose at home herself with a blood glucose monitor that she bought in her local pharmacy. Sharon was instructed in the principles of using the diabetic exchange diet. Although in Sharon's case diet alone was sufficient to control her condition, if it had not been, she would have been instructed how and when to inject insulin at home.

Infants of uncontrolled gestational diabetics often grow larger than full-term infants but are in other ways physically immature. The mother's placenta, the lifeline to the fetus, may not produce adequate nutrition for the infant to mature according to size. To monitor the growth and well-being of her fetus, Sharon was sent to the maternal-fetal radiologist for ultrasonic screening. Measurements of fetal movements and breathing patterns by the sonographer helped to ensure that the fetus was growing appropriately and appeared healthy.

During the last four weeks of her pregnancy, Sharon's perinatal team met weekly to discuss her case. They talked about the possibility of inducing labor if her fetus began to grow too large. Sharon had carefully followed her prescribed diet and had gained only 22 pounds. She had also monitored her blood glucose levels daily and adhered to a moderate exercise program throughout her pregnancy.

At 39 weeks gestation, one week before her expected delivery date, Sharon went into spontaneous labor. After a normal six-hour labor and vaginal delivery, she gave birth to a healthy 8-pound, 2-ounce son.

Like most women with gestational diabetes, Sharon's blood sugar levels returned to normal after she gave birth. On the third day after the birth, Sharon went home with her newborn son.

Almost all pregnant women are now screened for gestational diabetes during their second trimester, usually between 24 and 28 weeks gestation, because normal pregnancy causes a "diabetic-like" state in all pregnant women.

Some pregnant women can handle the imbalance of glucose and insulin while others cannot. When a pregnant woman develops diabetes during pregnancy, this medical condition is superimposed on the added stresses and physiologic changes that a normal pregnancy produces. Women with gestational diabetes must be carefully monitored for possible additional medical problems such as high blood pressure, vascular problems, and pre-term labor.

Research Progress in Gestational Diabetes

Many women who develop gestational diabetes mellitus during a pregnancy may become diabetic later in life. Few of these women, however, have in their blood the pancreatic islet cell antibodies (ICA's) that are considered markers for patients at risk for insulin-dependent diabetes mellitus, according to researchers at Case Western Reserve University and the University of Vermont in Burlington.

"In our study of 187 Vermont women with a history of gestational diabetes, islet cell antibodies were found in only 3 women (1.6 percent), a result in sharp contrast to earlier studies that suggested an ICA incidence of 10 to 38 percent," says principal investigator Dr. Patrick Catalano of Case Western Reserve University in Cleveland, Ohio.

Understanding Gestational Diabetes

Dr. Catalano and his colleagues were studying ICA's in women who had had gestational diabetes to determine the incidence of ICA in women with gestational diabetes and whether monitoring these antibodies would provide an early indication of developing diabetes. The appearance of antibodies against the beta-cells of the islets of Langerhans of the pancreas appears to signal ongoing destruction of these cells, the producers of insulin, eventually resulting in insulin-dependent diabetes mellitus (IDDM). According to medical authorities, approximately 10 percent of all diabetics in the United States have IDDM, also known as type I diabetes. The other 90 percent have non-insulin-dependent diabetes mellitus (NIDDM or type II diabetes), which often affects older, overweight persons. In NIDDM the pancreas produces some insulin but there is still a failure to regulate blood glucose for reasons that are not well-understood. The American Diabetes Association estimates that half of all diabetic Americans do not know that they are ill.

Gestational diabetes mellitus—glucose intolerance in pregnant women who never have had diabetes—occurs in approximately 2.5 to 5 percent of pregnancies, according to the investigators. Most of these women revert to a normal carbohydrate metabolism some time after giving birth, but have a high incidence of diabetes later in life. In one study, for example, 26 percent of nonobese women with prior gestational diabetes and 47 percent of obese women with prior gestational diabetes developed diabetes. In contrast, only 2 and 5 percent of nonobese and obese women, respectively, who did not have a history of gestational diabetes developed diabetes.

The women's risk of developing diabetes at some time after a pregnancy may be a greater risk of gestational diabetes than any immediate risk to their infants. In the United States the risk of perinatal mortality among offspring of women with gestational diabetes does not appear to differ from that of the nondiabetic population, according to Dr. Catalano. This may result at least partly from treatment to normalize blood glucose levels in gestational diabetes patients and close obstetrical followup. Development of type I diabetes in these children does not correlate with their mothers' prior gestational diabetes, although children of mothers with gestational diabetes have an increased risk of obesity as adolescents; the obesity places them at a higher risk for type II diabetes.

For the measurement of ICA's in serum, Dr. Catalano and his colleagues relied on an assay that was developed earlier by researchers at the Joslin Diabetes Center in Boston. The Joslin Diabetes Center cooperated in the study by performing the assay on serum samples sent from Vermont.

Like previous ICA assays, the Joslin monoclonal antibody method relies on immunofluorescence to detect antibodies to the beta-cells. In addition, the assay uses monoclonal antibody conjugated to the dye rhodamine to rapidly identify islets. "This test is a very specific test that decreases the chance of false positive results," Dr. Catalano says. According to Joslin researchers, the test procedure also decreases the number of false negative readings, resulting in more reliable data than the indirect immunofluorescence assays used in the earlier studies.

The incidence of ICA in a control population indicated by the protein A MoAb method is only 0.45 percent.

Because so few women with previous gestational diabetes had developed ICA's, the researchers have decided to eliminate the ICA assay as a predictor of future diabetes mellitus in women with a history of gestational diabetes. The rarity of ICA's also alleviates concerns that they might pose a widespread threat to fetal health.

Nevertheless, the three women in the study whose serum contained ICA's all had impaired glucose tolerance when tested several months after delivery of their infants. Oral glucose tolerance was normal for the 11 ICA-negative women in two control groups chosen for detailed comparisons; five women had had normal pregnancies, and six had developed gestational diabetes during the pregnancy. The ICA-positive women also had significantly higher fasting plasma glucose levels than the women in the other two groups. Only the fasting plasma glucose levels were significantly elevated when the ICA-positive women were compared retrospectively with the ICA-negative group for glucose testing during their pregnancies. The ICA-positive women also produced significantly less insulin immediately after an injection of glucose. Their total insulin production capacity was not impaired compared with the two control groups.

In their report the researchers suggested additional studies to determine whether the prevalence of ICA's increases over time after gestational diabetes and to search for a possible effect of ICA's on fetal islet cells. However, according to the investigators, such studies would be difficult to carry out because the number of women with gestational diabetes who are ICA-positive is too low (approximately 0.07 to 0.15 percent of all pregnancies) to provide sufficient subjects for the proposed studies unless a very large-scale study is conducted.

Instead, Dr. Catalano has begun to investigate various aspects of carbohydrate metabolism, comparing pregnant women with and without gestational diabetes, using pregravid studies of each woman as her own baseline, to detect any changes with the passage of time. "None of the metabolic tests I am using is unique, but there are differences in my approach," says Dr. Catalano. Specifically, he is using two techniques relatively new to obstetrical research, and he is searching for patterns in a combined analysis of the results of several tests rather than looking at each test separately.

One of Dr. Catalano's techniques employs stable isotopes to measure hepatic glucose production. In the other technique he uses the glucose clamp procedure to measure changes in insulin resistance. The glucose clamp technique involves a continuous infusion of insulin to achieve a high physiological level of insulin while the plasma glucose level is maintained (clamped) at a set level by variable infusions of glucose. A lower rate of glucose infusion means a lower rate of glucose disposal, implying insulin resistance. Conversely, a higher rate of glucose infusion is associated with greater insulin sensitivity.

Other techniques Dr. Catalano uses to study carbohydrate metabolism include the intravenous glucose tolerance test to measure insulin release, underwater weighing for percentage of body fat in body composition studies, and indirect calorimetry to examine energy expenditure.

So far 20 women have participated in these studies; 10 to 15 additional women are expected to participate.

In preliminary results Dr. Catalano reports that the combination of tests appears to be more sensitive in detecting differences in carbohydrate metabolism than any individual test. When test results for women who are 12 to 14 weeks pregnant are compared with the results obtained before conception, signs of gestational diabetes can already be detected. "This is earlier than previously thought possible," says Dr. Catalano.

By detecting gestational diabetes earlier and understanding the metabolic changes better, scientists expect to find ways to improve the health of both mother and child, according to Dr. Catalano.

Additional reading

Catalano, P. M., Tyzbir, E. D., and Sims, E. A. H., Incidence and significance of islet cell antibodies in women with previous gestational diabetes. *Diabetes Care* 13:478-482, 1990.

The research on islet cell antibodies described in this article was supported by the General Clinical Research Centers Program of the NIH National Center for Research Resources and a Diabetes Treatment Centers of America Clinical Research Award. The research on carbohydrate metabolism is supported by the National Institute of Child Health and Human Development.

Figure 33.12. *Self Blood Glucose Monitoring Diary*

DATE	Before eating am	2 hr. after breakfast	2 hr. after lunch	2 hr. after dinner	Amount of insulin	NOTES

Understanding Gestational Diabetes

Figure 33.13. *Food and Exercise Record Sheet*

The following chart is intended to help you and your health care providers keep track of your food and exercise habits and enable you to plan a regimen tailored to your particular needs.

1) Write down everything you eat or drink.
2) Write down items added to foods (e.g., sugar, butter).
3) Write down how your food was prepared (e.g., broiled, fried, baked).
4) Write down the amount you eat in household measures (e.g., 1/2 cup or 2 tbsp.).
5) Write down any exercising you have done, type of exercise, and time spent.

DAY	TIME	FOOD AND TYPE OF PREPARATION	AMOUNT	EXERCISE

Chapter 34

Gestational Hypertension and Preeclampsia-Eclampsia

Introduction

The hypertensive disorders during pregnancy are important causes of maternal death throughout the world, and most of these deaths are attributed to eclampsia. The hypertensive disorders also extensively contribute to stillbirths and neonatal morbidity and mortality. Hypertensive expectant mothers (or gravidas) are predisposed to the development of potentially lethal complications, notably abruptio placentae, disseminated intravascular coagulation (DIC), cerebral hemorrhage, hepatic failure, and acute renal failure.

The number of women who become hypertensive during pregnancy (preeclamptic) is also unclear, but one estimate from an indigent population is calculated to be about 13 percent, and incidences ranging from 10 to 20 percent have been noted in nulliparous women.

Preeclampsia (pure or superimposed) represents the greatest danger for the fetus and is associated with life-threatening maternal syndromes, while transient hypertension is a fairly benign disorder characterized by mild to moderate elevations of blood pressure late in pregnancy which return to normal postpartum.

Preeclampsia, a disease peculiar to pregnancy, mainly in nulliparas, presents primarily after gestational week 20, most frequently near term.

Preeclampsia can lead to two life-threatening complications. The first is a rapidly developing syndrome characterized by microangiopathic

Excerpts from NIH Publication No. 91-3029, August 1991

hemolytic anemia and marked signs of liver dysfunction as well as coagulation changes. This variant, termed HELLP (hemolysis elevated liver enzymes low platelet count), constitutes an emergency requiring prompt pregnancy termination. The second complication is progression of preeclampsia to a convulsive phase termed eclampsia, at one time the major cause of cerebral bleeding and maternal mortality in this disorder. Pending or frank eclampsia also requires immediate termination of gestation.

Classification of Preeclampsia-Eclampsia

The pregnancy-specific condition is termed preeclampsia in the ACOG classification and usually occurs after 20 weeks gestation (or earlier with trophoblastic diseases such as hydatidiform mole or hydrops). It is determined by increased blood pressure accompanied by proteinuria, edema, or both. Either of the following criteria suffice for the diagnosis of hypertension in this situation:

1. systolic blood pressure increases of 30 mm Hg or greater or
2. diastolic blood pressure increases of 15 mm Hg or greater from early values (average of values prior to 20 weeks gestation).

If prior blood pressure is not known, readings of greater than or equal to 140/90 mm Hg after 20 weeks gestation are considered sufficiently elevated to satisfy the blood pressure criteria of preeclampsia. Note, however, that many young pregnant women will show the blood pressure increase required for the diagnosis of preeclampsia without increasing their pressure to 140/90 mm Hg.

In preeclampsia and eclampsia, the blood pressure often is widely variable from moment to moment, and two observers measuring the blood pressure successively may obtain very different readings.

Proteinuria is defined as the excretion of 0.3 gm or greater in a 24-hour specimen. This will usually correlate with 30 mg/dL ("1+ dipstick") or greater in a random urine determination. Proteinuria usually is a late sign in the course of preeclampsia; although it is nonspecific, its appearance greatly bolsters the diagnosis of preeclampsia.

Edema is diagnosed as clinically evident swelling, but fluid retention may also be manifested as a rapid increase of weight without evident swelling.

Preeclampsia always presents potential danger to mother and baby. However, certain signs are particularly ominous:

Gestational Hypertension and Preeclampsia-Eclampsia

- Blood pressure of 160 mm Hg or more systolic, or 110 mm Hg or more diastolic.

- Proteinuria of 2.0 gm or more in 24 hours. The proteinuria should occur for the first time in pregnancy and regress after delivery.

- Increased serum creatinine (greater than 1.2 mg/dL unless known to be previously elevated).

- Platelet count less than 100,000 microliters and/or evidence of microangiopathic hemolytic anemia (with increased lactic acid dehydrogenase).

- Elevated hepatic enzymes (ALT or AST).

- Headache or other cerebral or visual disturbances.

- Epigastric pain.

- Retinal hemorrhage, exudates, or papilledema. These are extremely rare. It is most unlikely that they would occur in the absence of other major signs of severe disease. When present, these signs almost always denote underlying chronic hypertension.

- Pulmonary edema.

Eclampsia is the occurrence of seizures, in a preeclamptic patient, that cannot be attributed to other causes.

Preeclampsia Superimposed Upon Chronic Hypertension

There is ample evidence that preeclampsia may occur in women already hypertensive (i.e., who have chronic hypertension) and that the prognosis for mother and fetus is much worse than with either condition alone. The Committee on Terminology recommended that the diagnosis be made on the basis of increases of blood pressure (30 mm Hg systolic or 15 mm Hg diastolic, or 20 mm Hg mean arterial pressure) together with the appearance of proteinuria or generalized edema.

Risk Factors for Preeclampsia-Eclampsia

The following factors predispose to preeclampsia-eclampsia:

- Primigravidas are from six to eight times more susceptible than are multiparas.

- About one-third of primigravidas who have had eclampsia develop hypertension in about 20 percent of later pregnancies, but generally they have mere rises in blood pressure alone (transient hypertension) rather than preeclampsia. Only 10 to 15 percent have proteinuric hypertension. Transient hypertension, usually miscalled mild preeclampsia in the past as well as in some current classifications, recurs in 80 percent to 88 percent of women pregnant again and often portends ultimate chronic hypertension.

- Women who have had preeclampsia or eclampsia as multiparas usually have some predisposing factor, often chronic hypertension; in these women the recurrence of superimposed preeclampsia may be as high as 70 percent.

- The tendency for preeclampsia is inherited.

- Twin pregnancy increases the risk five times.

- Diabetes is a potent factor, but relative risk cannot be specified because diabetics often have other forms of hypertension that confuse the diagnosis.

- Large, rapidly growing hydatidiform moles increase the risk 10 times in both primigravidas and multiparas.

- Fetal hydrops increases the risk 10 times in both primigravidas and multiparas.

Contrary to popular belief, hydramnios alone and social class do not predispose to preeclampsia, which has the same incidence in white and black American women. Lack of prenatal care may lead to failure to recognize this condition in its early stages. Black women in the childbearing age have two to three times the prevalence of essential hypertension than white women. In blacks, frank and latent chronic hypertension and transient hypertension often are misdiagnosed as preeclampsia.

Gestational Hypertension and Preeclampsia-Eclampsia

Pregnancy can be considered a screening test for ultimate chronic hypertension because women having normotensive pregnancies, especially after age 25, have a low likelihood of developing later chronic hypertension; women with transient hypertension have high probability of ultimate essential hypertension. Preeclamptic and eclamptic hypertension predict nothing, because the disorder does not permit the screening. Had it not been for the intercurrent and unrelated preeclampsia, the pregnancy could have been either normotensive or complicated by transient hypertension.

The Pathology and Pathophysiology of Preeclampsia

Vasospasm

Vasospasm is presumed basic to the pathophysiology of preeclampsia-eclampsia. Vascular constriction causes resistance to blood flow and subsequent arterial hypertension. In some presentations the cardiac output is not maintained, and the resulting absent or mild hypertension underestimates the severity of the disorder. In this context it should be noted that there is good evidence for the condition of "normotensive preeclampsia." Vasospasm and associated vascular damage which cause endothelial cell leaks, together with local hypoxia of surrounding tissues, presumably lead to hemorrhage, necrosis, and other end-organ disturbances of severe preeclampsia.

Vascular reactivity to infused angiotensin II and catecholamines is decreased in normal pregnancy. There is an increased pressor response to some vasoactive hormones in early preeclampsia, and this increased response clearly precedes the onset of hypertension. Angiotensin II refractoriness, observed in normal pregnancy, may be mediated by vascular endothelial synthesis of vasodilatory prostaglandins—for example, prostacyclin or prostaglandin E2 or a prostaglandin-like substance. There are data suggestive that preeclampsia may be associated with inappropriately increased production of a prostaglandin with vasoconstrictor properties or either increased inactivation or diminished synthesis or release of another with vasodilator properties or a combination of these events.

Cardiovascular Changes

Values obtained by invasive cardiovascular monitoring in women with severe preeclampsia and eclampsia have helped to define cardiovascular status. At least five general observations can be made.

1. Before treatment, myocardial contractility is rarely impaired.
2. Cardiac afterload is elevated in the absence of therapeutic interventions.
3. Cardiac output varies inversely with vascular resistance.
4. Medications that reduce vascular resistance (for example, hydralazine) result in increased cardiac output.
5. Ventricular preload, measured by central venous and pulmonary capillary wedge pressures, is usually normal or even low in severe preeclampsia and eclampsia, unless substantial volumes of fluids are administered.

Hemoconcentration is common in women with severe preeclampsia or eclampsia, and the intravascular volume expansion that is normal for pregnancy is not present or is reduced significantly. The woman of average size usually has a blood volume of nearly 5,000 mL during the last several weeks of a normal pregnancy, compared with about 3,500 mL when nonpregnant. With preeclampsia or eclampsia, however, pregnancy-induced hypervolemia either never develops or is reduced significantly after vasospasm ensues. In the absence of hemorrhage, the intravascular compartment in these women usually is not "underfilled," since vasospasm has contracted the space to be filled. Hemoconcentration usually persists a few hours to a few days after delivery when typically the vascular system dilates, the blood volume increases, and the hematocrit falls. In the woman with severe preeclampsia or eclampsia, therefore, hypertension may be exacerbated and the risk for pulmonary edema increased as the result of vigorous fluid therapy administered in an attempt to expand the contracted blood volume to normal pregnancy levels. Likewise she can become hypovolemic even with normal blood loss at delivery.

Hematological Changes

Thrombocytopenia, while infrequently severe, is the most commonly found hematological aberration (by routine clinical testing) associated with hypertension in pregnancy. Fibrin degradation products in serum are elevated only occasionally. Unless there is some degree of placental abruption, plasma fibrinogen does not differ remarkably from levels found late in normal pregnancy.

Antithrombin III levels are lower and fibronectin levels higher in women with preeclampsia compared with normal pregnant women; these levels are consistent with vascular endothelial injury. The clinical utility of serial antithrombin III or fibronectin measurements for the diagnosis and management of preeclampsia awaits further evaluation.

The development of overt thrombocytopenia, that is, a platelet count less than 100,000 per microliter, is an ominous sign in women with preeclampsia. Without delivery, the platelet count most often continues to decrease and may reach levels that can result in cerebral or subcapsular hepatic bleeding as well as excessive blood loss during and after delivery, especially by cesarean section. Maternal thrombocytopenia is not an indication for cesarean delivery.

The cause of the thrombocytopenia is not firmly established. It has been ascribed to platelet deposition at sites of endothelial damage or to an immunological process. There is no firm evidence that the fetuses—infants born to women with severe preeclampsia—eclampsia will develop thrombocytopenia, despite severe maternal thrombocytopenia.

Renal Changes

The majority of women with preeclampsia experience mild to moderately diminished renal perfusion and glomerular filtration with correspondingly elevated plasma creatinine and uric acid levels. An elevated plasma creatinine is a late development in the evolution of preeclampsia and is often discerned only in the range that would be considered normal for nonpregnant individuals, for example, 0.8 to 1.0 mg/dL. In some cases of severe preeclampsia, renal involvement may be profound, and plasma creatinine may be elevated two- to threefold over normal values in nonpregnant women. This probably is due to intrinsic renal changes. In unusual instances, preeclampsia may lead to acute tubular, and even cortical, necrosis.

Although some degree of proteinuria should be found for the diagnosis of preeclampsia-eclampsia to be reliable, proteinuria usually develops late in the course of the disease, so some women may be delivered before it appears. Thus, they may have "true preeclampsia" without proteinuria. This type of proteinuria is nonselective; the increased permeability includes proportionally more of larger molecular weight proteins, such as transferrin and several globulins, than in renal diseases with selective proteinuria. Thus, abnormal albumin excretion is accompanied by increased quantities of many other proteins. Proteinuria usually recedes within a week following delivery and resolution of hypertension, but in exceptional cases the protein leak may take over a month to heal.

Renal changes identifiable by light and electron microscopy include those in the capillary loops, which are variably dilated and contracted.

The endothelial cells are swollen; deposited within and beneath these cells are fibrils, which have been mistaken for thickening and reduplication of the basement membrane. Electron-microscopic studies are consistent with the view that the characteristic changes are caused by swelling of intraglomerular cells, primarily of endothelial cells but on occasion mesangial cells. These changes, which may be accompanied by subendothelial deposits of a fibrin-like protein material, are termed glomerular capillary endotheliosis.

Hepatic Changes

Severe preeclampsia may result in alterations in tests of hepatic function and integrity, including elevation of serum aspartate aminotransferase levels. The lesion most likely to account for hepatic impairment is periportal hemorrhagic necrosis. Bleeding from these lesions may extend beneath the hepatic capsule to form a subcapsular hematoma. Hepatic involvement in preeclampsia-eclampsia is serious, and it frequently is accompanied by evidence of involvement of other organs, especially the kidney and brain, along with hemolysis and thrombocytopenia.

Changes in the Brain

The principal postmortem lesions described in the brains of women who died with eclampsia are hyperemia, focal anemia, thrombosis, and hemorrhage. Cerebral blood flow, oxygen consumption, and vascular resistance were reported as not altered in women with preeclampsia, but the possibility of focal blood flow changes could not be excluded. However, cerebral oxygen consumption is reported to be decreased by 20 percent in eclampsia with normal blood flow, such that McCall alluded to it as "histotoxic hypoxia." Nonspecific abnormalities in the electroencephalogram are common in eclamptic women within 48 hours of seizures, but the tracings are usually normal by 3 months.

Until recently, cranial computed tomographic scans usually were reported to be normal in women with otherwise uncomplicated eclampsia. However, with more advanced equipment, nearly half of eclamptic women have abnormal radiographic findings. The most common of these findings are hypodense areas, frequently seen in the cortical areas, that correspond to areas of petechial hemorrhage and infarction.

While visual disturbances are common with severe preeclampsia, blindness—either alone or accompanying convulsions—is uncommon.

Women with amaurosis of varying degrees usually have computerized tomographic evidence of extensive occipital lobe hypodensities. These women completely recover within a week. Retinal detachment also may cause altered vision, although it is usually one-sided and seldom causes total vision loss. Even without surgical treatment, vision usually returns to normal within approximately a week.

Uteroplacental Perfusion

Compromised placental perfusion due to placental pathology (failure of trophoblastic invasion of spiral arteries) and vasospasm is almost certainly a major culprit in the genesis of increased perinatal morbidity and mortality associated with preeclampsia. However, there are formidable problems to measuring uteroplacental blood flow in humans with preeclampsia. In an earlier study, it was observed that Na injected into the intervillous space was cleared two to three times more rapidly in normotensive pregnant women than in preeclamptic women, implying decreased uteroplacental perfusion.

These findings are supported indirectly by studies of the clearance rate of dehydroisoandrosterone sulfate through placental conversion to estradiol-17beta. More recently, measurement of the velocity of blood flowing through the uterine arteries has been used to estimate uteroplacental blood flow. Using arterial velocity waveforms obtained by Doppler ultrasound, vascular resistance is estimated by comparing systolic and diastolic waveforms. Normally, the uterine vascular bed is a low-resistance circuit and flow continues throughout diastole. As resistance increases, diastolic velocity diminishes in relation to systolic velocity, and this relationship is used to estimate decreased flow. Some investigators report an increased systolic-diastolic ratio in uterine arteries of women with preeclampsia. It should be emphasized that the aforementioned methods do not measure perfusion.

Management of Preeclampsia

Prevention of Preeclampsia

Our ability to prevent preeclampsia is limited by lack of knowledge regarding its cause. The cornerstone of "prevention" in preeclamptic patients has been identification of the high-risk individual, followed by close clinical and laboratory monitoring so that the disease process can be recognized in its early stages. Women can then be hospitalized for more intensive monitoring or delivery. While these measures do not enable us to prevent preeclampsia, they do help to prevent its catastrophic maternal and fetal sequelae.

Although various dietary and pharmacologic strategies (low-salt, high- or low-protein diet; diuretics) have been employed with the hope of preventing preeclampsia or minimizing its severity, none have proved effective so far. Many obstetricians consider daily rest to be effective in preventing preeclampsia or minimizing its severity in high-risk individuals, although this has not been proven.

One preventive strategy that is currently receiving a great deal of attention is the use of low-dose aspirin. At the present time many centers around the world are investigating the ability of low-dose aspirin to prevent preeclampsia. These clinical trials have been prompted by two initial encouraging reports. In both trials, low-dose aspirin or low-dose aspirin plus dipyridamole were successful in reducing the incidence of preeclampsia in the groups studied. There were no fetal or maternal complications attributable to aspirin in either study; however, the total number of women who received aspirin was fewer than 100. Two recently published trials of low-dose aspirin in moderate- and high-risk pregnant women support these earlier encouraging reports and provide evidence that the beneficial effects of aspirin are associated with selective inhibition of platelet thromboxane A2 generation, with preservation of vascular prostacyclin generation. However, since aspirin in large doses is associated with hemorrhagic complications in the newborn, and since prostaglandins play a major role in maternal-fetal physiology, we do not recommend treatment of women at risk for preeclampsia with low-dose aspirin until large clinical trials have conclusively documented the safety and efficacy of this therapy.

Rationale for Treatment

The objectives of therapy for preeclampsia are based on a philosophy of management arising from the knowledge of the pathology and pathophysiology and the prognosis of the disorder for mother and baby.

- Delivery is always appropriate therapy for the mother but may not be so for the fetus. For maternal health, the goal of therapy is to prevent eclampsia as well as other severe complications of preeclampsia. Preeclampsia is the precursor of eclampsia, and careful antepartum observation can identify the woman at risk. Preeclampsia is completely reversible and begins to abate with delivery. Thus, if only maternal well-being were considered, the delivery of all preeclamptic women, regardless of severity of the process or stage of gestation, would be appropriate. Considering the fetus, however, one ought not induce delivery in mildly preeclamptic women whose fetuses are immature but have no signs of fetal compromise. There are two important corollaries of this statement. First, any therapy for preeclampsia other than delivery must have as its successful endpoint the reduction of perinatal mortality and morbidity. Second, the cornerstone of obstetric management of preeclampsia is based on a decision as to whether the infant is more likely to survive in utero or in the nursery.

- The signs and symptoms of preeclampsia are not of pathogenetic importance. The pathologic and pathophysiologic changes of preeclampsia indicate that poor perfusion is the major factor leading to the derangement of maternal physiologic function and to increased perinatal mortality and morbidity rates. Attempts to treat preeclampsia by natriuresis or by the lowering of blood pressure do not alleviate the important pathophysiologic changes. In fact, natriuresis may be counterproductive and may adversely affect fetal outcome because plasma volume is already reduced in preeclamptic women.

- The pathogenetic changes of preeclampsia are present long before clinical criteria leading to the diagnosis are manifest. Several studies indicate that changes in vascular reactivity, plasma volume, and renal function antedate, in some cases by months, the increases in blood pressure, protein excretion, and sodium retention. These findings suggest that irreversible changes affecting fetal well-being may be present prior to the clinical diagnosis. This possibility probably explains why dietary, pharmacologic, and postural therapy are not successful when avoidance of perinatal morbidity and mortality is taken as the endpoint. If a rationale for modes of therapy other than delivery of the fetus exists, it would be to palliate the maternal condition in order to allow fetal maturation. However, even this rationale is controversial. Accelerated and severe hypertension can complicate any phase of gestation. Fortunately, most of these crises occur late in pregnancy and are associated with preeclampsia; the challenge to the physician is to maintain maternal blood pressure at safe levels while effecting a delivery.

Nonpharmacological Management

Antepartum monitoring of the mother has two goals. The first is the early recognition of the condition because infants of mothers with even mild preeclampsia are at increased risk, and the second is to gauge the rate of progression of the condition, both to prevent eclampsia by delivery and to determine whether fetal well-being can be safely monitored by the usual intermittent observations. Ideally, identification of early changes would allow intervention prior to the advent of clinical symptoms. At present, other than the early increased sensitivity to angiotensin II, which is not practical for application to widespread screening, no test has a predictive value sufficient to use clinically. Notably unsuccessful are the "rollover test" and elevated second trimester blood pressures.

At present, clinical management is dictated by the overt clinical signs of preeclampsia. Unfortunately, proteinuria—the most valid clinical indicator of preeclampsia—is often a late change, sometimes even preceded by seizures, and so is not a useful sign for early recognition. Although rapid weight increase and facial and digital edema indicate the fluid and sodium retention characteristic of preeclampsia, they are neither universally present nor uniquely characteristic of preeclampsia. These signs are, at most, a reason for closer observation of blood pressure and monitoring of urinary protein. Early recognition of preeclampsia is based primarily on diagnostic blood pressure increases in the late second and early third trimesters relative to early pregnancy. Using blood pressure changes without evidence of proteinuria as an indicator does, undoubtedly, result in the diagnosis of preeclampsia in some normal women as well as in some with underlying renal or vascular disease. Because the goal of early diagnosis is to identify patients requiring more careful observation, however, overdiagnosis is preferable to underdiagnosis.

Once the blood pressure changes suggestive of preeclampsia appear, an office examination within 24 to 48 hours is strongly recommended, or with selected patients, blood pressure and urinary protein must be checked at home. These measures are directed at determining how fast the condition is progressing in order to ensure that it is not following a fulminant course. Frequency of subsequent observations is determined by these initial observations and the ensuing clinical progression. If the condition appears stable, weekly observations may be appropriate. If it appears to be accelerating, more frequent observations, usually in hospital, are required. The initial appearance of proteinuria is an especially

Gestational Hypertension and Preeclampsia-Eclampsia

important sign of progression and dictates frequent observation, which is best accomplished in hospital.

If an increasing rate of deterioration is noted, as determined by laboratory findings, symptoms, and clinical signs, the decision to continue the pregnancy is determined day by day. Important clinical signs are blood pressure, urinary output, and fluid retention as evidenced by daily weight increase. Laboratory studies are performed at intervals of no more than 48 hours. These include examination for possible activation of the coagulation system as determined by platelet count, and evaluation of renal function as measured by urinary protein excretion and serum creatinine and urate levels. In addition, subjective evidence of central nervous system involvement—such as headache, disorientation, and visual symptoms—and the presence of hepatic distention, as indicated by abdominal pain and hepatic tenderness, are equally important indicators of worsening preeclampsia.

Antepartum Management of Preeclampsia

There is little to suggest that therapeutic efforts alter the underlying pathophysiology of preeclampsia. Therapeutic intervention is palliative. At best, it may slow the progression of the condition, but more likely, it merely allows continuation of the pregnancy. Bed rest is a usual and reasonable recommendation for the woman with mild preeclampsia, although its efficacy is not clearly established. Strict sodium restriction or diuretic therapy has no role in the prevention or therapy of preeclampsia. In women with marked sodium retention as manifested by significant edema, modest sodium restriction may not alter the course of the disease but may reduce discomfort.

Indications for Delivery

Prolonged antepartum management of women with severe preeclampsia is not practiced in most centers. With improvements in neonatal care, many investigators regard delivery of women with severe preeclampsia beyond 30 weeks gestation to be in the best interest of not only the mother but also the fetus. When gestational age is critical (between 25 and 30 weeks), one might consider controlling maternal blood pressure along with meticulous observation of the maternal and fetal condition. Delivery is then indicated by worsening maternal symptoms, laboratory evidence of end-organ dysfunction, or deterioration of fetal condition. Whether this plan of action can effect a decrease in perinatal morbidity and mortality rates is not clear. The use of this approach with even very immature fetuses may only replace a nonviable neonate with an extremely premature one, with the attendant risk of long-range neurologic disability. Such an approach should therefore be attempted only in centers equipped to provide meticulous maternal observation and daily assessment of fetal and maternal condition.

Fetal Indications. The major consideration in decisions for delivery should usually be fetal well-being, for the reasons cited. Thus, if the maternal condition is stable, delivery is indicated by signs of abnormal fetal function. If fetal growth and well-being remain normal, pregnancy should proceed to spontaneous labor. If the maternal condition is rapidly deteriorating, however, delivery is indicated for fetal well-being. With maternal deterioration, a reflection of increasingly poor perfusion of brain, kidney, and liver, uteroplacental blood flow is also likely to be compromised. In addition, the predictive value of all tests of fetal well-being is invalidated by rapid changes in the maternal and, hence, fetal condition.

Maternal Indications. Although fetal considerations usually dictate the timing of delivery, there are important exceptions. In the rare case in which a choice is made to palliate maternal signs and symptoms in order to allow fetal growth or maturation, such efforts must be abandoned if the maternal condition worsens. Also, a potentially lethal complication of preeclampsia, hepatic rupture, cannot be prevented by any mode of therapy other than delivery. It has a mortality rate of 65 percent. Thus, the woman with hepatic capsular distention manifested by hepatomegaly, tenderness of the liver, and abnormal hepatic function values should be delivered regardless of fetal well-being or maturity.

Route of Delivery

Vaginal delivery is preferable to cesarean delivery for preeclamptic women. It is desirable, if possible, to avoid the added stress of surgery because of multiple physiologic abnormalities. Palliation for several hours should not increase maternal risk if performed appropriately. Induction should be carried out aggressively and expeditiously once the decision for delivery is made. In gestation remote from term in which delivery is indicated but fetal and maternal condition are stable enough to permit pregnancy to be prolonged 36 hours, glucocorticoids can be safely administered to accelerate fetal pulmonary maturity.

Gestational Hypertension and Preeclampsia-Eclampsia

The aggressive approach to induction indicates that amniotomy be performed as soon as possible and a clear endpoint be formulated at the initiation of therapy, usually within 8 to 12 hours of the decision to induce delivery. A trial of induction is warranted regardless of cervical condition. Obviously, if vaginal delivery cannot be effected within the predetermined time frame, cesarean delivery should be considered. Likewise, cesarean delivery is performed for other usual obstetrical indications.

Regional anesthesia such as epidural analgesia offers its usual advantages for vaginal and cesarean delivery but does carry the possibility of extensive sympatholysis with consequent decreased cardiac output, hypotension, and impairment of already compromised uteroplacental perfusion. This is a common problem with spinal anesthesia, which is felt by most experts to be contraindicated in the preeclamptic woman. This problem can be avoided by meticulous attention to anesthetic technique and volume expansion. Regional anesthesia is not a rational means to lower blood pressure because it does so at the expense of cardiac output. Likewise, although analgesia with narcotics is not contraindicated and should be used when necessary, there is abundant evidence that attempting to manage or prevent eclampsia with profound maternal sedation is dangerous and ineffective.

Maternal-Fetal Surveillance

Whether the patient has acute or chronic hypertension, fetal surveillance is indicated. The methodology for fetal surveillance is the same in both cases and the interpretation is similar. If the fetus is compromised, then decision making and judgment are necessary. If intrauterine growth retardation is identified by fundal measurements and documented by ultrasound, biophysical testing should be implemented. The amount of amniotic fluid is significant, since a decreased amount of fluid may be associated with cord problems during labor.

Nonstress testing, oxytocin challenge testing, ultrasound, and fetal movement counts constitute the most common fetal surveillance techniques. If determination of pulmonary maturity would influence management, amniocentesis should be done to determine this prior to the interruption of pregnancy.

Fetal surveillance involves determining if the fetus is growing appropriately. When fundal height measurements are inappropriate, other investigative avenues such as ultrasound biophysical testing should then be pursued. As long as the fetus continues to grow in an appropriate manner, it can be inferred that the placenta and/or uterine blood flow are appropriate.

Drug Treatment of Hypertension Related to Preeclampsia

Disagreement exists on whether, and how efficiently, the uteroplacental blood flow is autoregulated. Those who liken the uterine circulation to a rigid conduit incapable of autoregulation caution against precipitous decrements in mean arterial pressure because placental perfusion is already compromised in preeclampsia. Others prefer a more aggressive approach when treating hypertension. Resolution of this problem awaits perfection of reliable and safe methodology to measure placental perfusion, followed by appropriately designed therapeutic trials. In the interim the following guidelines are recommended.

Treatment of Hypertension Remote From Delivery

The palliative management of preeclampsia remote from delivery is controversial. The sole rationale is to allow maturation of the fetus and, if attempted, it must not subject the mother to undue risk. An important part of safe management is control of elevated blood pressure. In the woman with diastolic blood pressure equal to or greater than 100 mm Hg, risk is sufficient to warrant pharmacological therapy. The therapy is solely for maternal benefit; there is neither theoretical basis nor empiric evidence that such therapy is beneficial to the fetus. If therapy is elected, methyldopa is the drug of choice. If this is not tolerated or is unsuccessful, calcium channel blockers, beta-blockers, or hydralazine are reasonable additions or alternatives. Successful control of blood pressure should not be interpreted as eliminating risk for mother or baby. No evidence indicates therapy improves fetal well-being or reduces the risk of abruption, disseminated intravascular coagulation, seizures, or other maternal risk. Both maternal and fetal assessment must be meticulously carried out regardless of the degree of blood pressure control.

Treatment of Acute Hypertension During Delivery

In the more usual situation, antihypertensive therapy may occasionally be indicated as acute palliative therapy in the woman in whom delivery is indicated. Antihypertensive agents can be withheld

Gestational Hypertension and Preeclampsia-Eclampsia

as long as maternal pressure is only mildly elevated. However, persistent diastolic levels of 105 mm Hg or higher should be treated. (It may, however, be prudent to treat lower levels in certain situations: e.g., the young gravida whose recent diastolic levels were below 75 mm Hg, or the woman with chronic hypertension for many years and in whom hypertensive heart disease may be present.) When treatment is required, the ideal drug that reduces pressures to a safe level should:

- Act quickly
- Reduce pressure in a controlled manner
- Not lower cardiac output
- Reverse uteroplacental vascular constriction
- Result in no adverse maternal or fetal effects.

The medications used to treat hypertensive crises in pregnancy are summarized below. The degree to which blood pressure should be decreased is disputed. Levels between 90 and 105 mm Hg diastolic are recommended.

- Hydralazine administered intravenously is the drug of choice. Use low doses (start with a 5-mg I.V. bolus, then give 5 to 10 mg every 20 to 30 minutes) in order to avoid precipitous decreases. Side effects include tachycardia and headache. Neonatal thrombocytopenia has been reported.

- Diazoxide is recommended for the occasional patient whose hypertension is refractory to hydralazine. Use 30-mg miniboluses, since maternal vascular collapse and death have been associated with the customary 300-mg dose. Side effects include arrest of labor and neonatal hyperglycemia.

- Experience with parenteral labetalol is growing, and this drug may replace diazoxide as the second-line drug.

- Favorable results have been reported with calcium channel blockers. However, if magnesium sulfate is being infused, the magnesium ion may potentiate the effect of calcium channel blockers, resulting in precipitous and severe hypotension.

- Do not use sodium nitroprusside (fetal cyanide poisoning has been reported in animal models) or diuretics (e.g., furosemide;

see text). However, in the final analysis, maternal well-being will dictate the choice of therapy.

The current drug of first choice is intravenous hydralazine, which if given cautiously is successful in most instances. It has been shown to be effective against preeclamptic hypertension. Although this is sometimes used as an intravenous (I.V.) infusion, the pharmacokinetics (maximal effect at 20 minutes, duration of action 6 to 8 hours), indicate intermittent bolus injections as more sensible. A 5-mg bolus is given intravenously over 1 to 2 minutes. Twenty minutes later, subsequent doses are dictated by the initial response. Once the desired effect is obtained, the drug is repeated as necessary (frequently in several hours). If a total of 20 mg is administered without therapeutic response, other agents should be considered.

Diazoxide is restricted to the occasional resistant case and should be administered in small doses (30-mg boluses). Preliminary successes have been recorded when calcium channel blockers (e.g., nifedipine) have been used, and in 1989 this group of drugs was undergoing testing.

One concern about calcium channel blockers, however, is that most patients with acute hypertension during delivery will also be receiving magnesium sulfate (vida infra). Magnesium may potentiate the effects of calcium channel blockers and lead to precipitous decreases in blood pressure. Nifedipine acts rapidly, causing significant reduction in arterial blood pressure within 10 to 20 minutes of oral administration. The onset of antihypertensive activity can possibly be shortened by chewing the capsule or puncturing it with several needle holes before it is swallowed. The principal side effects are headache and cutaneous flushing, but minimal reflex tachycardia may occur. Like vasodilators, calcium channel blockers may cause cessation of uterine contractions. They are used to stop premature labor without maternal or fetal side effects.

Limited data are available on the use of parenteral labetalol (which some advocate as a second-line drug), starting with 10 mg and not to exceed 1 mg/kg, or clonidine. Neither labetalol nor clonidine appears to be more effective than hydralazine. Sodium nitroprusside is chosen only after the failure of hydralazine, diazoxide, calcium channel blockers, labetalol, and clonidine because of cyanide poisoning and fetal death reported in laboratory animals.

Finally, the use of potent saluretic agents such as furosemide in treating hypertensive crises at term, as adjunct therapy to the vasodilators just discussed, is condemned by most authorities but still has its advocates. Given the hemoconcentration and cardiovascular hemodynamics of preeclampsia and the susceptibility of some women with this disease to either intrapartal hypotension or puerperal vascular collapse, many counsel against the use of potent diuretics and care must be taken with all antihypertensive agents. In the last analysis, however, the mother's well-being should take precedence, even if the therapy necessary to control pressure may potentially harm the fetus.

Anti-Eclamptic Therapy

It is a mistake to equate the eclamptic convulsion with hypertensive encephalopathy since the convulsion can arise in a seemingly stable patient manifesting only minimal blood pressure elevation. For this reason, many clinicians initiate prophylactic therapy when women with suspected preeclampsia are in labor, even if premonitory signs are absent.

Since the pathogenesis of the eclamptic convulsion is still poorly understood, it is not surprising to find disagreements on how to treat women with impending convulsions or frank eclampsia. Most authorities, especially in North America, use parenterally administered magnesium sulfate; others prefer conventional anticonvulsant drugs such as diazepam and phenytoin. Critics of the use of magnesium sulfate stress that it crosses the blood-brain barrier very slowly and has no effect on electroencephalographic abnormalities. Defense of magnesium sulfate therapy has been mainly empiric, but of interest are recent observations of the effect of magnesium ions on prostaglandin metabolism. For example, Watson et al. have demonstrated that magnesium at levels measured in treated preeclamptics increases prostacyclin release by cultured endothelial cells from human umbilical veins, and that plasma from preeclamptic women treated with magnesium sulfate had similar actions. The preference for magnesium sulfate, especially in the United States, is documented by its successful use in several large series, but it has never undergone a definitive controlled trial. Similarly, there is a need for more extensive data regarding the effect of both magnesium and standard anticonvulsant drugs on the neonate. Preliminary data on the effects of magnesium sulfate on fetuses are encouraging.

Volume Expansion Therapy

Just as there are advocates of saluretic agents, there are claims that volume expansion may reduce blood pressure in selected patients with preeclampsia. This approach derives from observations that plasma volume, cardiac output, and pulmonary capillary wedge pressure (PCWP) may be decreased in this condition, as well as from reports that infusion of colloids decreased blood pressure and peripheral vascular resistance, despite increments in intravascular volume. However, the effects of colloid infusion are usually transient, probably because the vasculature in preeclampsia is "leaky," whereas infusion of crystalloids alone decreases oncotic pressure, which is already depressed in preeclampsia. Such decrements can lead to pulmonary or cerebral edema, especially in the immediate puerperium, when oncotic pressure levels decrease further while central volume and PCWP tend to rise. Thus, one should be cautious concerning crystalloid infusions into preeclamptic women during labor, and until a postpartum diuresis is established. Signs suggesting poor renal perfusion (i.e., oliguria) resolve quickly after delivery, and acute renal failure is an unusual complication, even in severe preeclampsia.

Other Treatment Considerations

Invasive cardiovascular monitoring may be required in severe or complicated cases, especially during operative procedures. Criteria have recently been proposed for pulmonary artery catheterization in the patient with severe preeclampsia. Many experts, however, believe that these criteria are too broad, and find the indications for Swan-Ganz catheterization (a procedure associated with a certain morbidity) relatively uncommon.

Treating Hypertension Persisting Postpartum

The potential problems of serious compromise of placental perfusion and, in turn, fetal well-being that can be induced by antihypertensive agents are obviated by delivery. If there is a problem after delivery controlling persisting severe hypertension, intermittent intravenous hydralazine can be used repeatedly early in the puerperium to control it. Once repeated blood pressure readings remain near normal, the hydralazine is stopped and treatment with standard oral regimens should be started.

Several other regimens are effective for control of severe postpartum hypertension. These include infusion of nitroprusside (0.5 to 10 mg/kg/min). Labetalol, 20 to 80 mg by intravenous bolus, lowers blood pressure in 5 to 10 minutes and may be repeated at 10-minute intervals.

Acute hypertensive changes induced by pregnancy usually dissipate rapidly after delivery, certainly within the first several days. If severe hypertension persists more than 3 to 5 days, then the likelihood of underlying chronic hypertension is greatly increased. In these cases, oral antihypertensive therapy is begun before discharge and the woman evaluated in 1 week. For women who were hypertensive before pregnancy, chronic treatment is likely to be necessary. If prepregnancy blood pressure was normal or unknown, it is reasonable to stop oral medication after 3 to 4 weeks and observe the blood pressure at weekly intervals for a month, and at monthly intervals for a year. If hypertension recurs, treatment should be resumed.

Lactation

Many women who have been chronically hypertensive during pregnancy will have the desire to breast-feed their infant for a period of several weeks to 1 year. The concentrations of most of the antihypertensive drugs have been assessed in human breast milk and plasma after single or multiple dosings, and all agents studied have been detectable in the milk. However, only a few reports have evaluated whether the drug is detectable in the plasma of the breast-fed infant or if there is any hemodynamic or adverse effect of the agent on the infant. Furthermore, there have been no clinical trials involving several subjects which have studied the cardiovascular effects of any antihypertensive agent on the breast-fed infant.

In mildly hypertensive mothers who wish to breast-feed for a few months, the clinician may consider withholding medication with close observation of the maternal blood pressure. Following discontinuation of the nursing period, the antihypertensive therapy should be reinstituted as appropriate. For those patients with more severe blood pressure elevation on a single antihypertensive agent, the clinician may consider reducing antihypertensive drug dosage with close observation of both the mother and breast-fed infant. If the mother requires multiple agents for controlling her hypertension, breast-feeding is not advisable.

References

Chesley LC: Hypertensive Disorders In Pregnancy. New York: Appleton-Century-Crofts, 1978.

Cunningham FG, Leveno KJ: Management of pregnancy-induced hypertension. In: Rubin PC (ed), Handbook of Hypertension, vol. 10, Hypertension in Pregnancy. Amsterdam: Elsevier, 1988, pp 290-319.

Pollak VE: Pre-eclampsia and kidney disease. Ch. 4. In: Coggins CH, Cummings NB (eds), Prevention of Kidney and Urinary Tract Diseases. DHEW Publication No. (NIH) 78-855, 1978, pp 95-129.

Robinson N: Salt in pregnancy. Lancet 1958;1:178-181.

MacGillivray I: Some observations on the incidence of preeclampsia. J Obstet Gynaecol Br Emp 1958;65:536-539.

Thompson AM, Chun D, Baird D: Perinatal mortality in Hong Kong and in Aberdeen, Scotland. J Obstet Gynaecol Br Common 1963;70: 871-877.

Hughes EC (ed): Obstetric-Gynecologic Terminology. Philadelphia: Davis, 1972, pp 422-423.

Herrick WW, Tillman AJB: The mild toxemias of late pregnancy: their relation to cardiovascular and renal disease. Am J Obstet Gynecol 1936;31: 832-844.

Berman S: Observations in the toxemia clinic, Boston Lying-in Hospital, 1923-1930. N Engl J Med 1930;203: 361-363.

Hinselmann H: Allgemeine Krankheitslehre. In: Hinselmann H (ed), Die Eklampsie. Bonn: Cohen, 1924, pp 1-87.

Chesley LC, Cooper DW: Genetics of hypertension in pregnancy: possible single gene control of pre-eclampsia and eclampsia in the descendants of eclamptic women. Br J Obstet Gynaecol 1986;93(9):898-908.

White P: Pregnancy complicating diabetes. Surg Gynecol Obstet 1935;61: 324-332.

Page EW: The relation between hydatid moles, relative ischemia of the gravid uterus, and the placental origin of eclampsia. Am J Obstet Gynecol 1939;37: 291-293.

Jann R: Spatgestosen bei hydrops fetus et placentae infolge rhesusinkompatibilitat. Arch Gynaekol 1954;184:731-748.

Scott JS: Pregnancy toxaemia associated with hydrops foetalis, hydatidiform mole, and hydramnios. J Obstet Gynaecol Br Emp 1958;65: 689-701.

Nelson TR: A clinical study of pre-eclampsia, pts I and II. J Obstet Gynaecol Br Emp 1955;62: 48-66.

Redman CW: Eclampsia still kills. Br Med J 1988;296: 1209-1210.

Talledo OE, Chesley LC, Zuspan FP: Renin-angiotensin system in normal and toxemic pregnancies. III. Differential sensitivity to angiotensin II and norepinephrine in toxemia of pregnancy. Am J Obstet Gynecol 1968;100: 218-221.

Gant NF, Daley GL, Chand S, Whalley PJ, MacDonald PC: A study of angiotensin II pressor response throughout primigravid pregnancy. J Clin Invest 1973;52: 2682-2689.

Hankins GD, Wendel GD Jr, Cunningham FG, Leveno KJ: Longitudinal evaluation of hemodynamic changes in eclampsia. Am J Obstet Gynecol 1984;150: 506-512.

Groenendijk R, Trimbros JB, Wallenburg HC: Hemodynamic measurements in preeclampsia: preliminary observations. Am J Obstet Gynecol 1984;150:232-236.

Wallenburg HCS: Hemodynamics in hypertensive pregnancy. In: Ruben PC (ed), Handbook of Hypertension, vol. 10, Hypertension in Pregnancy. Amsterdam: Elsevier, 1988, pp 66-101.

Pritchard JA, Cunningham FG, Pritchard SA: The Parkland Memorial Hospital protocol for treatment of eclampsia: evaluation of 245 cases. Am J Obstet Gynecol 1984;148: 951-963.

Pritchard JA, Cunningham FG, Mason RA: Coagulation changes in eclampsia: their frequency and pathogenesis. Am J Obstet Gynecol 1976;124: 855-859.

Roberts JM, Taylor RN, Musci TJ, Rodgers GM, Hubel CA, McLaughlin MK: Preeclampsia: An endothelial cell disorder. Am J Obstet Gynecol 1989;161: 1200-1204.

Saleh AA, Bottoms SF, Welch RA, Ali AM, Mariona FG, Mammen EF: Preeclampsia, delivery, and the hemostatic system. Am J Obstet Gynecol 1987;157: 331-336.

Burrows RF, Hunter DJ, Andrew M, Kelton JG: A prospective study investigating the mechanism of thrombocytopenia in preeclampsia. Obstet Gynecol 1987;70: 334-338.

Pritchard JA, Cunningham FG, Pritchard SA, Mason RA: How often does maternal preeclampsia-eclampsia incite thrombocytopenia in the fetus? Obstet Gynecol 1987;69: 292-295.

Gaber LW, Spargo BH, Lindheimer MD: Renal pathology in preeclampsia. Clin Obstet Gynaecol (Bailliére) 1987;1:971-995.

Chesley LC: Diagnosis of preeclampsia. Obstet Gynecol 1985;65: 423-425.

Spargo B, McCartney CP, Winemiller R: Glomerular capillary endotheliosis in toxemia of pregnancy. Arch Pathol 1959;68: 593-599.

Sibai BM, Taslimi MM, el Nazer A, Amon E, Mabie BC, Ryan GM: Maternal-perinatal outcome associated with the syndrome of hemolysis, elevated liver enzymes and low platelets in severe preeclampsia-eclampsia. Am J Obstet Gynecol 1986;155: 501-509.

Sheehan HL: Pathologic lesions in the hypertensive toxaemias of pregnancy. In: Hammond J, Browne FJ, Wolstenholm GEW (eds), Toxaemias of Pregnancy, Human and Veterinary. Philadelphia: Blakiston, 1950, pp 16-22.

McCall ML: Cerebral circulation and metabolism in toxemia of pregnancy. Observations on the effects of veratrum viride and Apresoline (1-hydrazinophthalazine). Am J Obstet Gynecol 1953;66: 1015-1030.

Sibai BM, Spinnato JA, Watson DL, Lewis JA, Anderson GD: Eclampsia. IV. Neurological findings and future outcome. Am J Obstet Gynecol 1985;152: 184-192.

Brown CE, Purdy P, Cunningham FG: Head computed tomographic scans in women with eclampsia. Am J Obstet Gynecol 1988;159: 915-920.

Sheehan HL, Lynch JB (eds): Cerebral lesions, Ch. 32. In: Pathology of Toxaemia of Pregnancy. Baltimore: Williams and Wilkins, 1973: 524-553.

Browne JCM, Veall N: The maternal placental blood flow in normotensive and hypertensive women. J Obstet Gynaecol Br Emp 1953;60: 141-147.

Fleischer A, Schulman H, Farmakides G, et al: Uterine artery Doppler velocimetry in pregnant women with hypertension. Am J Obstet Gynecol 1986;154: 806-813.

Trudinger BJ, Giles WB, Cook CM: Flow velocity waveforms in the maternal utero-placental and fetal umbilical placental circulations. Am J Obstet Gynecol 1985;152: 155-163.

Beaufils M, Uzan S, Donsimoni R, Colau JC: Prevention of preeclampsia by early antiplatelet therapy. Lancet 1985;1: 840-842.

Wallenburg HC, Dekker GA, Makovitz JW, Rotmans P: Low-dose aspirin prevents pregnancy-induced hypertension and pre-eclampsia in angiotensin-sensitive primigravidae. Lancet 1986;1: 1-3.

Schiff E, Peleg E, Goldenberg M, et al: The use of aspirin to prevent pregnancy-induced hypertension and lower the ratio of thromboxane A2 to prostacyclin in relatively high-risk pregnancies. N Engl J Med 1989;321: 351-356.

Benigni A, Gregorini G, Frusca T, et al: Effect of low-dose aspirin on fetal and maternal generation of thromboxane by platelets in women at risk for pregnancy-induced hypertension. N Engl J Med 1989;321: 357-362.

Stuart MJ, Gross SJ, Elrad H, Graeber JE: Effects of acetylsalicylic-acid ingestion on maternal and neonatal hemostasis. N Engl J Med 1982;307: 909-912.

Davison JM, Lindheimer MD: Hypertension and pregnancy. In: Schrier RW, Gottschalk CW (eds), Diseases of the Kidney. 4th ed., vol. 2, Boston: Little Brown & Company, 1988, pp 1653-1686.

Ferris TF: How should hypertension during pregnancy be managed? An internist's approach. Med Clin North Am 1984;68: 491-503.

Walters BN, Redman CW: Treatment of severe pregnancy-associated hypertension with the calcium antagonist nifedipine. Br J Obstet Gynaecol 1984;91: 330-336.

Naulty J, Cefalo RC, Lewis PE: Fetal toxicity of nitroprusside in the pregnant ewe. Am J Obstet Gynecol 1981;139: 708-711.

Ferris TF: Prostanoids in normal and hypertensive pregnancy. In: Rubin PC (ed), Hypertension in Pregnancy. New York: Elsevier, 1988, pp 102-117.

Dinsdale HB: Does magnesium sulfate treat eclamptic seizures? Yes. Arch Neurol 1988;45: 1360-1361.

Kaplan PW, Lesser RP, Fisher RS, Repke JT, Hanley DF: No, magnesium sulfate should not be used in treating eclamptic seizures. Arch Neurol 1988;45: 1361-1364.

Thurnau GR, Kemp DB, Jarvis A: Cerebrospinal fluid levels of magnesium in patients with preeclampsia after treatment with intravenous magnesium sulfate. A preliminary report. Am J Obstet Gynecol 1987;157: 1435-1438.

Sibai BM, Spinnato JA, Watson DL, Lewis JA, Anderson GD: Effect of magnesium sulfate on electroencephalographic findings in preeclampsia-eclampsia. Obstet Gynecol 1984;64: 261-266.

Watson KV, Moldow CF, Ogburn PL, Jacob HS: Magnesium sulfate: Rationale for its use in preeclampsia. Proc Natl Acad Sci USA 1986;83: 1075-1078.

Sibai BM, Anderson GD: Pregnancy outcome of intensive therapy in severe hypertension in first trimester. Obstet Gynecol 1986;67: 517-522.

Pruett KM, Kirshon B, Cotton DB, Adam K, Doody KJ: The effects of magnesium sulfate therapy on Apgar scores. Am J Obstet Gynecol 1988;159: 1047-1048.

Gallery ED, Delprado W, Gyory AZ: Antihypertensive effect of plasma volume expansion in pregnancy-associated hypertension. Aust NZ J Med 1981;11: 20-24.

Oian P, Maltau JM, Noddeland H, Fadnes HO: Transcapillary fluid balance in pre-eclampsia. Br J Obstet Gynaecol 1986;93: 235-239.

Zinaman M, Rubin J, Lindheimer MD: Serial plasma oncotic pressure levels and echoencephalography during and after delivery in severe pre-eclampsia. Lancet 1985;1: 1245-1247.

Gestational Hypertension and Preeclampsia-Eclampsia

Clark SL, Cotton DB: Clinical indications for pulmonary artery catheterization in the patient with severe preeclampsia. Am J Obstet Gynecol 1988;158: 453-458.

American College of Obstetricians and Gynecologists: Invasive hemodynamic monitoring in obstetrics and gynecology. ACOG Technical Bulletin October 1988; No. 121.

White WB: Management of hypertension during lactation. Hypertension 1984;6: 297-300.

White WB, Andreoli JW, Cohn RD: Alpha-methyldopa disposition in mothers with hypertension and in their breast-fed infants. Clin Pharmacol Ther 1985;37: 387-390.

Miller ME, Cohn RD, Burghart PH: Hydrochlorothiazide disposition in a mother and her breast-fed infant. J Pediatrics 1982;101: 789-791.

Krause W, Stopelli I, Milia S, Rainer E: Transfer of mepindolol to newborns by breast-feeding mothers after single and repeated daily doses. Eur J Clin Pharmacol 1982;22: 53-55.

Chapter 35

Disorders of the Placenta

The placenta is an organ unique to pregnancy. Throughout pregnancy, it acts as a transport service between the mother and the baby. The placenta transfers oxygen and nutrients from the mother's bloodstream to the baby and carries fetal waste products in the opposite direction.

In the third trimester, the two main problems that can occur with the placenta are often signaled by the same symptom: vaginal bleeding. Any amount of bleeding in late pregnancy should be reported to your doctor immediately.

Placental Abruption

Causes and Risk Factors

Abruption, or separation, of the placenta refers to the separation of the placenta from the inner wall of the uterus before labor begins. It can decrease or interrupt the flow of oxygen-rich blood to the baby.

Placental abruption is one of the leading causes of fetal death in the third trimester. It can also cause the mother to go into shock as a result of hemorrhage or to have severe circulatory problems. Fortunately, with close monitoring of the mother and baby and prompt delivery at signs of trouble, the outlook for both is good.

Reprinted by permission of William Morrow & Company, Inc. from *Mayo Clinic Complete Book of Pregnancy and Baby's First Year.* Copyright 1994 by Mayo Foundation for Medical Education and Research.

Separation of the placenta may be partial, involving only a part of the placenta, such as an edge. Or it may be complete, in which the entire placenta is separated from the inside of the uterus. Although placental abruption always causes some bleeding, the blood may not always be apparent. Sometimes the middle portion of the placenta pulls away from the uterine wall, leaving the outer margins and membranes attached. Blood can thus be trapped and concealed in a "pocket." At other times, the baby's head or another body part may be so tightly pressed against the wall of the uterus that the blood cannot make its way past.

Placental abruption occurs in about one of every 150 births. Its cause is unknown, but it appears to be more common in black women, in women who are older (especially those older than 40), in women who have had many children and in women who smoke.

By far, however, the most common condition associated with placental abruption is hypertension in pregnancy. Women who have high blood pressure during their pregnancy—whether the condition first developed while they were pregnant or was present before—are more prone to placental abruption.

The risk of abruption also seems to be higher with premature rupture of the membranes. This is a condition in which the membranes that surround the fetus break too early in pregnancy, before labor begins. Very rarely, trauma or injury to the mother may cause placental abruption.

Signs and Symptoms

In the early stages of placental abruption, there may be no indication that it is happening. When symptoms do occur, the most common is bleeding from the vagina. The bleeding may be scant, heavy or somewhere in between, but the amount does not necessarily correspond to how much of the placenta has separated from the inside of the uterus. Other symptoms that may be caused by placental abruption include back or abdominal pain, uterine tenderness and rapid contractions. The uterus may feel hard and rigid.

Diagnosis

When a woman has vaginal bleeding in the third trimester, her doctor will usually try to exclude causes such as placenta previa (see below). Placental abruption is diagnosed through a process of elimination of other possible causes of the bleeding. An ultrasound exam

Disorders of the Placenta

may be done to try to detect a separated placenta, but often the condition is not detectable by this technique.

Management

When placental abruption is suspected, the steps taken depend largely on the condition of both the baby and the mother. Electronic monitoring is usually used to look at patterns of the baby's heart rate. If monitoring shows no signs that the baby is in immediate trouble, the mother may be hospitalized so that her condition can be monitored closely. This may be the chosen course if the pregnancy has not yet reached term.

Signs that the baby is in jeopardy will prompt immediate delivery. If there is severe bleeding, the mother may need blood transfusions. Cesarean delivery may be necessary, although in some situations vaginal birth may be possible.

Outlook For the Future

Unfortunately, there is an increased risk (about one in 10) that placental abruption will recur in a woman's subsequent pregnancies. The good news is that, with close monitoring and prompt action at signs of danger to the baby, most of these mothers and babies get safely through birth with no long-term ill effects.

Placenta Previa

Causes and Risk Factors

At term, the placenta normally is located high up near the top (fundus) of the uterus. But in some pregnancies, the placenta lies low in the uterus and may partly or completely cover the opening of the cervix. This condition, called placenta previa, poses a potential danger to mother and baby because of the risk of hemorrhage (excessive blood loss) before or during delivery.

Placenta previa may take one of several forms:

1. **Marginal.** The edge of the placenta is at the margin of the cervical opening. As the cervix dilates during labor, more of the placenta may move upward. Vaginal delivery may be possible under certain conditions.

2. **Partial.** The placenta partly covers the cervical opening. Vaginal delivery is likely to result in hemorrhage as the blood vessels in the placenta rupture during labor.

3. **Total.** The placenta completely covers the cervical opening, making vaginal delivery impossible because of the risk of massive bleeding.

Although the placenta may lie close to the cervical opening in the second or early third trimester, it almost always migrates up toward the top of the uterus as term approaches. This is referred to as low-lying placenta.

The cause of placenta previa is not known for certain. Like placental abruption, it is more common in women who have had children before, in older women and in women who smoke. A previous cesarean birth or induced abortion also seems to increase the risk of placenta previa. And when there's a large placenta, the risk of placenta previa is increased because it is more likely for the edge of the placenta to lie near or over the cervical opening.

Signs and Symptoms

The main symptom of placenta previa is painless vaginal bleeding. Most often this occurs near the end of the second trimester or the beginning of the third. The blood from placenta previa is usually bright red, and the amount may range from scant to heavy. The bleeding may stop on its own at some point after it starts, but it nearly always recurs days or weeks later.

If you notice bleeding in late pregnancy, don't assume it's harmless, even if it goes away on its own. Any bleeding in the third trimester should be reported to your doctor right away.

Diagnosis

An ultrasound exam is effective for detecting the location of the placenta. Up to 98 percent of cases of placenta previa may be detected in this way. A cervical exam, in which the entrance of the cervix is gently probed, is done only under certain circumstances when placenta previa is suspected. Because even the gentlest cervical exam can cause hemorrhage, it is done only when delivery is planned, and only when an immediate cesarean delivery can be performed.

Management

How placenta previa is managed depends on two factors:

1. Whether the fetus is mature enough to be born and
2. Whether there is active bleeding from the mother's vagina.

Disorders of the Placenta

If the placenta is found to be close to, but not covering, the cervix and the woman has no bleeding, she may be allowed to rest at home—with instructions to call the doctor or hospital immediately if bleeding starts. Alternatively, bleeding that cannot be controlled will probably necessitate an immediate cesarean birth for the sake of the baby, even if the birth is preterm. Such a baby is probably better off in the hands of the skilled caregivers and the sophisticated equipment of a modern neonatal intensive care unit than inside the mother's uterus, where a bleeding placenta is no longer able to support it.

Outlook For the Future

Because in most cases placenta previa can be detected accurately before the fetus is in significant danger, it no longer poses the threat to babies and their mothers that it once did. Advances in technology such as the ultrasound test and other potentially life-saving measures, however, are useless without the prompt recognition of potential problems by the pregnant woman. Bleeding in the third trimester may not necessarily lead to serious problems if it is acted on, but it should never be ignored.

Chapter 36

Intrauterine Growth Retardation

What causes it and who's at risk?

Each year in the United States, as many as 40,000 babies are born at term with a birth weight of less than 2,500 grams (less than 5 1/2 pounds). Because of less-than-optimal conditions inside the uterus, these babies did not grow as rapidly as they should have during pregnancy, a problem known as intrauterine growth retardation (IUGR).

Advances in medicine have greatly reduced the risks for growth-retarded infants, but they are still at risk for numerous problems. These babies have low stores of body fat and glycogen (a type of carbohydrate that is readily transformed into glucose, an energy source). As a consequence, they are unable to conserve heat and may develop hypothermia. Stillbirth and fetal distress are also more common in growth-retarded fetuses. Because of their lower energy stores, these fetuses are less able to tolerate the stress of labor than an infant of normal size.

Possible causes of IUGR include problems with the placenta that prevent it from delivering enough oxygen and nutrients to the fetus. This may occur as the result of high blood pressure in the mother, but it can also occur without a known cause. Other causes of IUGR include the following:

- Cigarette smoking

Reprinted by permission of William Morrow & Company, Inc. from *Mayo Clinic Complete Book of Pregnancy and Baby's First Year.* Copyright 1994 by Mayo Foundation for Medical Education and Research

- Certain infections (such as rubella, cytomegalovirus or toxoplasmosis)
- Birth defects or chromosome abnormalities
- Severe malnutrition
- Drug or alcohol use
- Juvenile diabetes
- Rheumatologic diseases
- Other chronic diseases in the mother

Women who have had a growth-retarded infant in a previous pregnancy are at an increased risk to have another undersized baby. Fortunately, careful monitoring and early intervention often can help lessen some of the dangers posed to growth-retarded infants. In some cases, growth retardation can even be reversed.

How is it diagnosed?

A woman carrying a growth-retarded fetus usually has few, if any, symptoms to alert her to the problem. The careful measurements your doctor makes at each of your prenatal visits are partly intended to detect IUGR at an early stage.

This is one reason your doctor measures the fundal height of your uterus—the distance between your pubic bone and the fundus, or top, of your uterus. Between 18 and 34 weeks, this measurement in centimeters corresponds roughly to the number of weeks of pregnancy. By looking at how this measurement increases over time, the doctor may be alerted to IUGR if the size of the uterus does not seem to be increasing as it should.

Accurate dating of your pregnancy is important for making the diagnosis of IUGR. If this date is off by even one or two weeks, it may be impossible to diagnose the condition correctly. Before about 20 weeks of pregnancy, an ultrasound exam can be used to determine the gestational age as precisely as possible.

If IUGR is suspected because of low fundal height measurements, an ultrasound exam likely will be done to confirm the diagnosis. This test can be used to measure some of the physical features of the fetus. The circumference of the head and abdomen, and the ratio of one to the other, is one of the most useful of these measurements. Other measurements that may be taken include the width of the baby's head (called the biparietal diameter, or the distance between the two side bones of the skull), the length of the thigh bone (femur) and the amount of amniotic fluid.

Intrauterine Growth Retardation

How is it managed?

First steps in the management of a woman with a growth-retarded fetus consist of reversing any factors, such as smoking, drug use or poor nutrition, that may be contributing to the problem. Sometimes the mother is admitted to the hospital for bed rest. Non-stress tests, contraction stress tests or biophysical profiles are often done to check on the baby's condition. The expectant mother may be asked to keep a daily record of the baby's movements. Ultrasound exams are generally done every two weeks to track the baby's growth and the volume of amniotic fluid.

Amniocentesis might be performed to check for chromosome abnormalities or infection, two of the causes of IUGR. However, because it often takes about 10 days to obtain the results of amniocentesis, PUBS (percutaneous umbilical blood sampling) may be offered instead. In this procedure, ultrasound is used to guide a needle into the umbilical cord, and blood is withdrawn for analysis. Although the results are obtained more quickly with PUBS, there is a greater risk to the baby than with amniocentesis. Your doctor will discuss the pros and cons of these techniques with you if these tests are being considered.

If tests continue to show no evidence that the baby is in danger, and if the ultrasound exam shows that the baby is growing, the pregnancy may be continued until labor begins on its own. But signs that the fetus may be in danger or is not growing appropriately will prompt your doctor to consider early delivery. In weighing this decision, two questions are asked:

1. How mature is the baby?
2. How safe (or dangerous) is the uterine environment?

To answer the first question, amniocentesis may be performed to find out if the baby's lungs are fully mature. But some conditions may make it safer for the baby to be outside rather than inside the uterus, even if the baby is born early or the lungs are not mature. The expert care that can be given in a neonatal intensive care unit may be a better option for the baby than remaining inside the uterus under unfavorable conditions.

Depending on individual circumstances, birth may be accomplished by inducing labor and having the baby born vaginally or by cesarean. During labor, the baby will be monitored closely. If the fetal heart rate pattern or other tests indicate that the baby is not tolerating labor, a cesarean birth might be necessary.

Whether a growth-retarded infant is born vaginally or by cesarean, there are still risks posed to the infant's health. You may be temporarily separated from your baby soon after birth so that she or he can be watched carefully for any complications, such as low blood sugar. A growth-retarded baby may need fluid with glucose (sugar) soon after birth. This may be given by bottle or through an intravenous line. The baby's temperature will also be monitored to make sure she or he remains warm enough.

What about the future?

Despite the many risks posed to the growth-retarded newborn, almost all of these babies go on to develop normally. The size of your baby at birth may not necessarily be an indication of how well she or he will grow and develop.

Most growth-retarded babies tend to catch up with their normal counterparts by 18 to 24 months. Unless there are serious birth defects, the chances are good for most of these babies to have normal intellectual and physical development in the long term.

If you have had one growth-retarded baby, you are more likely to have another baby with this problem in a future pregnancy. Good prenatal care, excellent nutrition and elimination of smoking and alcohol and drug use will increase your chances of having a healthy baby.

Chapter 37

Post-Term Pregnancy

What causes it and who's at risk?

In about 80 percent of all pregnancies, birth takes place between 38 and 42 weeks. About half of the remainder, or 10 percent, are preterm (end before 37 weeks), and the other 10 percent or so last beyond 42 weeks. These latter pregnancies—those lasting beyond the end of the 42nd week—are considered to be post-term.

Many of these pregnancies, however, may turn out not to be post-term after all. Often, a miscalculated due date is responsible for a pregnancy being considered post-term. When early ultrasound testing is used to confirm the due date, the actual frequency of post-term pregnancy turns out to be about 2 percent of all pregnancies.

The causes of post-term pregnancy are largely unknown. Heredity and hormonal factors may play a role.

Concerns in a post-term pregnancy center on the risks posed to the baby. After 41 weeks, the amount of amniotic fluid inside the uterus may decrease dramatically. This can increase the risk that the umbilical cord will become compressed during labor or delivery, interrupting the flow of oxygen to the baby.

Post-term pregnancies also increase the risk of meconium in the amniotic fluid. Meconium is the fetus's stool, and its presence means that the baby has had its first bowel movement while in the uterus.

Reprinted by permission of William Morrow & Company, Inc. from *Mayo Clinic Complete Book of Pregnancy and Baby's First Year*. Copyright 1994 by Mayo Foundation for Medical Education and Research

A type of pneumonia may develop if the baby inhales the meconium into the lungs while still in the uterus. For this reason, your doctor will suction the nose, mouth and back of the baby's throat as soon as the head is delivered. A pediatrician or other caregiver will then immediately pass a tube into the baby's windpipe to quickly suction out the meconium before it has a chance to reach the baby's lungs. You might not hear your baby cry until after this suctioning has been completed.

Another concern in a post-term pregnancy is macrosomia, or a baby weighing more than 4,500 grams (9 pounds 14 ounces). Such large babies may have a hard time getting safely through the birth canal during delivery. This is one of the reasons why cesarean birth is more common in post-term pregnancies. But despite the increased risks to the baby in a post-term pregnancy, most of these babies are born safely with careful management.

How is it managed?

If your pregnancy progresses beyond 41 or 42 weeks, one of your doctor's first concerns will be to find out whether the due date is accurate. Going back over the findings of previous exams and tests will help her or him pin down the true length of gestation. Knowing when you first felt the baby move, when the first fetal heart sounds were heard, how well the size of the baby correlated with the date of the pregnancy, the height of the uterus at 20 weeks (normally at the level of the mother's navel) and the results of early ultrasound exams all provide measures of how far along gestation was at various points during the pregnancy.

If your doctor determines that your pregnancy is truly post-term, the approach she or he takes will depend on your individual circumstances. Tests to find out the condition of the fetus, such as non-stress tests, contraction stress tests or biophysical profiles, will yield useful information. An ultrasound exam will be used to determine how much amniotic fluid surrounds the fetus. At signs that the baby's condition may be worsening, or that the amniotic fluid volume is low, the decision will be made to deliver the baby.

In addition, the cervix may be checked weekly after 40 weeks to find out whether it is beginning to dilate. Many doctors decide to induce labor when the cervix becomes "ripe" (softened, effaced and starting to dilate) after 41 weeks. In a woman whose cervix has not yet begun to dilate, but in whom delivery is the best course, agents can be used to ripen the cervix. These include gels containing the hormone prostaglandin or small inserts called laminaria, which are placed inside the cervix and expand as they absorb moisture.

Many doctors may adopt a wait-and-see attitude if the cervix is not dilated and there are no signs that the baby is in danger. Others feel it's best to deliver a post-term baby if labor has not begun by the end of 42 weeks, regardless of the condition of the cervix. Generally, a pregnancy will not be allowed to go beyond 43 or 44 weeks, because the risks to the baby are significantly increased after that time.

If delivery is decided on, how the baby is born—vaginally or by cesarean—will depend on many factors. A baby who is too large to pass through the mother's pelvis must be born by cesarean. A woman whose cervix is ripe and whose baby has shown no signs of problems is a candidate for vaginal delivery. The baby's heart rate, as well as contractions of the mother's uterus, will be monitored closely during a vaginal birth of a post-term infant. A cesarean birth may be necessary if there are signs that the baby is not tolerating the stress of labor.

Post-term babies may have long, thin bodies, without the whitish coating of vernix found on normal newborns. Because of the longer time they've spent in the uterus, they are frequently born with long fingernails, lots of hair and wrinkled palms and soles.

What about the future?

Even with the risks of post-term pregnancy, most post-term babies come safely into the world. How to best handle your own post-term pregnancy and birth is best decided by you and your doctor, weighing the benefits and risks of the available options. Despite the risks to the baby in a post-term pregnancy, the long-term outlook for most post-term babies is excellent.

Chapter 38

Maternal Death

From 1935 to 1993, the maternal mortality rate dropped from 582 maternal deaths per 100,000 live births to 7.5. Though all causes of maternal mortality declined dramatically over that period, the overall decline was largely due to marked decreases in maternal deaths from infection, toxemia, and hemorrhage.

Significant improvements in the care of women during labor, delivery, and the postpartum period have been made over the last 60 years.

Technical improvements (including sterile techniques) in the management of vaginal and cesarean deliveries and the advent of effective antibiotics probably accounted for much of the decrease in maternal morbidity. It is also likely that the development of widely used prenatal care protocols contributed to the decline in mortality from chronic or pregnancy-induced conditions.

Although maternal mortality has decreased significantly over the past 60 years, it is still a serious problem. Many of these deaths might be preventable if the health care system worked more effectively.

In 1992, there were 318 maternal deaths which resulted from complications of pregnancy, childbirth, or the postpartum period.

The maternal mortality rate for black women (20.8 per 100,000 live births) is more than four times the rate for white women (5.0 per 100,000 live births).

Excerpts from DHSS Publication No's. HRSA-M-DSEA-96-5, September 1996 and HRSA-MCH-9591, July 1995 and Morbidity and Mortality Weekly Report, January 13, 1995

Pregnancy and Birth Sourcebook

Regardless of race, the risk of maternal death increases for women over 30; women 35-39 years old have more than twice the risk of those aged 20-24 years.

Differences in Maternal Mortality Among Black and White Women—United States, 1990

The risk for maternal mortality has consistently been higher among black women than white women. The 1990 national health objective of reducing maternal mortality to no more than five deaths per 100,000 live births for any racial/ethnic group was nearly achieved for white women, for whom the maternal mortality ratio was 5.7 in

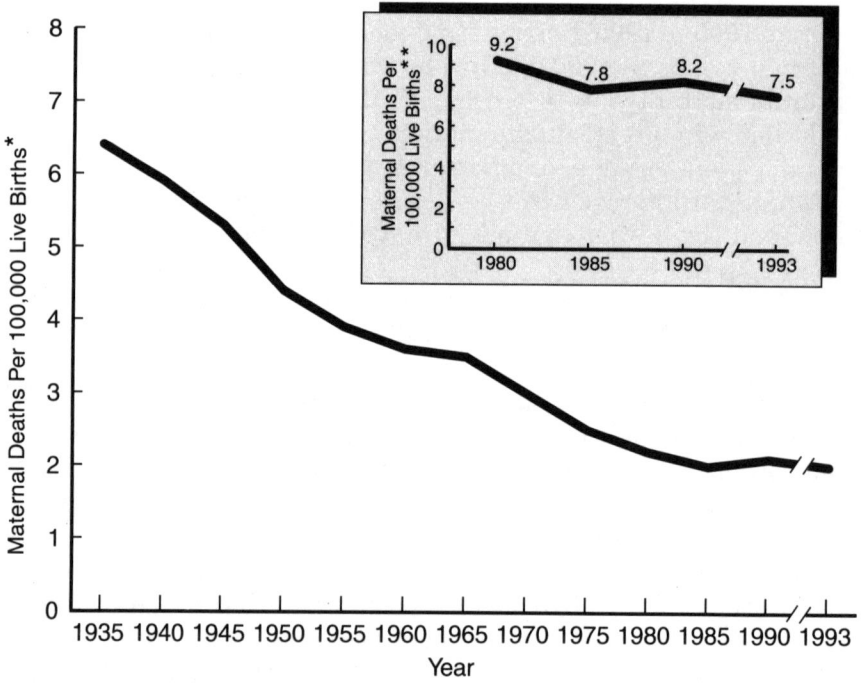

* *Data values represented on a log scale.*
** *Actual data values.*

Figure 38.1. *Maternal Mortality; 1935-1993. Source: National Center for Health Statistics*

Maternal Death

1990. (The maternal mortality ratio is the number of maternal deaths per 100,000 live births. CDC's National Center for Health Statistics (NCHS) uses the term maternal mortality rate as required by the World Health Organization. In this text, the term "ratio" is used because the numerator includes some maternal deaths that were not related to live births, and thus were not included in the denominator. For this analysis, 3 years of data were combined to calculate maternal mortality ratios to promote statistical reliability and stability in the estimates. For example, 1990 ratios are based on data from 1989 through 1991. In addition, beginning with the 1989 data year, NCHS began using race of mother instead of race of child to tabulate live birth and fetal death data by race. In this analysis, race for live births

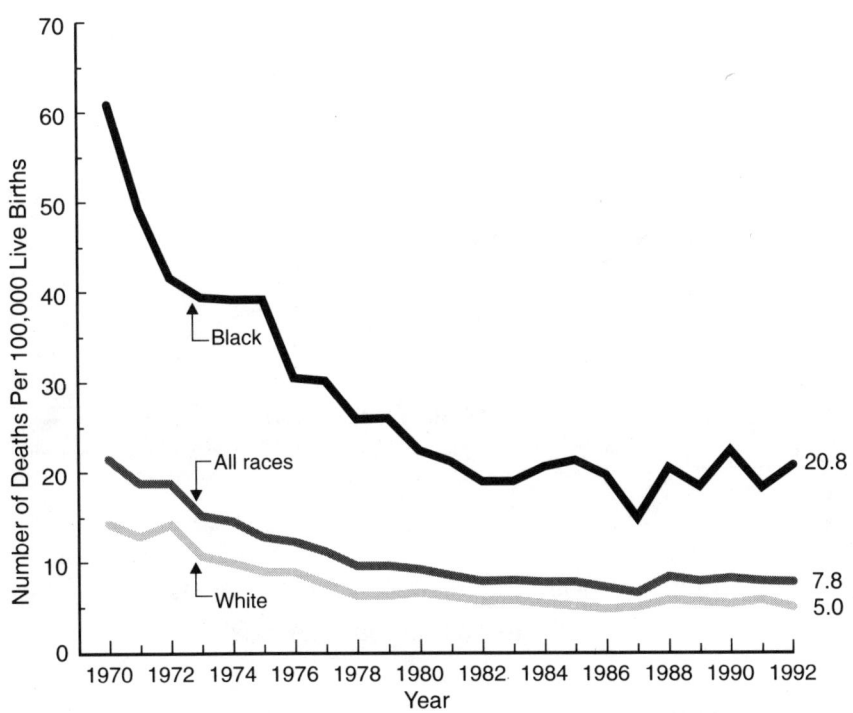

Figure 38.2. Maternal Mortality by Race: 1970-1992. Source: National Center for Health Statistics

is tabulated by the race of the child for maternal mortality to maintain comparability of ratios.) For black women, however, the ratio was 18.6. The year 2000 national health objectives include reducing the overall maternal mortality ratio to no more than 3.3 deaths per 100,000 live births and to no more than five for blacks. This text summarizes race-specific differences in maternal mortality among black and white women for 1990 and compares these with trends in mortality from 1940-1990.

Maternal mortality ratios were calculated at 10-year intervals from 1940 to 1990 using data contained on death certificates filed in state vital statistics offices and compiled by CDC in a national database. Maternal deaths were defined as those for which a maternal condition was designated as the underlying cause of death, as recorded on the death certificate by the attending physician, medical examiner, or coroner. This report compares maternal mortality only for black and white women because data for other racial/ethnic groups were not available for all years; data for Hispanic women are included in the totals for both blacks and whites.

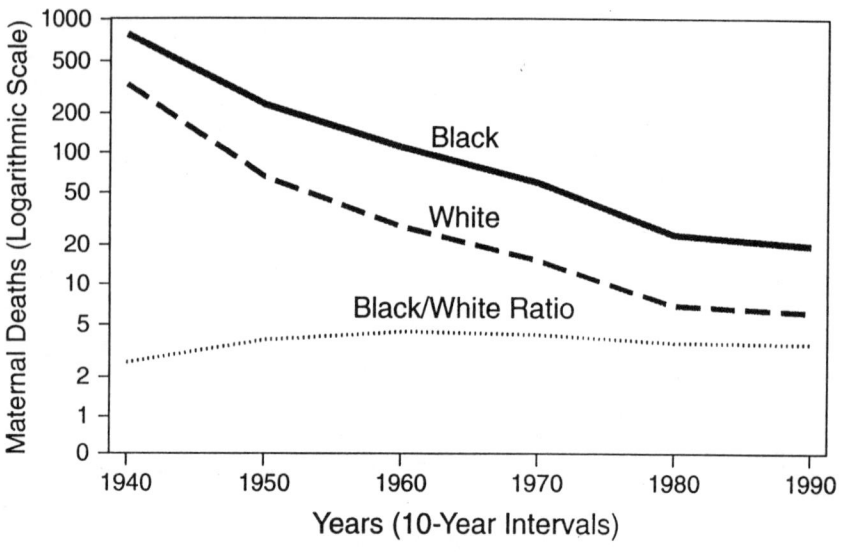

Figure 38.3. Maternal mortality ratio, by race—United States, 1940-1990. The maternal mortality ratio is the number of maternal deaths per 100,000 live births. For live births, maternal race is derived from the race of the child. Data for races other than black and white were not available for analysis.

Maternal Death

In 1990, the overall maternal mortality ratio was 8.0 deaths per 100,000 live births, a 98% decline from 363.9 in 1940. From 1940 to 1990, race-specific ratios declined substantially, from 319.8 to 5.7 for white women and from 781.7 to 18.6 for black women. Although the percentage decline was similar for black women and white women (97.6% and 98.2%, respectively), the ratios for black women were consistently two to four times higher than those for white women. For example, compared with that for white women, the maternal mortality ratio for black women was 2.4 times greater in 1940, 3.6 times greater in 1950, 4.1 times greater in 1960, 3.9 times greater in 1970, 3.4 times greater in 1980, and 3.3 times greater in 1990.

From 1960 through 1990 (years for which more detailed data were available), the maternal mortality ratio was higher for black women in all age groups and for each of the major causes of death. The black-white differential was greatest for pregnancies that did not end in a live birth, such as ectopic pregnancy, spontaneous abortion, induced abortion, and gestational trophoblastic disease.

Despite overall improved maternal survival during 1940-1990, black women were more than three times more likely than white women to die from complications of pregnancy, childbirth, and the puerperium. Although the reasons for this disparity are unclear, possible explanations include differences in pregnancy-related morbidity, access to and use of health-care services, and content and quality of care.

Maternal hospitalization, except when associated with delivery, can serve as a marker for severe maternal morbidity. For example, during 1987-1988, a study of pregnancy-related hospitalizations indicated the ratio for black women was 1.4 times that for white women. During the same period, the black-white maternal mortality ratio was 3.1. However, in a study of women in the military—who have unrestricted access to prenatal care—there was virtually no difference between black and white women in the overall prevalence of antenatal hospitalization and in the indications for hospitalization.

Early entry into prenatal care (i.e., during the first trimester)— one indicator of access to and use of pregnancy-related health care— has been assessed for women whose pregnancies ended in a live birth. During 1980-1990, although 76% of all mothers received early prenatal care, the percentage of black women who did not receive early prenatal care was nearly twice that for white women. In 1990, 39.4% of black mothers did not receive early prenatal care, compared with 20.8% of white mothers. Once women enter prenatal care, studies indicate differences between black and white women in the advice given to them and use of technology.

Data describing access to pregnancy-related health care other than prenatal care (e.g., gynecologic services) or the content and quality of health care once women obtain these services are limited. Narrowing discrepancies in maternal mortality between black and white women will require evaluating and addressing race-specific differences in morbidity and in access to and use and content of pregnancy-related care. Addressing discrepancies in maternal mortality also may improve maternal morbidity and infant survival.

References

Public Health Service. Promoting health/preventing disease: objectives for the nation. Washington, DC: US Department of Health and Human Services, Public Health Service, 1980.

Public Health Service. Healthy people 2000: national health promotion and disease prevention objectives. Washington, DC: US Department of Health and Human Services, Public Health Service, 1991, DHHS publication no. (PHS)91-50213.

NCHS. Vital statistics of the United States, for years 1939-1991. Vol l-natality. Hyattsville, Maryland: US Department of Health and Human Services. Public Health Service, CDC.

NCHS. Vital statistics of the United States, for years 1939-1991. Vol II-mortality, part A. Hyattsville, Maryland: US Department of Health and Human Services, Public Health Service, CDC.

NCHS. Estimates of selected comparability ratios based on dual coding of 1976 death certificates by the eighth and ninth revisions of the International Classification of Diseases. Hyattsville, Maryland: US Department of Health and Human Services, Public Health Service, CDC, 1980. (Monthly vital statistics report; vol 28, no. 11, suppl).

Franks AL, Kendrick JS, Olson DR, Atrash HK, Saftlas AF, Moein M. Hospitalization for pregnancy complications, United States, 1986-1987. Am J Obstet Gynecol 1992; 166:1339-44.

Adams MM, Harlass FE, Sarno AP, Read JA, Rawlings JS. Antenatal hospitalization among enlisted servicewomen, 1987-1990. Obstet Gynecol 1994; 84:35-9.

NCHS. Health, United States, 1993. Hyattsville, Maryland: US Department of Health and Human Services, Public Health Service, CDC, 1994; DHHS publication no. (PHS)94-1232.

Kogan MD, Kotelchuck M, Alexander GR, Johnson WE. Racial disparities in reported prenatal care advice from health care providers. Am J Public Health 1994; 84:82-8.

Brett KM, Schoendod KC, Kiely JK. Differences between black and white women in the use of prenatal care technologies. Am J Obstet Gynecol 1994; 170:41-6.

Chapter 39

Pregnancy Loss

Chapter Contents

Section 39.1—Infant Mortality 644
Section 39.2—Miscarriage (Spontaneous Abortion) 651
Section 39.3—Early Pregnancy Loss 656
Section 39.4—Grieving Your Loss 660

Section 39.1

Infant Mortality

Excerpts from DHSS Publication No. HRSA-M-DSEA-96-5 and DHSS Fact Sheet, Preventing Infant Mortality, Feb 1997

In 1993, 33,466 babies died before their first birthday. The infant mortality rate was 8.4 deaths per 1,000 live births. This figure represents a decline of 1% from the rate of 8.5 for the previous year.

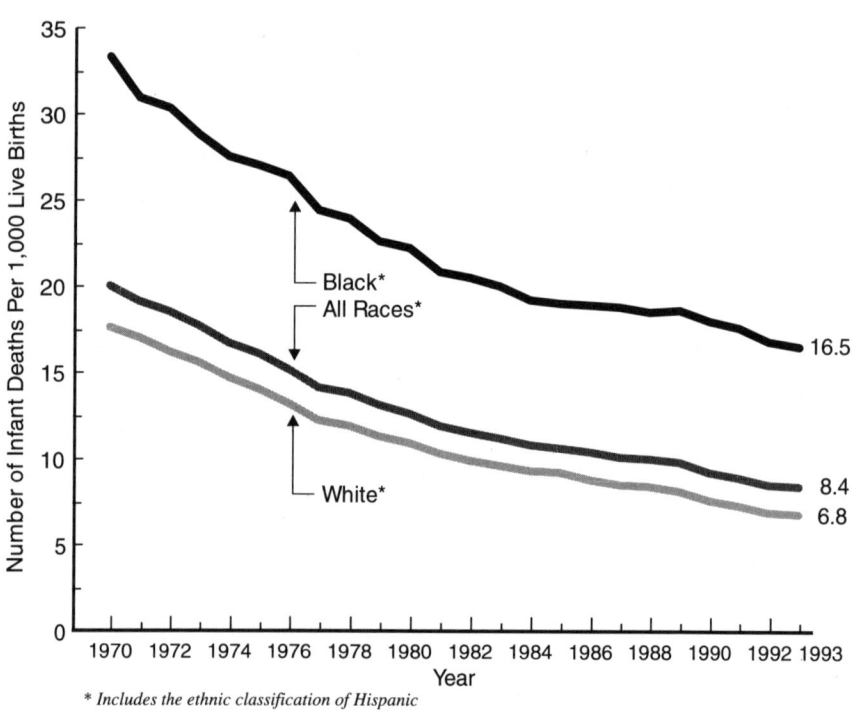

Figure 39.1. *U.S. Infant Mortality Rates by Race of Mother: 1970-1993*

Pregnancy Loss

The rapid decline in infant mortality, which began in the mid 1960's, slowed for both blacks and whites during the 1980's.

The 1993 infant mortality rate for black infants was 2.4 times the rate for white infants. Although the trend in infant mortality rates among blacks and whites has ben on a continual decline throughout the 20th century, the proportional discrepancy between black and white rates has remained unchanged.

Neonatal Mortality

In 1993, 21,174 infants younger than 28 days died; putting the neonatal mortality rate at 529.3 deaths per 100,000 live births. Both the overall mortality rate and rates by leading causes of mortality decreased from 1991 to 1993.

Blacks have the highest rates of neonatal mortality in all categories. Disorders related to short gestation and low birth weight are the primary causes of neonatal mortality for blacks, while congenital anomalies are the leading cause for whites.

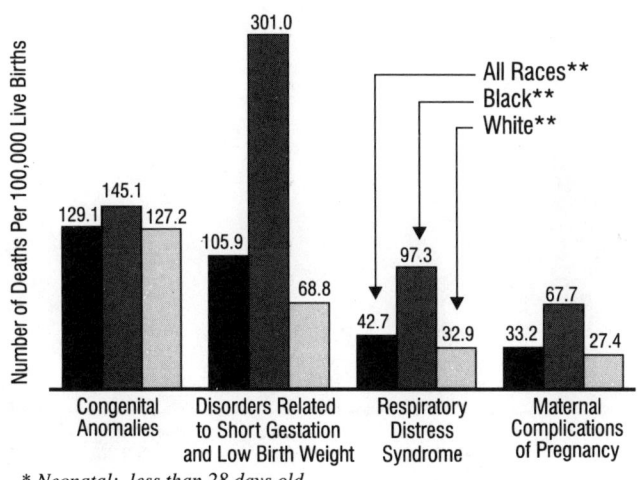

Figure 39.2. Leading Causes of Neonatal Mortality: 1993

Postneonatal Mortality

In 1993, 12,292 infants 28 days to 11 months old died; the postneonatal mortality rate was 307.3 deaths per 100,000 live births, a decrease of 7.1 deaths per 100,000 live births from 1992.

The postneonatal mortality rate for blacks is at least two times that for whites in all leading causes of postneonatal mortality (three times greater when homicide is the cause, with the exception of congenital anomalies).

Thanks to an intensified national commitment to giving babies a healthy start in life, the preliminary estimate for the U.S. infant mortality rate, which is the rate at which babies die before their first birthday, is at an historic low of less than 8 deaths per 1,000 live births in 1995, and the proportion of mothers getting early prenatal care is at a record high of 81.2 percent.

According to this estimate, the infant mortality rate has dropped 6 percent since 1994 and 18 percent since 1990. We've also seen declines in some of the risk factors for low birthweight and infant mortality: teen births dropped for the fourth straight year in 1995 and smoking among pregnant women has been decreasing in recent years. Nevertheless, the United States continues to have unacceptably high infant mortality rates with significant disparities among racial and ethnic groups.

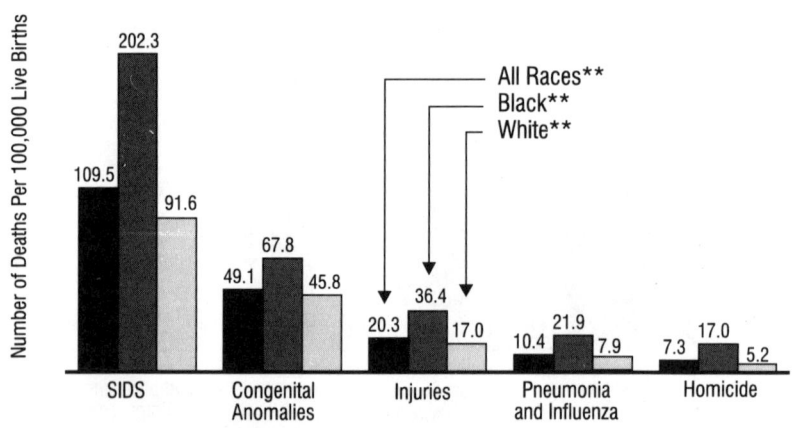

* Postneonatal: 28 days to less than one year old
** Includes Hispanic

Figure 39.3. Leading Causes of Postneonatal Mortality: 1993

Pregnancy Loss

The Clinton Administration supports a comprehensive national strategy to increase access to prenatal care and to help families care for infants. Early and continuous prenatal care helps prevent low birthweight and identify conditions and behavioral factors that often cause or aggravate low birthweight, such as smoking, drug and alcohol abuse, inadequate weight gain during pregnancy, and repeat pregnancy in six months or less.

To further help assure that women have proper prenatal care, DHHS today announced the nation's first toll-free referral and information service to help women obtain proper prenatal care throughout their pregnancies. Callers in all 50 states will be able to telephone 1-800-311-BABY (2229) for pregnancy and prenatal care information, including referral to local clinics and physicians. A separate phone number is available for Spanish speakers: 1-800-504-7081. The new service is supported by the Healthy Start program in DHHS' Health Resources and Services Administration.

The Administration's strategy is reflected in all of DHHS' infant mortality prevention activities. For example:

1. The new "Back to Sleep" campaign has contributed to a 30 percent decline in the death rate from Sudden Infant Death Syndrome (SIDS) in the U.S. between 1992 and 1995. Led by the National Institutes of Health (NIH) and other DHHS agencies, and co-sponsored by the American Academy of Pediatrics and other groups, the "Back to Sleep" campaign encourages parents both to place babies on their backs to sleep and to provide a smoke-free environment to reduce the risk of SIDS.

2. Based on emerging evidence from epidemiological and clinical studies, including studies funded by the Centers for Disease Control and Prevention (CDC) and NIH's National Institute of Child Health and Human Development (NICHD), in September 1992, the Public Health Service issued a recommendation that all women of childbearing age consume 400 micrograms of folic acid daily to reduce their risk of having a pregnancy affected by a neural tube defect (e.g., spina bifida or anencephaly). To aid in implementing this recommendation, DHHS' Food and Drug Administration promulgated regulations to require the mandatory addition of folic acid to all cereal grain products labeled as enriched (e.g., breads, pastas, rice) and authorized the use of a health claim that communicated the relationship between dietary folate and risk of neural tube defects on foods that were

good sources of folate. Neural tube birth defects affect about 4,000 pregnancies each year.

3. The Healthy Start Initiative, a demonstration effort in 22 communities with high infant mortality rates administered by the Health Resources and Services Administration (HRSA), has developed promising replicable models for collaborative community-based interventions to reduce infant mortality.

   DHHS has expanded perinatal services and service hours at community health centers in communities with the highest infant mortality rates through programs administered by HRSA's Healthy Start Initiative and Bureau of Primary Health Care. These programs also provide counseling on the dangers of cigarette smoking during pregnancy and smoking cessation services.

4. DHHS has expanded Medicaid eligibility and services for pregnant women and their infants. Individual states have tailored the implementation of these expansions to their residents' needs, adding, for example, provisions for outreach and perinatal/parenting education, more providers, and streamlined application procedures to facilitate early and continuous prenatal care. Families are encouraged and offered assistance to obtain well-child screenings that can identify and treat health problems and further reduce infant mortality.

5. DHHS provides information to women and their physicians on HIV testing and treatment with the anti-HIV drug zidovudine (AZT) to reduce transmission of HIV from mother to child. New guidelines and educational materials have been produced by DHHS, in collaboration with the Columbia University School of Public Health.

6. DHHS helps fund high-quality treatment programs for pregnant and postpartum women through the Center for Substance Abuse Treatment (CSAT) in the Substance Abuse and Mental Health Services Administration. Of the women treated in CSAT-funded programs, 95 percent reported uncomplicated, drug-free births and 75 percent who successfully completed treatment remained drug free for at least one to three months.

Pregnancy Loss

7. DHHS supports the provision of reproductive health and family planning services through the Title X program. Each year, some 5 million persons receive Title X-supported services, nearly a third of whom are under 20 years of age. Abstinence counseling and education are an important part of the Title X service protocol for adolescent clients. DHHS also encourages states to provide a wide array of family planning services under Medicaid by reimbursing states for 90 percent of the costs expended on these services.

8. DHHS also supports medical research to prevent birth defects, premature birth, sudden infant death syndrome and other life-threatening conditions. For example:

   - The wider use of corticosteroid treatments during premature labor, a clinical practice endorsed by the NIH Consensus Development Conference based on research supported by NICHD, has reduced deaths of premature infants, respiratory distress syndrome, and internal hemorrhage in the infant.

   - Treatment with surfactant, discovered and developed through research supported by NICHD and the National Heart, Lung and Blood Institute, has also reduced deaths of premature infants from respiratory distress syndrome.

   - NICHD-supported research has shown that treatment of a common condition known as bacterial vaginosis with specific antibiotics can reduce the risk of a premature delivery. Clinical trials are in progress to determine which precise treatment would be most effective.

   - NICHD-supported research is examining intrauterine drug exposure to accurately assess the impact on the infant and to facilitate effective interventions to promote healthy development.

   - The CDC is examining sociocultural, behavioral, and environmental factors, including stress and social support, related to preterm births among African-American women in Harlem, New York and Los Angeles, California.

- HHS also works in partnership with many civic and business organizations in efforts to reduce infant mortality, including Johnson & Johnson, March of Dimes, Robert Wood Johnson Foundation, Colgate Palmolive, Carnegie Corporation, Kellogg Foundation, and many more.

Recent Trends

Due in part to long-standing medical research and social services supported by DHHS, infant mortality has declined considerably in recent decades. Over the past twenty-five years alone, the infant mortality rate has dropped from 20 deaths per 1,000 live births in 1970 to less than 8 deaths per 1,000 live births in 1995.

According to preliminary estimates, infant mortality dropped to 7.5 deaths per 1,000 live births in 1995, down 6 percent since 1994 and 18 percent since 1990. Declines occurred among both neonates (infants under 28 days of age) and postneonates (infants aged 28 days to 12 months).

Between 1994 and 1995, the white infant mortality rate declined 5 percent, to 6.3 deaths per 1,000 live births, while the black infant mortality rate declined 6 percent, to 14.9 deaths per 1,000 live births. While the gap did not widen in 1995, the black infant mortality rate remains more than twice as high as the white infant mortality rate.

Compared to the white infant mortality rate, the American Indian/Alaska Native infant mortality rate is 70 percent higher, and the Asian/Pacific Islander rate is 11 percent lower. The infant mortality rate for Hispanic-origin infants is nearly 3 percent higher than for non-Hispanic white infants (based on linked birth/infant death data from 1989-91).

In 1995, the leading causes of infant mortality in the U.S. were: congenital anomalies, disorders related to immaturity (short gestation and unspecified low birthweight), SIDS, and respiratory distress syndrome.

In 1995, a record-high 81.2 percent of mothers began prenatal care within the first trimester of pregnancy, the sixth consecutive year of increase from 75.5 percent in 1989. However, in 1994, more than a third of teen mothers ages 15 to 19 (35.7 percent) did not begin prenatal care in the first trimester.

Disparities in the timely receipt of prenatal care between white mothers and black and Hispanic mothers still exist, but have narrowed. From 1989 to 1995, first trimester prenatal care increased 17 to 18 percent for black and Hispanic mothers (to 70.3 percent and 70.4 percent, respectively) and 6 percent for white mothers (to 83.5 percent).

Pregnancy Loss

The incidence of low birthweight was unchanged in 1995, at 7.3 percent.

Cigarette smoking during pregnancy declined for the fifth consecutive year in 1994, to 14.6 percent of mothers. Over 12 percent of births to smokers were low birthweight (less than 2,500 grams or 5 pounds 8 ounces) compared with almost 7 percent of births to non-smokers.

Among industrialized countries in 1992, the U.S. had the 22nd lowest infant mortality rate, up from the U.S. rank of 24th in 1990.

Section 39.2

Miscarriage (Spontaneous Abortion)

Reprinted with permission from Information Network, Inc. copyright 1995-1997. Information obtained online at http://www.medicinenet.com.

Facts About Miscarriage

- Miscarriage is a pregnancy that is non-viable or is born before the 20th week.

- Exercise, working, and intercourse do **not** increase risk of miscarriage.

- Causes for miscarriage include genetic abnormalities, infection, medications, hormonal effects, structural abnormality of the uterus, and immune abnormalities.

- After an isolated miscarriage, the chance of having a normal term pregnancy in the future is near 90%.

- Treatment of recurrent miscarriage is directed toward the underlying cause.

What is a miscarriage?

A miscarriage (spontaneous abortion) is any pregnancy that is non-viable (wherein the fetus cannot survive) or is born before the 20th week of pregnancy. Miscarriage occurs in about 15-20% of all recognized pregnancies, and usually occurs before the 13th week of pregnancy. Of those miscarriages before the eighth week, 30% have no fetus associated with the sac or placenta. This condition is called blighted ovum and many women are surprised to learn that there was never an embryo inside the sac.

After an isolated spontaneous miscarriage, the chance of having a successful pregnancy in the future is quite high. Repeated miscarriages occur in 0.5-1.0% of all pregnancies. In those women with repeated miscarriages, medical evaluation is advised to identify the reasons for these miscarriages. In women with two consecutive miscarriages, the risk of having another loss is between 35-40%. In those women with two non-consecutive losses, the risk of another miscarriage is between 15-20%.

What causes a miscarriage?

It must be emphasized that exercise, working, and intercourse do not increase the risk of pregnancy loss. Bed rest and staying off your feet probably do not prevent miscarriage although this advice is commonly given.

Chromosomal Abnormalities

Genetic (chromosomal) abnormalities represent the single most frequent reason for miscarriages. Chromosomes are microscopic components of every cell in the body that carry all of the genetic material that determine hair color, eye color and our overall appearance and makeup. These chromosomes duplicate themselves and divide many times during the process of development and there are numerous points along the way where a problem can occur. Genetic abnormalities account for up to 60% of early miscarriages. Chromosomal abnormalities are responsible for only 30% of losses after the 15th week of pregnancy. Certain genetic abnormalities are known to be more prevalent in couples that experience repeated losses. These genetic traits can be screened for by blood tests prior to attempting to become pregnant.

Infection

Infection of the uterus by bacteria and viruses has been associated with miscarriages. However, it is interesting to note that the same infections found at the time of miscarriage can also be present in normal pregnancies carried to completion. Therefore, the exact role infection plays in miscarriages is uncertain.

Drugs

Certain medications, alcohol and smoking, can increase the risk of miscarriage. When planning pregnancy, it is best to abstain from alcohol and tobacco. It is also important to be certain that your doctor or dentist is aware that you could be pregnant, especially if medications are prescribed. Certain drugs used to treat malaria, cancer and acne have been associated with an increased risk of miscarriage. On the other hand, video display terminals, like the one on your computer, as well as hair spray, dyes and coloring have not been shown to increase the risk of pregnancy loss.

Hormones

Hormones produced by the ovaries, such as progesterone, are known to play a role in maintaining an early pregnancy before the placenta takes over this important function. It is speculated that in some women, there may be abnormally low levels of these hormones and that oral hormone replacement early in the pregnancy may help avoid miscarriage. Although this theory has not been absolutely proven, providing hormone replacement is widely practiced in the medical community. Other hormone disturbances, such as in diabetes and thyroid disease, can be associated with recurrent miscarriage. Combined, hormonal and medical causes are responsible for about 15% of pregnancy losses.

Problems of the Uterus

Structural abnormalities of the uterus can also cause miscarriages. Fibroid tumors are benign growths of muscle cells in the uterus. While most fibroid tumors do not cause miscarriages, some can interfere with the embryo implantation and the embryo's blood supply, thereby causing miscarriage. In some women there can be a tissue bridge (uterine septum), that acts like a partial wall dividing the uterine cavity into sections. The septum usually has a very poor blood supply, and is not well suited for placental attachment and growth. Therefore, an embryo implanting on the septum would be at increased risk of miscarriage.

Immune System

Over the past several years, there has been a lot of interest focused on the role of the immune system in pregnancy and miscarriage. The immune system consists of cells and proteins that usually help the body fight infection and remove damaged or abnormal tissue. It consists in part of proteins called antibodies, that circulate through the blood looking for abnormal cells. Sometimes, in normal healthy women, antibodies are produced that attack seemingly normal cells and body tissue. The presence of these antibodies has been associated with compromise of an otherwise healthy placenta. Since the placenta is critical for nutrient support to the baby, severe compromise can cause an early pregnancy loss.

How can the cause of a miscarriage be determined?

Currently, most practitioners will not initiate an extensive medical evaluation for a single pregnancy loss since the chance of having a normal pregnancy subsequent to an isolated miscarriage is 80-90%. For women with recurrent pregnancy loss, an evaluation will focus on the pattern and history of the prior miscarriages.

Blood testing can be done to identify chromosomal abnormalities in the couple that could be transmitted to the fetus. The couple can each appear completely normal but still carry chromosomal defects, which, when combined, can be lethal to the embryo. The blood can also be tested for hormone levels to assess the degree to which hormone imbalance could play a role. Blood samples can also be tested for the antibodies that interfere with implantation and growth of the fertilized egg.

Evaluation of the uterus includes cultures taken from the cervix and vagina for infections. The structure of the uterus and the uterine cavity can be evaluated by ultrasound and other radiological imaging techniques, such as an MRI or CAT scan. The internal uterine cavity can be further assessed using direct vision through an instrument called a hysteroscope.

Chromosomal evaluation of the miscarried fetus can determine if genetics played a role in the miscarriage. Even after extensive testing, fully one-half to two-thirds of recurrent pregnancy losses occur for unknown reasons.

Can something be done to prevent future miscarriages?

The treatment of recurrent miscarriage depends on what is believed to be the underlying cause. This often is not as simple as it sounds. Careful evaluation may turn up several potential factors which alone or together may be responsible for the losses. If a chromosomal problem is found in one or both spouses, then counseling as to future risks is the only option. There is currently no method to correct genetic problems. If a structural problem is encountered with the uterus, surgical correction could be contemplated. It should be emphasized that just because a structural abnormality is found, it does not necessarily mean that it caused the miscarriage. Removal of a fibroid or uterine septum does not guarantee a future successful pregnancy.

Adequate control of diabetes and thyroid disease is critical in trying to prevent recurrent pregnancy loss in women with those conditions. For women with antibody problems, certain medications have been found to be useful in achieving successful pregnancy outcomes. Blood thinners, such as heparin, baby aspirin, and even the addition of steroids can, in some cases, prevent further pregnancy loss.

The use of progesterone to increase the blood levels of this hormone is commonly used for patients with recurrent pregnancy loss. This is especially true if it is found that the hormone concentration is low during the critical time of implantation. Some practitioners may even give this medication when the progesterone level has been tested and found to be normal. This is done because it has been shown that the progesterone level can fluctuate from month to month.

In dealing with recurrent pregnancy loss, it is important to realize that even though apparently obvious problems can be corrected, a miscarriage can still occur. In other patients, nothing may be done and a healthy baby is born. This is not to say that attempts should not be taken to correct identified abnormalities that have been historically associated with miscarriage. However, no treatment can be guaranteed. Even with repeated miscarriages, there is still a very good chance of achieving a successful pregnancy. Early pregnancy and prepregnancy counseling can help identify risk factors and allow the practitioner to provide any special care that may be needed.

Section 39.3

Early Pregnancy Loss

Reprinted by permission of Group Health Cooperative of Puget Sound, copyright, 1997. *Disclaimer of Warranties:* This publication was developed by Group Health for use in communicating with our enrollees. Group Health specifically disclaims any warranties, implied or expressed, including the warranty of merchantability and the warranty of fitness for a particular purpose.

Types of Early Pregnancy Loss

- **Blighted ovum**—In some cases, only placental tissue forms and there is no embryo or fetus. This is known as a blighted ovum (egg).

- **Missed abortion**—Sometimes the embryo or fetus stops growing and dies, but the tissue remains in the uterus and a spontaneous miscarriage doesn't take place. This is called a missed abortion.

- **Miscarriage (spontaneous abortion)**—In other cases, an embryo may be present, but cramping and heavy bleeding occur and the pregnancy tissue is expelled from the uterus. This is what most people call a miscarriage or spontaneous abortion.

Diagnosis

Ultrasound and/or blood tests for pregnancy hormone levels (beta HCG) can diagnose a missed abortion or blighted ovum. In other cases, a woman may have heavy bleeding and lots of cramping and it is obvious from these symptoms that she is going to have a miscarriage. Sometimes a woman may have a little bleeding or cramping but ultrasound shows a normal embryo and the pregnancy progresses normally.

Treatment

In most cases the uterus is able to expel the pregnancy tissue on its own. It may be several weeks before the miscarriage occurs. If there is excessive bleeding or a risk of infection, we may recommend a suction curettage to remove the pregnancy tissue. If you do not want to wait, you can schedule a pregnancy termination.

If you are Rh-negative and have an early miscarriage, you should receive MicRhoGam to prevent future Rh complications.

What are my chances for a successful pregnancy next time?

The chances are excellent that you will eventually have a successful pregnancy. Having one or even two miscarriages in a row doesn't affect your statistical chances for a perfectly normal pregnancy next time. Persistence seems to be the best advice. Even women who have had two or more miscarriages in a row have a good chance of carrying the next pregnancy to term.

Rarely, a woman may have many miscarriages and no successful pregnancies. This is called "habitual abortion". Your doctor may recommend special tests if you have had more than three miscarriages in a row.

Counseling and Support

Emotional healing is as important as physical healing after a miscarriage. It is normal to grieve over your loss. Some women and couples find their support during this time from family and friends. Others value the understanding that comes from people who have had a similar loss. Community groups of parents who have experienced miscarriage meet regularly.

If I want another pregnancy, how long should I wait?

It would be best to wait until you have had at least one normal menstrual period after your miscarriage before you become pregnant again. This will allow time for the lining of the uterus to heal completely. (If, however, you should become pregnant during the cycle immediately following your miscarriage, don't worry about it.)

Some couples need more time than others to heal emotionally. One sign that you may be ready to try again is when you feel you could face the possibility of another pregnancy loss. If this is taking longer than you wish, we encourage you to join a support group or to seek counseling.

Please remember that the majority (90%) of women who miscarry go on to have a successful pregnancy in future.

Care After a Miscarriage

Your bleeding may range from virtually none to as heavy as a normal menstrual period. You may have spotting on and off for up to four weeks after your miscarriage. Mild cramping may persist for a day or two. Your next menstrual period will probably be normal, but it may be up to two weeks late (in other words, 4-6 weeks from now). Watch for pain, fever and excessive bleeding:

1. Take your temperature in the evening for the next 5 days. If it is 100 degrees or higher, call your doctor's office.

2. Report bleeding heavier than a normal period. If you are using more than a regular sized pad every 2 hours, call your doctor's office. If you are using tampons and bleeding heavily, switch to a pad for a few hours to measure your bleeding.

3. Report increasing or persistent cramping.

More information:

- *Food:* You may eat as soon as you feel hungry.

- *Baths:* You may bathe or shower at any time.

- *Tampons:* Use regular pads for the next 24 hours. Then, if you are not bleeding heavily, you may begin to use tampons. Be sure to change them at least every 8 hours.

- *Swimming, hot tubs:* You may swim or use a hot tub as soon as you are able to use tampons or when the bleeding has stopped.

- *Intercourse:* No intercourse for one week after your miscarriage or termination procedure. Then, if you have no bleeding or minimal bleeding, you may have intercourse. Be sure to use contraception if you do not wish to become pregnant.

Pregnancy Loss

- *Douches:* None at all for at least a week after your miscarriage or termination procedure and then only if you have stopped bleeding. (Most women don't need to douche.)

- *Birth control pills:* If you will be taking birth control pills, start them the Sunday after your miscarriage/procedure. They will be effective immediately if you start them at the proper time.

- *Breast problems:* If you were more than three months pregnant at the time of your miscarriage, your breasts may become full and may actually begin to produce milk. To stop lactation (production of milk), keep a tight brassiere on 24 hours a day or bind your breasts until the engorgement has stopped. Don't try to express the milk. You can use ice packs and/or aspirin or ibuprofen (Motrin, Advil) for discomfort.

- *Checkup:* You should make an appointment for a checkup one month after your miscarriage or termination procedure. This can be with your family doctor, a Women's Health Care Specialist, or with your obstetrician (if you have been seeing him or her for this pregnancy).

Section 39.4

Grieving a Loss

Fact Sheets produced by National SIDS Clearinghouse and the National SHARE Office (Reprinted with permission).

Grief is an intense, lonely, and personal experience.

Grief is the emotions we feel following the loss of a significant person, thing or event in our lives.

Mourning is the process by which we work through those feelings and emotions following the loss.

Everyone learns about grief and grieving in the course of natural separations that occur during infancy and childhood and through their encounters with the deaths of loved ones. The death of an elderly loved one is mourned, but is usually expected. The death of a child, however, especially the death of an apparently healthy child, is an unexpected event. When a child dies not only does the death destroy the dreams and the hopes of the parents, but it also forces all family members to face an event for which they are unprepared. Most parents who experience the death of a child describe the pain that follows as the most intense they have ever experienced. Many parents wonder if they will be able to tolerate the pain, to survive it, and to be able to feel that life has meaning again.

The intense pain that parents experience when their child dies may be eased somewhat if they have insight into what has helped other parents overcome a similar grief. For example, one of the most important things for parents to realize is that recovery from the loss of a child takes time. Each person will have to establish his or her own method for recovery. There is no right or wrong way to grieve, but there is a pattern to the resolution of grief, and there is help available to family members. It is crucial that parents realize that they are not alone and that others have experienced such grief and have survived.

Often the first reaction of a parent after the death of a child is one of shock, disbelief denial, or numbness. These reactions are instinctive and soften the impact of the death until the parent is better prepared to face the reality and the finality of the child's death. These reactions, as normal as they are, can be deceptive to others who are unacquainted with the grieving process. They may incorrectly assume that the parent either is strong and holding up well, or is insensitive and incapable of expressing his or her feelings about the loss. What they fail to realize is that shock, disbelief, denial, and numbness allow the parent to begin to face the tragic occurrence without losing control. Many parents have said that they seem to be "functioning in a fog" during the first few weeks after their child's death. "Some parents describe their experience at the wake or funeral as 'being an observer' or 'not really (being) emotionally involved.'" All of these reactions are natures way of helping the parents confront the death of their child. These reactions may last minutes, hours, days, or weeks. The parent will determine subconsciously when he or she is better able to face the death. Crying, or some similar emotional release, usually marks the end of this initial period of grief.

When the child's death becomes a reality to the family, intense suffering and pain usually begin. During the weeks and months that follow, many parents say that they are frightened by the intensity and the variety of the feelings that they experience. Crying, weeping, and incessant talking are all normal reactions. The parent may find that he or she feels very much alone. Parents may express their grief differently and may have difficulty sharing their feelings. Relatives and friends may be uncomfortable with the actuality of death, may be busy with their own lives, or may be unable to meet the parents' needs for comfort and support. For some parents, help may be obtained from the clergy, physicians, counselors, other bereaved parents, or willing friends and relatives. It is important to remember, however, that no one can resolve the parents' grief but the parents themselves. Resolution can be achieved only by experiencing and working through these emotions.

It is important for the parents to allow themselves full expression of the emotions they feel. Margaret S. Miles and others have concluded that it is essential for these emotional feelings to be expressed at the time when an emotion is first experienced. It is vital that emotions not be held in for a "correct time." It is necessary for parents to express their emotions, though not necessarily in words, to gain a resolution to their child's death.

Emotions

Emotions that parents may experience include:

- **Guilt**—As the parents try to understand the reason their child died, they may develop feelings of guilt. Parents may blame themselves for something they did in the present or the past, or for something they neglected to do. Also, each parent might blame the other. "If only" becomes a familiar phrase. Many times parents feel guilty when thinking of all the things that they wish they had done with their child. For instance, a father may feel guilty for not having spent more time with his child. Guilty feelings may also arise in the mother who thinks, "If only I hadn't returned to work." And either parent could feel regret for not having given the child something that he or she wanted. In most instances there is no rational basis for these feelings. It can be extremely beneficial for parents to talk with people who will encourage the expression of these feelings, and who can help them to understand these feelings more clearly.

- **Anger**—Depending on his or her personality, a parent may express feelings ranging from mild anger to rage. Parents can feel angry at themselves, their spouse, the physician, or the child for having died. Religious beliefs may be questioned and parents may find themselves angry at a God who allows children to die. These thoughts, though normal and experienced by many grieving parents, may cause an extreme amount of anxiety. Anger that is left unreleased may be suppressed and may manifest itself at an inappropriate time or place or in an inappropriate manner. Anger can be expressed healthily and worked through in a number of ways: screaming in private, hitting something, or strenuous exercise.

- **Fear**—After the death of their child many parents experience an overall sense of fear that something else horrible is going to happen. Often, parents with older children become extremely overprotective of them. At the same time they may find themselves fearful of their responsibilities. After the death of their child, many parents find it is difficult to concentrate for any length of time. Their minds wander, making it difficult to read, write, or make decisions. Sleep may be disrupted, leaving parents overtired and edgy. Even in getting enough sleep, parents may still feel exhausted. Those in grief may experience physical symptoms centering around the heart, in the stomach, or throughout muscles. Many times parents feel an irresistible urge to escape. As normal as all these reactions are, grieving parents often fear that they are going crazy. Talking about these feelings with other parents who have experienced a similar loss can be extremely helpful for some grieving parents.

- **Depression**—As the parents continue to work through their grief, depression often occurs. Depression can take different forms for different parents. Some parents may feel constantly "down," unhappy, or sad; others may feel worthless or as though somehow they heave failed. Many are continually lethargic, tired, or listless. This may be an ideal time for parents, with the help of family or friends, to become involved in some type of activity. Caution should be taken to avoid frantic activity which, like running away, avoids facing the reality of the child's death. Grieved parents, in the midst of deep depression, may feel that life has little meaning for them. Occasionally thoughts of suicide may arise. Many parents say that thoughts of their child are constantly in the forefront of their minds. Aching arms, hearing the child cry, or continuing with routine tasks of caring for the child are all normal experiences for grieving parents. As the parents begin to recover, depression will lift slowly. "Down" times will come and go, but the time between the "downs" will become longer. It's a long, slow process that may take years. But resolution and recovery will come.

Resolution and Recovery

As the finality of the child's death becomes a reality for the parents, recovery occurs. Parents begin to take an active part in life and their lives begin to have meaning once again. The pain of their child's death becomes less intense but not forgotten. Birthdays, holidays, and the anniversary of the child's death can trigger periods of intense pain and suffering. As time passes, the painful days become less frequent. There is no set time in which recovery takes place after a child dies. The only comforting thought that one can give a parent is that it does occur. The process is slow, but it will happen. Parents need to be patient and loving with themselves, their spouses, and their families.

Signs of grief before the 1960's were considered pathological. The average person seems to expect that grief be completed or resolved within 48 hours or two weeks—according to polls taken on the street. This is an indication of the lack of understanding of the bereavement process and the reason for lack of support beyond the initial period. Bowly, Parkes and Holmes conducted a 10 year study of 1,200 bereaved adults to determine normal responses. They found that there were four phases of bereavement.

Phases of Mourning

1. **Shock and Numbness.** This happens initially and may last 48 hours to two weeks. The numbness is a healthy and normal defense. During this time the emotions may be uncontrollable. Often, it is difficult to "take in" information. The appetite may disappear. They often feel completely exhausted, yet unable to sleep. The reverse may occur where they sleep most of the time. Feelings may range from fear and anxiety to guilt and depression. There are times that they may feel they are going crazy. It is healthy to express their true feelings in this stage.

2. **Searching and Yearning.** This phase may last for months. During this time, the bereaved search for what was lost. It is during this period that the most bizarre behavior occurs. Guilt and anger are often a part of this phase, as they search for answers. They test what is real, become restless and impatient, along with the experience of a rising sensitivity to stimuli. For parents with a newborn death it is helpful to see, hold and touch the baby at the time of loss. Pictures of the baby are comforting and help them to perceptually confirm what it was they lost. It is important that the bereaved express feelings, including anger at God—if they have those feelings—jealousy and other strong emotions. They need not be ashamed of their feelings. Anger inward becomes guilt, and this leads to depression.

3. **Disorientation and Disorganization.** This is the longest phase for mourners. During the 4th to 6th months it becomes the most severe. The dominant emotion is depression. The appetite is poor, they lack motivation, have impaired judgement and experience insomnia. Once they do get to sleep, it can be difficult to awaken them. A physical examination is encouraged during the 4th to 6th month to diagnose any disease process in the early phases, because of lowered resistance to disease at this time. Tranquilizers and sedatives delay the process and cloud thinking. As the bereaved struggle to be relieved of disorientation there is a search to find the answer that feels right to them. By the 18th or 24th month they begin to resolve some of those questions. Our tendency is to try to answer questions that aren't even being asked. Cliches cause more disorientation.

Pregnancy Loss

A listening ear is our greatest gift to the bereaved. Anniversaries are very difficult. Society expect mourners to be healed quickly, and support is often lacking after a short time. Others tend to avoid talking about the person who has died, when that is the thing that helps the bereaved most. During disorientation the self-image is lowered and the mourner often isolates himself/herself from others.

4. **Reorganization.** This phase does not occur quickly. It begins around the 18th to the 24th month. Here they begin to sort out suspicions and attempt to identify what was lost. There is a sense of release, renewed energy, more socialization, better judgments and more stable eating and sleeping habits. It is at this time that they begin to enjoy themselves and have a good time without guilt feelings. There will still be momentary crisis and reliving of the loss, especially at anniversaries and holidays. Readaptation to the loss does not mean forgetting.

The normal degree of disorientation diminishes in duration and intensity gradually. Disorientation is facilitated by companionship with others who help the bereaved sort through what happened as they work toward reorientation. Mutual help groups can be important, however the best time for directing a mourner to a group is in the searching and yearning phase.

It is important to give permission for a wide range of emotions. Each person responds differently to bereavement and it is important that we not put expectations of the bereaved to imply that they need to go through various phases. Each emotion has a function. Joy is related to the creative impulse, depression protects the major organs by slowing us down, guilt occurs when we are beyond our capacity to cope and beyond the sense of what is right, while anger serves to warn others that they are intruding on one's ability to survive and that they are violated by the system. As stated earlier, mentally healthy mourners have a wide range of emotions and appropriate ways need to be found to express those feelings.

Typical Behaviors of Grief

- **Expressed frustration**—either direct such as couldn't see the baby, or indirect such as picking clothing, and other signs of restlessness and insomnia.

- **Bizarre searching**—playing with doll, cucumber, hear baby cry from grave. This reaches intensity by 2-4 months

- **Preoccupation with the experience**—delivery, prenatal period and how they feel they were treated prior to delivery.

- **Disorganized**—unable to accomplish ordinary activities.

- **Residual anger**—anger focuses on spouse and they won't talk about the baby to others. Hostility toward the dead person may be present.

Signs of Normal Grief

- Sighing
- Tightness of throat
- Dullness of perception (touch them to keep them aware of reality)
- Volatile emotions (those who don't cry need more attention)
- Guilt feelings
- Aloofness (do insignificant things to avoid contacts and distract themselves.
- A marked change in behavior and/or taking on the behavior of the deceased.

Bereavement and the Couple's Relationship

- Your marital relationship is the most important relationship, let it take precedence over all others.

- When a baby dies, the grief affects the couple at the same time. Other stresses in marriages usually don't impact on both simultaneously. Therefore, your closest support is not always able to respond to you as he/she is trying to deal with their own grief.

- Each person in the relationship will grieve in their own individual way. Learning to accept your spouses way can be difficult.

- Difficulties can arise in the best of marriages. Keep working at communicating your needs emotionally.

- Your spouse doesn't have to be your sole supporter.

Pregnancy Loss

- There could be stresses on your sexual relationship. Communicate openly your feelings. Remember human touch and hugs can be healing.

- Each person in a relationship may need some privacy with their feelings. Respect each other and give the space needed.

- Each person who has experienced a loss is not the same person they were before their baby died. This may take time to accept and understand the changes.

- Each of you will search for a meaning of your loss, one may turn to faith, the other may not.

- It is okay to enjoy life. Your baby doesn't expect you to be sad all the time. Sharing laughter and tears together helps you to heal. Search for some relaxing things to do, it helps give you a new perspective.

- This is a difficult time for both. Remember if your relationship was secure prior to your loss it can become a deeper relationship during your healing.

- Each may feel different regarding the choices of your child's memorabilia. Talk about your differences and work out compromise if able.

- Your losses are from broken hopes and dreams. Each person may have different dreams for this special baby. Sharing your dreams could give you some insights into each others feelings.

Ways to Survive as a Couple

- Seek outside support such as support group, clergy or professional help.

- Take time for each other alone.

- Set a time to talk each day.

- Work on your communication skills

- Pray together.

- Give yourselves the time to adjust to your loss.

What to do for Yourself after the loss of a baby

Suggestions from bereavement experts and support group leaders for parents facing pregnancy loss include:

- *Be human:* Admit it when you feel lonely or in pain. Allow yourself to ask for help, and accept it when family and friends extend a hand. If necessary, contact a local support group for grieving parents.

- *Communicate:* Talk about the baby and your feelings with your partner, family and friends.

- *Read:* Refer to books, articles and poems that provide comfort, understanding and the sense you're not alone.

- *Write:* Record your thoughts in a diary or journal. Write letters, notes or poems to or about the baby.

- *Physical exam:* Because your body also may respond to the grief, schedule a physical examination about four months after experiencing a loss.

- *Stay stable:* Wait at least a year before making any major job or relationship changes. Avoid new or uncertain trips and don't let others make decisions for you.

- *Faith:* Seek spiritual bonds, whether by renewing ties with clergy or setting aside quite time for reflecting.

- *Nutrition:* Eat a balanced diet that includes milk, protein, vegetables, fruit and whole grains. Avoid junk food.

- *Fluid intake:* Drink eight glasses of liquids (juice, water, soda) per day. Avoid caffeine or alcohol.

- *Exercise:* Do something active every day. Even a walk around the block can be useful.

- *Rest:* Avoid increased work activity. Maintain stable rest patterns, even if you're unable to sleep.

Supporting a Grieving Family

How to Help:

1. Be supportive—visit or call to say, "I care and want to help."
2. Treat the bereaved couple equally. Men need as much support as women.
3. Be available. Parents need direct help—providing a meal, doing errands, babysitting their other children.
4. Allow the parents to talk about their child; ask but don't pry.
5. Learn about the grieving process. There are many books available.
6. Don't be afraid of reminding the parents about the child. They have never forgotten. And letting them know you remember is comforting.
7. Be liberal with touching grieving parents. They often have a need for contact.

What to Say:

1. "I'm sorry."
2. "I'm so sad for your loss."
3. "I know this must be terribly hard for you."
4. "How are you managing all of this?"
5. "What can I do for you?"
6. "I'm here, and I want to listen."
7. "Talk as long as you want. I have plenty of time."
8. "You don't have to say anything at all."

What NOT to Say:

1. "It's all happened for the best."
2. "You're young. You can have others."
3. "Now you'll have an angel in heaven."
4. "You're better off having this happen now, before you knew the baby."
5. "This was God's way of saying something was wrong."
6. "You should feel lucky that you are alive."
7. "Forget it. Put it behind you and get on with your life."
8. "I understand." (if you have not had a similar experience).

For More Information

The following bibliography lists sources of further information.

Arnold, Joan Hagan & Gemma, Penelope Bushman. A Child Dies—A Portrait of Family Grief. The Charles Press, Philadelphia, PA. 1994.

Allen, Marie, PhD, & Marks, Shelly, MS. Miscarriage—Women Sharing From the Heart, John Wiley & Sons, NY. 1993.

Borg, Susan, & Lasker, Judith. In Search of Parenthood. Beacon Press, 25 Beacon Street, Boston, MA 02108. 1987.

Borg, Susan, & Lasker, Judith. When Pregnancy Fails: Families Coping With Miscarriage, Stillbirth and Infant Death. Bantam Press. 1989.

Bridwell, Debra. The Ache For a Child. Victor Books, Wheaton, IL. 1994.

Compassionate Friends. We Need Not Walk Alone After The Death of a Child, The Compassionate Friends National Office, Oak Brook, IL. 1992.

Creel, Mary-Jane. A Little Death. Vantage Press, Inc., 516 W. 34th Street, New York, NY 10001. 1987.

Davidson, Glen, PhD. Understanding Mourning. Augsburg Publishing House, 426 South Fifth Street, Box 1209, Minneapolis, MN 55440. 1984.

Davis, Deborah L., PhD. Empty Cradle, Broken Heart—Surviving the Death of Your Baby. Fulcrum Publishing, 350 Indiana St., Golden, CO 80401. 1991.

De Frain, John. Stillborn—The Invisible Death. Lexington Books. 1986.

Dodge, Nancy C. Thumpy's Story, A Story of Love and Grief Shared. National SHARE Office, St. Joseph Health Center, 300 First Capitol Drive, St. Charles, MO 63301.

Donnelly, Katherine Fair. Recovering From The Loss of a Child. Berkley Books, New York 1994.

Pregnancy Loss

Fritsch, Julie, & Ilse, Sherokee. The Anguish of Loss. Wintergreen Press, 3630 Eileen St., Maple Plain, MN 55359, or Pregnancy & Infant Loss Center, 1421 E. Wayzata Blvd., Ste. 30, Wayzata, MN 55391. 1988.

Gilbert, Kathleen R. PhD. & Smart, Laura S., PhD. Coping With Infant Loss, The Couple's Healing Process. Brunner/Mazel Publishers, 19 Union Square West, New York, NY 10003. 1992.

Gold, Michael. And Hanna Wept. The Jewish Publications Society, Philadelphia. 1988.

Grollman, Earl A. Straight Talk About Death For Teenagers: How to Cope With Losing Someone You Love. Beacon Press, Boston 1993.

Hales, Diane, & Creasy, Robert K., MD. New Hope for Problem Pregnancies. Harper & Row Publishers, Inc., 10 E. 53rd St., New York, NY 10002. 1982.

Hanson, Michelle Fryer. Infertility—The Emotional Journey. Deaconess Press.

Heavilin, Marylin Willett. When Your Dreams Die—Finding Strength and Hope Through Life's Disappointments. Here's Life's Publishers. Inc. San Bernardino, CA 1990.

Harkness, Carla. The Infertility Book, A Comprehensive Medical & Emotional Guide. Celestial Arts Publishing Berkeley, CA 94707. 1992.

Ilse, Sherokee. Empty Arms. Wintergreen Press, 3630 Eileen St., Maple Plain, MN 55359 or Pregnancy & Infant Loss Center, 1421 E. Wayzata Blvd, Suite #30, Wayzata, MN 55391. 1985.

Ilse, Sherokee, & Burns, Linda Hammer. Miscarriage—A Shattered Dream. Wintergreen Press, 3630 Eileen St., Maple Plain, 55359 or Pregnancy & Infant Loss Center, 1421 E. Wayzata Blvd, Suite #30, Wayzata, MN 55391. 1985.

Jeminez, Sherry Lynn Mims. The Other Side of Pregnancy. A Spectrum Book. 1982.

Johnson, Joy & Johnson, Marv, Editors. Dear Parents: Letters to Bereaved Parents. Centering Corporation, Box 3367, Omaha, NE 68103-0367. 1989.

Kohn, Ingrid, MSW & Moffit, Perry-Lyn & Wilkins, Isabelle, MD. A Silent Sorrow. Bantam Doubleday Dell Publishing Group, Inc., 666 Fifth Ave. New York, NY 10103. 1992.

Lamb, Sister Jane Marie, OSF. Bittersweet...hellogoodbye: A Resource in Planning Farewell Rituals When A Baby Dies. National SHARE Office, St. Joseph Health Center, 300 First Capitol Drive, St. Charles, MO 63301. 1988.

Leon, Irving G., PhD. When A Baby Dies: Psychotherapy for Pregnancy and Newborn Loss. Yale University Press, New Haven. 1990.

Levang, Elizabeth, PhD & Ilse, Sherokee. Remembering With Love—Messages of Hope for the First Year of Grieving and Beyond. Wintergreen Press, 3630 Eileen St., Maple Plain, MN 55359 or Pregnancy & Infant Loss Center, 1421 E. Wayzata Blvd. Suite #30, Wayzata, MN 55391. 1993.

Limbo, Rana & Wheeler, Sara. When A Baby Dies: A Handbook for Healing and Helping. RTS, LaCrosse Lutheran Hospital, 1910 South Ave. LaCrosse, WI 54601. 1985.

Loizeaux, William. Anna, A Daughter's Life, Little Brown & Co.

Manning, Doug. Don't Take My Grief Away From Me. Creative Marketing, Box 2423, Springfield, IL 62705. 1974.

Morrow, Judy Gordon, & DeHamer, Nancy Gordon. Good Mourning: Help and Understanding in Time of Pregnancy Loss. Word Publishing, Dallas, TX. 1989.

Neeld, Elizabeth Harper, PhD. Seven Choices: Taking the Steps to New Life After Losing Someone You Love. Crown Publishers, Inc., 201 East 50th Street, New York, NY 10022. 1990.

Nelson, James D., Editor, The Rocking Horse Is Lonely—and other stories of fathers' grief, Pregnancy & Infant Loss Center, 1421 E. Wayzata Blvd. Suite #30, Wayzata, MN 55391. 1994.

Pregnancy Loss

Page, Carole Gift. Misty, Our Momentary Child. Crossway Books, Division of Good News Publishing, Westchester, NY 60153. 1987.

Peppers, Larry, PhD. & Knapp, Ronald, PhD. How To Go On Living After the Death of a Baby. Peachtree Publishers. 1985.

Raab, Diana, BS RN. Getting Pregnant and Staying Pregnant: A Guide to Infertility and High-risk Pregnancy. Sirdan Publishing, Montreal, Canada. 1988.

Rank, Maureen. Free to Grieve: Healing & Encouragement for Those Who Have Experienced the Physical Mental & Emotional Trauma of Miscarriage & Stillbirth. Bethany House Publishers, 6820 Auto Club Road, Minneapolis, MN 55438. 1985.

Reid, Joanie. LIFELINE A Journal For Parents Grieving a Miscarriage Stillbirth or Early Infant Death, Pineapple Press, Muliett Lake, MI. 1994

Rue, Nancy. Handling the Heartbreak of Miscarriage. Here's Life Publishers, Inc., P.O. Box 1576, San Bernardino, CA 92402 1987.

Savage, Judith A. Mourning Unlived Lives: A Psychological Study of Childbearing Loss. Chiron Press, 400 Linden Ave. Wilmette, IL 60091. 1988.

Scher, Jonathon MD & Dix, Carol. Preventing Miscarriage. Harper & Row Publishers, NY 1990.

Schweibert, P. & Kirk, Paul MD. When Hello Means Goodbye. Perinatal Loss, 2116 NE 18th Ave. Portland, OR 97212. 1986.

Semchyshyn, Stefan, MD. How to Prevent Miscarriages and Other Crises of Pregnancy. Birth & Life Bookstore, 7001 Alonza Ave NW, P.O. Box 70625, Seattle, WA 98107-0625, 1990.

Staudacher, Carol. Beyond Grief: A Guide for Recovering From the Death of a Loved One. New Harbinger Publications, Inc., 2200 Adeline St. Suite 305, Oakland, CA 94640. 1987.

Wheeler, Sara Rich, RN, MS & Pike, Margaret. Goodbye My Child. Centering Corporation, 1531 N. Saddle Creek Rd. Omaha, NE 68104-5064. 1992

Williamson, Walter. Miscarriage. Walker & Company, NY 1988.

Wolfert, Alan D. PhD. Understanding Grief. Helping Yourself Heal. Accelerated Development Inc. Publishers, 3808 West Kilgore Ave. Muncie, IN 47304. 1992.

Woods, James R. Jr., MD & Esposito, Jenifer L. Pregnancy Loss: Medical Therapeutics and Practical Considerations. Williams and Wilkins. Baltimore. 1987.

For local references and assistance, bereaved parents may wish to contact the mutual help groups for parents listed below.

RESOLVE
1310 Broadway
Summerville, MA 02144
617-623-0744

A.M.E.N.D.
4324 Berrywick Terrace
St.Louis, MO 63128
314-487-7582

H.O.P.I.N.G.
contact Ellen Felton 714-858-5958

The National SIDS Foundation
10500 Little Patuxent
Parkway, Suite 420
Columbia, MD 21044
1-800-221-7437

SHARE National Headquarters
St. Elizabeth's Hospital
211 South Third Street
Belleville, IL 62222
618-234-2415

Pregnancy Loss

The Compassionate Friends National Headquarters
P.O. Box 3696
Oak Brook
IL 60522-3696
312-990-0010

Pregnancy and Infant Loss Center
1415 East Wayzata Boulevard
Suite 22
Wayzata, MN 55391
612-473-9372

Part Eight

Glossary

Chapter 40

Glossary of Medical Terms

This glossary contains many of the terms used throughout this volume of the Health Reference Series. The definitions given are not dictionary definitions but are those most applicable to usage relating to pregnancy and birth.

A

Abruptio placentae. Premature detachment of a normally situated placenta.

Adjudicate. To pronounce or decree by judicial sentence.

AIDS. Acquired immunodeficiency syndrome. A disease characterized by opportunistic infections (e.g., Pneumocystis carinii pneumonia, candidiasis, Kaposi's sarcoma) in immunocompromised persons; caused by the human immunodeficiency virus (HIV) and transmitted by exchange of body fluids.

Amniocentesis. A procedure whereby fluid is aspirated from the amniotic sac through the abdomen.

Anergy. Absence of demonstrable sensitivity reaction in a subject to substances that would be antigenic (immunogenic, allergenic) in most other subjects.

Excerpts from NIH Publication No. 93-2788, FDA Consumer, March 1992, DHSS Publication No. 93-1988

Anergia. Lack of energy.

Anomaly. Deviation from the average or norm; anything structurally unusual or irregular or contrary to a general rule.

Anorexia. Diminished appetite, aversion to food.

Antenatal. Refers to the period before birth. (Also see prenatal).

Asthma. A genetically linked problem, believed to cause airway obstruction, that is associated with narrowing of air passages, airway inflammation, and airway hypersensitivity to multiple stimuli.

Asymptomatic. Without signs or symptoms.

B

Bacteremia. The presence of viable bacteria in the circulating blood.

Birth Defect. Any defect present when a child is born. Birth defects are disorders of body structure, function, or chemistry which may be inherited or may result from environmental interference during embryonic or fetal life.

Blood Pressure. Force exerted by the heart in pumping blood from its chambers. The pressure of blood against the walls of a blood vessel or heart chamber. Unless there is reference to another location, such as the pulmonary artery or one of the heart chambers. it refers to the pressure in the systemic arteries, as measured, for example, in the forearm.

Booting. Any drug solution, such as cocaine or heroin, mixed with blood aspirated into a syringe and then injected into a vein, repeated one or more times to clear the syringe barrel and tip of any of the drug residue. Heavy blood contamination of the syringe may contribute to colonization with bacterial pathogens and to the more likely transmission of the human immunodeficiency virus (HIV).

Braxton Hicks contractions. Intermittent contractions that occur throughout pregnancy. When these contractions do not cause cervical changes they are called "false labor" contractions.

Glossary of Medical Terms

C

Carbohydrates. A type of food, usually from plants versus animals. Carbohydrates include simple carbohydrates (sugar, fruit) and complex carbohydrates (vegetables, starches). One of three nutrients that supply calories to the body. (See fat and protein.)

Case manager. One who defines, initiates, and monitors the medical, drug treatment, psychosocial, and social services provided for the woman and her family.

Cervical dysplasia. Abnormal tissue development of the uterine cervix.

Cervix. The lowermost portion of the uterus that dilates during labor, permitting the fetus to pass from the uterus through the vagina or birth canal during birth.

Chancroid. An acute bacterial infection characterized by single or multiple ulcers or sores in the genital area: an infectious venereal ulcer with a soft base.

Chlamydia. A sexually transmitted disease manifested by mucopurulent endocervical discharge and inflammation of the endocervical columnar epithelium. Symptoms may be moderate or scanty discharge, urethral itching, and burning on urination, but patients are often asymptomatic.

Chorionic Villus Biopsy. Biopsy of a very small portion of the placenta. this is done during the early stages of pregnancy to obtain tissue for genetic diagnosis. Prenatal diagnosis of cystic fibrosis can be made on examination of this tissue if there is a child with cystic fibrosis already in the family. The tissue is obtained by inserting a hollow needle into the womb and taking a very small piece of the placenta.

Chromosomes. Physical structures in the cell's nucleus that house the genes; each human cell has 23 pairs of chromosomes.

Condylomata. A wart-like excrescence at the anus, vulva, or on the glans penis caused by the human papilloma virus (HPV).

Congenital. Existing at birth. Refers to certain mental or physical traits, anomalies, malformations, or diseases which may be either hereditary or due to an influence occurring during gestation up to the moment of birth.

Contractions. The rhythmic firming of the uterine muscle, which may or may not be painful. Contractions associated with labor usually cause the cervix to open.

Corticosteroids. A group of hormones produced by adrenal glands.

Cross training. To be trained in several disciplines to facilitate broader coverage in a treatment unit.

D

Diabetes mellitus. A disorder that prevents the body from converting digested food into the energy needed for daily activities.

Diaphoresis. Increased perspiration.

Diastolic pressure. The lowest pressure to which blood pressure falls between contractions of the ventricles.

DNA (deoxyribonucleic acid). A nucleic acid that is found in the cell nucleus and is the carrier of genetic information.

Dysuria. Difficulty or pain in urination.

Dyspnea. Shortness of breath.

E

Edema. Swelling of tissue due to injury or disease.

Embryo. The developing organism from conception until approximately the end of the second month.

Endocarditis. Inflammation of the lining of the heart.

Glossary of Medical Terms

Epidemiology. The study of the relationship between various factors that determine the frequency and distribution of diseases in human and other animal populations.

F

Fat. One of three nutrients that supply calories to the body. Included are vegetable oil, lard, margarine, butter, shortening, mayonnaise, and salad dressing. (See carbohydrates and protein.)

Fetus. The unborn young from the end of the eighth week to the moment of birth.

Folliculitis. An inflammation of the hair follicles. The lesions may be papules (small skin elevations) or pustules.

Fungal infections. A general term used to describe those diseases caused by diverse morphological forms of yeasts and molds.

G

Gene. A unit of genetic material (DNA) that occupies a definite locus on a chromosome and contains the plan a cell uses to perform a specific function (e.g., making a given protein).

Genitourinary. Pertaining to the organs of reproduction and urination.

Gestation. The process, state, or period of pregnancy.

Gestational diabetes. A form of diabetes which begins during pregnancy when the woman's body is unable to properly process glucose, a form of sugar. It usually disappears following delivery.

Glucose tolerance test. A blood test used to make the diagnosis of diabetes, including gestational diabetes. After drinking a liquid containing 100 grams of glucose, blood is drawn every hour for 3 hours. Two or more abnormally elevated blood sugar levels indicate gestational diabetes.

Gonorrhea. A sexually transmitted disease manifested by an inflammation of the genital mucus membrane.

H

Hairy leukoplakia. A white lesion appearing on the tongue of patients with AIDS. The lesion appears raised, with a corrugated or "hairy" surface, due to keratin projections (a substance found in the dead outer corneal skin layer and in hair and nails).

Health care providers. Health care professionals who specialize in the management of certain conditions. In the case of gestational diabetes, the health care providers may include an obstetrician, an internist, a diabetologist, a registered dietitian, a qualified nutritionist, a diabetes educator, and a neonatologist.

Hemangiomas. A congenital anomaly in which a proliferation of vascular endothelium leads to a mass that resembles neoplastic tissue. It can occur anywhere in the body, but is most frequently noticed in the skin and subcutaneous tissue.

Hepatitis. Inflammation of the liver, usually from a viral infection, but sometimes from toxic agents.

Hepatomegaly. Enlargement of the liver.

Hereditary Traits. Or conditions that genetically passed on from parents to children.

Herpes simplex. A virus that in humans causes fever blisters, usually on the lips and external nares (nose), and also on the genitalia. This virus may also cause acute stomatitis and meningoencephalitis.

High-risk pregnancy. A pregnancy in which the woman or fetus has a higher than-average chance of experiencing medical complications or death.

Histoplasmosis. Darling's disease. An infectious disease manifested by a primary benign pneumonitis similar to primary tuberculosis.

Glossary of Medical Terms

HIV. Human immunodeficiency virus. The virus occurring in humans that causes a condition that results in a defective immunological mechanism, opportunistic infections, and eventually in the disease process know as AIDS (acquired immunodeficiency syndrome).

Hormone. A chemical substance produced within the body which has a "regulatory" effect on the activity of a certain tissue in the body. Estrogen, cortisol, and human placental lactogen are hormones produced by the placenta which cause changes in the mother's body to prepare her for the pregnancy and birth. These hormones also have a contra-insulin effect.

Hyperpnea. Breathing that is deeper and more rapid than is normal at rest.

Hyperpyrexia. An abnormally high fever.

Hypertension. Abnormally high blood pressure.

Hypoglycemia. A condition where the blood sugar is lower than normal. This Is a dangerous condition and should be avoided or treated rapidly.

Hypotonia. Having a lesser degree of tension in any part of the body.

I

Icterus. Relating to or marked by jaundice.

Incidence. the number of new cases of a condition occurring in a given population during a specified time, such as a year.

Infant. A child under the age of 1 year.

Insulin. A hormone manufactured by the pancreas. Insulin helps glucose leave the blood and enter the muscles and other tissues of the body.

Insulin-resistance. A partial blocking of the effect of insulin. This interference can be caused by hormones produced by the placenta or by excessive weight gain.

K

Kaposi's sarcoma (K.S.). Malignant neoplasm occurring in the skin and sometimes in lymph nodes, manifested by cutaneous lesions consisting of reddish-purple to dark blue macules, plaques, or nodules. It is seen mostly in men and as an opportunistic disease in AIDS patients.

Ketoacidosis. Enhanced production of ketone bodies due to alcohol or diabetes.

Ketone. A break-down product of fat that accumulates in the blood as a result of inadequate insulin or inadequate calorie intake.

L

Legumes. Beans, peas. and lentils which supply fiber and nutrients and are high in vegetable protein.

Lymphadenopathy. Any disease process affecting a lymph node or nodes; clinically refers to enlargement of nodes.

Macrosomia. A term meaning "large body:' This refers to a baby that is considerably larger than normal. This condition occurs when the mother's blood sugar levels have been higher than normal during the pregnancy. This is a preventable complication of gestational diabetes.

M

Meconium. The first intestinal discharge of the newborn infant.

Microcephaly. Pertaining to abnormal smallness of the head.

Morbidity. Pertaining to severe illness.

Mortality. Pertaining to death.

Mucopurulent. Containing or composed of mucus and pus.

Myoclonic. Spasm or twitching of a muscle.

Glossary of Medical Terms

N

Neonatal. Refers to the period directly after birth, Period up to the first 4 weeks after birth.

Neonate. A newborn. Refers to the period immediately following birth and continuing through the first 28 days of life.

Neurotropic. A virus or drug that has an affinity for nerve cells or tissue.

Nosocomial. Denotes a new disorder not related to patient's original condition that is associated with being treated in a hospital. e.g.. a hospital-acquired infection.

Nutrients. Proteins, carbohydrates, fats, vitamins, and minerals. These are provided by food and are necessary for growth and the maintenance of life.

O

Ocular. Pertaining to the eyes.

Odynophagia. Pain on swallowing.

P

Pancreas. A long gland that lies behind the stomach. The pancreas manufactures insulin and digestive enzymes.

Paresthesia. An abnormal sensation, such as burning, pricking, tickling, and tingling.

Perinatal. Occurring during, or pertaining to, the periods before, during, or after the time of birth, i.e., from the 28th week of gestation through the first seven days after delivery.

Pertussis. Whooping cough.

Placenta. A special tissue that joins the mother and fetus. It provides hormones necessary for a successful pregnancy, and supplies the fetus with water and nutrients (food) from the mother's blood.

Postnatal. Occurring after birth.

Prenatal. Occurring before birth.

Pre-term labor. Labor that occurs after 20 weeks but before 37 completed weeks of pregnancy.

Prophylaxis. To guard against or take precautions that will prevent either disease or a process that can lead to disease.

Protein. A substance found in many parts of the body that helps the body to resist disease. Protein often, but not always, comes from animal products. High protein foods include meat, poultry, fish, eggs, hard cheese, cottage cheese, yogurt, and milk. Non-animal sources of protein are nuts and seeds, peanut butter, legumes, whole grains, and tofu. One of three nutrients that supply calories to the body. (See carbohydrates and fat.)

Pruritus. Itching.

Psychotropic. Pertaining to drugs used in the treatment of mental illness; affecting the mind.

Pyoderma. Skin infection characterized by the formation of pus.

R

Recommended Dietary Allowances. Recommendations for daily intake of specific nutrients for groups of healthy individuals. There is a specific recommendation for pregnant and for lactating women. These recommendations are set by the Food and Nutrition Board of the National Research Council of the National Academy of Science.

Retinitis. Inflammation of the retina, which may be caused by the cytomegalovirus (CMV).

Rh antigen. Rhesus antigen; a red blood cell surface antigen.

Glossary of Medical Terms

S

Seborrheic dermatitis. Over-activity of the sebaceous glands resulting in a scaly macular eruption that occurs primarily on the face, scalp (dandruff), and pubic and anal areas.

Self(or home) blood glucose monitoring. A process by which blood sugars can be determined at home by pricking the finger, putting a drop of blood on a chemically treated test strip. and comparing the color changes to a chart.

Septicemia. Systemic disease caused by the spread of microorganisms and their toxins via the bloodstream.

Sonogram. An image made through ultrasound scanning technology. When done during pregnancy, the image can give information about the fetus.

Splenomegaly. Enlargement of the spleen.

Spontaneous abortion. The loss of an embryo or fetus prior to the stage of viability at about 20 weeks of gestation as a result of natural causes (not artificially induced).

Stabilization. The accomplishment of a steady, non-varying physical state.

Sudden infant death syndrome (SIDS). The unexpected death of an apparently healthy baby, usually occurring during sleep, without apparent cause.

Syndrome. The combination of signs and symptoms associated with any morbid process, which together constitute the picture of the disease.

Syphilis. An acute and chronic infectious, sexually transmitted disease. Syphilis is manifested first by a chancre, followed by a slight fever, and progresses through several stags that include skin eruptions and functional abnormalities resulting from cardiovascular and nervous system lesions.

Systolic pressure. The highest pressure to which blood pressure rises with the contraction of the ventricles.

T

Tachypnea. Rapid breathing.

Tenesmus. The urgent feeling of a need to urinate or defecate without the ability to do so.

Teratogen. A drug or other agent that causes abnormal fetal development.

Thrombocytosis. An increase in the number of platelets in the circulating blood.

Thrush. Infection of the oral (mouth) tissues with Candida albicans.

Tocolytic medication. A drug that inhibits labor.

Toxemia. A metabolic disorder of pregnancy characterized by hypertension, edema, and albumin in the urine. Also known as pregnancy-induced hypertension (PIH) or pre-eclampsia.

Toxoplasmosis. Disease caused by protozoan parasite. This prenatally acquired human infection from cat litter boxes can result in an infant with microcephalus or hydrocephalus at birth as well as other abnormalities.

Trimester. A period of 3 months. Pregnancy is divided into three trimesters. The first trimester is 0-13 weeks gestation. The second trimester is 14-26 weeks gestation. The third trimester is 27 weeks gestation until birth.

U

Urine toxicology. The science dealing with the detection of drugs in the urine.

Uterus. A hollow muscular organ that nourishes and houses the developing fetus until birth. It is sometimes called the womb.

Glossary of Medical Terms

V

Vaccine. A substance that contains antigenic components from an infectious organism; by stimulating an immune response (but not disease), it protects against subsequent infection by that organism.

Vaginal candidiasis. Infection in the vagina manifested by yeast-like fungi.

Vas Deferens. A duct in the reproductive system of the male. Carries sperm form the testes to the prostate gland.

Vitamins. Substances that occur in foods in small amounts and are necessary for the normal functioning of the body.

Index

Index

Page numbers in *italics* refer to tables and illustrations; the letter "n" following a page number refers to a note.

A

AAP *see* American Academy of Pediatrics (AAP)
Abbott Laboratories *333*
Abboud, T. K. 417
abortions, complications of 107–8
　see also induced abortions; miscarriage; spontaneous abortions
abruptio placentae 172, 298, 679
　cocaine and 188
　ultrasound and 100
abstinence *328–29*
　see also sexual activity
access to care
　drug dependency and 163–64
　drug rehabilitation and 181
Accutane (acne medication)
　birth defects and 138, 140
　warning about 141–45
ACE inhibitors 459–60
acid elution (Kleihauer-Betke) test 380
acne 141–42, 144
ACOG *see* American College of Obstetricians and Gynecologists (ACOG)
active management, labor and 236–38
acupuncture 121, 174
acute chest syndrome 493–94
acute splenic sequestration crisis 363
ADA *see* American Diabetes Association (ADA)
Adam, K. 618
Adams, M. M. 384, 640
Adamson, K. 418
addictions 159
　see also drug use
adhesions 538
adipose tissues 355
adjudicate 679
adult polycystic kidney disease 25
adults, chickenpox and 8
AFP *see* alpha-fetoprotein (AFP)
afterpains 307
age factor
　chromosomal analysis during 107
　Down syndrome and 106
　folic acid and 68–70
　miscarriage risk and 104–5
　pregnancy and 3
　prenatal care and 91

age factor, continued
 vaccines and 15
 see also gestational age; pregnancy, first trimester; pregnancy, second trimester; pregnancy, third trimester
Agency for Health Care Policy and Research (AHCPR) 240, 485n, 495–96
Agnew, J. A. 426
AIDS (Acquired Immune Deficiency Syndrome) 206, 209–10, 516–34, 679
 listeriosis and 226
 toxoplasmosis and 213
AIUM/NEMA Safety Standard for Diagnostic Ultrasound Equipment 97
Akerlund, M. 418
Albert Einstein College of Medicine 274, 278
Albright, G. A. 424
alcohol and other drug interview 182–83
alcohol use 628
 hypertension and 454
 during pregnancy 42, 44, 147, 151–56, 572
 prenatal care and 84–90
 preterm labor and 240
 prior to pregnancy 4
 withdrawal from 153–55
Aldridge, A. 403, 418
Alexander, G. R. 641
Alexander, T. P. 479
Alexandre, G. P. 427
Alfin-Slater, Arthur 58
Alfin-Slater, Roslyn B., PhD 51, 54
Ali, A. M. 615
Ali, N. J. 424
Allen, Marie, PhD 670
Aller, J. 431
allergies 353
alpha-adrenergic inhibitors 458
alpha-fetoprotein (AFP)
 amniotic fluid and 107
 neural tube defects and 116
 ultrasound and 100
Alzheimer's disease 32
Ameda Egnell Mother's Touch 349

A.M.E.N.D. 674
American Academy of Dermatology 142, 144
American Academy of Pediatrics (AAP) 44, 142, 338, 339, 351, 352, 647
 Committee on Drugs 404, 418
 Committee on Nutrition 336
 publications 289
American Academy of Pediatrics/Pediatric AIDS Coalition 530
American Association of Blood Banks 384, 386
American College of Obstetricians and Gynecologists (ACOG) 44, 57, 78, 96, 284, 382
 publications 289, 290, 384, 385, 583, 619
 publications of Committee on Obstetric Practice 286
 recommendations of 275
American Diabetes Association (ADA) 577, 587
 Council on Diabetes in pregnancy 556
American Journal of Clinical Nutrition 337
American Journal of Clinical Oncology 513
American Journal of Diseases of Children 180
American Journal of Emergency Medicine 419
American Journal of Epidemiology 71
American Journal of Hematology 512
American Journal of Obstetrics and Gynecology 286, 287, 288, 383, 385, 386, 387, 388, 418, 419, 420, 421, 422, 423, 425, 426, 427, 428, 429, 430, 431, 448, 449, 462, 463, 464, 545, 614, 615, 616, 617, 618, 619, 640, 641
The American Journal of Public Health 384
American Medical Association (AMA) 576
The American Red Cross 8
American Social Health Association (ASHA) 206, 211–12

Index

American Society of
Psychoprophylaxis in Obstetrics,
Inc. (ASPO/Lamaze) 351
American Thoracic Society 418
amino acids 28
see also proteins
aminophylline 401, 404
amniocentesis 378, 379, 382, 629, 679
described 104–5
diabetes and 564
miscarriage risk from 108–9
ultrasound and 98
use of 106–8
amnion 104
amniotic fluid 378, 381
see also amniocentesis
amniotomy 283, 607
Amon, E. 616
amoxicillin 416
amphetamines 158
ampicillin 222, 403–4
Ananth, U. 387
anaphylaxis 223, 417
Anderson, G. D. 463, 616, 618
Anderson, I. 288
Anderson, J. C. 427, 429
Andreoli, J. W. 619
Andrew, M. 616
anemia 27, 486, 494, 594
fetal test for 35
pica substances and 51–53
Rh-immunoglobulin and 381
test for 94
treatment for 4
see also sickle-cell disease
anencephaly 61, 68, 116
anergia 680
anergy 679
anesthesia 272, 299
see also epidural
Anesthesiology 420, 421, 423, 427, 429
aneuploidy, risk of 106, 107
angiotensins 456–57, 459
animal studies
caffeine and 148
cholesterol levels and 358
corticosteroids and 261
pregnancy and 37

animal studies, continued
prescription medications and 139
ultrasound and 102, 103
Annals of Internal Medicine 423, 463, 513
anorexia 680
anti-anxiety medications 148
antibiotic medications 649
asthma and 416
bacterial vaginosis and 249
birth defects and 139
pregnancy and 146
streptococcal infections and 222–24
antibody tests 377, 497, 502–3
anti-cancer drugs 146
anticoagulant medications 146, 503
anti-convulsant drugs 146
antidepressants 172, 173
antihistamines 415
antihypertensive medication 455–59, 608–9
anti-nausea drugs 120–21
anti-seizure medications 63, 175
antithrombin levels 598–99
Antsaklis, A. 288
AOD see alcohol and other drug interview
Apgar, B. S. 545
aplastic crisis 486, 494
Appel, L. L. 427, 429
Appleton-Century-Crofts 461, 545, 613
Apter, A. J. 400, 418
Arcuri, P. A. 418
Arias, F. 464
Arkansas Children's Hospital 340
Arnold, Joan Hagan 670
artificial sweeteners 576
Arwood, L. L. 418
Ascari, W. K. 386
Aselton, P. 418
ASHA see American Social Health Association (ASHA)
Ashikari, R. 509
asphyxia 278, 282
aspirin 147, 502, 503, 602
ASPO/Lamaze see American Society of Psychoprophylaxis in Obstetrics, Inc. (ASPO/Lamaze)

Asrat, T 430
Association of Asian/Pacific Community Health Organizations 231n
Association of Reproductive Health Professionals 321
asthma 389–417, 431–34, 680
  described 389
  medications for,433 391–93, 401–4, 405
Atkinson, A. J., Jr. 403, 404, 421, 423
Atrash, H. K. 545, 640
atropine 393
attention deficit disorder 177
auscultation 85, 279, 280, 282–83
Aviles, A. 512
azathioprine (Imuran) 502
AZT (zidovudine) 516, 530–34, 648

B

baby bottle tooth decay 354
Back, K. C. 418
bacteremia 680
bacterial vaginosis (BV) 247
bacteria vaccines 15
Bahna, S. L. 397, 418
Bailey, J. 403, 418
Baillie, P. 418
Baird, D. 614
Bajtai, G. 386
Baker, P. 462
Baldwin, M. L. 386
Bamford, D. G. 420
Banerjee, B. N. 419
Bantam Books 479
barbiturate abstinence syndrome 174–75
Barbour, Dennis 321
Barnavon, Y. 509
Barrier, G. 426
Barron, W. M. 463
bases (gene building blocks) 28, 31
Bash, Deborah 240
Baskett, T. F. 384
Bates, J. N. 420
Baudin, J. C. 386
Baumgarten, A. 385
Baumgarten, K. V. 289

Baxi, L. V. 419
Bayliss, K. M. 386
Baylor College of Medicine 334, 359
Beach, J. E. 421
Beaufils, M. 617
Beaulieu, M. D. 287
beclomethasone 392
bed rest 452–53, 652
Beevers, D. G. 463
Beilin, L. G. 462
Belizan, J. M. 462
Bende, M. 415, 419
Bendectin 120
Benedetti, T. J. 388
Bengtsson, L. P. 418
Benigni, A. 617
Bennett, F. C. 289
Bennett, P. N. 404, 419
Bennett, P. R. 387
Benowitz, L. 404, 427
benzodiazepines 147, 174
Berendes, H. 397, 398, 423
Berlin, C. M., Jr. 419
Berman, S. 614
Bertrand, J. M. 398, 419
Best Start-Kentucky 346, 352
beta-adrenergic blocking agents 457
beta2-agonists 392, 393, 414, 417
betamethasone 256, 260
beta-methasone (Celestone) 502
beta-mimetic tocolytics 258–59
bicornuate uterus 99
biopsy 506
biotinidase deficiency test 27, 361
bipolar disorder 319
Birth 290
birth canal
  abnormalities of 296
  exercises and 74
  size of 632
  see also vaginal delivery
birth control 3–4, 207, 309
  guide for *328–29*
birth control pills 659
  estrogen in 147
  twins and 467
  see also contraceptives; family planning

Index

birth defects 3, 628, 680
  alpha-fetoprotein and 116
  Bendectin and 120–21
  from chickenpox 8
  chorionic villus sampling and 105, 109–14
  congenital rubella syndrome and 11
  diagnosis of 55
  folate and 60
  multivitamins and 59
  mumps and 12
  prescription medications and 136–38
  from rubella 10
  sexually transmitted diseases and 206
  spina bifida and 63
  statistical risk of 8–9
  vitamin A and 141, 145–46
Birth Defects Monitoring Program (BDMP) 155, *156*
birth weight 55, 56
  see also low birth weight
Bittersweet 479
Bjerkedal, T. 397, 418
Bjorkhem, I. 426
Blackwell Scientific Publications 383
Blackwood, W. 417, 422
bladder, fetal, blocked 35
bladder control 313–16
  see also Kegel squeeze exercise; urination
bladder infections 63
Blair, A. M. 421
Blakemore, K. J. 385
blighted ovum 656
Block, G. 71
blood
  changes in 18
  hepatitis B virus and 13–14
  sexually transmitted diseases and 208
  volume of 598, 611–12
blood gases, asthma and 394–95
blood pressure 682
  diastolic 680
  systolic 690

blood pressure tests 453–54
  preeclampsia and 594
  prenatal care and 86, 87
  see also high blood pressure; hypertension
blood sugar levels 584
  gestational diabetes and 557, 560–62, 576
  during pregnancy 54
  see also diabetes mellitus; hyperglycemia; hypoglycemia
blood tests 532, 548
  DNA (deoxyribonucleic acid) and 20, 371
  for fetus 35
  hepatitis B virus 14–15
  for lupus 498
  miscarriage and 656
  during pregnancy 94
  prenatal care and 84
blood types 377–83
Bock, Robert 245
Boehm, F. H. 287
Boike, G. M. 398, 422
bone meal 54
Bongiovanni, A. M. 419
Bonica, J. 419
Bonnar, J. 462
boosters *see* immunizations; vaccines
booting 680
Bopp, Deborah 120
Borg, Susan 670
Bosco, L. A. 463
Boston City Hospital 159
Boston University School of Medicine 159
Bottoms, S. F. 398, 422, 615
Bove, J. R. 388
Bowen, Rosellen 341
Bowen, T. 383
Bowes, W. A., Jr. 425
Bowly, Parkes and Holmes study 663
Bowman, J. M. 383, 384, 385, 386, 387, 388
BPD *see* bronchopulmonary dysplasia (BPD)
bradycardia 395
Brandenburg, H. 385

699

Braxton Hicks contractions 241, 680
breakfast cereals, folic acid and 68–70
breast cancer 505–8
   oral contraceptives and 324
breast feeding 312
   age factor and 332
   cocaine exposure and 191-193
   versus cow's milk 334
   diabetes and 354, 582
   health benefits of 352
   versus infant formula 335
   infant infections and 334, 352
   lactation suppression and 341–345
   prenatal care and 86
   psychotherapeutic medications and 147
   racial factor and 332
   and vitamin supplements 338–339
   weight loss and 58
   and work environment 346–351
breast pumps 348–49
breast tenderness 309
   contraceptives and 324, 325
breathing techniques, labor and 233–36
breech position 295
Brenner, B. E. 419
Brenner, B. M. 463
Brett, K. M. 641
Bridwell, Debra 670
Briggs, G. G. 419, 430
Brigham and Women's Hospital 236
Bristol-Myers Squibb 459
British Journal of Cancer 513
British Journal of Clinical Pharmacology 422
British Journal of Obstetrics and Gynaecology 385, 386, 429
British Medical Journal 288, 354, 384, 387, 388, 418, 464, 615
Brojer, E. 387
bromocriptine 173, 343–44
bronchitis 353
bronchopulmonary dysplasia (BPD) 240, 258, 265–66
Brooks, P. M. 426
Brossard, Y. 388
Brown, C. E. 616

Brown, Judith E. *567, 568*
Browne, F. J. 616
Browne, J. C. M. 616
Bruskin/Goldring Research 497
Bruyere, H. J., Jr. 419, 420
Bueker, E. D. 420
Bullen, M. 464
Bulpitt, C. J. 462
Bunnell Inc. 265
Bureau of Radiological Health 101
Burghart, P. H. 619
Burns, K. A. 180
Burns, Linda Hammer 671
Burns, W. J. 180
Burroughs Wellcome Company 264
Burrows, R. F. 616
Buster, J. E. 545
Butte, Nancy F. 359
Butters, L. 457, 462, 463
Butz, R. F. 422
BV *see* bacterial vaginosis (BV)

C

Caesarean section *see* cesarean delivery
caffeine
   breast feeding and 350
   postpartum 310
   pregnancy and 148, 572, *575*
   prior to pregnancy 4
   sources of 148
calcium
   pregnancy and 53–54
   recommended daily allowance of *52*
   sources of 53–54
calcium channel blockers 457, 609, 610
calcium deficiency 53
California Department of Health Services 480
California Medical Center, San Francisco 481
California State Department of Health 492
calories *see* diet and nutrition
Canada Communication Group 388
Canadian Medical Association Journal 287, 383, 384, 385

Index

Canadian Task Force on the Periodic Health Examination 252, 284, 382
  publications 290, 388
Cancer 509, 512
candidiasis 691
Capella-Pavlovsky, M. 385
Capsules 157
carbohydrates 681
Carcelen, A. 429
cardiotocography 279, 280
cardiovascular concerns
  preeclampsia and 597–98, 612
  during pregnancy 391–97
Carnegie Corporation 650
carriers
  colonized 221–22
  for cystic fibrosis 33
  DNA (deoxyribonucleic acid) testing and 23, 24
  hepatitis B virus 14
  parents as 26
  sickle-cell disease and 21, 27
Carson, S. A. 545
Carter, A. M. 418
case management 164–65, 681
Case Western Reserve University 586
Cassinelli, M. T. 429
Catalano, Patrick 586–87, 588–89
cat feces
  pregnancy and 4
  toxoplasmosis and 212, 216–17, 218
catheter, chorionic villus sampling and 106
CDC *see* Centers for Disease Control and Prevention (CDC)
CD4 cells 532
Cederqvist, L. L. 420
Cefalo, R. C. 617
cefuroxime 403–4
cells, nucleus of *19*
Center for Substance Abuse Treatment (CSAT) 648
Centers for Disease Control and Prevention (CDC) 10, 59, 139, 140, 142, 276, 383, 387, 398, 420, 481, 638, 647, 649
  Division for Viral and Rickettsial Diseases 13

Centers for Disease Control and Prevention (CDC), continued
  Hepatitis Hotline 15
  National AIDS Clearinghouse 534
  National Center for Health Statistics (NCHS) *636, 637, 637,* 640, 641
  National Center for Infectious Diseases 221
    homepage of 221
  National Hospital Ambulatory Medical Care Survey (NHAMCS) 542, 543–44
  National Hospital Discharge Survey (NHDS) 542–44
  publications 8, 10, 12, 15, 16, 70, 71, 545
  revised guidelines 521
  surveillance data of 108
  unpublished data of 518
central nervous system (CNS)
  cocaine exposure and 189, 190–91
  fetal alcohol syndrome and 152
  neonatal abstinence syndrome and 184
cephalosporin 416
cerclage 99, 245
cereals 68–70, 339
cerebral hemorrhage 593
cerebral palsy 277–78
  electronic fetal monitoring and 283
cerebrospinal fluid
  birth defects and 63
cervical caps 322, *328–29*
cervical dysplasia 681
cervix 681
  dilation of 623
    morning sickness and 123
    preterm labor and 243
  length of 245–46
  ripeness of 632
"Cesarean Childbirth Consensus Statement" 301
cesarean delivery 291–301, 629
  active management and 236–37
  electronic fetal monitoring and 277–78, 283–84
  versus forceps delivery 274

cesarean delivery, continued
  incisions for *292*, 294
  lupus and 504
  preeclampsia and 599, 607
  prenatal care and 87
  ultrasound and 98
Chadd, M. A. 462
Chalmers, I. 289, 290
chancroid 681
Chand, S. 615
Chang, A. 288
charcoal 51
Chasnoff, I. J. 159, 180
chemicals
  pica substances and 51
  pregnancy and 4, 43
chemotherapy 506–7, 511–12, 549, 550
Chen, T. 417
Chesley, L. C. 461, 613, 614, 615, 616
Chester, S. W. 420
Chestnut, D. H. 420
Cheung, M. O. 420
chickenpox 8–9
childbirth classes 86, 87–88
children
  cancers in 31
  chickenpox and 8
  drug addiction and 161
  drug exposure and 201–4
  illnesses of 353–54
  prenatal care and 80
Childrens Defense Fund 44
Childrens Hospital of Los Angeles 178
chlamydia 208, 544, 681
chlordiazepoxide (Librium) 177
  alcohol withdrawal and 154
  cocaine withdrawal and 173
Choi, W. W. 420
cholesterol levels
  in human milk 357
  pregnancy and 51
choriocarcinoma 547
chorionic villus sampling (CVS) 379, 382, 681
  cystic fibrosis 33
  described 104
  limb deficiencies and 109–14

chorionic villus sampling (CVS), continued
  miscarriage risk from 108–9
  ultrasound and 99
  use of 106–8
Chow, M. J. 403, 404, 423
Chowers, I. 461
Chown, B. 384, 385
Christianson, R. 462
chromosomal abnormalities
  amniocentesis and 104, 107
  chorionic villus sampling and 107
  risk of 106
  ultrasound and 102
chromosome abnormalities 628
chromosomes *19*, 681
  described 31
  DNA (deoxyribonucleic acid) and 18
  polymorphisms and 21–22
chromosome walking technique 31
Chua, T. 508
Chun, D. 614
Churgay, C. A. 545
Ciba-Geigy 459
cigarettes *see* smoking; tobacco use
Cincinnati Comprehensive Sickle Cell Center 492
Ciocca, D. R. 506, 509
Clark, B. 420
Clark, D. M. 462
Clark, E. B. 420
Clark, K. E. 180
Clark, N. C. 420
Clark, N. M. 422
Clark, R. 430
Clark, R. M. 508
Clark, S. L. 287, 395, 396, 397, 420, 421, 619
Clarke, A. J. 420
Clarke, C. A. 384
clay consumption 51
Clearblue Easy home pregnancy test 38
Clegg, A. 479
Clinical Center Communications 492
Clinical Laboratory Improvement Act (1988) 34
Clinical Obstetrics and Gynecology 290, 448, 449, 461, 616

Index

Clinical Oncology 508
Clinical Practice Guideline on Sickle Cell Disease 495
Clinton Administration 647
Cloherty, J. P. 448
clonazepam 175
clonidine 171, 610
Coates, A. L. 398, 419
cocaine 157–59
　effects on fetus of 159–60
　infants and 178–79, 187–91
　pregnancy and 44, 180
　withdrawal from 171–74
"Cochrane Updates on Disk" 288, 289
Cockburn, J. 464
Coggins, C. H. 614
cognitive impairments 177
Cohen, A. B. 287
Cohen, R. M. 448
Cohen, Wayne R., MD 274, 278
Cohn, R. D. 619
coitus interruptus 326
Colau, J. C. 617
cold medicines 4
Colgate Palmolive 650
Colin, Y. 387
Collins, Francis, PhD, MD 33
Collins, Jane 157
Collins, R. 464
colonized carriers 221–23
color chart 560
Columbia Hospital for Women 271, 272
Columbia University 50, 648
Committee on terminology 595
Compassionate Friends National Headquarters 670, 675
compensatory hyperinsulinemia 436
complex carbohydrates 577
computer imaging 95
computerized chromosome sorters 105
conception date determination 95, 98, 631
condoms 207, 321–22, *328–29*
condylomata 681
confidentiality
　sickle-cell disease and 369
confined placental mosaicism 109
congenital, defined 682
congenital adrenal hyperplasia
　test for 362
congenital defects
　drug exposure and 191
　of extremities 109
　ultrasound and 100
congenital heart disease 11
congenital rubella syndrome (CRS) 10, 11
　see also rubella
congenital syphilis 221
　see also syphilis
congenital varicella syndrome 8–9
　see also chickenpox
Conneally, P. Michael, PhD 33
Connelly, T. J. 403, 421
Constantine, G. 463
constipation
　postpartum 307–8
　treatment for 474
Contraception 324
contraceptives 321–29
　diabetes and 447
　see also birth control; family planning
Contraceptive Technology 323, *328*
contractions *see* uterine contractions
Contreras, M. 383
Cook, C. M. 617
Coombs test 378
Cooper, D. W. 614
Corbascio, A. N. 429
cordocentesis 379, 382
Correa-Villasenor, A. 428
Corry, M. 290
Corssen, G. 421
corticosteroids 649, 682
　asthma and 392, 393, 414
　preterm labor and 250–62
Cote, C. J. 421
Cottle, M. K. 421
Cotton, D. B. 395, 396, 397, 421, 618, 619
cough medicines 4
counseling
　DNA (deoxyribonucleic acid) testing and 18
　for HIV (human immunodeficiency virus) 516–29

counseling, continued
  for hypertension 451–52
  miscarriage and 657
  prenatal care and 82–84, 84–91
  for sickle-cell disease 489–90
  sickle-cell disease and 368
Cousins, L. 403, 404, 423
Coutts, I. I. 400, 430
cow's milk formula 336, 337
  allergies and 352
  versus human milk 358
Cox, C. 71
Cox, J. S. 421
crack cocaine 157–58
  pregnancy and 44, 188
  see also cocaine; drug use
Crane, J. P. 385
Craparo, Frank, MD 35
Crawford, J. S. 421
Creamer, J. 463
Creasy, Robert K., MD 240, 671
Creel, Mary-Jane 670
Creighton University School of Medicine 116
Crenin, M. D. 545
Crews, Paula 157–58
cromolyn sodium 392
Crown Publishers 479
CRS *see* congenital rubella syndrome (CRS)
Cruikshank, D. P. 464
Crying Baby, Sleepless Nights (Jones) 310
C-section *see* cesarean delivery
culdocentesis 540
Cummings, M. B. 614
Cundiff, J. H. 512
Cunningham, A. S. 290
Cunningham, F. G. 288, 545, 613, 615, 616
CVS *see* chorionic villus sampling (CVS)
cyclophosphamide (Cytoxan) 502
cystic acne 141–42, 144
cystic fibrosis 30
  cow enzymes and 36
  diagnosis of 107
  DNA (deoxyribonucleic acid) studies and 25

cystic fibrosis, continued
  genetic screening for 32–34
  mode of inheritance 29
  test for 362
cytomegalovirus 628, 688
Czeizel, A. 401, 421

D

Daffos, F. 385, 387
daily food guide 572, *573–74*
Daily Values (FDA) 64, 66
  see also recommended daily dietary allowances
Daley, G. L. 615
Dalkon Shield 326
Dana, Nancy 351
Daniel, E. E. 400, 424
Darling's disease 684
Dasta, J. F. 418
dAthis, P. 426
Davey, M. G. 385
Davidson, Glen, PhD 670
Davidson, J. K. 449
Davies, Robertson 137
Davis, Deborah L., PhD 670
Davis, S. A. 427
Davison, J. M. 617
day care centers, breast feeding and 347, 350
deafness, congenital rubella syndrome and 11
Dean, M. 403, 421
De Frain, John 670
Degendorfer, P. 513
DeHamer, Nancy Gordon 672
dehydration
  caffeine and 148
  exercise and 74, 78
  morning sickness and 121
Dekker, G. A. 617
delirium, alcohol withdrawal and 154
delivery *see* cesarean delivery; labor and delivery; vaginal delivery
Delprado, W. 618
delusions, alcohol withdrawal and 154
Demedeiros, N. 388

Index

Demerol (pain killer) 271
dental care 43
Department of Health and Human Services (DHHS) 42, 46, 50, 56, 59, 79n, 94, 119n, 129n, 136, 141, 149, 151, 157, 225, 231n, 312, 320, 332, 530, 635n, 644, 649, 650, 679n
  Bureau of Primary Care 648
  Health Resources and Services Administration 647, 648
  Healthy People 2000 236–37
  National Heart, Lung, and Blood Institute 426
  publications of 183, 204n, 286, 640, 641
  Substance Abuse and Mental Health Services Administration 648
  Web page for 149
Department of Health Education and Welfare (DHEW) 614
Depo-Provera 324, *329*
depression
  postpartum 312, 317–19
  pregnancy loss and 663
Derbes, V. J. 421
DES *see* diethylstilbestrol (DES)
desipramine (Norpramin) 173
DeSwiet, M. 464
dexamethasone 256, 260, 502
Diabetes Care 448, *557*, 589
diabetes mellitus 354, 596, 628, 682
  causes of 553–55
  cesarean delivery and 297
  corticosteroids and 252, 255, 258
  gestational 241, 435, 553–91, 683
  pre-gestational 435–47
  pregnancy and 54
  spina bifida and 63
  treatment prior to pregnancy 4
  ultrasound and 98
Diabetes Treatment Centers of America 589
diaphoresis 682
diaphragm 322
diarrhea 353
Diaz, D. M. 422
Diaz, S. F. 422

diazepam (Valium) 175
  alcohol withdrawal and 154
  cocaine withdrawal and 173
Diaz-Maqueo, J. C. 512
diazoxide 609, 610
diet and nutrition 668
  breast milk and 334
  cheese and 225–28
  constipation and 307–8
  diabetes and 438
  folate and 60–61
  gestational diabetes and 566–67, 571–75
  hypertension and 453
  for infants 356–59
  lactation and 355–56
  morning sickness and 120
  postpartum 313
  pregnancy and 43, 50–55
  prenatal care and 66
  prior to pregnancy 4, 55
  twins and 468–73
  see also breast feeding; infant formula; recommended daily dietary allowances (RDA)
dietary supplements 64, 67
  see also vitamin supplements
diethylstilbestrol (DES) 139
Dignan, P. S. J. 448
DiGuiseppi, Carolyn, MD, MPH 277, 377n
dilantin 175
dilation and curettage (D and C) 550
Dillard, Jim 266
Dinsdale, H. B. 618
diphenhydramine 417
diphtheria toxoid 16
diphtheria vaccine 15, 16
direct detection 20–21
dirt consumption 51
discoid lupus 498
disease transmission, polymorphisms and 22
disseminated intravascular coagulation (DIC) 593
disulfiram (Antabuse) 154
diuretics 458–59, 602, 609–11
Dix, Carol 673

Dixon, S. D. 180
dizygotic twins 481
dizziness
  ectopic pregnancy and 539
  exercise and 74, 78
DMD *see* Duchenne's muscular dystrophy (DMD)
DNA (deoxyribonucleic acid) 105, 371, 682
  described 18–19
  genetic diseases and 28–31
  testing and 18–25
Dodge, Nancy, C. 670
dolomite 54
Dombrowski, M. P. 398, 422
Donaldson, S. S. 513
Donnelly, Katherine Fair 670
Donsimoni, R. 617
Doody, K. J. 618
Dooley, J. B. 420
Dooley, S. L. 447
dopamine 178–79
Doppler ultrasound 96–97, 99, 279
  preeclampsia and 601
  see also ultrasound examinations
Double Talk 479
douches 659
Down syndrome
  alpha-fetoprotein and 116
  chorionic villus sampling and 114
  chromosome 21 and 104, 105
  human chorionic gonadotropin and 116
  risk of 106
  test for 95
doxepin (Sinequan) 173
Doyle, L. W. 422
Dreis, M. 463
Driscoll, S. G. 448
drug-induced lupus 498
drug use 628
  children and 201–204
  infant exposure and 180–201
  miscarriage and 653
  during pregnancy 136–140
    age factor and 158
    continuum of care and 164–165
    fetal effects of 159–160, 168–169, 178–180, 185

drug use, continued
  guidelines for 161–164
  maternal effects of 159–160, 168, 185
  mental health and 176–178
  withdrawal from 165–168, 170–175, 177
  pregnancy and 42, 44
  prenatal care and 84–90
  preterm labor and 240
  prior to pregnancy 4
  see also alcohol use; over-the-counter medications; prescription medications
DTP (diphtheria, tetanis, pertussis) vaccine 15
Duchenne's muscular dystrophy (DMD) *30, 35*
  DNA (deoxyribonucleic acid) studies and 25
  genetic testing and 31
  mode of inheritance *29*
Duckworth, A. F. 429
Duff, A. M. 384
Dukoff, R. 509
Duncan, B. R. 425
Dunlop, J. C. H. 462
Dunn, L. J. 464
Duy, Nick 336
dyspnea 390, 394, 682
dystocia 293, 296
dystrophin *30, 31, 35*
dysuria 682

E

ear infections 353
eclampsia 79, 593–613
ectopic pregnancy 379, 538–44
  sexually transmitted diseases and 207
  ultrasound and 95, 99
edema 682
Eden Foods 340
Edensoy 340
education
  for childbirth 237
  diabetes and 440–41

Index

education, continued
  folic acid and 70
  prenatal care and 82–83
  sickle-cell disease and 365, 368, 485, 490
  smoking and 150
  Tay Sachs disease and 28
Education Programs Associates 492
Einarson, T. R. 422
electrocardiograms 244, 280
electrolytes 51
electronic fetal monitoring 277–86, 297, 391, 623
electrophoresis 365–66
Elephant Man disease *see* neurofibromatosis
Elledge, R. M. 506, 509
Ellenberg, J. H. 286
Ellison, A. C. 425
Ellison, G. T. 461
el Nazer, A. 616
Elrad, H. 617
Elsevier 613, 615, 618
embryo 18, 682
embryo transfer 99
Emetral 120
emotional changes
  after pregnancy 317
  pregnancy and 44, 85–90
emotional health
  pregnancy loss and 661–69
  treatment prior to pregnancy 5
  twins and 477
endocarditis 682
endometriosis 538
endometritis 299
endothelial cells 600
Engelfriet, C. P. 383
Engle, William A., MD 264, 266
Enkin, M. W. 288, 289, 290
Entman, S. S. 417, 422
enzyme inhibitors 456–57
enzymes
  hexosaminidase 28
  phenylalanine hydroxylase 26
epicanthal folds 152
epidemiology 139, 682
epidural 272–73, 274, 299

epidural, continued
  asthma and 396 393
  see also anesthesia
epilepsy 4, 146
epinephrine 178, 417
episiotomy 235, 273, 275–76
  postpartum concerns 309
e.p.t home pregnancy test 37
Erasmus, C. 417, 422
erythremia 445
erythroblastosis fetalis 297, 378
erythromycin 416
Esposito, Jenifer L. 674
Establishing Criteria for Gestational Diabetes **557**
estrogens 323, 324
  birth defects and 139
  lactation and 343
  morning sickness and 119
ethnic factor, Tay Sachs disease and 28
Evans, D. 422
Every Child Deserves a Healthy Start 42
exercises 668
  diabetes and 582–84
  miscarriage and 651, 652
  postpartum 308
  during pregnancy 73–78, 86
  prior to pregnancy 4
Expert Panel on the Content of Prenatal Care 382
expression *see* breast feeding
eye problems, rubella and 11

F

F. A. Davis Company 419
Fabia, J. 287
facial abnormalities, fetal alcohol syndrome and 152
Facts about Cesarean Childbirth 291n
Fadnes, H. O. 618
FAE *see* fetal alcohol effects (FAE)
failure to thrive
  fetal alcohol syndrome and 152
  prenatal care and 80

Fairley, K. F. 461
Fallon, J. F. 419
fallopian tubes 538
  sterilization and 326
false labor 241, 680
false negative test results 33
false positive test results 116
family history
  DNA (deoxyribonucleic acid) and 21, 23–25
  spina bifida and 63
family issues
  asthma and 394
  DNA (deoxyribonucleic acid) testing and 18
  drug exposed infants and 194–96
  pregnancy loss and 666–69
  prenatal care and 79, 80
  twins and 468
family planning 3, 312, 320–29
  diabetes and 437
  see also birth control
Fanta, C. H. 422, 427
Farmakides, G. 617
FAS *see* fetal alcohol syndrome (FAS)
Fast Food Facts: Nutritive and Exchange Values for Fast Food Restaurants 581
Fayers, P. 464
Federal Register 71, 324
Feldman, C. H. 422
Feldman, N. 386
Ferencz, C. 428
Ferris, T. F. 462, 617, 618
fertility awareness 326
fertility drugs 467
  ultrasound and 98
fetal abnormalities
  diabetes and 435–36
  diagnostic procedures for 104
  ultrasound and 95, 100
fetal alcohol effects (FAE) 151–52, 155
fetal alcohol syndrome (FAS) 151–56
fetal distress
  asthma and 392
  cesarean delivery and 283, 297
  electronic fetal monitoring and 285

fetal growth and development 129–34
  diabetes and 437
  prenatal care and 86–90
  ultrasound and 98
fetal heart monitoring 96–97, 279–80, 391, 439, 467–68
fetal limbs 110
fetal lung maturity 250
fetal malnutrition 98
fetal monitoring 277–86
  asthma and 390–91
  diabetes and 563
  non-stress testing and 117
  stress testing and 117
fetal mortality
  ultrasound and 99
  see also infant mortality; neonatal mortality
fetal parasitism 50
fetal position
  cesarean delivery and 292
  ultrasound and 95, 98, 100
fetal size, cesarean delivery and 292
fetal weight, ultrasound and 100
fetal well-being
  hypertension and 456
  non-stress test 467–68
  ultrasound and 100
fetoscope 99, 245, 277–86
fetus 683
  cystic fibrosis test 33
  kidney damage in 35
  neurological development of 121
  prenatal care and 81–82
FEV *see* forced expiratory volume (FEV)
FHR (Doppler) test 85
fibronectin levels 598
Fidler, J. 464
Fields, L. M. 287
Findlay, J. W. 422
Finnegan, Loretta P., MD 159
Finnish Register of Congenital Malformations 139
First Response home pregnancy test 37
Fischer, M. 448
Fisher, R. S. 618

Index

Fitzsimons, R. 423
Fleischer, A. 617
Fletcher, A. E. 462
flow cytometry test 380
flow meters, asthma and 390
fluid retention 570, 594
fluoride
  in human milk 58
  in infant formula 339
Flury, G. 463
Flynt, J. W. 384
folacin 53
folate 60, 571
  birth defects and 63–64
  deficiency 53
  pregnancy and 51, 53
  recommended daily allowance of 52
  sources of 53, 60, 64–66, 65
folic acid 53, 60
  birth defects and 63
  fortification program 64
  see also vitamin B
folinic acid, toxoplasmosis and 215
Folkenberg, Judy 119n
folliculitis 683
Foman, Samuel J. 337
Fontanarosa, M. 387
food additives 64
Food and Drug Administration (FDA) 97, 120, 121, 138, 139, 140, 145, 271, 273, 341, 459, 460, 647
  Advisory Review Panel on OTC Internal Analgesic and Antirheumatic Drug Products 502
  approvals 242, 243, 244, 265, 266, 321, 322, 324, 325, 344, 345, 520, 576
  Center for Food Safety and Applied Nutrition 335
  Clinical Nutrition Branch 55
  Dermatologic Drugs Advisory Committee 142–44
  Division of Clinical Laboratory Devices 33
  Division of Regulatory Guidance 336
  Division of Urologic and Reproductive Products 325

Food and Drug Administration (FDA), continued
  Fertility and Maternal Health Drugs Advisory Committee 343
  folic acid fortification program of 64
  genetic screening and 26, 33–34, 36
  National Center for Devices and Radiological Health 96
  Office of Food Labeling 67
  Office of Special Nutritionals 60, 64, 65, 66, 67, 70
  publications of
    FDA Consumer 26, 37n, 56, 59, 60, 95, 104, 116, 119n, 141, 148, 240, 262, 270, 272, 273, 275, 277, 320, 334, 341, 502, 679n
    FDA Drug Bulletin 142
  reports by 101
  studies by 148
  surveys by 54
  warnings 502
food cravings 50
food groups 469–73, 572
food labels, folate and 64, 66
food poisoning, listeriosis and 225–28
foot deformities, spina bifida and 63
Foote, G. 387
forced expiratory volume (FEV) 390, 395
forceps 273–74, 284
Ford, G. W. 422
Forestier, F. 385
formula *see* infant formula
Forsythe, A. 400, 401, 428
Foundation for Blood Research 116
fragile X syndrome 25
Francis, V. 425
Franks, A. L. 640
Franz, Marion J. 581
Freda, V. J. 384
Frederiksen, M. C. 403, 404, 421, 423
Freeman, J. B. 286
Freeman, R. K. 419
Freinkel, N. 447
Friedman, C. 418
Friedman, E. A. 462
Friedrich, E. 479
Frigoletto, F. D., Jr., MD 236, 290

Fritsch, Julie 671
fructose 576
Frusca, T. 617
Fuchs, U. 424
Fuhrmann, K. 448
Fuller, L. M. 512
fundal height 85
Fung, D. L. 423
fungal infections 683
furosemide 610

G

Gabbe, S. G. 387, 448
Gaber, L. W. 616
Gaensler, E. A. 394, 427
Gail, Dorothy, PhD 265
galactosemia test 27, 361
Gallenberg, M. M. 509
Gallery, E. D. 461, 618
Gallup Organization 68
Gal T. J. 423
Gant, N. F. 287, 545, 615
Garcia, J. 290
Gardner, M. J. 403, 404, 423
Gaston, Marilyn, MD 27
Gautieri, R. F. 418
GBS *see* group B streptococcus (GBS); streptococcal infections
Geary, F. H., Jr. 386
Gelb, A. 429
Gemma, Penelope Bushman 670
gender factor, lupus and 499
Genentech Inc. 36
General Clinical Research Centers Program 589
genes 494, 683
  defective 26
  described 19
  disease-causing 31–32
  inherited traits and 18
  polymorphisms and 21–22
  sickle-cell disease and 488
genes, cancer-causing *see* oncogenes
genetic counseling
  chorionic villus sampling and 114–15
  DNA (deoxyribonucleic acid) testing and 24

genetic factors 26–36, 684
  DNA (deoxyribonucleic acid) and 20
  infant health and 66
  miscarriage and 652
  preeclampsia and 596
  and pregnancy 5
genetic markers 31–32
  for cystic fibrosis 32
  DNA (deoxyribonucleic acid) and 21, 23
genetic specialists 18, 24, 25
genital herpes *see* herpes infections
Georgetown University Hospital 263
Gerard, C. 481
German measles *see* rubella
gestational age
  corticosteroids and 252, *253*, 257
  risks and 107–8
  ultrasound and 98, 100
gestational diabetes *see under* diabetes mellitus
gestational hypertension *see under* hypertension
gestational trophoblastic tumor 547–51
Ghysen, J. 427
Gibbs, C. J. 400, 430
Gibson, G. 424
Gilbert, E. F. 419, 420
Gilbert, Kathleen R., PhD 671
Giles, W. B. 617
Gilstrap, L. C. 545
Gindoff, P. R. 419
Glinsmann, Walter H., MD 55
Glockner, E. 448
Gluck, E. H. 425
Gluck, J. C. 400, 423
Gluck, P. 400, 423
glucose 54, 630
  diabetes and 435, 436, 438, 445, 553–90
  monitoring of 560, *590,* 689
  pregnancy and 51
  tests for 467, 557
glucose tolerance test 683
glycohemoglobin 441–42
glycopyrrolate 393
Gold, Michael 671

Index

Goldberg, M. F. 384
Goldenberg, M. 617
Goldner, T. E. 545
Goldstein, D. H. 427
gonorrhea 208, 684
Gonzalez, A. R. 463
Good, Barbara 271, 278
Goodlin, R. C. 286
Gordon, M. 397, 398, 423
Goretex 34
Gorman, J. G. 384
Gozzi, E. K. 425
Graeber, G. E. 617
Graham, C. F. 463
Grant, A. 287, 289
Greenberger, P. 429
Greenberger, P. A. 400, 418, 423
Greene, M. F. 448
Greenwood, B. 420
Gregorini, G. 617
grief and mourning 660–69
Grimes, D. A. 386
Grobler, N. 417
Groenendijk, R. 615
Grollman, Earl A. 671
Gromada, K. 479
Gross, S. J. 617
Grossman, H. G. 464
Grossman, R. A. 464
Grossman, S. D. 461
group B streptococcus (GBS) 221–24
 see also streptococcal infections
Group Health Association 120
Group Health Cooperative 73n, 306, 656
Gruppo Italiano Diagnosi Embrio-Fetali *111*
Guinee, V. F. 509
Gunderson, Erica P., MS, MPH, RD 481
Gunton, P. 383
Gustafson, J. 384
Guthrie, Robert 361
Gutierrez, J. 421
Gutsche, B. B. 423
Guzman, E. R. 289
gynecologists 315
Gyory, A. Z. 461, 618

H

habitual abortion 657
haemophilus influenzae 494
Haesslein, H. c. 286
Hagerdal, M. 423
hairy leukoplakia 684
Hales, Diane 671
Hallgårde, U. 415, 419
hallucinations, alcohol withdrawal and 154
Hammond, J. 616
Hamod, K. A. 416, 423
hand-and-foot syndrome 486, 494
Hankins, G. D. 615
Hanley, D. F. 618
Hansen, J. M. 396, 430
Hansen, P. K. 288
Hanson, Michelle Fryer 671
Hara, T. 426
Harden, K. 400, 401, 428
Hare, J. W. 448
Hargreave, F. E. 400, 424
Harkness, Carla 671
Harlass, F. E. 640
Harman, C. R. 388
Harris, J. B. 424
Harrison, B. D. 424
Harrison, Michael, MD 34
Hart, G. J. 424
Hartikainen-Sorri, A. L. 416, 429
Harvard Community Health Foundation 236
Harvard Medical School 31, 236
Harvey, J. C. 509
Hatcher, R. A. 386
Haverkamp, A. D. 288, 289
Hawley, J. 509
Hays, P. M. 464
HBV (hepatitis B virus) *see* hepatitis B
HCG *see* human chorionic gonadotropin (HCG)
He, S. 513
headaches during pregnancy 125
Head Start 201
health care providers 684
 exercise and 73
 postpartum examination and 312

health care services
  drug dependency and 163–64
  drug exposed infants and 196–201
health maintenance organizations (HMO) 369
health promotion
  prenatal care and 84–91
health promotion, prenatal care and 81, 82–83
Health Research Group 344–45
Health Resources and Services Administration 364
Health Valley Foods 340
Healthy Mothers, Healthy Babies Coalition 45
Healthy people 2000 640
Healthy Start Initiative 648
Healthy Start Program 150, 197
Healthy Start programs 150, 647
healthy women
  before pregnancy 320–21
  pregnancy visits for 84–85
  prenatal care and 83–84
hearing loss, ultrasound and 102
heartburn 124–25, 474
heart diseases 4
Heavilin, Marylin Willett 671
Heinonen, O. P. 424
hemagglutination 378
hemangiomas 684
hematocrit 94, 598
  prenatal care and 84
hemoglobin *30*, 485–86, 494
  DNA (deoxyribonucleic acid) and 21
  prenatal care and 84
  test for 94, 365, 437
hemoglobinopathies
  diagnosis of 107
  test for 94, 362, 363–73
hemolysis elevated liver enzymes low platelet count 594
hemolytic anemia 377–78, 381
hemophilia 25, *29,* 107
Hendriksen, E. H. 417
heparin 503
hepatic changes 593
  preeclampsia and 600
  see also liver diseases

hepatitis 684
  treatment prior to pregnancy 4
hepatitis B
  immune globulin 14
  test for 94
  vaccine for 13–15, 200–201
Hepatitis Hotline (CDC) 15
hepatomegaly 684
heredity *see* genetic factors
heroin 157, 158
  infants and 179
herpes infections 209, 298, 684
  cesarean delivery and 297
  test for 94
Herrick, W. W. 614
hexosaminidase 28, *30*
high blood pressure
  during pregnancy 396
  treatment prior to pregnancy 4
  see also hypertension; pregnancy induced hypertension (PIH)
high pressure liquid chromatography (HPLC) 366
high-risk pregnancies 684
  electronic fetal monitoring and 281–83, 284
  ultrasound and 100
Hill, Washington, MD 116
Hillier, Sharon 247, 249
Hinselmann, H. 614
Hippocrates 137
histoplasmosis 684
HIV/AIDS Treatment Information Service 534
HIV (human immunodeficiency virus) 516–34, 648, 685
  breast feeding and 192
  cocaine use and 187
  electronic fetal monitoring and 283
  prenatal care and 183, 185
  Rh-immunoglobulin and 381
  test for 94
Hochberg, H. M. 287
Hochner-Celnikier, D. 427
Hodach. R. J. 420
Hodgkin's disease 511–12
Hoechst-Roussel Pharmaceuticals 459

Index

Hoffman, C. P. 428
Hoffmann-La Roche 142, 143–44
Hollmen, A. I. 424
Holmes, F. 395, 424
Home Exercise Program: Exercise During Pregnancy and the Postnatal Period 78, 583
home health care 242, 244–45
homocystinuria test 27, 361
Hoover, H. C. 508
H.O.P.I.N.G. 674
Horenstein, J. 387
hormonal contraception 323–25
hormones 685
    appetite and 473
    changes during pregnancy 53
    ectopic pregnancy and 539–40
    lactation and 343–44
    lupus and 499
    miscarriage and 653
Hormuth, Rudolf 361
Horowitz, D. A. 424
Hospital for Sick Children 33
hotlines
    Hepatitis Hotline 15
    National AIDS Hotline 211, 530
    National STD Hotline 207, 211
Hou, S. H. 461
Household Survey of the National Institute on Drug Abuse (1990) 180
Howard, Judy 161
Howard University Comprehensive Sickle Cell Center 492
Hu, N. 420
Hubel, C. A. 615
Huber, F. C., Jr. 421
Huchcroft, S. 383
Huengsburg, M. 398, 425
Hughes, E. C. 614
Hult, A. M. 481
human chorionic gonadotropin (HCG) 544, 548
    alpha-fetoprotein and 116
    home pregnancy tests and 37
    morning sickness and 120
human papilloma virus (HPV) 681
human placental lactogen (HPL) 436, 555

Humphreys, D. M. 462
Hunter, D. J. 616
Hunter, J. R. 418
Huntington disease 29, 32, 33
Hunyor, S. N. 461
Hurley, Candace 477
Hutchison, J. M. 287
hyaline membrane disease 263–64
hydatidiform moles 99, 547–51, 596
hydralazine 498, 609, 610
hydrocephalus
    spina bifida and 63
    treatment for 35
hydropic fetus 382, 596
hydroxychloroqine (Plaquenil) 502
hyperactive children, fetal alcohol syndrome and 152
hyperbilirubinemia 377, 381, 445
hyperemesis gravidarum 121
    asthma and 389, 397
hyperextended head 295
hyperglycemia 414, 436, 443
hyperphenylalaninemia (PKU) 361
hyperpnea 685
hyperpyrexia 685
hypertension 685
    asthma and 389, 397, 414
    cesarean delivery and 297
    coritcosteroids and 256, 258
    gestational 593–613
    pre-gestational 451–61
    ultrasound and 98, 99
    see also pregnancy induced hypertension (PIH)
Hypertension 619
hyperthermia 102
hyperthyroidism test 361, 362
hyperventilation, asthma and 394
hypnosis, morning sickness and 121
hypocalcemia 445
hypoglossia/hypodactyly 109
hypoglycemia 435, 439, 445, 559, 583, 584, 685
hypothyroidism test 27
hypotonia 685
hypoxemia 391
hypoxia 278, 282
    asthma and 390, 395, 397

hysterectomy 550
Hytten, Frank E., MD 50

I

IAGT *see* indirect antiglobulin test (IAGT)
Iannucci, Lisa 56, 59
ice consumption 51
ICI Pharmaceuticals Group 459
icterus 685
IDEA *see* Individuals with Disabilities Education Act (IDEA)
IFA test 526
Ihle, B. U. 461
Iisalo, E. 424
illegal drugs *see* drug use
illicit drug screen 94
Ilse, Sherokee 671, 672
Imamura, S. 426
immune system
  breast milk amd 334
  miscarriage and 654
  see also AIDS; HIV
immunizations 8–16
  prior to pregnancy 4
  schedule for 311
  see also vaccines
immunoglobulin 378–79, 380–83
immunosuppression 256
immunotherapy, asthma and 391
Improving Treatment for Drug-Exposed Infants 183, 204n
incompetent cervix 99
incontinence 61
Indiana University Medical Center 264
Indiana University Riley Hospital for Children 266
Indiana University School of Medicine 33
indirect antiglobulin test (IAGT) 378
indirect detection (linkage analysis) 21, 23
Individual Family Service Plan (IFSP) 199–200
Individuals with Disabilities Education Act (IDEA) 198–99

induced abortions 107, 382
induced labor 232, 389
infant formula 337–38, 356
  versus breast feeding 334, 335
  homemade 336–37
infant mortality 42, 644–51
  cesarean delivery and 293
  diabetes and 435
  preterm delivery and 240
  smoking and 150
  see also maternal mortality; neonatal mortality
infants
  drug exposure and 183–87, 196–98
  hospital discharge of 193–94
  medical screening of 361–73
  sleep cycle of 309
  testing of 361–73
infections
  amniocentesis and 108
  birth defects and 137
  breast feeding and 352
  cesarean delivery and 299
  chorionic villus sampling and 108
  contraceptives and 325
  miscarriage and 653
  opportunistic 519
  sickle-cell disease and 486
  treatment prior to pregnancy 4
infertility
  oral contraceptives and 323
  ultrasound and 99
Information Network Inc. 651
Infrasonics Inc. 265
inherited diseases 26, *29*
  cystic fibrosis 32
  DNA (deoxyribonucleic acid) testing and 18, 20, 24
  sickle-cell disease as 489
  see also genetic factors
inherited traits 18, 20
Institute of Medicine 59
insulin 436, 437, 439, 441, *554,* 555, 562, 583–84, 685
  see also diabetes
International Diabetes Center 581
International Journal of Radiation Oncology, Biology, Physics 512

Index

International Lactation Consultant Association 351
International Registry of CVS procedures 106
International Twins Association, Inc. 478
Internet addresses
  Department of Health and Human Services 149
  March of Dimes 67
  National Cancer Institute 505n, 511n
  National Center for Infectious Diseases 221
  National Institutes of Health 231n, 245, 247, 377n
intrapartum fetal asphyxia 278
intrauterine devices (IUD) 99, 325–26, *328–29*
intrauterine growth retardation (IUGR) 172, 627–33
  asthma and 389
  hypertension and 461
  prenatal care and 80
  ultrasound and 98, 99
intrauterine transfusion 99
intraventricular hemorrhage (IVH) 240, 250, 254, 257–58
inunction (anointing) 123–24
in-vitro fertilization 99, 467
iodine 52
iron 52, 53
iron deficiency anemia 51
iron supplements 51–53, 572
Ishikawa, S. 420
islet cell antibodies 586–88
isoimmunization 377–83
isotretinoin *see* Accutane (acne medication)
Italian Multicentric Birth Defects Registry 112
Ito, M. 462
IUD *see* intrauterine devices (IUD)
IUGR *see* intrauterine growth retardation (IUGR)
IVH *see* intraventricular hemorrhage (IVH)

J

Jablonski, W. J. 424
Jacob, H. S. 611, 618
Jacobs, C. 513
Jahoda, M. C. J. 385
James, J. 384
Jann, R. 614
Janz, D. 424
Jarvis, A. 618
Jelliffe and Jelliffe Advances in International Maternal and Child Health 354
Jeminez, Sherry Lynn Mims 671
Jensen, K. 424
Jick, H. 418
Johansson, H. 509
Johns Hopkins Medical Journal 425
Johns Hopkins University Press 428
Johnson, Joy 672
Johnson, Marv 672
Johnson, S. T. 386
Johnson, W. E. 641
Johnson & Johnson 650
Jones, Sandy 310
Josephson, G. W. 424
Joslin Diabetes Center 587, 588
Jouppila, P. 424
Jouppila, R. 424
Journal of Clinical Oncology 509
Journal of Reproductive Medicine 287
Journal of the American Medical Association 180, 384, 424, 428, 464, 545
Journal of the Medical Society of North Carolina 123
Joy, M-T 289
Joyce, T. H., 3rd 430
Juniper, E. F. 400, 424
Jusko, W. J. 403, 423, 430

K

Kaminski, M. 461
Kanto, J. 424
Kantor, A. G. 397, 398, 423
Kaplan, P. W. 618
Kaposi's sarcoma 686

Karja, J. 416, 429
Karlman, I. 464
karyotyping of cells 106
Katz, A. I. 461
Katz, F. H. 425
Katz, V. L. 425
Kawasaki, N. 462
Kegel squeeze exercise 74, 75, 310
Keirse, M. J. N. C. 288, 289, 290
Kellogg Foundation 650
Kelly, E. A. 422
Kelman, G. R. 394, 429
Kelsey, Frances O. 136
Kelso, I. M. 287
Kelton, J. G. 386, 616
Kemp, D. B. 618
Kendrick, J. S. 640
Kennedy, M. S. 386
Kennedy, S. 457, 463
Kessler, David A., MD 460
ketamine 393
ketoacidosis 436, 686
ketones 56, 121, 561–62, 686
Keuck, B. D. 386
Khouzomi, V. A. 416, 423
kidney diseases 25
    fetal 35
    spina bifida and 63
    treatment prior to pregnancy 4
    Wilm's tumor 31
    see also renal diseases
Kidroni, J. 427
Kiely, J. K. 641
Killen, M. J. 290
Kincaid-Smith, P. 461, 464
Kirk, Paul, MD 673
Kirshon, B. 618
Kitchen, W. H. 422
Kivalo, I. 425
Kiyohara, A. 426
Klapholz, H. 287
Klebanoff, Mark A. 119, 122
Kline, P. A. 400, 424
Knapp, Ronald, PhD 673
Knight, George J., PhD 116
Knopp, R. H. 448
Knott, P. D. 463
Knowles, H. C. 449

Kochesky, R. J. 386
Kogan, M. D. 641
Kohn, Ingrid, MSW 672
Koivula, A. 424
Kollantai, Jean 479
Konwinski, T. 481
Koren, G. A. 422
Korsch, B. M. 425
Kotelchuck, M. 641
Koyama, K. 426
Kraus, A. M. 425
Kraus, G. W. 464
Krause, W. 619
Kreek, M. J. 404, 427
Kubicek, M. 430
Kunkel, Louis, PhD 31
Kurtzweil, Paula 60

L

labeling
    prescription medication and 143–44
    see also food labels
labetalol 609, 610
labor and delivery
    asthma management during 393
    difficult 293
    gestational diabetes and 564–65
    hypertension and 608–11
    obstructions to 298
    pain management during 270–71, 272–73
    stages of 231–38
lactation 50, 307
    asthma medication during 404, 433
    breast cancer and 508
    caloric intake and 58
    diet and nutrition and 51
    preeclampsia and 612
    suppression of 341–45
Lactobacillus 247–48
lactose 337
lactose intolerance 54
La Leche League International 312, 335, 350, 351, 478, 479
Lamb, Sister Jane Marie, OSF 672
laminaria 633
Lamont, C. A. R. 463

Index

lancet 560
The Lancet 64, 123, 286, 289, 385, 424, 428, 429, 430, 462, 463, 509, 614, 617, 618
Landesman, R. 462
Landon, M. B. 448
Langendoerfer, S. 288, 289
Langone, G. 506, 509
language development, drug addiction and 161
Lao, T. T. 398, 425
laparoscopy 540
Laragh, J. H. 463
Larson, D. 385
Larson, E. B. 286
Lasker, Judith 670
Laszewski, L. J. 420
Latham, Jean 67
Lavin, J. P. 449
Law, Peter K., MD 35
Lawrence, G. F. 287
Lawrence, Ruth, MD 341, 345
Lawson, H. W. 545
Lea and Febiger 423
lead 54
Leather, H. M. 462
Lebherz, T. B. 385
Leduc, B. 287
Lee, W. 395, 396, 397, 421
Leeder, J. S. 422
legumes 686
Leon, Irving G., PhD 672
Lesser, R. P. 618
Levang, Elizabeth, PhD 672
Le Van Kim, C. 387
Leveno, K. J. 288, 545, 613, 615
Levy, G. 403, 421
Levy, W. 509
Lewis, Christine, PhD 64–65
Lewis, D. F. 430
Lewis, J. A. 616, 618
Lewis, M. 384, 385
Lewis, P. E. 617
Lewis, Ricki 36
LFA *see* Lupus Foundation of America (LFA)
Librium *see* chlordiazepoxide (Librium)

Lietman, P. S. 424
lifting during pregnancy 77
Liley, A. W. 387
limb deficiencies, chorionic villus sampling and 109–14
Limbo, Rana 672
Lind, T. 286
Lindheimer, M. D. 461, 463, 616, 617, 618
Ling, F. W. 545
linkage analysis
  DNA (deoxyribonucleic acid) and 21, 23
lipids 51
Lishner, M. 513
Listeria 225–28
listeriosis 225–28
lithium 146
Littenberg, B. 425
Little Brown & Company 427, 617
Litwin, S. D. 420
Liukko, P. 424
liver diseases 13, 684
  cirrhosis 13
  see also hepatitis; hepatitis B
liver dysfunction 594
Loffer, F. D. 545
Loffredo, C. 428
Loizeaux, William 672
Loman, Kaye 350–51
Loprinzi, C. L. 509
Los Angeles County/USC Medical Center 178
Los Angeles Department of Water and Power 352
low birth weight
  alpha-fetoprotein and 116
  asthma and 389–90, 397
  bacterial vaginosis and 247–48
  defined 42
  fetal alcohol syndrome and 152
  heroin and 184
  methadone exposure and 185–86
  surfactants and 263
  tobacco and 149–50
lower back pain
  postpartum 308
  during pregnancy 75–77

Loyd-B pump 349
lubricants 309, 321
Luesley, D. M. 463
Luke, B. 480
lupus 497–504
Lupus Foundation of America (LFA) 497, 497n
Luthy, D. A. 286, 288, 289, 388
lying down during pregnancy 76–77
lymphadenopathy 686
Lynch, J. B. 616

M

Mabie, B. C. 616
Mabie, W. C. 463
Mabry, R. L. 414, 425
MacDonald, D. 287, 290
MacDonald, P. C. 287, 545, 615
MacGillivray, I. 614
MacGregor, S. N. 387
MacIntyre, C. A. 400, 430
MacKenzie, E. J. 424
MacLean, William, MD 338
macrosomia 98, 435, 558–59, 632, 686
Madans, J. 71
Madias, N. E. 461
Madigan Army Medical Center 273
Maenpaa, K. 424
magaloblasic anemia 53
magnesium 52
magnesium sulfate 393, 609, 610, 611
  preterm labor and 244
Mahomed, K. 288
Maietta, A. L. 425
Make Room for Twins: A Complete Guide 479
Makovitz, J. W. 617
Malaga, J. M. 429
Malin, Murray, MD 272
malnutrition 628
Maltau, J. M. 618
Mammen, E. F. 615
mammograms 505
Manning, Doug 672
Manning, F. A. 388
Mansberger, A. R., Jr. 461
Mansberger, J. A. 461
maple syrup urine disease 361
Marchese, J. R. 464
March of Dimes Birth Defects Foundation 45, 67, 68, 137, 149, 492, 650
Maren, T. H. 425
marijuana 44, 157, 158–59, 162
  prior to pregnancy 4
  see also drug use
Mariona, F. G. 615
markers *see* genetic markers
Marks, J. S. 384
Marks, Shelly, MS 670
marriage licenses
  sickle-cell disease test and 27
Martin Luther King Hospital 178
Marx, G. F. 422
Mason, James, MD 150
Mason, R. A. 615, 616
Massachusetts General Hospital 236
Maternal and Child Health Clearinghouse 67
maternal malnourishment 50–51
maternal mortality 635–40
  asthma and 398
  cesarean delivery and 299
  diabetes and 435
  prenatal care and 80
  see also infant mortality; neonatal mortality
maternal oxygen tension 394
maternal substance abuse 182–83
  see also drug use
maternity leave 346
Matria Healthcare 466
Matsui, K. 462
Mayo Clinic Complete Book of Pregnancy and Baby's First Year 538, 621n, 627n, 631n
Mayo Foundation for Medical Education and Research 538, 621n, 627n, 631n
McCall, M. L. 600, 616
McCartney, C. P. 616
McCartney, Marion 270, 272, 274, 276
McFadden, E. R., Jr. 422, 425, 427
McFee, J. G. 288
McKenzie, S. A. 426

Index

McLarn, W. D. 462
McLaughlin, M. K. 615
McNellis, Donald, MD 237
McPadden, A. J. 419
meconium 686
meconium aspiration 184, 631–32
Medela Manualectric 349
Medical Decision Making 287
Medical Research Council **111,** 385
medicines *see* drug use; over-the-counter medications; prescription medications
Meehan, F. P. 418
Mehta, K. A. 424
Melam, H. 428
Mellin, G. W. 426
Mellins, R. B. 426
Menczel, J. 427
mendelian (single-gene) conditions 107
Mendelsohn, B. 462
meningitis 221, 222, 354, 486
meningocele 61
meningomyelocele 61
Menon, R. K. 448
menstrual period
　fertility awareness and 326
　oral contraceptives and 323
　postpartum 307
　pregnancy and 5
mental health, substance abuse and 176–78
mental retardation
　congenital rubella syndrome and 11
　costs of 363
　Down syndrome and 153
　fetal alcohol syndrome and 152–53
　ketones and 56
　spina bifida and 63, 153
Merck-Sharp & Dohme 459
Merkatz, I. R. 420
Merrell Dow Pharmaceuticals 120
mesangial cells 600
metabolism errors 366
　amniocentesis and 104
　see also phenylketonuria (PKU)
metal exposure 4
Metcalfe, J. 396, 430

methadone 158, 177, 403–4
　children and 161
　infants and 179, 185–86
　opium dependency and 166, 168, 169–71
methotrexate 541, 544
methyldopa 456, 458
methylprednisolone (MEDROL) 256
methylprednisolone (Medrol) 502
methylxanthine 403, 404
metronidazole 249
Metzger, B. E. 447
Metzger, W. J. 426
Meuwissen, H. J. 421
Mibashan, R. S. 387
microcephaly 152, 686
microphthalmia 152
Middleton, E. 403, 404, 423
Mid-South Sickle Cell Center 493
Mijagawa, A. 426
Milavetz, G. 424
Miles, Margaret S. 661
Milia, S. 619
Miller, F. 417
Miller, M. E. 619
Mills, J. 464
Mills, J. L. 448
Milstien, J. B. 463
Milunsky, A. 418
Mimouni, F. 448, 449
Mimouni, Francis, MD 442, 443, 444
mini-pills 324, *328–29*
Miodovnik, Menachem, MD 441–43, 444, 448, 449
miscarriage 651–55
　Accutane and 142
　alcohol use and 153
　alpha-fetoprotein and 116
　amniocentesis and 105, 106
　chorionic villus sampling and 105, 114
　congenital rubella syndrome and 11
　defined 651
　morning sickness and 121–22
　mumps and 12
　risk of 104–5
missed abortion 656
Mississippi State Department of Health 493

MMWR publications 387, 420, 545
Moar, V. A. 464
Moein, M. 640
Moffit, Perry-Lyn 672
Mohun, M. 415, 426
Moise, K. J. 417, 422
molar pregnancy 547–51
Moldow, C. F. 611, 618
Moller, T. 509
Mollison, P. L. 383
monoclonal antibodies 371
  home pregnancy tests and 37–38
monozygotic twins 481
Morbidity and Mortality Weekly Report 68, 104, 151, 481, 516, 542, 635n
Moretti, M. 463
Morgan, C. W. 423
Morganti, A. A. 396, 430
morning after pills *see* oral contraceptives
morning sickness
  during pregnancy 119–24
  see also nausea; vomiting
Morrow, Judy Gordon 672
mosaicism 108–9
Mothering Multiples: Breastfeeding and Caring for Twins 479
Mothers of Supertwins (M.O.S.T.) 478
Mothers of Twins Club (MOTC) 478
motor development, drug addiction and 161
MSAFP test 85
MTP Press, Limited 429
Mueller-Heibach, E. 418
Mulambo, T. 288
multiple pregnancy 466–83
  ultrasound and 95, 98, 101
  see also twins
multivitamins 59, 64, 575
  folic acid and 68
  twins and 469
  see also *individual vitamins*
mumps 12
Murphy, J. 289
Murphy, M. D. 463
Musci, T. J. 615

muscle strain 74
muscular dystrophy
  diagnosis of 107
  DNA (deoxyribonucleic acid) studies and 25
  see also Duchenne's muscular dystrophy; myotonic muscular dystrophy
myelocele 61
Myers, R. E. 418
myoblasts 35
myoclonic 686
myotonic muscular dystrophy 25

N

Nadel, A. S. 290
Nageotte, M. P. 430
nalaxone 187
Nance, S. J. 387
narcotic addictions 159, 160
  see also drug use
NAS *see* National Academy of Sciences (NAS); neonatal abstinence syndrome (NAS)
Nassif, E. 424
National Academy of Sciences (NAS) 56, 343, 344
  and dietary allowances 575
  Food and Nutrition Board 51
  Institute of Medicine 480
National Academy Press 480
National AIDS Hotline 211, 530
National Association for Perinatal Addiction Research and Education 158
National Association for Sickle Cell Disease 492
National Asthma Education Program 426
National Cancer Institute (NCI) 505n, 511n, 547n
National Center for Education in Maternal and Child Health 351
National Center for Health Statistics (NCHS) 79, *91*, *92*, 245, 286, 356, *357*
  publications 545

Index

National Center for Research Resources 444, 589
National Coalition of Hispanic Service Organizations (COSSMHO) 45
National Commission to Prevent Infant Mortality 45
National Council on Radiation Protection and Measurements 101
National Healthy Mothers, Healthy Babies Coalition 351
National Heart, Lung, and Blood Institute 27, 250
National Information Center for Children and Youth with Disabilities 61
National Institute of Allergy and Infectious Diseases (NIAID) 121, 212, 219–20, 247
National Institute of Child Health and Human Development (NICHHD) *111,* 119, 121, 122, *122,* 231n, 250, 291, 300, 364, 444, 445, 529, 589, 647, 649
  amniocentesis and 105
  funding by 236, 246, 247
  Maternal-Fetal Medicine Network 245, 246, 249
  Pregnancy and Perinatology Branch 237
  ultrasound and 96
National Institute of Diabetes and Kidney Diseases 316
National Institute of Nursing Research 250
National Institute on Drug Abuse (NIDA) 169, 174, 180
  program funding by 158, 159, 160, 162
  publications of 157
National Institutes of Health (NIH) 34, 647
  Consensus Development Conference 250, 649
  Consensus Development Conference Statement (1987) 361n
  consensus statements 95, 250
  Division of Research Resources 96
  National Center for Health Statistics 149

National Institutes of Health (NIH), continued
  National Heart, Lung, and Blood Institute 27, 364, 649
  Cell and Developmental Biology Branch 265, 266
  Web page of 231n, 245, 247, 377n
National Kidney and Urologic Diseases Information Clearinghouse 316
National Maternal and Child Health Clearinghouse 45, 493
National Maternity Hospital, Dublin 237
National Natality Survey (1980) 96
National Newborn Screening Report (1992) 361n, 364
The National Organization of Mothers of Twins Clubs, Inc. (NOMOTC) 479
National Pediatric and Family HIV Resource Center 521
The National Pediatric HIV Resource Center 529
National Pregnancy and Health Survey 162
National Research Council (NRC) 51, 343, 344, 575
National SHARE Office 660, 670, 672
National SIDS Clearinghouse 660
National SIDS Foundation 674
National STD Hotline 207, 211
National Survey of Childbearing Women 518
natriuresis 603
Naulty, J. 617
nausea
  during pregnancy 54, 119
  treatment for 473
  see also morning sickness
NCHS *see* National Center for Health Statistics (NCHS)
NEC *see* necrotizing entercolitis (NEC)
necrotizing entercolitis (NEC) 240, 250, 254
needle sharing, hepatitis B virus and 13
Needs, C. J. 426
Neeld, Elizabeth Harper, PhD 672

Neff, R. K. 462
Neilsen, J. P. 288, 289
Neims, A. H. 403, 418
Neldam, S. 288
Nelson, J. M. 387
Nelson, James D. 672
Nelson, K. B. 286
Nelson, S. 288
Nelson, T. R. 615
neonatal abstinence syndrome (NAS) 160, 168, 184, 187
neonatal lupus 503
neonatal methadone abstinence syndrome 186
neonatal mortality 645
  asthma and 397, 398
  electronic fetal monitoring and 281
  hypertension and 593
  preterm labor and 240
  sickle-cell disease and 363
  see also infant mortality; maternal mortality
neonatal neurotoxicity assessment 190
neonates 687
  drug exposure and 183–87
  see also infants
neoplasms
  ultrasound and 99
nephropathy 437
Ness, P. M. 386
neural tube defects
  alpha-fetoprotein and 116
  diagnosis of 107
  folate and 60, 61–63, 64
  food labels and 66
  multivitamins and 59
  vitamin-mineral supplements and 55
neurofibromatosis 29, 31, 32
neurologic abnormalities 178–80, 188, 241
neurotransmitters 178–79
neurotropic 687
Newberne, J. W. 418
The New England Journal of Medicine 105, 180, 236, 245, 247, 249, 286, 288, 289, 384, 387, 388, 419, 425, 427, 447, 448, 461, 464, 545, 614, 617

Newhouse, M. T. 400, 424
New York State Department of Health 493
niacin 52
NICHHD see National Institutes of Health (NIH), National Institute of Child Health and Human Development (NICHHD)
Nickelsen, C. 287
Nicolaides, K. H. 387
nicotine 149
  see also smoking; tobacco use
NIDA see National Institutes of Health (NIH), National Institute on Drug Abuse (NIDA)
Niebyl, J. R. 386, 423, 480
Nielsen, P. V. 287
nifedipine 610
Nisce, L. Z. 513
Niswander, K. R. 397, 398, 423
Nochimson, D. J. 289
Noddeland, H. 618
Noguchi, Y. 428
nonoxynol-9 spermicide 321
non-stress test (NST) 467–68, 563–64
norepinephrine 178–79, 188
Norman, P. S. 415, 426
Norplant 325, *329*
Norpramin see desipramine (Norpramin)
North California Comprehensive Sickle Cell Center 493
Northwestern University Perinatal Center for Chemical Dependence 159
nosocomial 687
Novotny, P. P. 479
Novy, M. J. 396, 430
NRC see National Research Council (NRC)
NST see non-stress test (NST)
Nubain (pain killer) 271
nulliparous women
  hypertension and 593
  pregnancy visits for 85–91
nurse midwives 272, 278
nursery environment, drug exposure and 187, 190

Index

nurses, home health care and 244–45
Nusbacher, J. 388
Nussberger, J. 463
nutrition *see* diet and nutrition
Nutrition: Eating for Good Health 355
Nutritional Disorders of American Women 50
Nutritional Impacts on Women 50, 55
Nutrition and Motherhood 51, 54
Nutrition for Your Pregnancy 567, 568
Nyoni, R. 288

O

Oats, J. 287
O'Brien, N. 289
Obstetrics and Gynecology 273, 448, 449
odynophagia 687
Of Cradles and Careers: A Guide to Reshaping Your Job to Include A Baby In Your Life 350
Office of Medical Applications of Research (OMAR) 96, 250, 364
Ogburn, P. L. 611, 618
Ohguro Y. 426
Oian, P. 618
oligohydramnios 99
Olive, G. 426
Ollstein, R. N. 462
Olson, D. R. 640
Olsson, H. 509
oncogenes 32
Online Journal of Current Clinical Trials 275
Onnen, I. 426
oocysts 216–17
opiate abstinence syndrome 184
opioid withdrawal syndrome 167–68
opium withdrawal 166–71
opportunistic infections 519
  see also AIDS; HIV
oral contraceptives 323–25, *328–29*
  estrogen as 344
organ formation, during pregnancy 3
Orleans, M. 288

orofacial defects 110
oromandibular hypogenesis 110
oromandibular-limb hypogenesis 109
O'Rourke, J. 428
Ory, S. J. 545
Osler, M. 288
Ost, L. 426
osteopenia 53
O'Sullivan, J. B. *557*
Ounsted, M. 464
Ounsted, M. K. 462
"Our Newsletter" and Network 479
ovarian cysts 99
ovarian follicle development surveillance 99
over-the-counter medications 141–48
  asthma and 432
  prior to pregnancy 4
Owaki, Y. 428
Oxford University Press 354
oxygen starvation
  asthma and 394–95
  cerebral palsy and 277–78
oxymetazoline 416
oxytocin 232, 272–73, 282
  challenge test 117, 564
  hormone 117

P

pacifiers 335
Packham, D. K. 461
Page, C. 387
Page, Carole Gift 673
Page, E. W. 462, 614
painful episode 486, 494
pain killers 270–71
  see also epidural
Palomaki, J. F. 461
Palti, Z. 427
pancreas 32, 687
PaO_2 392
Papiernik, E. 461
Papiernik-Berkhauer, E. 481
Pap smear 208
  prenatal care and 84
Paragard CopperT 380A 325
paralysis, spina bifida and 61

paregoric, neonatal abstinence syndrome and 186
Pareja, G. 462
parental karotype test 94
Parent Care, Inc. 478
parenting skills 311–12
  prenatal care and 80, 84, 86, 87
paresthesia 687
Parke-Davis 459
parous women, pregnancy visits for 85–91
Parras, M. K. 419
Parsons, M. L. 384
Parsons, R. J. 287
Pass, Kenneth, PhD 28
patent ductus arteriosus (PDA) 240
paternity testing 25
Patterson, R. 400, 418, 423, 426, 428
Patterson, R. J. 403, 421
Paul, R. H. 287
PCP *see* phencyclidine (PCP); pneumocystis carinii pneumonia (PCP)
PCR *see* polymerase chain reaction (PCR)
PDA *see* patent ductus arteriosus (PDA)
peak expiratory flow rate (PEFR) 390, 392, 393
Pearson, J. 290
Peckham, M. J. 512
The Pediatric AIDS Foundation 529
Pediatrics 286, 418, 425, 430
pedigrees (family history) 23
PEFR *see* peak expiratory flow rate (PEFR)
Peleg, E. 617
pelvic examinations 99, 548
pelvic floor exercise 314–15
pelvic inflammatory disease (PID) 539
  intrauterine devices and 326
  oral contraceptives and 323
pelvic organ injury 108
pelvic size
  cesarean delivery and 296
  ultrasound and 99
pelvic tilt exercise 74–75
pelvic tumors 298

penicillin
  sickle-cell disease and 27–28, 363, 365, 372
  streptococcal infections and 222
Pennington, Jean 55
Pennsylvania Hospital 35
pentazocine (Talwin) 168
Peppers, Larry, PhD 673
percutaneous umbilical blood sampling (PUBS) 35
perinatal, described 687
Perinatal Medicine 289
perinatal mortality
  asthma and 389
  diabetes and 444
  see also fetal mortality; infant mortality; neonatal mortality
perineum, cutting of *see* episiotomy
period *see* menstrual period
Perkins, R. P. 287
pertussis 687
  vaccine for 15
Peterson, E. N. 396, 430
Peto, R. 464
Petrek, J. A. 509
phencyclidine (PCP) 44, 158
phenobarbital 175
  alcohol withdrawal and 154
  cocaine exposure and 190
  cocaine withdrawal and 173
  neonatal abstinence syndrome and 187
phenylalanine hydroxylase 26–27, *30*
phenylketonuria (PKU) 26–27, *30*
  mode of inheritance *29*
  test for 362, 363
Philip, J. 386
Philipson, A. 403, 404, 427
phosphorus *52*
pH tests, bacterial vaginosis and 248
physical examinations
  diabetes and 437
  of neonates 183
  prenatal care and 84–91
  prior to pregnancy 3–4
pica 51
Pickering, R. J. 421
Piehl, E. J. 462

Index

Pielet, B. W. 387
PIH *see* pregnancy induced hypertension (PIH)
Piirila, P. 398, 400, 429
Pijpers, L. 385
Pike, Margaret 674
Pildes, R. S. 430
the pill *see* oral contraceptives
Pirson, Y. 427
Pitkin, Roy M., MD 55
Pitocin (oxytocin) 232, 272–73
Pivarnik, J. M. 396, 421
PKU *see* hyperphenylalaninemia (PKU); phenylketonuria (PKU)
placenta 503, 687
  biopsy of 106
  calcium and 53
  described 129
  diabetes and 555
  disorders of 621–25
  drugs and 138
  fetal nourishment and 50–51
  preeclampsia and 601
  removal of 100
  see also chorionic villus sampling (CVS)
placental abruption 621–23
placental hemorrhage, chorionic villus sampling and 113
placental-site trophoblastic disease 547, 548
placenta previa 298, 623–25
  ultrasound and 100
plasma fibrinogen 598
plasmapheresis 503
Platner, W. S. 420
Plessinger, M. A. 180
pneumocystis carinii pneumonia (PCP) 521
pneumonia 353, 372, 486
  fetal 632
  in infants 363
  streptococcal infections and 221, 495
pneumothorax, defined 266
Poissonier, M. H. 388
Pollack, K. L. 420
Pollack, W. 384, 386
Pollak, A. 289

Pollak, V. E. 614
Pollock, J. 384
Pollock, J. M. 386
polyhydramnios 99, 556
polymerase chain reaction (PCR) 33
polymorphisms 21–24
Pond, S. M. 404, 427
Popkin, J. 398, 419
postpartum concerns 306–29
  diabetes and 440
  mood disorders and 318–19
  preeclampsia and 602–3, 612–13
post-term pregnancy 631–32
PPROM *see* preterm premature rupture of membranes (PPROM)
prednisolone 502
prednisone 502, 503
preeclampsia 252, 437, 452, 455, 570, 593–613, 690
  asthma and 389, 398
  ultrasound and 98
  see also hypertension
Pregenzer, G. J. 419
pregnancy
  chickenpox during 8
  length of 240
  planning for 3–5
  signs of 5
  symptoms of 48
  tests for 37–38
pregnancy, first trimester
  blood sugar levels during 558
  caloric intake during 56, 57
  chorionic villus sampling and 105
  chromosomal abnormality detection during 107
  chromosomal analysis during 107
  congenital rubella syndrome and 11
  fetal growth and development and 129, 130, *131*
  hyperventilation during 394
  morning sickness and 119
  mumps during 12
  prenatal care and 91
  prenatal care during 79
  teratogenic medications during 147
  toxoplasmosis and 213
  weight gain during 570

pregnancy, second trimester
  amniocentesis and 104
  bacterial vaginosis and 247
  caloric intake during 56
  fetal growth and development and 129, 130, *131, 132*
  low back pain prevention during 75–77
  Td vaccine and 15, 16
  toxemia and 56
  weight gain during 58, 570
pregnancy, third trimester
  amniotic fluid spectrophotometry and 381
  bleeding during 252
  caloric intake during 56, 57
  childbirth classes during 88
  diabetes and 439
  fetal growth and development and 131, *132, 133, 134*
  fetal iron absorption during 53
  hypertension and 455
  megaloblastic anemia during 53
  placental disorders during 621
  Td vaccine and 16
  toxoplasmosis and 214
  vaginal bleeding during 622
  weight gain during 58, 570
Pregnancy and Infant Loss Center 672, 675
pregnancy induced hypertension (PIH) 56
  see also preeclampsia; toxemia
premature labor and delivery 172
  alpha-fetoprotein and 116
  chickenpox risk and 9
  ultrasound and 100
  see also labor and delivery
prenatal care 639
  basic components of 81
  described 42
  folate and 60
  information about 45
  obstetrics and 79–92
  vitamin recommendations and 59
prenatal diagnostic centers 106
prenatal exercise 73–78
Prentice, A. 286

prescription medications 141–48
  birth defects and 136–38
  for lupus 502
  pregnancy and 42, 44, 47
  pregnancy categorization of 140, 145
  preterm labor and 243–44
  prior to pregnancy 4
  zidovudine (AZT) 516–34, 648
  see also drug use; over-the-counter medications
preterm birth 240, 262–67, 503
  asthma and 389, 397
  infant nutrition and 356–59
  prenatal care and 80
  twins and 475–76
preterm labor 240–67, 688
  prenatal care and 86, 87
preterm premature rupture of membranes (PPROM) 255, 257–58, 260
Price, Anne 351
Price, Phil, MD 120, 121
Price, Phill, MD 270–71, 272, 274, 277
Print, C. G. 429
Pritchard, J. A. 287, 615, 616
Pritchard, S. A. 615, 616
prochloroperazine 121
Progestasert Progesterone T 325
progesterone 394
progestin 323, 324–25
prolactin 343
promethazine hydrochloride 121
prostacyclin 597
prostaglandins 393, 597, 633
proteins
  cystic fibrosis 32
  dystrophin *30*, 31
  equivalents for *571*
  genetic diseases and *30*, 31
  hemoglobin *30*, 485–86
  hexosaminidase *30*
  phenylalanine hydroxylase *30*
  during pregnancy 58, 403
  pregnancy and 51
  recommended daily allowance of *52*
  transmembrane *30*
proteinuria 594, 595, 604
  ultrasound and 99

Index

Prowse, C. M. 394, 427
Pruett, K. M. 618
pruritus 688
PSG Publishing Company 462
psoriasis 145–46
psychiatric illness 176–78
psychosocial factors
  opium withdrawal 166
  prenatal care and 81, 82, 85
psychotropic drugs 177
ptosis 152
publications 286
Public Health Service (PHS) 64, 68, 69, 219, 316, 388, 647
  see also Department of Health and Human Services (DHHS)
Publishing Sciences Group 424
PUBS see percutaneous umbilical blood sampling (PUBS)
pulmonary edema 598
Purdy, P. 616
Purohit, D. M. 463
pyoderma 688
pyrimethamine 215, 216

Q

Queenan, J. T. 387

R

Raab, Diana, BS RN 673
racial factor
  asthma and 398
  breast feeding and 332, *333*
  cystic fibrosis and 32, 33
  infant mortality and 645, 646
  listeriosis and 226
  maternal mortality and 635–40
  phenylketonuria and 27
  pica and 51
  preeclampsia and 596
  prenatal care and 91
  sickle-cell disease and 488
  smoking and 150
Racz, J. 401, 421
Rader, Jeanne, PhD 67

radiation therapy 506–7, 549, 550
radiology 47
  see also X-rays
Raghunath, J. 404, 427
Rainer, E. 619
Rane, A. 426
Rank, Maureen 673
rapid assay delivery system 38
Rarick, Lisa, MD 325, 326, 327, 345
Raven Press 463
Rawlings, J. S. 640
raw meats during pregnancy 4
Raya, J. 417
Rayburn, W. F. 427, 429, 462
RDA see recommended daily dietary allowances (RDA)
RDS see respiratory distress syndrome (RDS)
Read, J. 417
Read, J. A. 640
recombination, described 25
recommended daily dietary allowances (RDA) 51, *52,* 59, 688
record keeping
  food and exercise *591*
  glucose monitoring *590*
  prenatal care and 83
  ultrasound examinations and 103
  x-rays and 48
Redman, C. W. 462, 463, 464, 615, 617
Rees, G. 290
Reid, Joanie 673
Reiher, H. 448
renal diseases 593
  hypertension and 457
  preeclampsia and 599–600
  ultrasound and 98
  see also kidney diseases
Renfrew, M. J. 288, 289
Renou, P. 287, 288
Repke, J. 462
Repke, J. T. 618
Research Resources Reporter 157, 435n
RESOLVE 674
respiratory distress syndrome (RDS) 435, 649
  cesarean delivery and 299–300

respiratory distress syndrome (RDS), continued
   corticosteroids and 240, 250, 252, 254, 256–57
   diabetes and 445
   premature birth and 263–65
   smoking and 150
respiratory synctial virus (RSV) 353
resting arterial carbon dioxide tension (PCO_2) 394
restriction endonuclease 20
restriction enzymes 23
Retin-A (tretinoin) 145
retinitis 688
retinopathy 437
retinopathy of prematurity 240
Reves, J. G. 421
Reynolds, A. L. 463
Rh factor 688
   cesarean delivery and 297
   Rh-negative information 377–83, 657
   test for 84, 94
rhinitis 414–16
Rhinology 429
Rhoads, George G., MD 105
riboflavin 52
Richards, Y. 387
Rickards, A. L. 422
Riley, A. 463
Riley, S. P. 398, 419
risk assessment
   cesarean delivery and 299–300
   chorionic villus sampling and 115
   for diabetes 556–57
   for eclampsia 596–97
   electronic fetal monitoring and 285
   for miscarriage
      and amniocentesis 108–9
      and chorionic villus sampling 108–9
   for preeclampsia 596–97
   prenatal care and 81, 82–83, 84–91
   ultrasound and 101–2
   ultrasound examinations 96
ritodrine 258
ritodrine hydrochloride (Yutopar) 243–44
Roberts, J. M. 615

Roberts, R. S. 400, 424
Robert Wood Johnson Foundation 650
Robinson, A. A. 424
Robinson, N. 614
Robson, J. M. 427
Rochester Community Hospital 341
Rodeck, C. H. 383, 387
Rodgers, G. M. 615
Rogatko, A. 509
Rohland, B. 385
Rojas, J. A. 430
Ron, H. 427
Roodenburg, P. J. 427
Rosa, F. W. 463
Rose, N. 480
Rosen, P. P. 509
Rosenberg, S. A. 513
Ross, W. C. 386
Rossing, T. H. 422, 427
Ross Laboratories 264, 338
Rosso, Pedro, MD 50
Rotmans, P. 617
Rouse, D. 480
Rowland, C. 479
Royal College of Radiologists 508
RSV *see* respiratory synctial virus (RSV)
rubella (German measles) 4, 221, 312, 628
   test for 94
   vaccine for 10–11
Rubin, J. 618
Rubin, J. D. 428
Rubin, P. 457, 463
Rubin, P. C. 462, 613, 618
Rue, Nancy 673
Ruo, T. I. 403, 404, 421, 423, 429
Ryan, G. M. 616

S

Saarikoski, S. 425
Sadri, S. 417
safety concerns
   see also risk assessment
safety concerns, ultrasound and 101–2, 103–4
Saftlas, A. F. 640

Index

Sahakian, V. 480
Sailstad, J. M. 422
Sakai, T. 428
Saleh, A. A. 615
salpingostomy 544
Sanders, J. E. 509
Sarno, A. P. 640
Savage, Judith A. 673
Saxen, I. 428
scalp blood sampling 283–84
Schaak, Barbara, RN 479
Schaefer, G. 398, 428
Schanler, Richard, MD 334, 337, 339, 340
Schatz, M. 400, 401, 403, 404, 414, 423, 428
Schenker, J. G. 461
Scher, Jonathon, MD 673
Schiff, E. 617
Schnoll, S. H. 180
Schoendod, K. C. 641
Schoenfeld-Dimaio, M. 385
Schubiger, G. 463
Schuetz, S. 180
Schulman, B. A. 428
Schulman, H. 617
Schwartz, R. 449
Schweibert, P. 673
Science 266
Scool, M. L. 387
Scott, A. A. 463
Scott, J. R. 428
Scott, J. S. 614
Scripps Research Institute 266
Sears, M. R. 429
seatbelt usem prenatal care and 85
seborrheic dermatitis 689
seconal, alcohol withdrawal and 154
sedative-hypnotic drug withdrawal 174
seizures
　alcohol withdrawal and 154
　eclampsia and 595
　neonatal 282, 285
　neonatal abstinence syndrome and 184
　neonatal methadone abstinence syndrome 186
　preeclampsia and 611

selenium *52*
Selley, J. A. 426
Semchyshyn, Stefan, MD 673
Semmler, K. 448
SensorMedics Corporation 265
sepsis 221, 222, 240, 365, 486, 495
septicemia 689
septum 653–54
serum albumin 403
sexual activity
　bacterial vaginosis and 248
　drug use and 187
　hepatitis B virus and 13
　miscarriage and 651, 652
　postpartum 308–9
　prenatal care and 84
　see also abstinence
sexually transmitted diseases (STD) 517, 544
　contraceptives and *328–29*
　prenatal care and 183–87
　protection from 206–12
　treatment prior to pregnancy 5
Shady Grove Adventist Hospital 338
Shak, Steve 36
Shamsa, F. 463
Shapiro, S. 424
SHARE National Headquarters 674
Sharp Memorial Hospital 157
Sheehan, H. L. 616
Shephard, T. H. 428
Sheppard, D. 429
Sheridan-Pereira, M. 287
Shim, C. S. 429
shunt placement, ultrasound and 99
Shy, K. A. 290
Shy, K. K. 286, 288, 289
Sibai, B. 386
Sibai, B. M. 463, 464, 616, 618
sickle-cell disease *30*, 485–95
　DNA (deoxyribonucleic acid) and 20–21
　DNA (deoxyribonucleic acid) studies and 25
　genetic screening for 27–28
　mode of inheritance *29*
　newborn testing and 27
　test for 363–73

Siddiqi, T. A. 448
Sidelines National Support Network 477
SIDS *see* The National SIDS Foundation; sudden infant death syndrome (SIDS)
Siegel, D. 429
Silverman, F. 398, 428
Simonovits, I. 385, 386
Simpson, J. L. 448
Sims, E. A. H. 589
Sinequan *see* doxepin
sinusitis 414, 416–17
Sipes, S. 480
sister chromatid exchange frequency 102
Sjögren, C. 415, 419
Skoll, A. 386
Slone, D. 424
Smart, Laura S., PhD 671
Smidt-Jensen, S. 386
Smith, C. V. 427, 429
Smith, G. 424
Smith, N. T. 429
Smith, R. L. 427
Smith, Sandra 149
Smith, V. 464
smoking 627
  asthma and 398
  gestational diabetes and 575
  infant mortality and 651
  during pregnancy 147, 149–50, 158
  preterm labor and 240
  see also tobacco use
Snapper, J. R. 427
Soares de Moura, R. S. 429
Sobreville, L. A. 429
Sodeman, W. A. 421
sodium 54, 572
sodium nitroprusside 609
solid food for infants 339–40
sonar 95
sonogram 689
Soranus of Ephesus 123, 137
Sorri, M. 416, 429
Southeastern Region Genetics Group 18
soy formula 336, 337, 340–41

Soy Moo 340
Spargo, B. H. 616
speech development, drug addiction and 161
Sperling, M. A. 448
sperm, chromosomes in 18
spermicides 207, 321, 323, *328–29*
spina bifida 221
  alpha-fetoprotein and 116
  folate and 61
  folic acid and 68
spina bifida aperta 61, *62*
Spina Bifida Association of America 61
spina bifida occulta 61
Spinnato, J. A. 616, 618
spirometer, asthma and 390
splenic sequestrian crisis 487, 495
splenomegaly 689
sponge contraceptive 322–23, *328–29*
spontaneous abortions 172, 651–55, 689
  asthma and 401
  diabetes and 441–44
  lupus and 499
  see also miscarriage
sporozoites 217
sports activities during pregnancy 78
Squifflet, J. P. 427
St. Martin's Press 479
St. Mary's Hospital 33
starch consumption 51
starvation symptoms 56
State Family Planning Administrators 3n
state health departments 45
Staudacher, Carol 673
STD *see* sexually transmitted diseases (STD)
Stec, G. P. 429
Stedman, C. M. 386
Steel, J. M. 449
Stehlin, Dori 270, 272, 273, 275, 277, 341, 345
Stenius-Aamiala, B. 398, 400, 429
Stergachis, A. 418
sterilization 326–27, *328–29*, 544
steroids 502

Index

Stevenson, B. J. 385
Stewart, J. J. 429
Stiernstedt, G. 403, 404, 427
Stigsby, B. 287
stillbirths 379, 382
  congenital rubella syndrome and 11
  hypertension and 593
Stillerman, A. 424
Stine, L. 417
Stock, B. 403, 421
Stock, Julie 335
Stokes, T. C. 424
Stopelli, I. 619
Storsater, J. 464
Stovall, T. G. 545
strabismus
  fetal alcohol syndrome and 152
streptococcal infections 221–24, 363, 495
streptomycin 139
stress
  breast feeding and 352
  diabetes and 437
  postpartum 313
  twins and 468
stress test 564
stretch marks 307
stroke 488
Stuart, M. J. 617
Stuff, J. E. *357*
Subramanian, K. N. Siva, MD 263
substance abuse *see* alcohol use; drug use
Substance Abuse and Mental Health Services Administration 183, 204
sudden infant death syndrome (SIDS) 160, 172, 179, 185, 649, 689
  cocaine exposure and 191
  drug exposure and 186–87, 188
sugar *see* diabetes; glucose
Suidan, J. S. 287
sulfadiazine 215, 216
sulfisoxazole 416
Sullivan, F. M. 427
Sullivan, Louis W., MD 149
Sumner, A. E. 423
supine hypotensive syndrome 395
Suratt, P. M. 423

Sureau, C. 426
surfactants 263–65
  postnatal pulmonary 252, 258
Surgeon General of United States 332, 572
Surgery 461
surgery, experimental 34
Surgery, Gynecology and Obstetrics 509, 614
Surgical Clinics of North America 508
Symonds, E. M. 463
symptoms
  of breast cancer 505
  of congenital rubella syndrome 11
  of cystic fibrosis 32
  of hepatitis B virus 13–14
  of hypoglycemia 583
  postpartum depression 318
  salty perspiration 32
  of sexually transmitted diseases 210–11
  of toxoplasmosis 213, 214
syphilis 94, 209, 221, 689
systemic lupus 498

T

Tabsh, K. M. A. 385
tachypnea 394, 690
Taffel, S. M. 286
tailor stretch exercise 75
Talavera, A. 512
Talledo, O. E. 615
Tannirandorn, Y. 383
target heart rates 78
Taslimi, M. M. 616
Taylor, P. R. 429
Taylor, R. N. 615
Tay-Sachs disease *30*
  genetic screening for 28
  mode of inheritance *29*
  test for 94
T cells 532
Td (tetanus and diphtheria) vaccine 15
Tegison (etretinate)
  birth defects and 145–46

Templeton, A. 394, 429
tenesmus 690
Teramo, K. 398, 400, 429
teratogenic drugs
　alcohol withdrawal and 154
　avoidance of
　　prenatal care and 84–90
　birth defects and 138–40
　pregnancy and 146
teratogens 690
Teratology 420, 421, 428, 448
terbutaline 258
terbutaline sulfate, preterm labor and 244
Tessem, J. 430
testing
　see antibody tests; blood tests; pregnancy, tests for; and *individual diseases and tests*
testosterone, lactation and 343–44
tetanus toxoids 15, 16
tetanus vaccine 16
tetracycline 139
Texas Department of Health 493
Thacker, Stephen B., MD 276, 288
thalassemia 25, 364, 371–72, 486
Thalhammer, O. 289
thalidomide 147
thalidomide epidemic (1956-1963) 136–37
The Joy of Twins 479
theophylline 403, 404
The Parents Guide to Raising Twins 479
thiamine 52
Thomas, P. R. 512
Thomas Jefferson University 159
Thompson, A. M. 614
Thompson, H. E. 288
Thompson, M. S. 287
Thomson, Angus 50
Thornton, J. G. 387
Thorp, J. M., Jr. 425
Thorpe, S. S. 463
three-quarter lying position 77
thrombocytopenia 598–99
thrombocytosis 186
thromboembolism 344
thromocytosis 690

thrush 690
Thurnau, G. R. 618
thylprednisolone 393
thyroid hormones 258
Tillman, A. J. B. 614
Timar, I. 386
TIP *see* treatment improvement protocol (TIP)
Title X program 649
tobacco use
　asthma and 432–33
　hypertension and 454
　oral contraceptives and 323
　pregnancy and 42, 43–44, 149–50
　prenatal care and 84–90
　prior to pregnancy 4
tocolytic agents
　corticosteroids and 258–59, 260
　premature labor and 243, 252
tocolytic medication 690
Tome, M. A. 513
Tong, T. J. 404, 427
Torrance, G. W. 388
Tovey, L. A. D. 385, 386
Towers, C. V. 430
Townley, A. 385
toxemia 54, 298, 502, 690
　alpha-fetoprotein and 116
　asthma and 389, 397
　prevention of 79
　weight gain during pregnancy and 56
　see also pregnancy induced hypertension (PIH)
toxoic vaccines 15
Toxoplasma gondii 213
toxoplasmosis 212–20, 628, 690
　test for 94, 362
Tracy, M. Elizabeth 435n
transducers 95, 242–43, 540
Transfusion 384, 386
transfusion for infants 378, 381–82
transmembrane protein *30*
transverse terminal defects 109–14
treatment improvement protocol (TIP) 180–82
treatment programs
　for drug use 161–64
　for hypertension 608

Index

triggers for asthma 391, 432
triglicerides 51
Trimbros, J. B. 615
trimesters *see* pregnancy, first trimester; pregnancy, second trimester; pregnancy, third trimester
trimethobenzamide hydrochloride 121
triplesulfa drugs 215, 216
The Triplet Connection 478
Trolle, B. 385
Trudinger, B. J. 617
Tsakeris, Tom 33, 34
Tsang, R. C. 448, 449
Tsui, Lap-Chee, PhD, MD 33
tubal pregnancy *see* ectopic pregnancy
tube agglutination 37
tuboplasty 99
tumors 31
  molar pregnancy and 547–51
  morning sickness and 120
Turner, E. 426
twins 466–83
  identical *versus* fraternal 466
  preeclampsia and 596
  ultrasound and 100, 101
Twins 479
Twins: From Conception to Five Years 479
Twin Services 478
tyrosinemia test 362
Tyzack, A. J. 418
Tyzbir, E. D. 589

U

Ueland, K. 396, 430
Ulmsten, U. 464
ultrasonography 95, 246, 439
ultrasound examinations 34, 95–104, 391, 467, 629
  diabetes and 562–63
  ectopic pregnancy and,544 540
  indications for 102–3
  miscarriage and 656
  placenta previa and 624
  preeclampsia and 607
  see also Doppler ultrasound

umbilical cord, described 129
umbilical cord prolapse 283, 298
unconjugated estriol 116
undescended testes 139
University of Alabama, Birmingham 249
University of California, Los Angeles 161
University of California, San Francisco 34
University of Cincinnati College of Medicine 441
University of Iowa College of Medicine 55
University of Michigan, Ann Arbor 33
University of Minnesota Press 567, 568
University of Pittsburgh/Magee Women's Hospital 247
University of Rochester Medical School Hospital 341, 345
University of Southern California (USC) School of Medicine 178
University of Tennessee, Memphis 35
University of Texas Science Center, Houston 240–41
University of Utah 32
University of Vermont, Burlington 586
University of Washington Health Sciences Center, Seattle 152
Urbaniak, S. J. 388
urinalysis 84, 94
urination
  diabetes and 555
  frequent 126
  Kegel squeeze exercise and 75
  postpartum 307
urine 690
  changes in 18
  home pregnancy tests and 37
  phenylketonuria and 26
  protein in 56
urine tests
  for diabetes 556
  for drug use 159, 162
  during pregnancy 94
urogynecologists 315

urologists 315
U.S. Air Force Academy 27
U.S. Children's Bureau 361
U.S. Department of Agriculture (USDA) 64
    Children's Nutrition Research Center 355, 356, 358, 359
    publications 355
U.S. Dietary Guidelines 70
U.S. Multistate Case-Control Study 112, 113
U.S. Preventive Services Task Force 252, 277, 377n
uterine abnormalities
    miscarriage and 653
    ultrasound and 99
uterine contractions 682
    asthma and 393
    Braxton Hicks 241, 680
    fetal stress and 117
    hormones and 117
    timing of 231–36, 237, 241–42
    weak 296
uterine lining 324
uterine size
    cesarean delivery and 292
    ultrasound and 99
uteroplacental insufficiency 98
uterus 690
uterus didelphys
    ultrasound and 99
Uzan, S. 617

V

Vaccine in Pregnancy Registry (VIP) 10
vaccines 490, 691
    for diphtheria 16
    for hepatitis B virus 13–15, 200–201
    for mumps 12
    for pertussis 15
    for rubella 10–11
    for tetanus 16
    see also immunizations
VACTERL syndrome 154
vacuum extractor 273
vaginal bleeding 548
    after miscarriage 658
    asthma and 389, 397
    exercise and 78
    placental disorders and 621, 622
    prenatal care and 85
    ultrasound and 98
vaginal cancers 139
vaginal delivery
    versus cesarean delivery 294, 297, 300, 606–7
    see also cesarean delivery; labor and delivery
Vaginal Infections and Prematurity (VIP) Study 247, 248
Valium see diazepam (Valium)
Valle, R. 417
van Belle, G. 288
VanDenBerg, Jerry 478
Van Lierde 427
van Muyden, P. 421
Van Nostrand Rheinhold 479
Van Petten, G. R. 421
Van Weering, H. K. 427
van Ypersele de Strihou, C. 427
varicella test 94
Varicella-Zoster Immune Globulin (VZIG) 8
Varvarigos, I. 288
vascular disruption syndrome 172
vas deferens 691
vasectomy 327
vasodilators 459, 610
vasospasm 597
Vaughn, D. A. 424
Veall, N. 616
vegans 59
vegetarians 59
ventilators, premature birth and 265–66
vernix 130
viable fetus 95
Vierola, H. 424
Villar, J. 462
Villar, M. 463
villi cells 105
    see also chorionic villus sampling (CVS)
Vintzileos, A. M. 288, 289

Index

VIP *see* Vaccine in Pregnancy Registry (VIP)
Virtanen, R. 424
vitamin A 66
  birth defects and 141, 145–46
  in food groups 471–72
  recommended daily allowance of 52
  see also Accutane (acne medication)
vitamin and mineral supplements
  during pregnancy 138
vitamin B 68
  in food groups 470
vitamin B_6 473
  pregnancy and 51
  prenatal intake of 59
  recommended daily allowance of 52
vitamin B_{12}
  pregnancy and 51
  prenatal intake of 59
  recommended daily allowance of 52
vitamin B_{12} deficiency 59
vitamin C
  in food groups 471
  recommended daily allowance of 52
vitamin D 66
  infant formula and 339
  recommended daily allowance of 52
vitamin E
  in food groups 472–73
  recommended daily allowance of 52
vitamin megadosages 59, 66
vitamins 691
  in human milk 58
  in infant formula 336–37
vitamin supplements
  breast feeding and 338–39
  folic acid and 68–70
  vegetarians and 59
  vitamin A as 145–46
  see also dietary supplements
volume expansion 611–12
vomiting
  during pregnancy 119
  treatment for 473
von Schoultz, E. 509
Vrandall, B. F. 385
VZIG *see* Varicella-Zoster Immune Globulin (VZIG)

W

Wachsman, L. 180
Wald, J. 398, 422
Walker, R. H. 384
walking
  postpartum 310
  during pregnancy 78
Wallack, M. K. 509
Wallenberg, H. C. 615
Wallenburg, H. C. 617
Wallingford, John C., PhD 335, 336, 338
Walters, B. N. 617
Ward, Sally L. Davidson, MD 178–80
Warren, J. T. 422
Washington, A. E. 545
water breaking 231–32
water on the brain *see* hydrocephalus
water retention
  during pregnancy 56
water retention during pregnancy 54
Watson, Christine 338
Watson, D. L. 616, 618
Watson, K. V. 611, 618
Watts, D. H. 388
Weaver, L. C. 418
weight factor
  diabetes and 556
  Norplant and 325
  spina bifida and 63
weight gain 50, 56–58
  diabetes and 567–71, 579–81
  twins and 469, 475–76
weight gain chart *57, 567, 568, 569*
weight loss, postpartum 306–7
Weinberg, P. F. 429
Weinberger, M. M. 424
Weir, E. K. 462
Welch, R. A. 615
Welch, R. M. 422
Wendel, G. D., Jr. 615
Western blot test 526
Western Journal of Medicine 180
Wettrell, G. 426
Whalley, P. J. 615

What's Bred in the Bone (Davies) 137
Wheeler, Sara 672
Wheeler, Sara Rich, RN, MS 674
White, C. A. 386
White, P. 614
White, R. J. 400, 430
White, Ray, PhD 32
White, W. B. 619
Whitehall Laboratories 38
Whitwirth, J. A. 461
WHO *see* World Health Organization (WHO)
whooping cough 687
WIC *see* Women, Infants, and Children (WIC)
Widdicombe, J. G. 430
Widerlov, E. 464
Wilking, N. 509
Wilkins, Isabelle, MD 672
William Morrow & Company, Inc. 538, 621n, 627n, 631n
Williams, D. A. 398, 400, 430
Williams, M. H., Jr. 429
Williams, Rebecca 60, 267
Williams and Wilkins 616
Williams obstetrics 287, 545
Williamson, Robert, MD 33
Williamson, Walter 674
Willis, Judith 141
Willis, Judith Levine 55
Wilms' tumor 31
Wilson, J. 417, 422, 430
Wilson, J. T. 429
Wilson, M. 396, 430
Wilson, S. M. 386
Winemiller, R. 616
withdrawal before ejaculation 326
withdrawal symptoms
 alcohol use and 153–55
 from barbiturates 174–75
 from cocaine 171–72
 from methadone 166–67
 from opium 166–67
Wladimiroff, J. W. 427
Wolfert, Alan D., PhD 674
Wolstenholm, G. E. W. 616
Women, Infants, and Children (WIC) 163, 332

Woo, S. Y. 512
Wood, C. 287
Woodard, G. 419
Woods, J. R. 180
Woods, James R., Jr., MD 674
Woolcock, A. J. 430
Woollett, A. 479
woring mothers, breast feeding and 346–51
Working Group on Pregnancy and Asthma 390
The Working Woman's Guide to Breastfeeding 351
World Health Organization (WHO) 101, 106, 113, 404, 637
World Wide Web *see* Internet addresses
Wysowki, D. K. 384
Wysowski, Diane, PhD 344

X

X chromosomes 31
Xia, Z. 545
X-rays
 breast cancer and 506
 DNA (deoxyribonucleic acid) testing and 23
 pregnancy and 43, 46–48
 versus ultrasound 95

Y

Yaffe, S. J. 419
Yamaguchi Igaku 426
Yancey, Michael K., MD 273, 274
Y chromosomes 31
Yeh, T. F. 430
Yen, S. S. C. 464
Yetley, Elizabeth, PhD 60
Young, B. K. 287
Younker, D. 430
Yurchak, A. M. 430
Yusuf, S. 464
Yutopar (ritodrine hydrochloride) 243–44

Z

Zamora, J. 464
Zamula, Evelyn 136, 141, 151, 157
ZDV (zidovudine) 516, 520–21, 530–34
Zeiger, R. 403, 404, 423
Zeiger, R. S. 414, 428
Zeitz, S. 428
Zemlickis, D. 513
Zervoudakis, I. 396, 430
zidovudine *see* AZT
Zilianti, M. 431
Zinaman, M. 618
zinc 52
Zipursky, A. 385, 388
Zuckerman, Barry, MD 159
Zupanska, B. 387
Zuspan, F. P. 462, 615

32378 75

SOUTH COLLEGE
709 Mall Blvd.
Savannah, GA 31406

DO NOT REMOVE FROM LIBRARY

REFERENCE